Current Research in Hematology

Current Research in Hematology

Edited by Martha Roper

hayle
medical

New York

Hayle Medical,
750 Third Avenue, 9th Floor,
New York, NY 10017, USA

Visit us on the World Wide Web at:
www.haylemedical.com

ISBN: 978-1-63241-490-8

The publisher's policy is to use permanent paper from mills that operate a sustainable forestry policy. Furthermore, the publisher ensures that the text paper and cover boards used have met acceptable environmental accreditation standards.

Printed in China.

Cataloging-in-Publication Data

Current research in hematology / edited by Martha Roper.
p. cm.
Includes bibliographical references and index.
ISBN 978-1-63241-490-8
1. Hematology. 2. Blood--Diseases. I. Roper, Martha.
RC633 .C87 2018
616.15--dc23

Table of Contents

Preface

Hematology is the branch of medicine which studies blood and treats the disorders of the blood. Cholemia, blood hammer, pancytopenia, thalassemia are some prevalent blood disorders. The different types of treatments given to patients with blood disorders are blood transfusion, platelet transfusion, venesection, bone marrow transplant, etc. This book includes some of the vital pieces of work being conducted across the world, on various topics related to hematology. It will prove to be immensely beneficial to students and researchers in this field.

This book is a result of research of several months to collate the most relevant data in the field.

When I was approached with the idea of this book and the proposal to edit it, I was overwhelmed. It gave me an opportunity to reach out to all those who share a common interest with me in this field. I had 3 main parameters for editing this text:

1. Accuracy – The data and information provided in this book should be up-to-date and valuable to the readers.

2. Structure – The data must be presented in a structured format for easy understanding and better grasping of the readers.

3. Universal Approach – This book not only targets students but also experts and innovators in the field, thus my aim was to present topics which are of use to all.

Thus, it took me a couple of months to finish the editing of this book.

I would like to make a special mention of my publisher who considered me worthy of this opportunity and also supported me throughout the editing process. I would also like to thank the editing team at the back-end who extended their help whenever required.

Editor

A Multi-Compartment Single and Multiple Dose Pharmacokinetic Comparison of Rectally Applied Tenofovir 1% Gel and Oral Tenofovir Disoproxil Fumarate

Kuo-Hsiung Yang[1]*, Craig Hendrix[2], Namandje Bumpus[2], Julie Elliott[3], Karen Tanner[4], Christine Mauck[5], Ross Cranston[6], Ian McGowan[6], Nicola Richardson-Harman[7], Peter A. Anton[3], Angela D. M. Kashuba[1]

1 Division of Pharmacotherapy and Experimental Therapeutics, UNC Eshelman School of Pharmacy, Chapel Hill, North Carolina, United States of America, **2** Departments of Medicine and Pharmacology, Johns Hopkins University School of Medicine, Baltimore, Maryland, United States of America, **3** Center for HIV Prevention Research, David Geffen School of Medicine at UCLA, Los Angeles, California, United States of America, **4** Department of Biostatistics, UCLA School of Public Health, Los Angeles, California, United States of America, **5** CONRAD, Arlington, Virginia, United States of America, **6** Department of Medicine, University of Pittsburgh, Pittsburgh, Pennsylvania, United States of America, **7** Alpha StatConsult LLC, Damascus, Maryland, United States of America

Abstract

This Phase 1, randomized, two-site (United States), double-blind, placebo-controlled study enrolled 18 sexually abstinent men and women. All received a single 300-mg dose of oral tenofovir disoproxil fumarate (TDF) and were then randomized 2:1 to receive single and then seven daily rectal exposures of vaginally-formulated tenofovir (TFV) 1% gel or a hydroxyethyl cellulose (HEC) placebo gel. Blood, colonic biopsies and rectal and vaginal mucosal fluids were collected after the single oral TDF, the single topical TFV gel dose, and after 7 days of topical TFV gel dosing for extracellular analysis of TFV and intracellular analysis of the active metabolite tenofovir diphosphate (TFVdp) in peripheral blood mononuclear cells (PBMCs) and isolated mucosal mononuclear cells (MMC), including CD4+ and CD4- cell subsets. With a single rectal dose, TFV plasma concentrations were 24–33 fold lower and half-life was 5 h shorter compared to a single oral dose ($p = 0.02$). TFVdp concentrations were also undetectable in PBMCs with rectal dosing. Rectal tissue exposure to both TFV and TFVdp was 2 to 4-$\log_{10}$ higher after a single rectal dose compared to a single oral dose, and after 7 daily doses, TFVdp accumulated 4.5 fold in tissue. TFVdp in rectal tissue homogenate was predictive (residual standard error, RSE $= 0.47$) of tissue MMC intracellular TFVdp concentration, with the CD4+ cells having a 2-fold higher TFVdp concentration than CD4- cells. TFV concentrations from rectal sponges was a modest surrogate indicator for both rectal tissue TFV and TFVdp (RSE $= 0.67$, 0.66, respectively) and plasma TFV (RSE $= 0.38$). TFV penetrates into the vaginal cavity after oral and rectal dosing, with rectal dosing leading to higher vaginal TFV concentrations ($p < 0.01$).

Trial Registration: ClinicalTrials.gov NCT00984971

Editor: Alan Winston, Imperial College London, United Kingdom

Funding: The study was funded by a U19 grant under the Integrated Preclinical-Clinical Program for HIV Topical Microbicides (IPCP-HTM), Division of AIDS, National Institute of Allergy and Infectious Diseases, National Institutes of Health (NIH) (AI060614) and the NIAID's Microbicide Trials Network (5UM1AI068633). Additional support was provided by Gilead Sciences Inc.; the University of California, Los Angeles Center for AIDS Research (5P30 AI28697) Cores of Mucosal Immunology, Flow Cytometry and Biostatistics; the University of North Carolina-Chapel Hill Center for AIDS Research, Clinical Pharmacology/Analytical Chemistry Core (P30 AI50410); the Johns Hopkins Clinical Pharmacology Analytical Laboratory and CONRAD. The RMP-02/MTN-006 study was registered at www.ClinicalTrials.gov (NCT00984971) and the protocol can be http://www.mtnstopshiv.org. This analysis was supported by a contract with Advanced BioScience Laboratories, Inc., Rockville, Maryland, and its subcontractor, Alpha StatConsult LLC, through a NIH/NIAID/DAIDS contract: "Comprehensive Resources for HIV Microbicides and Biomedical Prevention" (#HHSN272201000001C). The funders had no role in study design, data collection and analysis, decision to publish, or preparation of the manuscript.

Competing Interests: The study was funded by a U19 grant under the Integrated Preclinical-Clinical Program for HIV Topical Microbicides (IPCP-HTM), Division of AIDS, National Institute of Allergy and Infectious Diseases, National Institutes of Health (NIH) (AI060614) and the NIAID's Microbicide Trials Network (5UM1AI068633). Additional support was provided by Gilead Sciences Inc.; the University of California, Los Angeles Center for AIDS Research (5P30 AI28697) Cores of Mucosal Immunology, Flow Cytometry and Biostatistics; the University of North Carolina-Chapel Hill Center for AIDS Research, Clinical Pharmacology/Analytical Chemistry Core (P30 AI50410); the Johns Hopkins Clinical Pharmacology Analytical Laboratory and CONRAD. The RMP-02/MTN-006 study was registered at www.ClinicalTrials.gov (NCT00984971) and the protocol can be found at http://www.mtnstopshiv.org. This analysis was supported by a contract with Advanced BioScience Laboratories, Inc., Rockville, MD, and its subcontractor, Alpha StatConsult LLC, through a NIH/NIAID/DAIDS contract: "Comprehensive Resources for HIV Microbicides and Biomedical Prevention" (#HHSN272201000001C).

* Email: kuohyang@email.unc.edu

Introduction

Both topical and oral tenofovir (TFV)-containing regimens have demonstrated efficacy in HIV prevention. TFV 1% gel demonstrated 39% protective efficacy in women using the gel within 12 hours before and after sexual activity in the Centre for the AIDS Programme of Research in South Africa (CAPRISA) 004 study [1]. The fixed dose combination of tenofovir disoproxil fumarate (TDF)/emtricitabine (Truvada) prescribed daily in a population of men who have sex with men in the iPrEx study provided 44% protection against HIV infection [2]. Daily dosing of TDF or Truvada provided 62 to 73% protection against HIV transmission in serodiscordant men and women enrolled in the Partners PrEP Study [3]. Furthermore, daily dosing of oral TDF provided 49% reduction in HIV incidence rates among IV drug users [4]. In both CAPRISA 004 and iPrEx, the level of protection was related to drug exposure and adherence [1,2,5,6].

The primary objective of the Phase 1 RMP-02/MTN-006 clinical trial was to evaluate the systemic safety of TFV 1% gel when applied rectally [7]. Built into this study was a comprehensive pharmacokinetic evaluation comparing systemic and compartmental pharmacokinetics among oral TDF and rectal TFV 1% gel users. These novel within-subject pharmacokinetic analyses were also used in an *ex-vivo* biopsy HIV challenge model to correlate TFVdp exposure with protection against *ex vivo* infection (*reported in accompanying paper: Richardson-Harman et al.*) [7]. This is the first study to quantify human rectal mucosal pharmacokinetics after topical administration of tenofovir in multiple compartments concurrently, to compare it to exposure after oral administration and to determine whether less-invasive indicators of TVFdp concentrations in tissue CD4+ cells emerge, potentially playing a future role in large clinical trials.

Materials and Methods

The protocol for this trial and supporting CONSORT checklist are available as supporting information; see Checklist S1 and Protocol S1.

Ethics Statement

The trial was IRB-approved at each site (UCLA IRB in Los Angeles, CA; University of Pittsburgh IRB, Committee C in Pittsburgh, PA); all participants provided written informed consent. RMP-02/MTN-006 is registered at ClinicalTrials.gov (#NCT00984971) and is in compliance with the CONSORT 2010 trial reporting recommendations (www.consortstatement.org).

Study Participants

Study participants were healthy HIV-1-seronegative men and women with a history of consensual rectal anal intercourse, willing to abstain from vaginal and rectal sex during active protocol phases. Female participants were required to be using an acceptable form of contraception (e.g., barrier method, IUD, hormonal contraception, surgical sterilization, or vasectomization of male partner).

Study Design

The pharmacokinetic component of the RMP-02/MTN-006 trial was designed to compare systemic and compartmental pharmacokinetics among single oral TDF dosing (300 mg), and single as well as multiple doses of rectally-applied vaginally-formulated TFV 1% gel. This was a Phase 1, double-blind, randomized, placebo-controlled comparison of oral TDF (300 mg), rectally applied TFV 1% gel, and the hydroxyethyl cellulose (HEC) placebo gel, the design of which has been previously published [7], and is illustrated in Figures 1, 2.

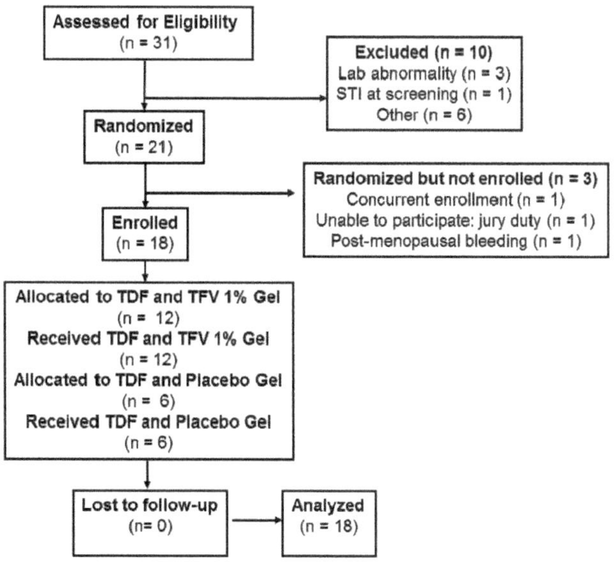

Figure 1. Study Design.

Briefly, in this three-stage trial, all participants received a single dose of oral TDF followed 4 weeks later by rectally applied TFV 1% gel or the HEC gel given as a single dose, and 4 weeks later, seven daily doses of the same product previously administered rectally. After enrollment, each subject was assigned to either the treatment or placebo arm (2:1; TFV 1% gel:HEC gel) and also to one of two post-exposure biopsy sampling arms (groups "A" and "B") to ensure mucosal safety. This limited the number of sigmoidoscopic procedures per participant to three sigmoidoscopic procedures in each of the first two study stages (single oral, single rectal) with several days delay between biopsy collections for mucosal healing. A single sigmoidoscopy biopsy collection point was used following the 3rd stage (7-day rectal exposures). All subjects provided biopsies (and other compartment samples) 0.5 h after their dose of oral TDF or single/7-day dose of TFV gel. For the single oral and single rectal exposures, in addition to all subjects being sampled at 0.5 h, Group "A" subjects were also biopsied on days 1 (24 hr) and 7; Group "B" subjects were also biopsied on days 4 and 10. Participants were allowed a 2 day visit window for this sampling but nearly all were seen on the first day of their 3-day window. Just prior to each biopsy sample, blood samples were obtained for plasma and peripheral blood mononuclear cell isolation, and rectal and vaginal mucosal fluids were collected by sponge. Each 2 weeks of biopsy sampling was followed by a 2-week resting period. The sample size (N = 18) was based on a similar phase 1 study of topical microbicide UC781. [8] The study was conducted from November 2009 to July 2010.

Pharmacokinetic Procedures for Single Oral and Topical Dosing. All participants had blood plasma, PBMCs, and vaginal and rectal fluid obtained before single oral and rectal dosing. Additionally, 30 minutes after the dose, blood plasma, PBMCs, rectal biopsies, rectal fluid and vaginal fluid samples were obtained. At 2, 4, and 24 h after the dose, blood plasma, PBMCs, and rectal/vaginal fluid samples were obtained. Subsequently, on either days 1 and 7 (Group A) or 4 and 10 (Group B) post-dose, blood plasma, PBMCs, rectal biopsies, rectal/vaginal fluid were obtained.

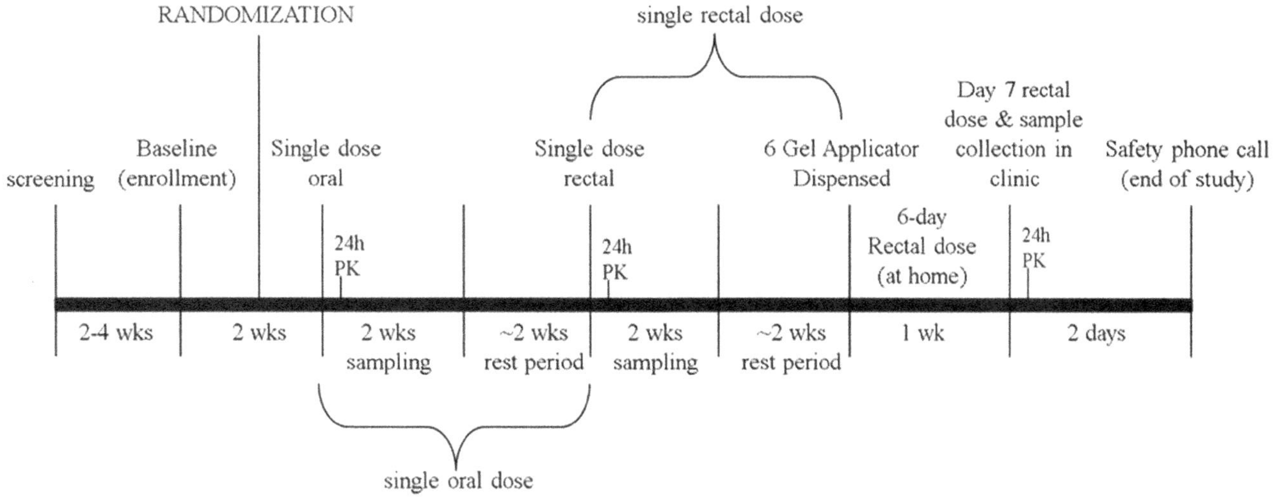

Figure 2. Sample Collection. All 18 trial participants received a single oral dose of 300 mg TDF followed by intensive 24 h PK. After ~2 week resting period, 12 subjects were randomized to receive a single rectal gel dose of 1% TFV gel with intensive 24 h PK followed, after ~2 week resting period, by 6 sequential, daily, self-administered rectal 1% TFV gel doses with the 7th dose administered in-clinic with subsequent 24 h intensive PK.

Pharmacokinetic Procedures for Multiple Topical Dosing. Thirty minutes after the 7th rectal dose of gel (observed), blood plasma, PBMCs, rectal biopsies, rectal fluid and vaginal fluid samples were obtained. At 2, 4, and 24 h after the dose, blood plasma, PBMCs, rectal fluid, and vaginal fluid samples were obtained.

Study Products

TDF tablets (300 mg) were supplied by Gilead Sciences (Foster City, CA). TFV 1% gel and HEC gel were supplied by CONRAD (Arlington, VA). TFV 1% gel (weight/weight) is tenofovir (PMPA, 9-[(R)-2-(phosphonomethoxy)propyl]adenine monohydrate), formulated in purified water with edetate disodium, citric acid, glycerin, methylparaben, propylparaben, and hydroxyethyl cellulose with pH adjusted to 4–5 with an osmolarity of 3111 mOsmol/kg. The HEC placebo gel contained hydroxyethyl cellulose as the gel thickener, purified water, sodium chloride, sorbic acid, and sodium hydroxide. The gel was isotonic with a pH of 4.4, osmolarity of 304 mOsmol/kg, 24 and viscosity similar to the other microbicide gel candidates. Both TFV and HEC gels were prefilled into single-use, opaque applicators (HTI Plastics, Lincoln, NE) containing 4 ml of gel.

Sample Processing

Plasma was collected in tubes containing EDTA anticoagulant. Samples were centrifuged at 800 g for 10 minutes at 4°C, plasma aliquoted into cryovials, and stored at −70°C. Peripheral blood mononuclear cells (PBMCs) were isolated via centrifugation from cell preparation tubes (CPT) at 1,800×g for 25 min at 28°C. PBMCs were collected from the buffy coat and washed twice with normal saline at room temperature (~21°C). Cells were resuspended in 1 ml normal saline for cell counting. Cell pellets were lysed with 70% methanol and stored at −80°C until analysis.

To release cells for intracellular analysis from colonic tissue, biopsies were incubated with a dissociative enzyme cocktail consisting of collagenase (0.5 mg/ml, Sigma-Aldrich, St. Louis, MO), DNase I (0.083 U/ml, Roche, Indianapolis, IN), elastase (0.07 U/ml, Worthington Biochemicals, Lakewood, NJ), and hyaluronidase (0.4 U/ml, Worthington Biochemicals, Lakewood, NJ). The digestions were carried out in RPMI with 7.5% FBS in 50 ml-conical tubes at 37°C with agitation (Invitrogen, Carlsbad, CA) as previously described. [9,10] Cells were counted using Guava/Millipore EasyCyte Plus (Millipore, Billerica, MA).

CD4+ T cells from tissue and PBMCs were isolated via positive selection with CD4 microbeads using magnetic affinity column separation (MACS) according to the manufacturer's recommended protocol (Miltenyi Biotec, Auburn, CA). CD4-positive and CD4-negative fractions were collected for cell counting and intracellular drug analysis. We used PBMCs to test for changes in intracellular TFV-DP concentrations as a result of tissue cell extraction and cell subset isolation compared to typical PBMC preparation. Compared to usual PBMC processing, there was no difference in PBMC TFV-DP concentrations resulting from the tissue digestion cocktail, monoclonal antibody incubation, or running cells over the MACS column.

Sample Analysis

All TFV and TFVdp concentrations were measured using validated LC–MS/MS methods. Total numbers of samples analyzed were as follows: 275 blood plasma, 460 PBMCs, 205 tissue homogenates, 98 isolated mononuclear cells, 99 CD4+ cells, 99 CD4- cells, 264 rectal sponges, 54 vaginal sponges [11]. Briefly, TFV and TFVdp concentrations were determined by previously described LC-MS/MS methods [12,13] validated for all matrices by the Johns Hopkins Clinical Pharmacology Analytical Laboratory. TFV and TFVdp assays meet the FDA bioanalysis guidance values of ≤ ±15% for precision and accuracy [14]. All calibrators were prepared using analyte calibrator stock solution diluted in the relevant human biological matrix corresponding to the samples to be assayed (plasma, PBMC lysate, cervicovaginal fluid, rectal fluid, homogenized colon or vaginal tissue). Thawed aliquots of plasma and tissue homogenate with ^{13}C-TFV internal standard were protein precipitated with methanol. Vaginal and rectal fluid sponges were eluted in 50:50 methanol:water mixture. Sponges were weighed both before and after. Aliquots, also with ^{13}C5-TFV internal standard, underwent solid phase extraction using HLB oasis cartridges. The supernatants and eluants were collected, dried, and reconstituted in 0.5% acetic acid for analysis. For chromatographic separation of samples, a gradient elution with a Zorbax Eclipse XDB-C18 column, with positive electrospray

Table 1. Demographics.

	Oral tenofovir	Tenofovir Gel	HEC placebo gel
N	18	12	6
Age (mean, STD)	42.1 (11.4)	41.3 (11.9)	43.7 (10.2)
Gender: M	14 (78%)	10 (83%)	4 (67%)
Gender: F	4 (22%)	2 (17%)	2 (33%)
Latino or Hispanic Origin: Y	5 (28%)	3 (25%)	2 (33%)
Latino or Hispanic Origin: N	13 (72%)	9 (75%)	4 (67%)
Race: Black or African-American	2 (11%)	1 (8%)	1 (17%)
Race: White	15 (83%)	10 (84%)	5 (83%)
Race: Other	1 (6%)	1 (8%)	0

ionization (ESI) was used, with detection via multiple reaction monitoring using a LC-MS/MS system (Waters Acquity UPLC and Agilent 1100 HPLC Applied Biosystems API4000 mass spectrometer). Calibration standards for the TFV assay ranged from 0.31 to 1,280 ng/ml (0.25–50 ng/sample for tissue).

For intracellular TFVdp analysis, tissue homogenates and isolated cell lysates were analyzed using an indirect assay [13].

Table 2. Noncompartmental Pharmacokinetic Parameters (*Insufficient data to perform NCA on CD4- and CD4+ PBMC; see companion publication Richardson-Harmon et.al for exposure-response analysis; **Composite Profile).

Matrix	Analyte, PK parameter	Single Oral Dose, median (min–max); N	Single Rectal Dose median (min–max); N	Multiple Rectal Dose median (min–max); N
Plasma	TFV T1/2 (h)	10.8 (6.82–19.2); 18	4.56 (2.61–62.9); 12	6.62 (4.55–32.1); 10
	TFV AUC24 h (ng/mL ×h)	2210 (1100–2940); 18	66.3 (12.4–114); 12	46.5 (17.1–178); 10
	TFV Cmax (ng/mL)	252 (76.8–387); 18	10.5 (5.08–33.4); 12	8.61 (2.37–11.2); 10
	TFV Tmax (h)	1.93 (0.267–3.92); 18	0.317 (0.183–1.98); 12	0.258 (0.183–2.03); 10
PBMC (total)[1]	TFVdp AUC24 h (fmol/10^6 cells ×h)	4.26 (0.240–389)	0.24 (0.24–0.24)	0.24 (0.24–0.24)
	TFVdp Cmax (fmol/10^6 cells)	0.375 (BLQ–38.6)	BLQ (BLQ–0.01)	BLQ (BLQ–0.01)
Rectal Tissue	TFV AUC24 h (ng/mg ×h)*	0.790	70.4	
	TFVdp AUC24 h (fmol/mg ×h)**	0.240	5470	
	TFV C24 h (ng/mg)	0.06 (BLQ–0.360)	0.06 (BLQ–12.6)	
	TFVdp C24 h (fmol/mg)	BLQ (BLQ–991)	285 (BLQ–490)	
	Accumulation Ratio, TFV			2.03
	Accumulation Ratio, TFdp			4.48
	TFV C30 min (ng/mg)		5.81 (BLQ–95.1); 12	11.8 (BLQ–430); 11
	TFVdp C30 min (fmol/mg)		176 (BLQ-1230); 12	789 (55.7–7190); 12
Rectal Mononuclear Cells	TFVdp C30 min (fmol/10^6 cells)	BLQ (BLQ–BLQ); 18	454 (BLQ–1460); 12	1324 (BLQ–13900); 11
	TFVdp C24 h (fmol/10^6 cells)	BLQ (BLQ–524); 8	228 (BLQ–290); 3	
	TFVdp CD4+ C30 min (fmol/10^6 cells)	BLQ (BLQ–BLQ); 18	266 (BLQ–3950); 12	1080 (BLQ–31200); 12
	TFVdp CD4+ C24 h (fmol/10^6 cells)	26.7 (BLQ–724); 18	250 (BLQ–1110); 3	
	TFVdp CD4- C30 min (fmol/10^6 cells)	BLQ (BLQ–20); 18	112 (BLQ–1340); 12	330 (BLQ–12000); 12
	TFVdp CD4- C24 h (fmol/10^6 cells)	28.4 (BLQ–157); 8	92.7 (BLQ–265); 3	
Rectal Fluid	TFV AUC24 h (ng/g ×h, ×10^5)	1.03 (0.00265–15.1); 16	11.0 (1.56–42.5); 12	7.03 (1.49–32.6); 7
	TFV Cmax (ng/g, ×10^4)	0.978 (0.00179–15.1); 17	73.9 (8.79–297); 12	41.6 (10.1–87.2); 7
	TFV Tmax (h)	24 (0.330–24.5); 4	0.380 (0.300–2.08); 12	0.330 (0.280–0.370); 7
Vaginal Fluid	TFV AUC24 h (ng/g ×h)	2.33 (0.979–2.72); 4	1.43 (0.587–2.27); 2	11.8; 1
	TFV Cmax (ng/g, ×10^4)	0.134 (0.0515–0.182); 4	0.313 (0.0432–0.582); 2	0.696; 1
	TFV Tmax (h)	3.01 (1.92–24); 4	2.74 (1.62–3.87); 2	3.58; 1

*Insufficient data to perform NCA on CD4- and CD4+ PBMC; see companion publication Richardson-Harmon et.al for exposure-response analysis.
**Composite Profile.

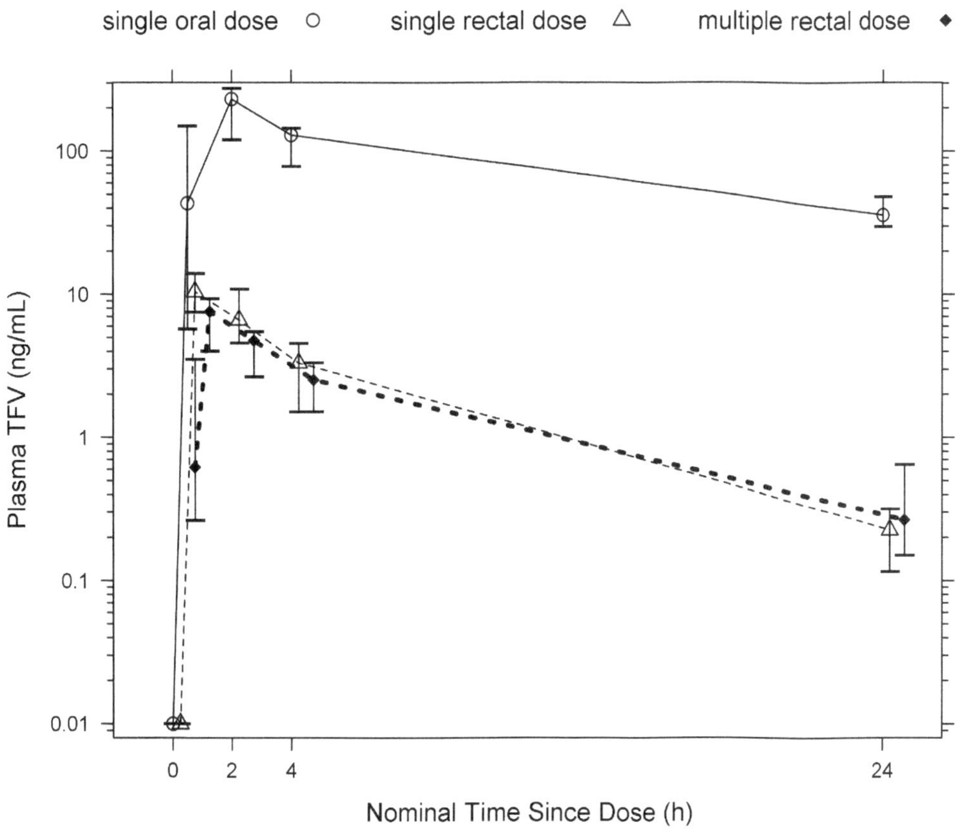

Figure 3. TFV Plasma Half-life is shorter (p = 0.02) during rectal administration. Plasma concentration-time profile is shown (median and interquartile range). Nominal time for single rectal dose was shifted right by 0.250 h and multiple rectal dose by 0.500 h for clarity. N = 18 for oral dose, 12 single rectal dose, 12 multiple rectal dose. (BLQ values are imputed as 0.01.)

TFVdp was isolated from cell lysates on a Waters QMA cartridge (Waters Corporation, Milford, MA) over a salt (KCl) gradient. TFV and tenofovir monophosphate (TFVmp) were separated from the cartridge under lower salt concentrations followed by elution of TFVdp with application of 1 M KCl to the cartridge. Isolated TFVdp was then enzymatically dephosphorylated to TFV via phosphatase digestion with incubation with phosphatase and ^{13}C-TFV internal standard. TFV was isolated from the KCl solution using trifluoroacetic acid and eluted in methanol. TFV with ^{13}C-TFV internal standard was analyzed via UPLC-MS/MS mass spectrometer as described above.

Pharmacokinetic and Statistical Analysis

Data Standardization

All values below the limit of quantification (BLQ) were imputed to be 0.01 for noncompartmental pharmacokinetic analysis (NCA) for all arms except rectal administration of placebo. Concentration data during rectal administration for the placebo arm is excluded from this report. All sponge concentrations (ng/sponge) were normalized to fluid weight on sponge (g) by division, resulting in units of ng/g. Data are presented as median (range) unless otherwise noted.

PK Parameter Calculations

Actual time after dosing was used for NCA. When calculating individual pharmacokinetic (PK) parameters (C_{max}, T_{max}, $AUC_{24\ h}$, half-life), only profiles with: a) greater than two data points, b) last concentration time point less than or equal to 24 h, and c) first concentration time point less than or equal to 12 h were used. A composite PK profile was constructed for rectal tissue homogenates using the median concentrations from all subjects at each nominal time point, regardless of the actual time. In this case, PK parameters were calculated based on this composite profile with nominal times. Composite profiles must be calculated with protocol-specified nominal times because descriptive statistics cannot be calculated with actual times; there were minor deviations in sample collection time during the trial, as it is impossible to collect at the exact protocol-specified time. For calculating $AUC_{24\ h}$, linear interpolation was used to interpolate the concentration at 24 h if the actual time was greater than 24 h. If actual time was between 22 h and 24 h, then that concentration was imputed to be the 24 h concentration. Half-life estimation was performed by choosing points during the beta-phase of the elimination slope. (3 single rectal dose plasma PK profiles contained an imputed value of 0.01 at the 24 h timepoint.)

Parameter calculation was performed with Phoenix WinNonlin 6.3.0.395 (Certara/Pharsight). Data manipulation and plotting was performed with R 2.15.10 [15] with libraries: lattice [16], latticeExtra [17], plyr [18] and reshape2 [19].

Accumulation ratio for rectal dosing was defined in one of two ways: either the $AUC_{24\ h}$ ratio of multiple dose gel to single dose gel, or if unavailable, the 0.5 h concentration ratio of multiple dose gel to single dose gel.

Statistical Analysis

Robust linear regression was carried out with robust package for R [20], and fitted to the model: $DV = \beta_0 + \beta_1 \times IV + \beta_2 \times CV + \beta_3 \times IV \times CV$. Dependent (DV) and independent variables (IV) are

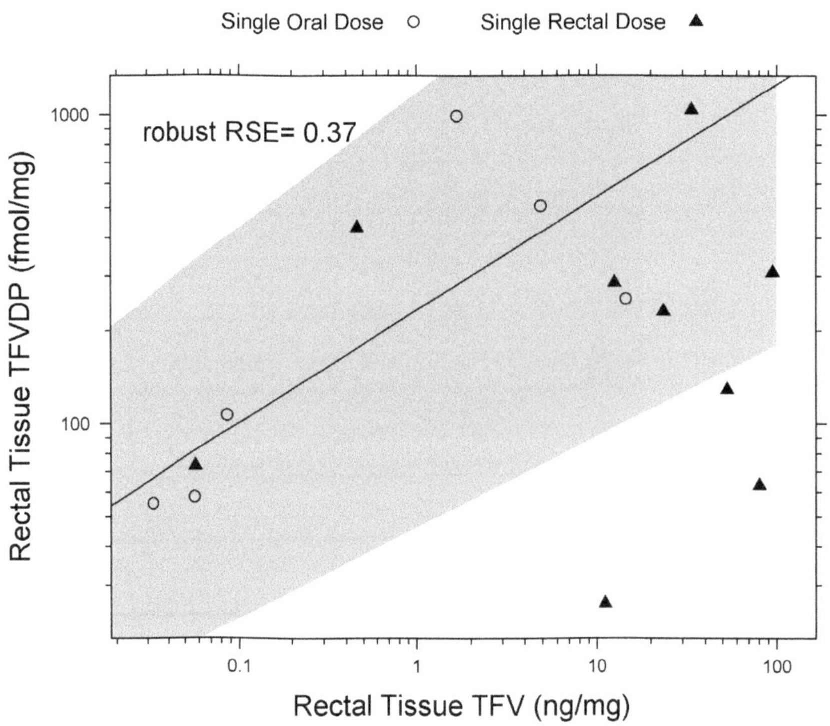

Figure 4. Increasing TFV in Rectal Tissue Homogenate results in increased TFVdp. There is a linear correlation between rectal tissue homogenate TFVdp and TFV ($p = 0.04$, robust RSE $= 0.37$) with oral dosing only (solid line is mean prediction of TFVdp in rectal tissue from oral dosing). Shaded regions are the 10–90% confidence intervals of the mean predictions from robust linear regression model. There is no correlation during rectal dosing.

continuous, while categorical variable (CV) is either 0 or 1. Any parameter terms with $p>0.05$ were dropped and excluded from the statistical model, and re-fitted with a simpler model (backward elimination). All robust linear regression was performed with $\log_{10}$-transformed concentration data. Robust linear regression allows for differential weights to datapoints in respect to outlier datapoint; outliers were given less weight. This results in a more stable model. [21] All statistical comparisons were performed using paired Wilcoxon signed-rank test with a bonferroni correction for 2 comparisons (oral to single rectal, single to multiple rectal), resulting in a critical p-value of 0.025 (0.05/2). Standard error (SE, standard deviation) was a measure of uncertainty around parameter estimates. Relative standard error (RSE) was a measure of overall goodness of fit (0 would be a perfect fit).

Results

Demographics

There were a total of 18 subjects included in this analysis. (Table 1) Mean age was 41, 78% were male, and 84% white. For oral dosing, the following data were used for pharmacokinetic analysis: 139 plasma samples, 131 PBMC samples, 149 rectal tissue homogenates, 72 rectal tissue isolated MMC samples, 31 vaginal sponges, and 135 rectal sponges. For topical dosing, the following data were used for pharmacokinetic analysis: 228 plasma samples, 210 PBMC samples, 144 rectal tissue homogenates, 69 rectal tissue isolate MMC sample, 46 vaginal sponges, and 224 rectal sponges. For the purpose of concentration correlation analysis across matrices only, BLQ samples were excluded. Thus, 163 plasma, 319 PBMC, 208 rectal tissue homogenate, 107 rectal tissue MMC, 42 vaginal sponge, and 130 rectal sponge samples were excluded. All pharmacokinetic data are summarized in Table 2 and Figures 2 and 3. Matrix comparisons are presented in Figures 4–8.

Plasma Pharmacokinetics

As expected, systemic TFV exposure, measured by both $AUC_{24\ h}$ and C_{max}, was 24–33 fold higher after a single oral dose (median $AUC_{24\ h}$ 2200 ng/mL ×h, median C_{max} 250 ng/mL) than after a single rectal dose (median $AUC_{24\ h}$ 66 ng/mL ×h, median C_{max} 11 ng/mL). An accumulation ratio of 0.73 demonstrated that there was no clinically relevant difference in plasma exposure between single and multiple rectal dosing. A 24-fold lower C_{max} was achieved approximately 1.5 h faster with rectal dosing than with oral dosing (median T_{max} single rectal $= 0.32$ h versus single oral $= 1.9$ h; Table 2). TFV half-life was noted to be at least 5 h shorter (paired t-test on log-transformed half-lives, $p = 0.02$) for single and multiple rectal dosing (4.6–6.6 h) compared to oral dosing (11 h). (Table 2; Figure 3) Inter-individual variability of the PK parameters (CV%) ranged from 31–100% during oral dosing, 55–106% during single rectal dosing, and 53–103% during multiple rectal dosing. T_{max} was the most variable PK parameter with CV% consistently above 100%.

PBMC

No detectable TFVdp was found in total PBMCs after single and multiple rectal dosing. (Table 2) In contrast, PBMC exposure after oral dosing was consistently detected in most (10/18) subjects (median $AUC_{24\ h}$ 4.3 fmol/10^6 cells ×h, median C_{max} 0.38 fmol/10^6 cells). There was insufficient data to perform NCA on CD4- and CD4+ cell subpopulations; please see companion paper (Richardson-Harmon et.al) for exposure-response analysis.

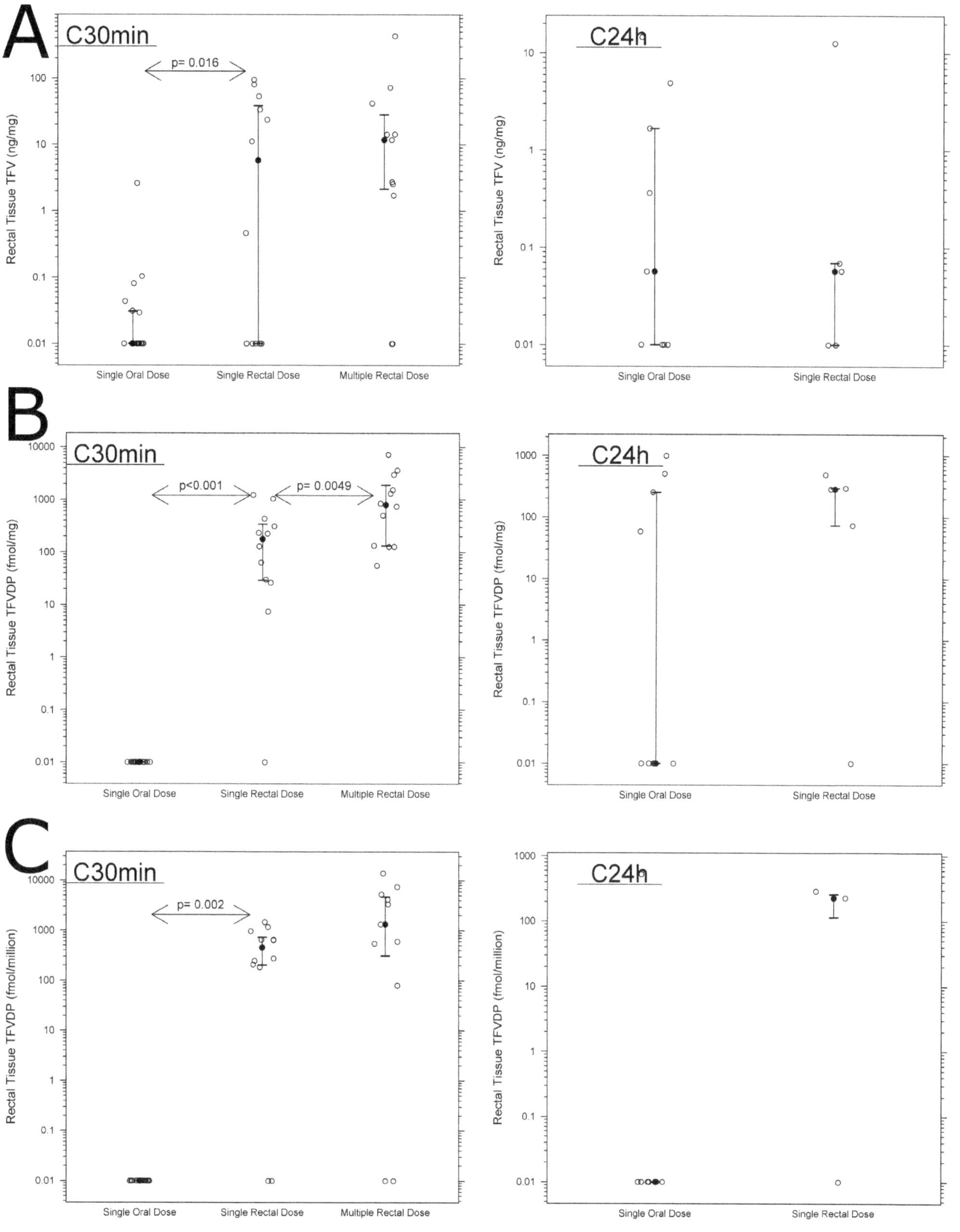

Figure 5. Rectal tissue exposure to TFV and TFVdp (median ± IQR) is higher during rectal dosing with multiple rectal dosing, resulting in accumulation of TFVdp. Each set of figures documents the 30 min drug quantification in the left-side graph and the 24 hr in the right side graph in rectal tissue biopsy homogenate (5A, 5B) and isolated mucosal mononuclear immune cells (MMC) (5C). Comparisons performed with paired Wilcoxon signed-rank test; only a subset of patients gave both $C_{30\ min}$ and $C_{24\ h}$ samples. Figure S5A = TFV_{Tissue}; Figure S5B = $TFVdp_{Tissue}$; Figure S5C = $TFVdp_{MMC}$. There is accumulation of TFV and TFVdp from multiple rectal dosing. Critical p for significance was 0.025 after Bonferroni correction.

Rectal Tissue

There was a linear relationship ($p = 0.04$) between TFVdp and TFV in rectal tissue homogenates during oral dosing. This relationship can be seen in Figure 4. The resulting model (± standard error) was as follows: Rectal Tissue homogenate TFVdp concentration (fmol/mg) = 2.37 (±0.168)+0.366 (±0.121)× rectal tissue homogenate TFV concentration (ng/mg). Although rectal data from topical dosing was excluded from the model due to nonsignificance, they are overlaid in Figure 4 for reference.

Population composite AUC showed that topical dosing resulted in 2-$\log_{10}$ higher rectal exposure to TFV (single oral vs. single rectal dose $AUC_{24\ h}$ = 0.79 vs. 70 ng/mg ×h, Table 2) and a 4-$\log_{10}$ higher rectal exposure to TFVdp (single oral vs. rectal dose $AUC_{24\ h}$ = 0.24 vs. 5500 fmol/mg ×h). When comparing tissue concentrations 30 minutes post-dose, single topical dosing resulted in 2-fold higher TFV (paired $p = 0.016$) and 4-fold higher (paired $p < 0.001$) TFVdp concentrations compared to oral dosing (Figures 4A, 4B). Multiple rectal dosing resulted in a non-statistically significant 2-fold accumulation in TFV concentrations compared to single dosing (paired $P > 0.8$), with TFVdp concentrations accumulating 4.5-fold (paired $p < 0.01$). Over 24 h, we observed TFV concentrations continuing to increase after oral dosing, such that 24 h concentrations post-dose were similar between oral and topical dosing: median TFV concentration at 24 h was 0.060 ng/mg after oral dosing vs 0.060 ng/mg after rectal dosing, paired $p > 0.8$). However, median TFVdp concentrations 24 h post topical rectal dose were almost 300-fold higher than after an oral dose, though not statistically significant. (paired $p = 0.125$). With 4 subjects having missing paired $C_{24\ h}$ rectal biopsy samples for rectal dosing in Figure 5B, this may have resulted in biased TFVdp concentrations after topical dosing.

Isolated total mucosal mononuclear cells yielded similar results to tissue homogenates. At 0.5 h post-dose, rectal dosing resulted in 4-$\log_{10}$ higher concentration (paired $p = 0.002$) of TFVdp (median 454 fmol/10^6 cells) compared to oral administration (median 0.010 fmol/10^6 cells), and remained 4-$\log_{10}$ higher 24 h post dose (median rectal: 230 fmol/10^6 cells, oral: 0.010 fmol/10^6 cells, Table 2, Figure 5C, paired $p = 0.5$). There was also accumulation of TFVdp in these isolated cells after multiple rectal dosing (accumulation ratio: 2.9, paired $p = 0.084$).

Regardless of dosing route, compared to plasma, there was large inter-individual variability in TFV and TFVdp tissue and cell concentrations at each nominal time. Although no dosing route was found to have more variable exposure than the other. In tissue homogenates, TFV CV% ranged from 112–364%, 0 to 220%, and 236% for single oral, single rectal, and multiple rectal dosing, respectively. The CV% of TFVdp ranged from 0–307%, 85–312%, and 132% for single oral, single rectal, and multiple rectal dosing. The lower CV% of 0 in these groups is a result of all measured values being below the limit of quantification. The variability of TFV and TFVdp in isolated mucosal mononuclear cells was also similarly high regardless of CD4 expression status, and ranged from 0 to 316%.

Robust linear regression analysis demonstrated that TFVdp in isolated mucosal mononuclear cells was positively and linearly correlated with TFVdp in rectal tissue homogenates (Figure 6). The β_3 term (see methods for the initial model) was dropped due to nonsignificance. Despite a large number of data points (85%) excluded from the analysis for concentrations below the limit of

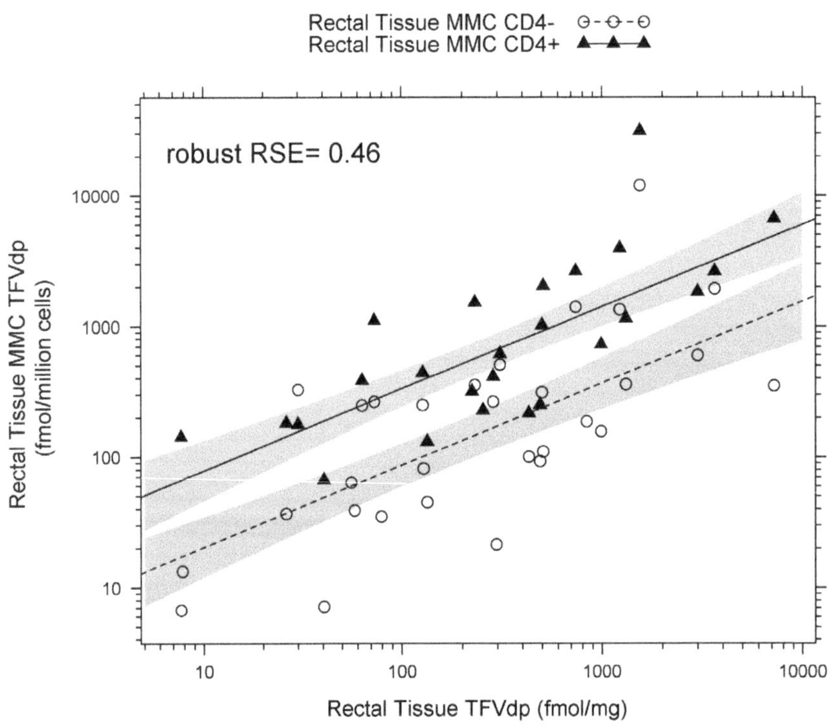

Figure 6. TFVdp in rectal tissue homogenate is predictive of intracellular TFVdp concentration in isolated rectal mucosal mononuclear cells (MMCs), with higher levels of phosphorylation in the CD4+ T cells compared to CD4- T cells. Intracellular TFVdp concentration in isolated rectal mucosal mononuclear cells increases linearly as TFVdp concentration in rectal tissue homogenate increases. ($p < 0.001$, robust RSE = 0.46) There is higher phosphorylation of TFV in CD4+ cells, seen in its higher y-intercept. The lines are the mean rectal tissue MMC TFVdp concentration predictions from robust linear regression model; solid is CD4+, dashed is CD4-. Shaded regions are the 10–90% confidence intervals of the mean prediction.

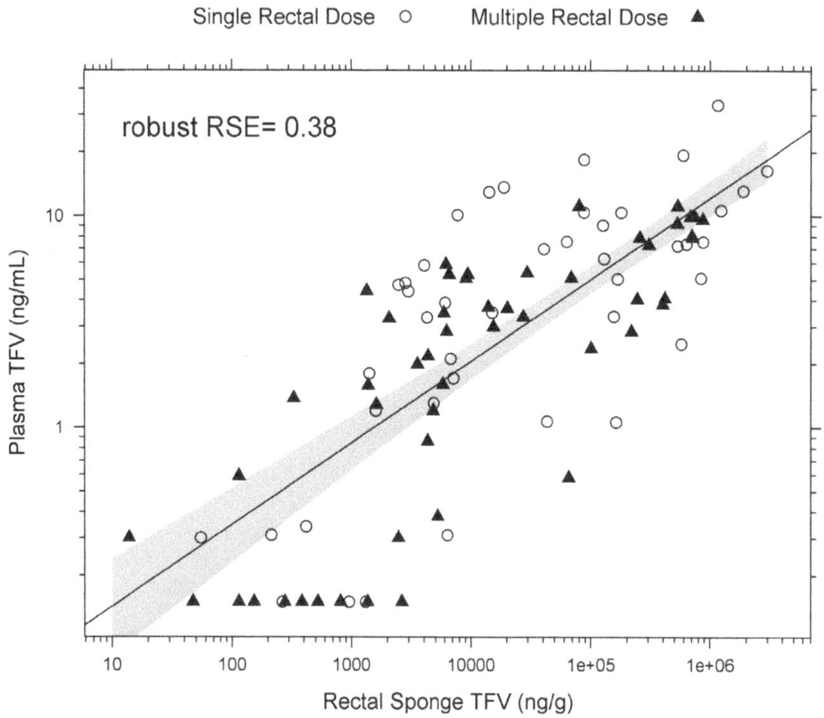

Figure 7. TFV quantification from rectal sponges is predictive of plasma TFV exposure during rectal dosing. Plasma TFV exposure is correlated linearly with rectal sponge TFV exposure. ($p<0.001$, robust RSE $=0.38$) The linear correlation is the same regardless of number of rectal doses. Shaded regions are the 10–90% confidence intervals of the mean predictions from robust linear regression model.

detection, the final model ($\pm$ standard error) still achieved statistical significance ($p<0.001$), and was as follows: Cellular TFVdp concentration $=0.680$ (±0.205) $+0.628$ ($\pm$ 0.0818) $\times$ homogenate TFVdp concentration $+0.586$ (±0.125) $\times$ cell type (cell type $=0$ for CD4- cells and cell type $=1$ for CD4+ cells). Though there is no interaction between cell type and TFVdp, the y-intercept of the CD4+ cells was significantly higher (0.680 vs 1.27; $p<0.01$) than that of the CD4- cells.

Rectal Sponge

TFV exposure in rectal fluid was 1–2 $\log_{10}$ higher during topical administration (single dose median $AUC_{0-24\ h}$: 1,100,000 ng/g $\times$h, C_{max} 740,000 ng/g, Table 2) compared to oral administration (median $AUC_{0-24\ h}$: 100,000 ng/g $\times$h, C_{max} 9,800 ng/g). As expected, topical administration achieved maximal concentrations nearest the time of application (C_{max} $=0.38$ h). However, oral administration achieved maximal concentrations 24 hours after dosing. There was no accumulation of TFV in rectal fluid after multiple rectal dosing (median $AUC_{24\ h}$ single dose 11.0×10^5 ng/g $\times$h, multiple dose 7.03×10^5 ng/g $\times$h). Inter-individual variability was higher for rectal sponge samples compared to direct sampling of other matrices. With oral dosing, single rectal dosing, and multiple rectal dosing, TFV concentration CV% ranged from 150–390%, 92–320%, and 56–150%, respectively.

Robust linear regression demonstrated that plasma TFV concentrations positively and linearly correlated with TFV in rectal fluid after topical dosing (Figure 7). No correlation between plasma concentrations and rectal fluid after oral dosing was noted. Both β_2 and β_3 terms were dropped due to nonsignificance, with the following model ($\pm$ standard error) achieving statistical significance ($p<0.001$): Plasma TFV $=-1.23$ (±0.170) $+0.386$ (±0.0328) $\times$ TFV rectal fluid concentration. The number of rectal doses did not significantly affect these concentration correlations.

Robust linear regression demonstrated that rectal tissue TFV and TFVdp concentrations positively and linearly correlated with TFV in rectal fluid, regardless of administration route (Figure 8). Thus, dose route was dropped as an interaction term. The following model ($\pm$ standard error) achieving statistical significance ($p<0.001$): [Rectal Tissue TFV or TFVdp] $=\beta_0+\beta_1\times$ [Rectal Fluid TFV] For predicting rectal tissue TFV, $\beta_{1,TFV}=0.634(\pm0.0777)$ ($p<0.001$) and $\beta_{0,TFV}=-2.43(\pm0.335)$. For predicting rectal tissue TFVdp, $\beta_{1,TFVdp}=0.197$ (±0.0612) ($p<0.001$), and $\beta_{0,TFVdp}=1.41$ (±0.272). Dose route and frequency was not found to be significant factors in the correlation.

Vaginal Sponge

TFV concentrations in the vaginal lumen peaked at approximately 3 hours regardless of route of administration. However, median TFV C_{max} in the vagina was approximately 2-fold higher after a single rectal dose than after a single oral dose (3100 ng/g vs. 1300 ng/g, Table 2). Additionally, from data in one subject only, there was evidence of accumulation in the vaginal lumen after multiple rectal dosing (accumulation ratio $=5$).

Less inter-individual variability was seen in the vaginal sponge data than the rectal sponge data. TFV concentration CV% at each nominal time from oral dosing, single rectal dosing, and multiple rectal dosing ranged from 50–140%, 40–120%, and 110–140%, respectively.

Robust linear regression demonstrated that TFV concentrations on vaginal sponges are positively and linearly correlated with TFV concentrations in plasma (Figure 9A). The final predictive model ($\pm$ std error) was: TFV in vaginal fluid $=1.32$ (±0.0948) $+0.778$ (±0.0704) $\times$ [plasma TFV] $+0.951$ (±0.169) $\times$ route. For oral

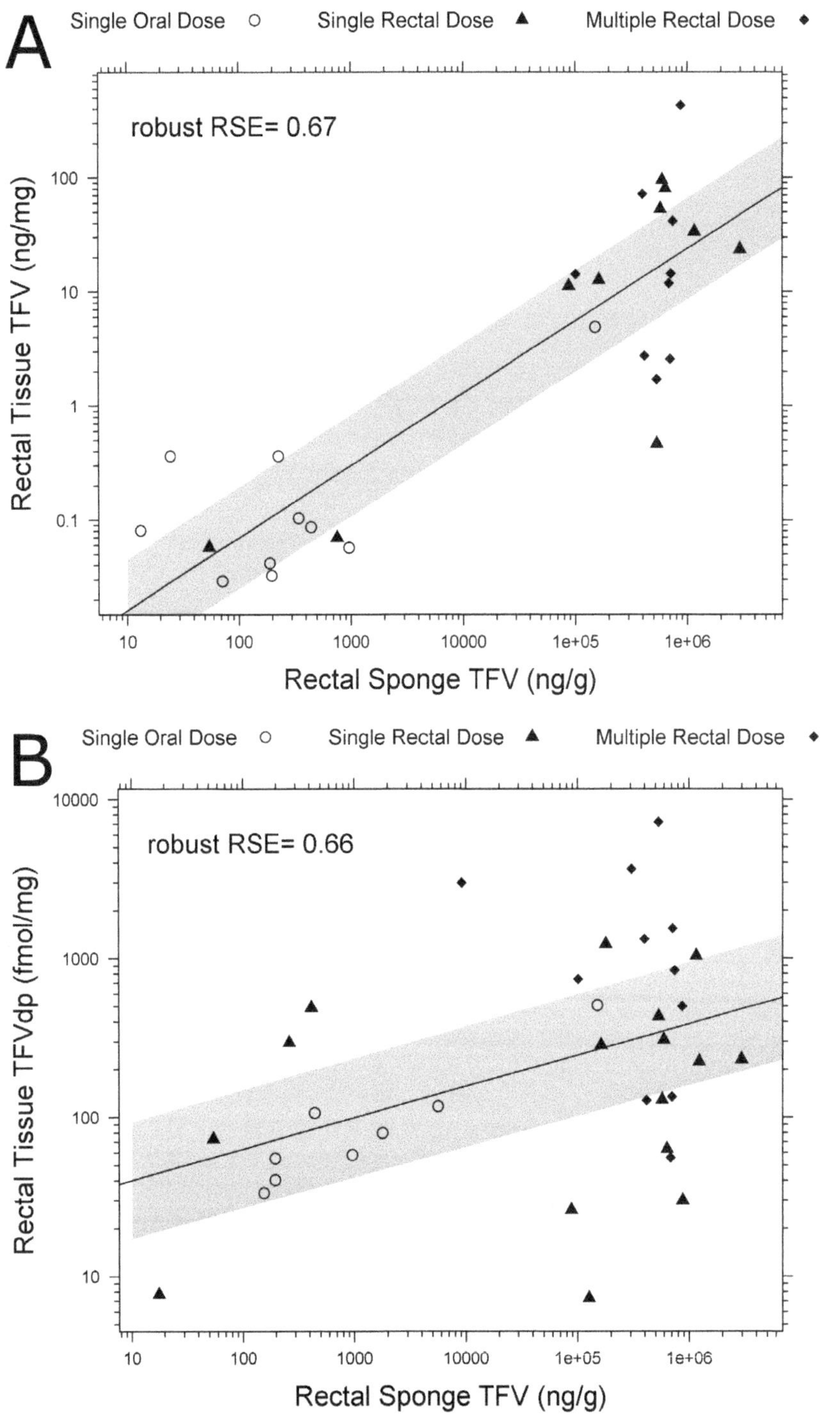

Figure 8. TFV (A) and TFVdp (B) concentrations in rectal tissue homogenate are predicted by Rectal Sponge TFV. ($p<0.001$, robust $RSE_{TFV} = 0.67$, $RSE_{TFVdp} = 0.66$) Shaded regions are the 10–90% confidence intervals of the mean predictions from robust linear regression model. The correlations are consistent regardless of administration route and number of doses.

dosing, route $= 0$, and for rectal dosing, route $= 1$. Though there was no interaction between dose route and TFV in vaginal fluid, the y-intercept of rectal administration was significantly higher (2.27 vs. 1.32; $p<0.01$) than that of oral administration.

Robust linear regression also demonstrated that TFV concentrations on vaginal sponges are positively and linearly correlated with TFV and TFVdp concentrations in rectal tissue. (Figure 9B) The final model ($\pm$ std error) was as follows: [vaginal fluid TFV] $= \beta_0 + \beta_1 \times$ [TFV or TFVdp in rectal tissue] For TFV in rectal tissue as an independent predictor of vaginal fluid concentrations, $\beta_{1,TFV} = 0.741$ (± 0.105, $p<0.001$) and $\beta_{0,TFV} = -0.37$ (± 0.402). For TFVdp in rectal tissue as an independent predictor of vaginal fluid concentrations, $\beta_{1,TFVdp} = 1.66$ (± 0.114, $p<0.001$), and $\beta_{0,TFVdp} = -6.91$ (± 0.649). TFV and TFVdp evaluations were performed as two separate analyses. The coefficients do not directly compare with each other since the predictor variables are independent and in different units. Nonetheless, this demonstrates that TFV vaginal fluid concentrations are significantly linearly correlated with rectal tissue TFV and TFVdp exposure within the concentration range of 0.10 to 10 ng/mg TFV and 30 to 1000 fmol/mg TFVdp.

Discussion

This is the first study examining the pharmacokinetic distribution of rectally applied tenofovir gel in various tissues and cells relevant to HIV infection. This study also compares compartment concentrations of rectally applied TFV kinetics to oral dosing. It is important and biologically relevant to quantify TFV and TFVdp exposures in tissues and cells targeted for HIV infection. Measuring these concentrations allows for a better understanding of how drug distributes from the sites of absorption to target tissues, what factors can impact this distribution, and the possible identification of less-invasive surrogate markers of exposure that could be useful in larger clinical trials.

In this study's intra-subject comparison, the TFV exposure ($AUC_{24\ h}$) in plasma was, expectedly, more than 30 times higher after oral administration of 136 mg of TFV equivalent than after rectal administration of 44 mg of TFV. Additionally, T_{max} was 1.6 h shorter with rectal administration than with oral dosing. Differences in absorption kinetics between the rectum/lower large intestine and upper small intestine may explain this discrepancy. The extent and rate of absorption is often lower in the rectum compared to the intestines. This can be due to the relatively smaller surface area of the rectum for drug absorption, the inherent differences in the formulation, and the environment surrounding the route of administration, such as pH and fluid content [22–24]. In the particular case of TFV gel, the major difference is the formulation. Oral TFV is administered as tenofovir disoproxil fumarate, a di-ester prodrug [25,26]. In contrast, TFV gel contains only the drug. Thus, TFV gel would not require the additional metabolism step, leading to a faster T_{max}. The lower plasma exposure after gel dosing is not completely explained by the lower dose, since the equivalent oral dose was only 3 times higher. This is most likely due to the lower extent of drug absorption in the rectum, and also possibly due to gel leakage.

The half-life of TFV in plasma was 4–6 h longer ($p = 0.02$) with oral dosing than with rectal administration, and consistently longer in all patients except for one. The plasma half-life observed was 1–3 hours shorter than typically reported [25,26] most likely due to lack of data in this study during the terminal elimination phase. Nonetheless, the relative difference in half-life between oral and rectal administration is significant. One possible explanation is that the kinetics with rectal dosing may be driven by absorption, leading to flip-flop kinetics [27]. If this is the true, then the half-life would be rate-limited by the rate of absorption instead of elimination. One other explanation may be the saturation of renal elimination processes [28] as a result of higher TFV plasma exposure. Tenofovir is eliminated by filtration and secretion [25]. Although renal filtration is not saturable, tubular secretion is carrier-protein mediated and can exhibit nonlinear, saturable behavior. During tubular secretion, tenofovir is a substrate for the MRP4 transporter in the tubular lumen [29–31]. Saturation of this excretion transporter could explain nonlinear elimination.

In the case of topical administration, the decreased half-life and lower plasma exposure during both single and multiple administrations can minimize systemic toxicity. C_{max} of TFVdp after a single oral dose was below limit of detection (LLOQ = 8 fmol/10^6 cells); this is significantly lower than what has been previously reported (20 fmol/10^6 cells [9]), but not unexpected based on inter-individual variability. This is probably also due to lower cell penetration of TFV compared to TFVdp. Due to the low plasma exposure following rectal dosing (median plasma $AUC_{24\ h}$ 66 ng/mL ×h), TFVdp exposure was undetectable in PBMCs of all subjects.

As expected, rectal tissue exposure to TFV and TFVdp was 2–4 $\log_{10}$ higher with topical administration than with oral dosing. After multiple dosing, TFV does not appear to significantly accumulate in the tissue. Although the accumulation ratio from the median profile showed an approximately 2-fold increase in $AUC_{24\ h}$, a paired analysis of concentration within individuals showed no statistically significant changes between the 30 min and 24 h post-dose samples. TFVdp, however, did show significant accumulation in rectal tissue (approximately 5-fold) and in isolated mucosal mononuclear cells (approximately 3-fold). The long intracellular half-life of TFVdp is likely the cause of this tissue accumulation [32].

It has previously been noted that an increase in TFV tissue homogenate concentration yields an increase in TFVdp concentration [9,32]. We confirmed this at 24 h after oral dosing (Figure 4). The correlation may have been stronger if there would have been more data to analyze. Furthermore, it is possible that the different absorption kinetics of the rectum compared to the intestines could cause variations in this correlation.

To address the question of whether TFVdp in tissue homogenates accurately reflect TFVdp concentrations in target cells for HIV transmission, or whether the heterogeneous mix of cells in mucosal tissue confounds the results, we compared homogenate results to those of isolated mucosal mononuclear cells. Encouragingly, a linear relationship was noted between TFVdp concentration in rectal tissue homogenate and isolated mucosal mononuclear cells. This linear relationship was not influenced by CD4 status: as TFVdp concentration in the homogenate increased by 100%, there was a 63% increase of TFVdp in the isolated mucosal mononuclear cells. However, the data did suggest that there may be differences in phosphorylation based on the CD4 expression status of the cell. When plotting the relationship between TFVdp in tissue homogenates and in CD4+ and CD4- cells, the Y intercept in CD4+ cells was 1.6-fold higher than in CD4- cells. That is, for every observed TFVdp concentration in the homogenate, the TFVdp concentration in the CD4+ cells was 1.6-fold higher than CD4- cells. This difference persisted throughout the 10–10,000 fmol/mg range of TFVdp concentrations, and achieved statistical significance ($p<0.01$), even with small numbers of samples. The source of this difference is unclear, as some studies suggest that tenofovir is phosphorylated to a similar extent between quiescent and stimulated cells, while others suggest higher phosphorylation in resting cells [33]. Although it is currently unknown whether these concentration differences are of clinical significance, these data are encouraging, as they suggest that TFVdp is found in higher concentrations in the cells that are targets for HIV infection.

In this study, rectal mucosal fluid was collected to determine whether it could be a surrogate for TFV and TFVdp concentration in rectal tissue. TFV concentrations in the rectal fluid linearly correlated with rectal tissue TFVdp. (Figure 8) This relationship remained consistent regardless of dose route or frequency. Despite dramatic differences between oral and rectal absorption characteristics, we still observe a similar linear relationship between these two matrices. Therefore, rectal fluid TFV concentrations collected by sponge are useful in estimating drug concentrations in the target rectal tissue.

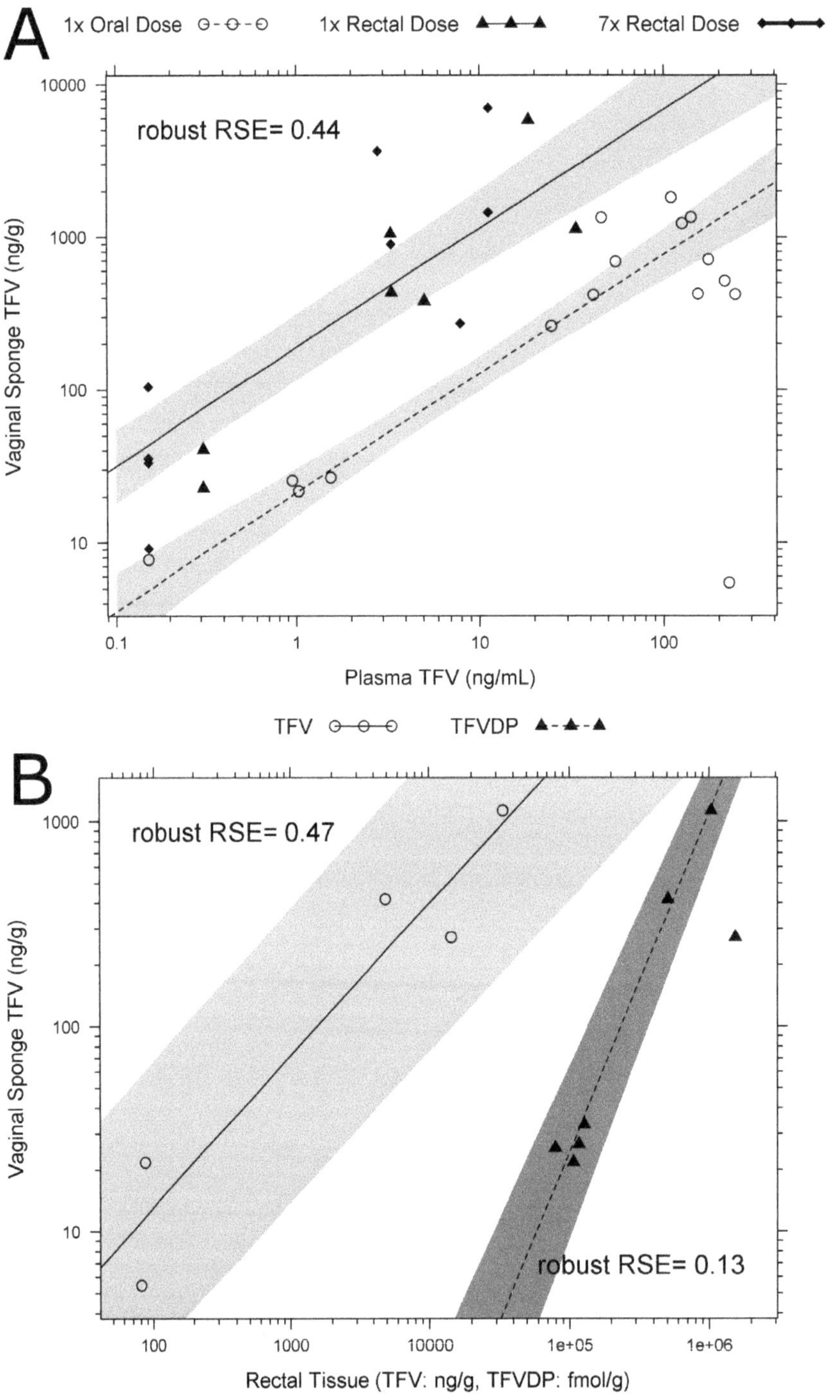

Figure 9. There is vaginal penetration of TFV from both oral and topical rectal exposures. (A) Vaginal fluid detection of both TFV and TFVdp concentration in vaginal fluid is higher following rectal dosing than following single oral dosing TFVdp. There is a linear correlation between vaginal fluid sponge TFV and plasma TFV concentrations ($p<0.001$, robust RSE $=0.44$). TFV penetration into vaginal fluid is 1-$\log_{10}$ higher with rectal administration than oral, seen with higher y-intercept. ($p<0.001$). (B) There is a linear correlation between vaginal fluid TFV and both rectal tissue TFV and TFVdp ($p<0.01$, robust $RSE_{TFV}=0.47$, $RSE_{TFVdp}=0.13$). Shaded regions are the 10–90% confidence intervals of the mean predictions from robust linear regression model. Solid line is mean vaginal fluid TFV concentration, dashed TFVdp.

We also attempted prediction of plasma TFV exposure from rectal mucosal concentrations. There was high variability in these predictions, so a precise prediction was not possible. However, our data suggest that a rough estimation of high or low plasma TFV based on rectal TFV concentration could be feasible. Therefore, rectal sponge TFV concentration could be used as a non-invasive surrogate for plasma TFV concentrations for safety and toxicity monitoring. With more patient data, prediction variability may be decreased using patient demographic covariates, which could potentially minimize the need for blood sampling in future trials of rectal dosing. We did not observe similar correlation with oral dosing; this is probably due to the high variability in the data compared to the possible strength of the correlation. If we had a higher range of rectal fluid concentration, through either different oral dose levels or sample collection times, then it is possible a correlation may be observed.

Previous data in macaques has demonstrated that 5–7% of tenofovir dosed rectally can be found in vaginal fluid [34]. We evaluated this phenomenon in 4 women, and found that vaginal concentrations were 8.7% of rectal secretion concentrations sampled at the same time, similar to the 1–2 $\log_{10}$ difference found previously in animals. Additionally, we noted a 1.6-fold higher exposure of TFV in vaginal secretions with rectal dosing than with oral dosing. Since the slopes of the relationship between vaginal fluid TFV and plasma TFV with the two administration routes are not significantly different, the rate of TFV penetration into the vagina does not vary with administration route. As plasma concentrations with oral dosing are much higher than with rectal dosing, systemic re-distribution into the vaginal fluid cannot be the only mechanism by which TFV reaches the vaginal lumen. Vaginal TFV penetration was further confirmed when we observed a linear relationship between vaginal TFV exposure and rectal tissue exposure. When rectal tissue TFV and TFVdp exposure increased, there was also a linear increase in vaginal exposure to TFV. Due to the low number of data points, we could not discern whether route of administration affected this relationship.

It is interesting to note that there was accumulation of TFV in the vaginal fluid (Table 2, single rectal dose AUC = 1.4 ng/g ×h, multiple rectal dose = 11), but not rectal fluid (single rectal dose AUC = 11 ng/g ×h, multiple rectal dose = 7.0). There are two possible explanations for this. One is that the rectal site is already saturated due to proximity to administration, whereas vaginal site is more distal and takes time to build up. Another is that there may be differences in fluid turnover between the two sites. Therefore, the kinetics is inherently different between the two sites.

One limitation of this analysis is the treatment of BLQ values and nominal times used for the composite PK profiles in Table 2. BLQ numbers are still valuable because there is a lot of information content in these numbers. Therefore, the treatment of BLQ values depended on the analysis performed. They are imputed as 0.01 for NCA, and ignored for correlation analysis due to statistical difficulties in treating these numbers. Since this was done systematically and consistently, there should be no impact on the overall conclusions. Also, the proportion of BLQ values for plasma was low (2.4%), so this should have little impact on the calculated plasma PK parameters. Similarly, since only datapoints that fell within a specific time window were included in the composite profiles, there should not have been a significant bias in PK parameter estimates.

Conclusion

This was the first comprehensive pharmacokinetic study of rectally administered tenofovir gel that describes the distribution of TFV and TFVdp into various tissue compartments relevant to HIV infection. The compartments included rectal fluid, rectal tissue and its isolated mucosal mononuclear cells, vaginal fluid, blood plasma and PBMCs. It was expected, and now confirmed, that rectally applied TFV would have lower systemic exposure and higher vaginal exposure compared to oral. There was accumulation of TFVdp in the rectal tissue, due to the long intracellular half-life. An unexpected yet biologically interesting finding was detecting a consistent difference in concentrations of TFVdp in rectal mucosal CD4+ cells, prime targets for new HIV infections. It is useful to know that TFV rectal fluid concentrations may be reasonable bio-indicators of plasma and, importantly, rectal tissue concentrations, making it easier to estimate adherence and TFV concentrations in the target tissue.

We were encouraged to see many concentration correlations across various relevant matrices, such as rectal mucosal mononuclear cells and rectal tissue homogenate TFVdp, and vaginal fluid and plasma. This will enable more advanced population pharmacokinetic modeling methods and developing a single mathematical model that describes the distribution of TFV with more accuracy. Furthermore, if target TFV and TFVdp concentrations are identified, then these data and models will assist in dose/regimen selection that maximizes efficacy and minimizes toxicity.

Supporting Information

Protocol S1 Trial Protocol.

Checklist S1 CONSORT Checklist.

Acknowledgments

Deep appreciation is offered to the dedicated participants who enrolled in this intensive study. Significant support at all stages of this study was provided by site staff and the study sponsors including UCLA (Elena Khanukhova, Charina McDonald, Terry Saunders, Karen Tanner, VaShira Rhodes, and Justin Akin), MWRI/University of Pittsburgh (Ross Cranston, Carol Oriss, Lorna Rabe, Kathryn Duffill, Lisa Rohan, and Sharon Hillier), JHU (Ed Fuchs, Nicolette Louissaint, Nicole Anders, and Jianmeng Chen), CONRAD (Henry Gabelnick, Timothy McCormick, Marianne Callahan, and David Friend), Gilead Sciences Inc. (Jim Rooney) and NIH/NIAID/DAIDS (Jim Turpin, Jeanna Piper, and Grace Chow).

Author Contributions

Wrote the paper: KY CH RC IM PA AK. Conceived and designed the experiments: PA. Performed the experiments: CH NB JE CM RC IM PA. Analyzed the data: KY KT NR AK. Contributed reagents/materials/analysis tools: CH.

References

1. Abdool Karim Q, Abdool Karim SS, Frohlich JA, Grobler AC, Baxter C, et al. (2010) Effectiveness and safety of tenofovir gel, an antiretroviral microbicide, for the prevention of HIV infection in women. Science 329: 1168–1174. Available: http://www.pubmedcentral.nih.gov/articlerender.fcgi?artid=3001187&tool=pmcentrez&rendertype=abstract Accessed 31 January 2013..
2. Grant RM, Lama JR, Anderson PL, McMahan V, Liu AY, et al. (2010) Preexposure chemoprophylaxis for HIV prevention in men who have sex with men. N Engl J Med 363: 2587–2599. Available: http://www.pubmedcentral.nih.gov/articlerender.fcgi?artid=3079639&tool=pmcentrez&rendertype=abstract. Accessed 29 January 2013.
3. Baeten JM, Donnell D, Ndase P, Mugo NR, Campbell JD, et al. (2012) Antiretroviral prophylaxis for HIV prevention in heterosexual men and women. N Engl J Med 367: 399–410. Available: http://www.ncbi.nlm.nih.gov/pubmed/22784037. Accessed 22 May 2013.
4. Choopanya K, Martin M, Suntharasamai P, Sangkum U, Mock PA, et al. (2013) Antiretroviral prophylaxis for HIV infection in injecting drug users in Bangkok, Thailand (the Bangkok Tenofovir Study): a randomised, double-blind, placebo-controlled phase 3 trial. Lancet 381: 2083–2090. Available: http://www.ncbi.nlm.nih.gov/pubmed/23769234. Accessed 30 October 2013.
5. Karim SSA, Kashuba ADM, Werner L, Karim QA (2011) Drug concentrations after topical and oral antiretroviral pre-exposure prophylaxis: implications for HIV prevention in women. Lancet 378: 279–281. Available: http://www.pubmedcentral.nih.gov/articlerender.fcgi?artid=3652579&tool=pmcentrez&rendertype=abstract. Accessed 27 May 2013.

6. Anderson PL, Glidden D V, Liu A, Buchbinder S, Lama JR, et al. (2012) Emtricitabine-tenofovir concentrations and pre-exposure prophylaxis efficacy in men who have sex with men. Sci Transl Med 4: 151ra125. Available: http://www.ncbi.nlm.nih.gov/pubmed/22972843. Accessed 18 July 2013.
7. Anton PA, Cranston RD, Kashuba A, Hendrix CW, Bumpus NN, et al. (2012) RMP-02/MTN-006: A phase 1 rectal safety, acceptability, pharmacokinetic, and pharmacodynamic study of tenofovir 1% gel compared with oral tenofovir disoproxil fumarate. AIDS Res Hum Retroviruses 28: 1412–1421. Available: http://www.ncbi.nlm.nih.gov/pubmed/22943559. Accessed 31 January 2013.
8. Anton PA, Saunders T, Elliott J, Khanukhova E, Dennis R, et al. (2011) First phase 1 double-blind, placebo-controlled, randomized rectal microbicide trial using UC781 gel with a novel index of ex vivo efficacy. PLoS One 6: e23243. Available: http://www.pubmedcentral.nih.gov/articlerender.fcgi?artid=3182160&tool=pmcentrez&rendertype=abstract. Accessed 2013 July 18.
9. Louissaint NA, Cao Y-J, Skipper PL, Liberman RG, Tannenbaum SR, et al. (2013) Single Dose Pharmacokinetics of Oral Tenofovir in Plasma, Peripheral Blood Mononuclear Cells, Colonic Tissue, and Vaginal Tissue. AIDS Res Hum Retroviruses. Available: http://www.ncbi.nlm.nih.gov/pubmed/23600365. Accessed 2013 July 18.
10. Louissaint NA, Fuchs EJ, Bakshi RP, Nimmagadda S, Du Y, et al. (2012) Distribution of cell-free and cell-associated HIV surrogates in the female genital tract after simulated vaginal intercourse. J Infect Dis 205: 725–732. Available: http://www.ncbi.nlm.nih.gov/pubmed/22279121. Accessed 2013 July 18.
11. Beigi R, Noguchi L, Parsons T, Macio I, Kunjara Na Ayudhya RP, et al. (2011) Pharmacokinetics and placental transfer of single-dose tenofovir 1% vaginal gel in term pregnancy. J Infect Dis 204: 1527–1531. Available: http://www.pubmedcentral.nih.gov/articlerender.fcgi?artid=3192189&tool=pmcentrez&rendertype=abstract. Accessed 2013 July 18.
12. Keller MJ, Madan RP, Torres NM, Fazzari MJ, Cho S, et al. (2011) A randomized trial to assess anti-HIV activity in female genital tract secretions and soluble mucosal immunity following application of 1% tenofovir gel. PLoS One 6: e16475. Available: http://www.pubmedcentral.nih.gov/articlerender.fcgi?artid=3026837&tool=pmcentrez&rendertype=abstract. Accessed 2 February 2013.
13. King T, Bushman L, Kiser J, Anderson PL, Ray M, et al. (2006) Liquid chromatography-tandem mass spectrometric determination of tenofovir-diphosphate in human peripheral blood mononuclear cells. J Chromatogr B Analyt Technol Biomed Life Sci 843: 147–156. Available: http://www.ncbi.nlm.nih.gov/pubmed/16828350. Accessed 2 February 2013.
14. Hendrix CW, Chen BA, Guddera V, Hoesley C, Justman J, et al. (2013) MTN-001: randomized pharmacokinetic cross-over study comparing tenofovir vaginal gel and oral tablets in vaginal tissue and other compartments. PLoS One 8: e55013. Available: http://www.pubmedcentral.nih.gov/articlerender.fcgi?artid=3559346&tool=pmcentrez&rendertype=abstract. Accessed 27 May 2013.
15. R Core Team (2013) R: A Language and Environment for Statistical Computing. Available: http://www.r-project.org/.
16. Sarkar D (n.d.) Lattice: Multivariate Data Visualization with R (Use R!). Springer. Available: http://www.amazon.com/Lattice-Multivariate-Data-Visualization-Use/dp/0387759689. Accessed 2 February 2013.
17. Sarkar D, Andrews F (2012) latticeExtra: Extra Graphical Utilities Based on Lattice. Available: http://cran.r-project.org/package=latticeExtra.
18. Wickham H (2011) The split-apply-combine strategy for data analysis. J Statis. Available: http://citeseerx.ist.psu.edu/viewdoc/download?doi=10.1.1.182.5667&rep=rep1&type=pdf. Accessed 2 February 2013.
19. Wickham H (2007) Reshaping data with the reshape package. J Stat Softw. Available: http://www.had.co.nz/reshape/introduction.pdf. Accessed 2 February 2013.
20. Wang J, Zamar R, Marazzi A, Yohai V, Salibian-Barrera M, et al. (2013) robust: Robust Library. Available: http://cran.r-project.org/package=robust.
21. Hampel FR, Ronchetti EM, Rousseeuw PJ, Stahel WA (2005) Robust Statistics. Hoboken, NJ, USA: John Wiley & Sons, Inc.
22. Van Hoogdalem E, de Boer AG, Breimer DD (1991) Pharmacokinetics of rectal drug administration, Part I. General considerations and clinical applications of centrally acting drugs. Clin Pharmacokinet 21: 11–26. Available: http://www.ncbi.nlm.nih.gov/pubmed/1717195. Accessed 17 July 2013.
23. Van Hoogdalem EJ, de Boer AG, Breimer DD (1991) Pharmacokinetics of rectal drug administration, Part II. Clinical applications of peripherally acting drugs, and conclusions. Clin Pharmacokinet 21: 110–128. Available: http://www.ncbi.nlm.nih.gov/pubmed/1884566. Accessed 17 July 2013.
24. De Boer AG, Moolenaar F, de Leede LG, Breimer DD (n.d.) Rectal drug administration: clinical pharmacokinetic considerations. Clin Pharmacokinet 7: 285–311. Available: http://www.ncbi.nlm.nih.gov/pubmed/6126289. Accessed 17 July 2013.
25. Fung HB, Stone EA, Piacenti FJ (2002) Tenofovir disoproxil fumarate: a nucleotide reverse transcriptase inhibitor for the treatment of HIV infection. Clin Ther 24: 1515–1548. Available: http://www.ncbi.nlm.nih.gov/pubmed/12462284. Accessed 18 July 2013.
26. Kearney BP, Flaherty JF, Shah J (2004) Tenofovir disoproxil fumarate: clinical pharmacology and pharmacokinetics. Clin Pharmacokinet 43: 595–612. Available: http://www.ncbi.nlm.nih.gov/pubmed/15217303. Accessed 18 July 2013.
27. Yáñez JA, Remsberg CM, Sayre CL, Forrest ML, Davies NM (2011) Flip-flop pharmacokinetics—delivering a reversal of disposition: challenges and opportunities during drug development. Ther Deliv 2: 643–672. Available: http://www.pubmedcentral.nih.gov/articlerender.fcgi?artid=3152312&tool=pmcentrez&rendertype=abstract. Accessed 16 December 2013.
28. Van Ginneken CA, Russel FG (1989) Saturable pharmacokinetics in the renal excretion of drugs. Clin Pharmacokinet 16: 38–54. Available: http://www.ncbi.nlm.nih.gov/pubmed/2650954. Accessed 17 July 2013.
29. Rodríguez-Nóvoa S, Labarga P, Soriano V, Egan D, Albalater M, et al. (2009) Predictors of kidney tubular dysfunction in HIV-infected patients treated with tenofovir: a pharmacogenetic study. Clin Infect Dis 48: e108–16. Available: http://www.ncbi.nlm.nih.gov/pubmed/19400747. Accessed 17 July 2013.
30. Imaoka T, Kusuhara H, Adachi M, Schuetz JD, Takeuchi K, et al. (2007) Functional involvement of multidrug resistance-associated protein 4 (MRP4/ABCC4) in the renal elimination of the antiviral drugs adefovir and tenofovir. Mol Pharmacol 71: 619–627. Available: http://www.ncbi.nlm.nih.gov/pubmed/17110501. Accessed 17 July 2013.
31. Ray AS, Cihlar T, Robinson KL, Tong L, Vela JE, et al. (2006) Mechanism of active renal tubular efflux of tenofovir. Antimicrob Agents Chemother 50: 3297–3304. Available: http://www.pubmedcentral.nih.gov/articlerender.fcgi?artid=1610069&tool=pmcentrez&rendertype=abstract. Accessed 30 May 2013.
32. Patterson KB, Prince HA, Kraft E, Jenkins AJ, Shaheen NJ, et al. (2011) Penetration of tenofovir and emtricitabine in mucosal tissues: implications for prevention of HIV-1 transmission. Sci Transl Med 3: 112re4. Available: http://www.pubmedcentral.nih.gov/articlerender.fcgi?artid=3483088&tool=pmcentrez&rendertype=abstract. Accessed 31 May 2013.
33. Robbins BL, Wilcox CK, Fridland A, Rodman JH (2003) Metabolism of tenofovir and didanosine in quiescent or stimulated human peripheral blood mononuclear cells. Pharmacotherapy 23: 695–701. Available: http://www.ncbi.nlm.nih.gov/pubmed/12820810. Accessed 18 July 2013.
34. Nuttall J, Kashuba A, Wang R, White N, Allen P, et al. (2012) Pharmacokinetics of tenofovir following intravaginal and intrarectal administration of tenofovir gel to rhesus macaques. Antimicrob Agents Chemother 56: 103–109. Available: http://www.pubmedcentral.nih.gov/articlerender.fcgi?artid=3256015&tool=pmcentrez&rendertype=abstract. Accessed 18 July 2013.

2

Establishment of a Humanized APL Model via the Transplantation of *PML-RARA*-Transduced Human Common Myeloid Progenitors into Immunodeficient Mice

Hiromichi Matsushita[1,2,3]*, Takashi Yahata[1,2,4], Yin Sheng[1], Yoshihiko Nakamura[1], Yukari Muguruma[1], Hideyuki Matsuzawa[1,5], Masayuki Tanaka[5], Hideki Hayashi[5], Tadayuki Sato[5], Anar Damdinsuren[3], Makoto Onizuka[6], Mamoru Ito[7], Hayato Miyachi[3], Pier Paolo Pandolfi[8], Kiyoshi Ando[1,2,6]*

1 Research Center for Cancer Stem Cell, Tokai University School of Medicine, Isehara, Kanagawa, Japan, **2** Medical Research Institute, Tokai University, Isehara, Kanagawa, Japan, **3** Department of Laboratory Medicine, Tokai University School of Medicine, Isehara, Kanagawa, Japan, **4** Department of Cell Transplantation, Tokai University School of Medicine, Isehara, Kanagawa, Japan, **5** Support Center for Medical Research and Education, Tokai University, Isehara, Kanagawa, Japan, **6** Division of Hematology and Oncology, Department of Internal Medicine, Tokai University School of Medicine, Isehara, Kanagawa, Japan, **7** Central Institute for Experimental Animals, Kawasaki, Kanagawa, Japan, **8** Cancer Research Institute, Beth Israel Deaconess Cancer Center, Departments of Medicine and Pathology, Beth Israel Deaconess Medical Center, Harvard Medical School, Boston, Massachusetts, United States of America

Abstract

Recent advances in cancer biology have revealed that many malignancies possess a hierarchal system, and leukemic stem cells (LSC) or leukemia-initiating cells (LIC) appear to be obligatory for disease progression. Acute promyelocytic leukemia (APL), a subtype of acute myeloid leukemia characterized by the formation of a PML-RARα fusion protein, leads to the accumulation of abnormal promyelocytes. In order to understand the precise mechanisms involved in human APL leukemogenesis, we established a humanized *in vivo* APL model involving retroviral transduction of *PML-RARA* into $CD34^+$ hematopoietic cells from human cord blood and transplantation of these cells into immunodeficient mice. The leukemia well recapitulated human APL, consisting of leukemic cells with abundant azurophilic abnormal granules in the cytoplasm, which expressed CD13, CD33 and CD117, but not HLA-DR and CD34, were clustered in the same category as human APL samples in the gene expression analysis, and demonstrated sensitivity to ATRA. As seen in human APL, the induced APL cells showed a low transplantation efficiency in the secondary recipients, which was also exhibited in the transplantations that were carried out using the sorted $CD34^-$ fraction. In order to analyze the mechanisms underlying APL initiation and development, fractionated human cord blood was transduced with *PML-RARA*. Common myeloid progenitors (CMP) from $CD34^+/CD38^+$ cells developed APL. These findings demonstrate that CMP are a target fraction for *PML-RARA* in APL, whereas the resultant $CD34^-$ APL cells may share the ability to maintain the tumor.

Editor: Marina Konopleva, University of Texas M.D. Anderson Cancer Center, United States of America

Funding: Hiromichi Matsushita received funding from a Grant-in-Aid for Scientific Research from The Ministry of Education, Culture, Sports, Science and Technology of Japan (#24591411, URL http://www.jsps.go.jp/english/e-grants/), Tokai University School of Medicine Project Research (http://www.med.u-tokai.ac.jp/web/international/about_us/message_from_the_dean.html), and the Takeda Science Foundation (http://www.takeda-sci.or.jp/index.html). Kiyoshi Ando received support from a Grant-in-Aid for Scientific Research from The Ministry of Education, Culture, Sports, Science and Technology of Japan (#24390248). The funders had no role in study design, data collection and analysis, decision to publish, or preparation of the manuscript.

Competing Interests: The authors have declared that no competing interests exist.

* Email: hmatsu@is.ic.cc.u-tokai.ac.jp (H. Matsushita); andok@keyaki.cc.u-tokai.ac.jp (KA)

Introduction

Acute myeloid leukemia (AML) constitutes a heterogeneous group of tumors in myeloid lineage cells characterized by the proliferation and accumulation of immature myeloblasts [1]. Recent advances in cancer biology have revealed that various genetic events result in the blockage of differentiation with subsequent uncontrolled cellular proliferation. In addition, *in vivo* analyses using a xenograft model with immunodeficient mice have shown that a very immature subset of AML cells called leukemic stem cells (LSC), which are typically characterized as $CD34^+/CD38^-$ cells, as observed in normal hematopoietic stem cells (HSCs), have been shown to slowly undergo cell division to both yield progenitor cells and sustain the LSC population, thus resulting in the maintenance of the tumor [2–6]. More recently, several reports have shown that $CD34^+/CD38^+$ hematopoietic progenitors are able to acquire the ability to maintain populations of LSC or leukemia-initiating cells (LIC) [7]. It is therefore possible that the phenotypes of LIC differ among the subtypes of AML.

Acute promyelocytic leukemia (APL) is a subset of AML defined by the formation of a chimeric gene, promyelocytic leukemia-retinoic acid receptor α (*PML-RARA*) [8]. It is characterized by the accumulation of abnormal promyelocytes with abundant large azurophilic granules, suggesting that APL cells undergo maturation arrest in the later steps of myeloid differentiation. The typical pattern of cellular surface markers of APL is positive for CD13,

CD33 and CD117, and negative for CD34, which is usually presumed to indicate cellular immaturity, and HLA-DR [9]. It is very difficult to engraft primary APL samples in immunodeficient mice. They did not become engrafted into the NOD/SCID mice to any degree [3]. In NOD/Shi-SCID/IL-2Rγ^{null} (NOG) mice, which are more profoundly immunocompromised than NOD/SCID mice [10,11], six out of eight APL samples were not engrafted or only very little engrafted [12]. It is therefore possible that the mechanisms underlying the development of APL differ from those involved in the pathogenesis of AML uncovered to date. Elucidating the pathogenesis of APL is important for improving the treatment of APL patients, and will provide clues to understand the development of other subtypes of AML.

In vivo analyses using transgenic APL mice models with *PML-RARA* have revealed that a population of committed myeloid progenitor cells (CD34$^+$, c-kit$^+$, FcγRIII/II$^+$, Gr1^{int}) was identified as the APL-LIC [13,14]. However, the cellular surface antigens and the gene expression pattern in humans are different from those in mice. In particularly, in transgenic systems, murine APL developed after a long latent period through a myelodysplastic/proliferative phase, which does not usually precede human APL [15–18]. There have been no *in vivo* models for exploring leukemogenesis of human APL to date; largely because human primary APL cells are difficult to engraft as a xenograft [3,12]. *PML-RARA*-retrovirally transduced human CD34$^+$ cells from cord blood have therefore only been evaluated *in vitro* [19].

Therefore, the aim of this study was to establish a humanized xenograft APL model using the retroviral transduction of *PML-RARA* into human CD34$^+$ cells and NOG mice in order to investigate the mechanisms of APL leukemogenesis, such as that involving disease initiation and maintenance in the model.

Materials and Methods

Fractionation of human hematopoietic cells from cord blood

Cord blood (CB) and patients' APL samples were obtained after written informed consent was provided in accordance with the Declaration of Helsinki and with approval from the Tokai University Committee on Clinical Investigation (Permit number: #12I-46 and #12I-49). CD34 positive and negative specimens were primarily prepared using the CD34 Progenitor Cell Isolation Kit (Miltenyi Biotec, Bergisch Gladbach, Germany). CD34$^+$ cells were then purified again using anti-human CD34 mAbs (Beckman Coulter, Brea, CA), in combination with or without an anti-CD38 antibody (BD, Franklin Lakes, NJ), with a FACS vantage instrument (BD). CD34$^-$/CD33$^+$ cells were also purified again using anti-human CD34 and CD33 mAbs (Beckman Coulter) and the FACS vantage instrument. The preparation of common myeloid progenitors (CMP), granulocyte-monocytic progenitors (GMP) and megakaryocyte-erythrocyte progenitors (MEP) was performed using an anti-CD123 antibody (BD) and anti-CD45RA (Biolegend, San Diego, CA) antibody, according to a previous report [20].

Retrovirus transduction of *PML-RARA* into human hematopoietic cells

The MIGR1 retroviral vector [21] or MIGR1-*PML-RARA* (bcr3/short form) [22] in combination with the vesicular stomatitis virus-G protein (VSV-G) envelope vector (pCMV-VSV-G) was transiently transfected into PLAT-gp cells using the Fugene 6 transfection reagent (Roche Diagnostics, Basel, Switzerland). The culture supernatant was concentrated 100 to 200 times by ultracentrifugation. After overnight culture of the fractionated cells in StemPro-34 (Life Technologies, Carlsbad, CA) with TPO, SCF, and FLT3 ligand (50 ng/ml each), they were incubated with the concentrated supernatant on retronectin-coated plates (Takara-Bio, Otsu, Japan). Retroviral transduction was performed twice, and then transplantation was performed the next day.

Colony-forming unit-cells assay

PML-RARA transduced cells were sorted by their EGFP, CD34 and CD38 expression by FACS vantage 48 h after infection. The colony-forming unit-cells (CFU-C) assay was performed as described previously [23]. The fluorescent images were captured using a HS All-in-One Fluorescence Microscope Biorevo 9000 (Keyence Corporation, Osaka, Japan) and were analyzed by the BZ II software program (Keyence Corporation).

RNA extraction and RT-PCR

Total RNA was isolated using the RNeasy micro kit (Qiagen, Hilden, Germany) or Isogen (Nippon gene, Tokyo, Japan), and the reverse-transcribed cDNA was amplified by qualitative PCR. The qualitative-PCR analysis was performed by SRL Inc. (Hachioji, Tokyo, Japan). The sequences of PCR primers and probes were shown in **Table S1**.

Transplantation, serial transplantation and ATRA treatment

Nine- to 20-week-old NOD/Shi-scid, IL-2Rγc^{null} (NOG) mice [10,11] were irradiated with 220 cGy of X-rays. On the following day, the whole infected cells or primary AML cells were intravenously injected. The EGFP-positive cells in the peripheral blood were monitored. The mice with induced APL were defined as those bearing more than 0.1% EGFP$^+$ cells which dominantly expressed CD33 (more than 70%) in their bone marrow at four months after transplantation. In the initial analysis, the occurrence of APL was confirmed by the morphological observations using cytospin slides after EGFP sorting. For serial transplantation, bone marrow cells were obtained from recipient mice, and the sorted EGFP-positive cells were injected intravenously or intramedullary into the irradiated mice [24]. The engrafted mice were treated intraperitoneally with 1.5 µg/g of body weight/day of all-*trans* retinoic acid (ATRA, Sigma) for 21 days [25], and were then sacrificed to collect the EGFP-positive cells in the bone marrow by sorting. All the experiments using animals were approved by the animal care committee of Tokai University (Permit number: #132028).

Flow cytometric analysis

The cells were stained with APC-conjugated anti-human CD45, CD33, CD34, HLA-DR (Beckman Coulter), CD13, and CD117 (BD) mAbs. They were subjected to flow cytometry using a FACSCalibur instrument (BD) and the CellQuest software program (BD).

Cell preparation, Wright-Giemsa staining and immunofluorescence microscopy

Cytospin slides were prepared using a Cytospin 4 Cytocentrifuge (Thermo Scientific, Waltham, MA) at 500 rounds per minute for 5 min. To observe the cellular morphology, Wright-Giemsa staining was performed. For the immunofluorescent study, cells were seeded onto poly-L-lysine coated slides and fixed with ice cold 70% ethanol for 15 min. After permeabilization with 0.2% Triton X-100 for 20 min, the slides were treated with PBS containing 5% normal goat serum for 1 hour to block the nonspecific binding of antibodies. The anti-PML antibody (Merck

Millipore, Billerica, MA) was applied overnight at 4°C. Cells were counterstained with DAPI. Images were captured with an LSM510 META confocal microscope (Carl Zeiss, Oberkochen, Germany) and processed using Adobe Photoshop 7.0 (Adobe Systems, San Jose, CA).

Southern blot analysis

Genomic DNA was extracted from the cells using a DNeasy kit (Qiagen). Ten micrograms of the DNA were electrophoresed and transferred to nylon membranes (Hybond-N+, GE Healthcare, Fairfield, CT). The DNA was then crosslinked to the membrane by ultraviolet light. The EGFP probe was prepared from MIGR1 vector by cutting it using NcoI and SalI, and was labeled with ^{32}P-dCTP using the Rediprime II DNA Labelling System (GE Healthcare). The membrane was hybridized with the probe in Rapid-hyb buffer (GE Healthcare), and was analyzed by a Phosphoimager (LAS1000, Fuji Film, Tokyo, Japan).

Microarray

Total RNA was labeled and hybridized to Affymetrix Human Genome U133 Plus 2.0 Array GeneChip microarrays (Affymetrix, Santa Clara, CA) using the manufacturer's protocols. The results were deposited in the Gene Expression Omnibus (GEO; http://www.ncbi.nlm.nih.gov/geo/; accession no. GSE49344). The microarray data from normal human promyelocytes and clinical samples bearing AML, including APL, were obtained from the deposited data on the GEO (GSE12662). The APL-specific expressed genes have been described in detail in a previous study [26]. The probe set data were generated using standard normalization algorithms included in the Affymetrix Microarray Suite software program, v.5 (MAS5.0). The clustering analysis was performed by the Gene spring GX software program, version 11 (Agilent technology, Santa Clara, CA).

To identify the genes that are differentially expressed in a specific cellular subset, all probe sets with fewer than 10% present calls in both groups and a coefficient of variation <0.5 across all samples were eliminated prior to the subsequent analysis; (i) The genes differently expressed in the induced APL cases among the AML cases were defined as genes whose expression change (upregulation or downregulation) was ≥2.0 fold in comparison to those in AML other than APL, (ii) The genes associated with immaturity in the induced APL cases were expressed at significantly higher levels in CD34$^+$ cells than the other normal cells (FDR <0.05, fold-change >2.0 upregulated), and were also expressed in the induced APL cells at similar levels (induced APL: CD34$^+$ ≥1:1), and moreover, these genes were expressed at higher levels in promyelocytes (induced APL: Pros ≥2:1). (iii) The genes upregulated during promyelocyte differentiation were expressed at significantly higher levels in promyelocytes than in the other normal cells (FDR <0.05, fold-change >2.0 upregulated), and were expressed at lower levels in the induced APL (induced APL: Pros ≤1:2), (iv) The genes induced by *PML-RARA* were expressed at higher levels in the induced APL than in all the normal cells (induced APL: normal ≥2:1), and were not expressed in any normal cells (more than 75% absent calls, as summarized by the MAS5.0). Statistical significance was assessed by the unpaired unequal variance Welch test (P<0.05), and correction for multiple testing was performed by the Benjamini and Hochberg False Discovery Rate (FDR), using a cutoff of 0.05.

The gene set specific for induced APL was defined to fulfill one or more of the above criteria (ii) to (iv) in the gene set identified in (i).

The integration site analysis of *PML-RARA* using linear amplification-mediated PCR

To identify the genomic-proviral junction sequence, linear amplification-mediated polymerase chain reaction (LAM-PCR) was performed as described previously, with minor modifications [27,28]. In brief, genomic DNA from bone marrow cells was first digested with Tsp509I. A linear amplification of target DNA in the digested genome was performed by repeated primer extension using a vector-specific 5′-biotinylated primer, LTR1.5, and Taq polymerase. After selection with Dynabeads MyOne Streptavidin C1 (Life Technologies), a double-stranded asymmetrical linker cassette was ligated to the Tsp509I-digested site using T4 DNA Ligase. The DNA products were then amplified by PCR using a vector-specific primer, LTR3, and linker cassette primer, LC1. The nested PCR was performed using internal primers LTR5 and LC2. The final products were sequenced after cloning them into the TOPO TA cloning vector (Life Technologies). The primer sequences are shown in **Table S1**.

Statistical analyses

The Kaplan-Meier method was used to estimate the leukemia-free survival (LFS) of mice. Log-rank p values were used for comparisons of the LFS among three subgroups. The analyses were conducted using the GraphPad Prism software package (GraphPad Software, La Jolla, CA). The other statistical analyses were performed using the Mann-Whitney U Test with the IBM SPSS Statistics software program (New York, NY). Values of $p < 0.05$ were considered to be statistically significant.

Results

Functions of PML-RARα in human CD34 cells *in vitro*

To examine the functions of PML-RARα *in vitro*, a MIGR1-*PML-RARA* or MIGR1 control vector was retrovirally infected into human CD34$^+$ cells from cord blood. The transduction efficiency evaluated by EGFP positivity was 0.5% to 18.6% (n = 10, median: 5.7%) and 2.1% to 19.7% (n = 25, median: 6.8%), respectively. The expression of *PML-RARA* in these cells was confirmed by RT-PCR (**Figure S1**). The induction of *PML-RARA* in CD34$^+$ cells disrupted PML nuclear bodies by interacting with wild-type PML via the PML portion of the chimeric transcript, and the distribution of PML in the nucleus was altered to show a microspeckled pattern in these cells [29–31] (**Figure 1A**). Additionally, the induction of *PML-RARA* reduced all the colony formation capacity (**Figure 1B**). The *PML-RARA* expression was confirmed in these colonies by EGFP fluorescence (**Figure S1 and S2**) and RT-PCR, although the expression levels were 37 times lower compared to those in the CD34$^+$ cells 48 hours after *PML-RARA* transduction (**Figure S3**). Regarding the content of colonies, MIGR1-infected CD34$^+$ cells mainly generated the erythroid lineage-containing colonies, such as CFU-mix and BFU-E, whereas more than half of the colonies from the CD34$^+$ cells with *PML-RARA* were of the myeloid lineage, like CFU-GM (**Figures 1C**). These data demonstrate that *PML-RARA* induces the myeloid commitment of human CD34$^+$ cells.

Establishment of a humanized *in vivo* APL model

The cells transduced with *PML-RARA* or the MIGR1 control vector were then transplanted into NOG mice. The EGFP$^+$ cells survived and proliferated three to four months after transplantation only in the NOG mice transplanted with *PML-RARA*-, not control vector at all, infected human CD34$^+$ cells. The median proportion of EGFP$^+$/CD45$^+$ cells in the bone marrow obtained from the transplanted mice was 23.7% (0.95% to 96.5%, n = 24)

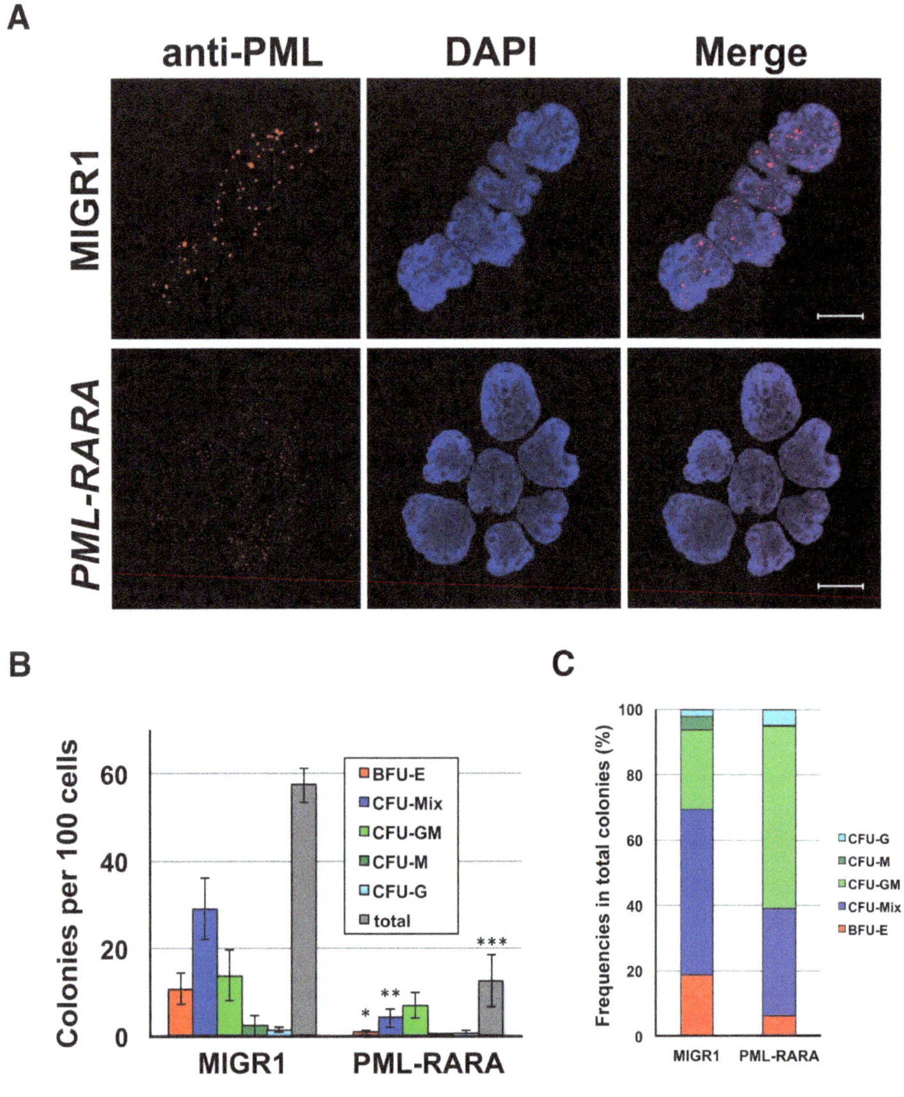

Figure 1. The function of *PML-RARA* in human CD34$^+$ cells *in vitro*. (**A**) The results of an immunofluorescent analysis of PML distribution in human CD34$^+$ cells transduced with *PML-RARA*. The images were captured with an LSM510 META confocal microscope (Carl Zeiss). The bars indicate 10 μm. (**B**) The colony-forming assay using *PML-RARA*-transduced CD34$^+$ cells. The cells were sorted by EGFP expression 48 h after infection. Colony formation was evaluated on days 10 to 12 after plating the cells. The average numbers of colonies from three independent experiments are shown. Data represent the means ± SD. The asterisks (*) indicate $p<0.05$. (**C**) The proportion of each kind of colony was calculated from the results of the colony-forming assay shown in (B). The percentages of CFU-GM are higher in *PML-RARA*-infected cells than in control (MIGR1) cells ($p=0.013$).

(**Figure 2A**). The majority of the engrafted EGFP$^+$/human CD45$^+$ cells expressed human CD33 (70.2% to 100%, median 90.6%, n = 24) (**Figure 2B**), thus suggesting that they were of the myeloid lineage. The *PML-RARA* expression was detected only in the EGFP$^+$ fraction and not in the EGFP$^-$ fraction of the sorted human CD45$^+$/CD33$^+$ cells from the NOG mice (**Figure 2C**). The expression levels of *PML-RARA* were decreased about 17-fold in comparison to those in the CD34$^+$ cells 48 hours after *PML-RARA* transduction (**Figure S3**), but the presence of *PML-RARA* in the human myeloid cells, recognized as EGFP$^+$ cells, caused marked accumulation of promyelocytes, in comparison to the control EGFP$^-$ human myeloid cells (52.8% in EGFP$^+$ cells vs 19.4% EGFP$^-$ cells in the 13 paired samples, $p<0.0001$). On the other hand, the proportions of myeloblasts, mature neutrophils and monocytes were decreased (5.2% vs 14.4%, $p=0.010$; 2.5% vs 12.7%, $p=0.005$; 4.0% vs 10.1%, $p=0.016$) (**Figure 2D**). These findings confirmed that the expression of *PML-RARA* induced the myeloid differentiation of human CD34$^+$ cells and blocked them at the promyelocytic stage. Morphologically, the promyelocytes had abundant large azurophilic granules and round nuclei with a high nucleocytoplasmic ratio. Some of them had a number of Auer bodies and looked like Faggot cells, which are the typical morphological features of APL cells, and were not seen in the previous murine models (**Figure 2E**). A Southern blot analysis using an EGFP probe revealed that the EGFP$^+$/CD45$^+$/CD33$^+$ cells oligoclonally proliferated *in vivo* (**Figure 2F**).

The induced APL cells were detected in 24 out of the 34 mice (71%) transplanted with *PML-RARA*-transduced CD34 cells ($p=0.0184$ in comparison to the control). They were detected in all 16 mice when the calculated number of the transplanted EGFP$^+$/CD34$^+$ cells per mouse was more than 3,000 (4,655 to 29,728 cells, median: 11,085 cells) ($p=0.0006$ in comparison to the control). On the other hand, they were only detected in eight out of 18 mice (44%) transplanted with EGFP$^+$/CD34$^+$ cells at a

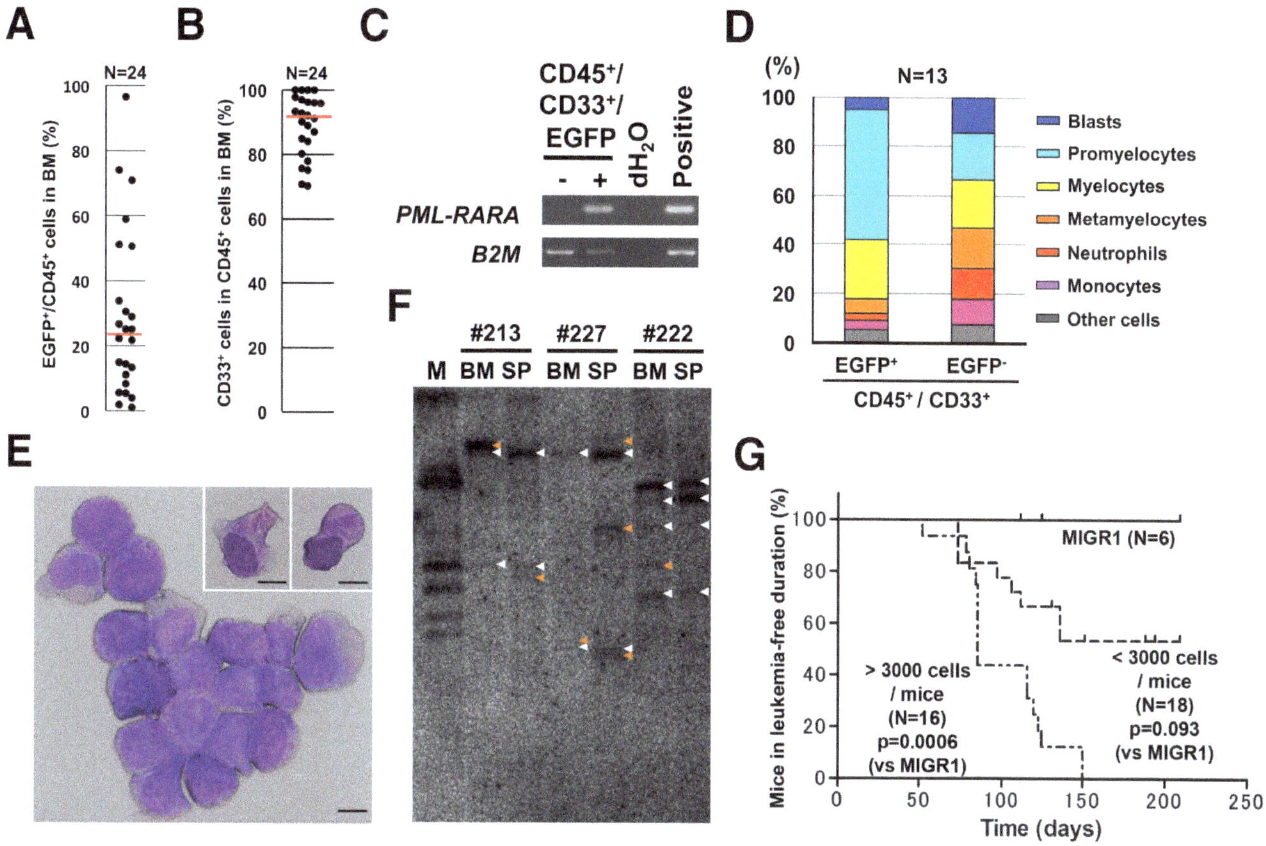

Figure 2. Establishment of humanized APL *in vivo*. (**A**) The proportion of EGFP$^+$/human CD45$^+$ cells in the bone marrow of leukemic NOG mice. Each dot represents a single mouse. The horizontal line represents the median value. (**B**) The proportion of CD33$^+$ cells among the EGFP$^+$/human CD45$^+$ cells in the bone marrow of the leukemic NOG mice. Each dot represents a single mouse. The horizontal line represents the median value. (**C**) The expression of *PML-RARA* in RT-PCR was detected only in the EGFP$^+$ fraction obtained from the engrafted human CD45$^+$/CD33$^+$ cells. The cells were obtained from bone marrow 16 weeks after transplantation. *B2M, beta 2 microglobulin*. The *PML-RARA* expression vector and human CD34$^+$ cells were used as a positive control for the *PML-RARA* and *B2M* analysis, respectively. (**D**) The differential counts of the engrafted CD45$^+$/CD33$^+$/EGFP$^+$ and EGFP$^-$ cells from the mice transplanted with *PML-RARA*-induced human CD34$^+$ cells. They were obtained from bone marrow 16 to 20 weeks after transplantation. The data represent the means. (**E**) A representative photograph of the resulting leukemic cells which morphologically recapitulated APL. Faggot cells were recognized, as seen in the right top corner. The images were captured with a BX41 microscope (Olympus). The bar indicates 10 μm. (**F**) The results of a Southern blot analysis of the genomic DNA from induced APL cells with an EGFP probe. Clonal bands are shown by arrow heads: white, seen in both BM and SP; orange, seen only in BM or SP. BM, bone marrow; SP, spleen. (**G**) The leukemia-free duration in NOG mice transplanted with *PML-RARA*-transduced CD34$^+$ cells.

density of less than 3,000 (480 to 2,660 cells, median: 1,861 cells) (p = 0.093 in comparison to the control) (**Figure 2G**). This proportion was not dependent on the number of transplanted EGFP$^+$/CD34$^+$ cells.

These findings demonstrate that a humanized APL model can be successfully established by the transplantation of *PML-RARA*-transduced human CD34 cells into NOG mice.

Characteristics of the induced APL cells obtained from the humanized *in vivo* model

The induced APL cells were positive for human myeloid markers such as CD13, CD33 and CD117, and were negative for CD34 and HLA-DR, as seen in typical human APL [32]. *PML-RARA* did not contribute to the development of lymphocytes. Human CD19$^+$ B-cells in the spleen and human CD4$^+$/CD8$^+$ T-cells in the thymus were negative for EGFP (**Figure 3A**).

To evaluate the gene expression of the induced APL cells, a microarray analysis was performed, and the expression of the 510 APL-specific genes identified in a previous study was compared with that observed in the clinical AML samples [26]. Two clinical APL samples from our patients were simultaneously evaluated and were aligned in the APL category defined in the study, suggesting that our microarray results were comparable with those in the previous study. The induced APL cells from our models were also classified into the APL category when compared to normal promyelocytes and AML samples other than APL (**Figure 3B**).

In common with this previous study [26], the 3,439 probes (3278 genes) differentially expressed in the induced APL and the AML other than APL ((i) in the Materials and Methods) grouped the induced APL and human primary APL together, separately from the other types of AML (**Figure S4**). The gene sets whose expression in the induced APL cases was not dependent on the myeloid differentiation were also filtered by comparison with the data for normal myeloid cells. They included the genes for immaturity expressed in the induced APL (1,782 probes, including 1,720 genes), the genes upregulated in promyelocyte differentiation not in the induced APL (447 probes, including 427 genes) and the genes specifically induced by *PML-RARA* (466 probes, including 429 genes) ((ii), (iii) and (iv) in the Materials and Methods). Each gene set was analyzed using the DAVID website

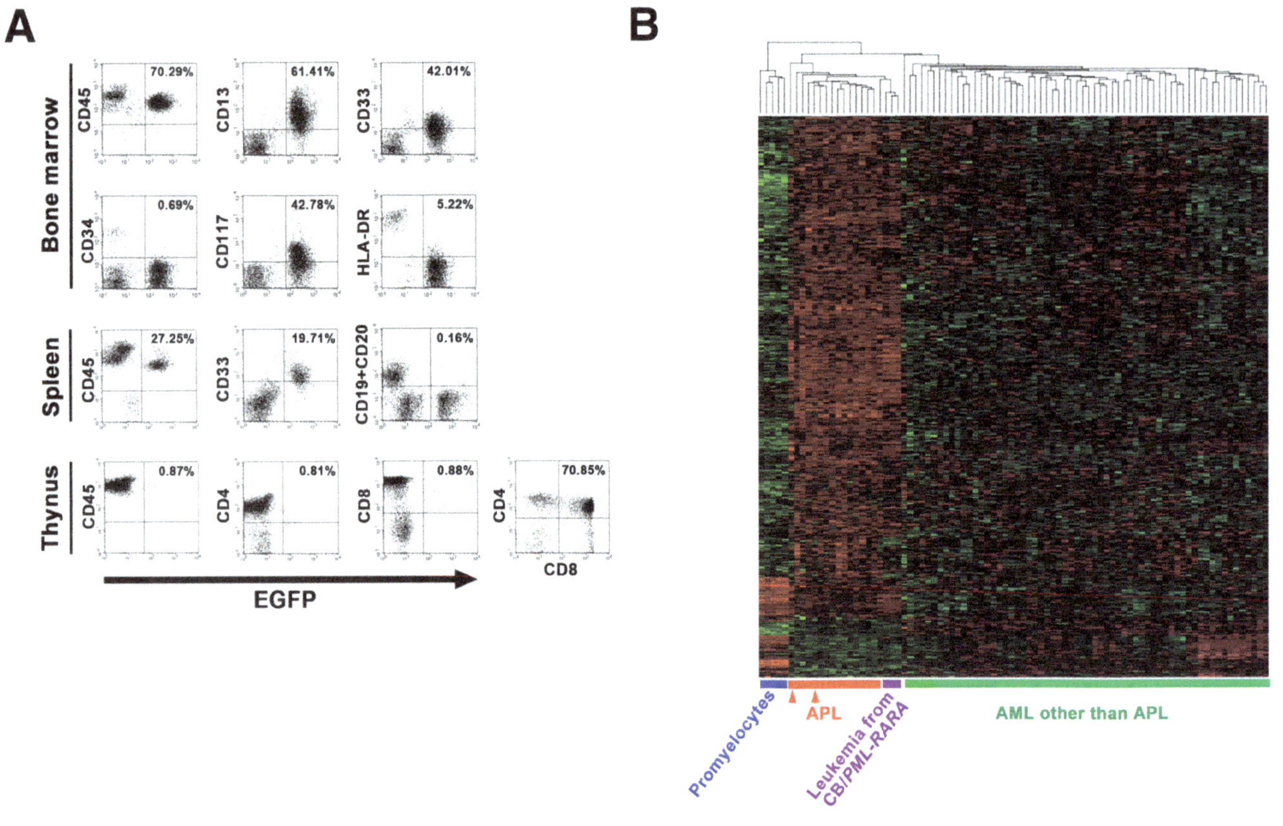

Figure 3. Characteristics of the induced APL *in vivo*. (A) The representative expression pattern of cell surface markers in the induced APL cells determined by a flow cytometric analysis. All the scatter plots show the relationships between the EGFP positivity and cell surface marker expression. The whole living cells gated as a propidium iodide-negative fraction in the bone marrow were analyzed. The induced APL cells were recognized as $EGFP^+$ cells. A few murine hematopoietic cells, recognized as a human $CD45^-$ fraction, were detected in this mouse. **(B)** The heat map of the microarray analysis using the 510 APL-specific genes for the comparison of the induced APL cells (purple, n = 3) with APL (red, n = 16), other types of AML (M0, 1, 2 and 4 in FAB classification, green, n = 62) and normal promyelocytes (blue, n = 5) in a previous study [26]. The red triangles (n = 2) for a total 16 APL cases show the clinical APL samples whose microarray data were obtained in this study.

(david.abcc.ncifcrf.gov/). In the induced APL cases, the genes related to N-Glycan, steroid and heparan sulfate biosynthesis, the spliceosome and pyrimidine metabolism were expressed similar to the levels in normal $CD34^+$ cells, and those related to the MAPK signaling pathway were exclusively expressed in comparison to normal myeloid cells, including normal $CD34^+$ cells. On the other hand, the genes related to neurotrophin signaling and the cell cycle, as well as those associated with metabolic processes, such as glycolysis/gluconeogenesis, the pentose phosphate pathway and sphingolipid metabolism were downregulated (**Table S2**), thus suggesting that the induced APL exhibited dysregulated signaling and metabolism as differentiated myeloid cells. Additionally, the gene set composed of 573 probes including 547 genes, which fulfilled one or more above criteria (ii) to (iv) in the gene set identified in (i), clearly separated the normal and malignant promyelocytes, such as those of induced and human primary APL (**Figure S5 and Table S3**), as described in the previous study using primary APL cases [26].

To evaluate the additional genetic events that accompanied the integration of *PML-RARA* in the genome, the insertion sites of *PML-RARA* were analyzed. Some of the integration sites of *PML-RARA* were in the introns or exons of genes (**Table S4**). However, they were neither recurrent nor found in the previous whole genome sequence analysis of the APL patients [33]. These findings suggest that *PML-RARA* was a common key event, but that there were various additional genetic events in these induced APL cells, and this finding was compatible with the previous analysis using human primary APL [33].

The induced APL cells differentiated into mature neutrophils following treatment with all-*trans* retinoic acid (ATRA) *in vitro* (**Figures 4A and 4B**), which was accompanied by alterations in the PML distribution in the nucleus, from a microspeckled to a speckled pattern (**Figure 4C**). Similarly, ATRA induced transient myeloid differentiation *in vivo* (n = 4), as has been seen in APL patients (**Figures 4D and 4E**).

These findings demonstrate that our induced APL cells recapitulate human APL both phenotypically and functionally.

Re-transplantable cellular fraction in the induced APL cells

It is necessary to prove that the resultant induced APL cells possess the reproducibility of APL in the secondary recipients in order to demonstrate their capacity for leukemogenesis. However, previous studies have revealed that primary APL cells exhibit difficultly in engrafting in immunodeficient mice [3,12]. When the induced APL cells were transplanted into the second recipients, they were proven to be re-transplantable intravenously; 500,000 to 1,000,000 leukemic cells, but not 50,000 cells, were required, and the frequency of APL cells in the secondary recipients was low (0.04% to 1.41%, n = 6). The frequency was still low, even though

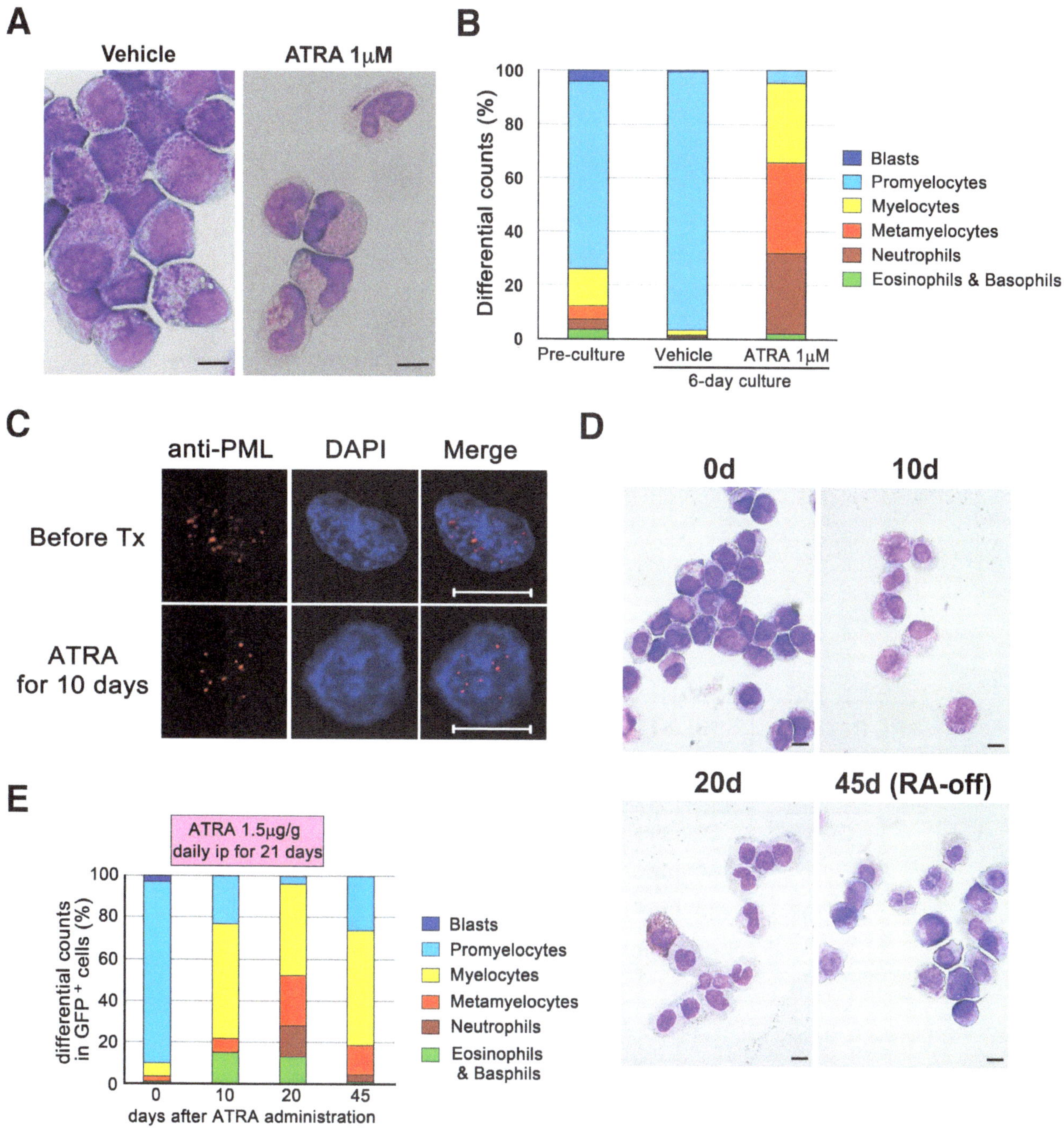

Figure 4. The induction of myeloid differentiation in the APL cells induced by ATRA treatment *in vitro* and *in vivo*. (**A**) Cytospin slides of the induced APL cells cultured with or without 1 μM ATRA for 6 days. The mature neutrophils with Auer rods are seen in the ATRA-treated group. The images were captured with a BX41 microscope (Olympus). The bar indicates 10 μm. (**B**) The differential cellular counts of the induced APL cells cultured with or without ATRA. The average leukocyte differentiation in three independent experiments is shown. (**C**) The results of an immunofluorescent analysis of the PML distribution in the induced APL cells before and after treatment with ATRA. The images were captured with an LSM510 META confocal microscope (Carl Zeiss). All the bars indicate 10 μm. (**D, E**) The induction of myeloid differentiation in the induced APL cells by ATRA *in vivo*. The secondary recipients transplanted with the induced APL cells were then intraperitoneally treated with ATRA for 21 days. Cytospin slides of $EGFP^+/hCD45^+/hCD33^+$ cells from the secondary recipients transplanted with the induced APL cells are shown (**D**). The images were captured with a BX41 microscope (Olympus). The bar indicates 10 μm. Their differentiated cellular counts were evaluated, and the representative series data are indicated (**E**).

they were transplanted intramedullary (iBM, 2.00% to 5.98%, n = 2) (**Figure 5A**). The immunophenotype of the engrafted cells was the same as that seen in the primary induced APL cells: they were positive for CD13 and CD33, without the expression of CD34 or HLA-DR (**Figure 5B**), demonstrating that the induced APL retains self-renewal capacity with a low level of transplan-

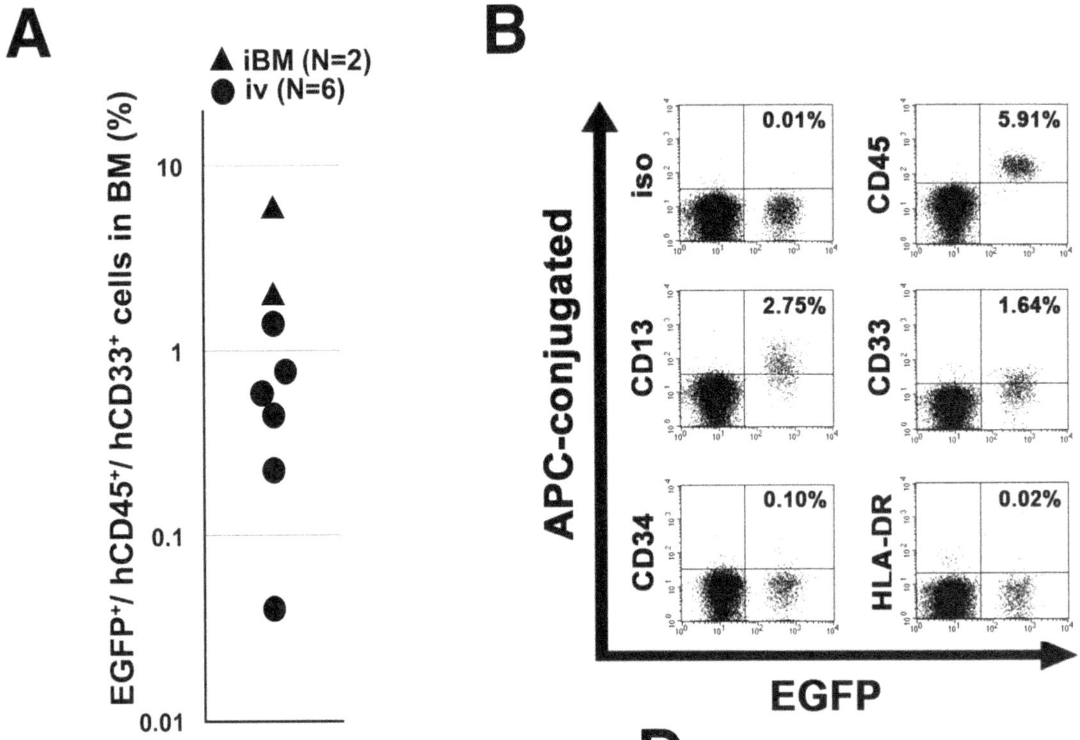

C

APL fractions for secondary transplantation		No. of cells per mouse	Detection of engraftment
EGFP+	CD34+	50 000	0 / 4
	CD34-	50 000	0 / 4
		500 000	0 / 1
		1 000 000	4 / 4

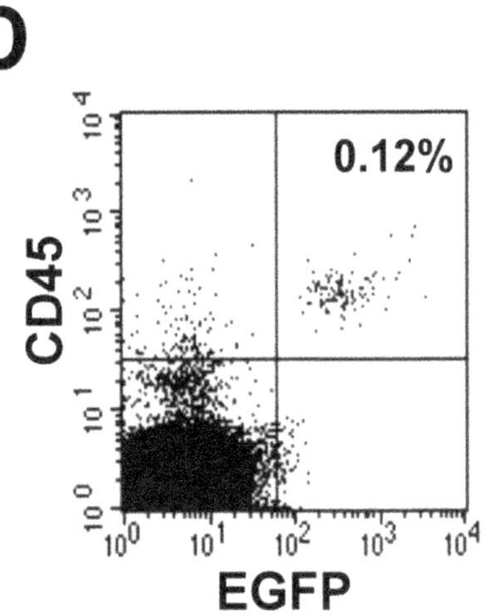

Figure 5. APL-LIC in the humanized APL *in vivo* model. (**A**) The engraftment of the induced APL cells in the secondary recipients. The bone marrow cells were obtained 16 weeks after transplantation and evaluated. Each dot represents a single mouse. (**B**) The immunophenotype of the induced APL cells in the secondary recipients. The representative pattern is shown. (**C**) The engraftment capacity in each fraction from the induced APL cells in the secondary recipients. The bone marrow cells were obtained 16 weeks after transplantation and evaluated. (**D**) The engraftment of the $CD34^-$ fraction in the secondary recipients. The engrafted cells are shown as $EGFP^+/CD45^+$ cells.

tation efficiency. In addition, the results suggested that the capacity for engraftment in this xenograft model differed between the $CD34^+$ cells transduced with *PML-RARA* and the APL cells mostly composed of the $CD34^-$ fraction.

To identify a fraction responsible for the APL maintenance in the induced APL cases, $CD34^+$ and $CD34^-$ APL fractions were separately collected and transplanted intravenously. The $CD34^+$ fraction was pooled because there were very few $CD34^+$ cells in each induced APL case (**Figures 3A and 5B**). The $CD34^-$ fraction was sorted twice to exclude the $CD34^+$ fraction completely. Fifty thousand APL cells in both the $CD34^+$ and $CD34^-$ fractions failed to engraft in the secondary recipients (0 out of 4 mice in each fraction). Similar to the unsorted cells, one million $CD34^-$ fraction cells were able to engraft in recipient mice (4 out of 4 mice) (**Figures 5C and 5D**).

These findings revealed that $CD34^-$ induced APL cells exhibit the ability to function as APL-LIC *in vivo*, although the LIC function was not excluded in the $CD34^+$ APL fraction.

The $CD34^+/CD38^+$ progenitors trigger APL by *PML-RARA* induction *in vivo*

The findings that the *PML-RARA* transduced-$CD34^+$ cells developed APL while the resultant $CD34^-$ APL cells exhibited transplantability indicate the possibility that the initiation and maintenance of APL arise at different steps of differentiation, which are not likely to involve the $CD34^+/CD38^-$ fraction, as originally reported in human AML. Therefore, in order to identify a cellular target for *PML-RARA* that effectively develops APL, *PML-RARA* was transduced into fractionated cells: CD34$^+$/CD38$^-$, CD34$^+$/CD38$^+$ and CD34$^-$/CD33$^+$ cells from the cord blood (**Figures 6A and 6B**). The transduction efficiency, as evaluated by EGFP expression, ranged from 1.9% to 5.0% (median: 3.53%, n = 6) in CD34$^+$/CD38$^-$ cells, 4.5% to 10.6% (median: 10.07%, n = 6) in CD34$^+$/CD38$^+$ cells and 19.1% to 22.1% (median: 20.63%, n = 4) in CD34$^-$/CD33$^+$ cells. Because the CD34$^+$ fraction from human cord blood possessed a higher proportion of CD34$^+$/CD38$^+$ (74.5% to 94.2%) than that of CD34$^+$/CD38$^-$ cells, the presumed absolute number of *PML-RARA* transplanted cells was higher in CD34$^+$/CD38$^+$ cells than in CD34$^+$/CD38$^-$ cells (3,430 to 31,800 cells vs 140 to 450 cells per mouse; 22,900 to 27,700 CD34$^-$/CD33$^+$ cells). One hundred unfractionated human CD34$^+$ cells, including both CD34$^+$/CD38$^-$ and CD34$^+$/CD38$^+$ cells, were engrafted with multi-lineage differentiation in our previous study [10], thus suggesting that the transplanted cell numbers were adequate for engraftment in the NOG mice. The induction of *PML-RARA* in CD34$^+$/CD38$^+$ cells reduced the colony formation capacity and favored the formation of myeloid colonies, as seen in CD34$^+$ cells (**Figures 1B and 1C**). On the other hand, the induction of *PML-RARA* in CD34$^+$/CD38$^-$ cells generated very few colonies in comparison to the MIGR1 control vector-infected CD34$^+$/CD38$^-$ cells (**Figures 6C and 6D**). Consistent with the results, the induced APL cells were detected mostly in the mice transplanted with CD34$^+$/CD38$^+$ cells (median, 16.4% in the whole bone marrow cells) (**Figure 6E**). These findings suggest that CD34$^+$/CD38$^+$ progenitors proliferate and survive more efficiently than CD34$^+$/CD38$^-$ cells *in vitro* and trigger APL *in vivo* by inducing *PML-RARA*.

Human common myeloid progenitors develop into APL by inducing *PML-RARA* among CD34$^+$/CD38$^+$ progenitors

In order to identify the detailed target fraction in CD34$^+$/CD38$^+$ cells that generates APL with *PML-RARA*, the CD34$^+$/CD38$^+$ cells were then divided into three fractions based on their expression of CD123 and CD45RA; CMP, GMP and MEP (**Figure 6F**). The retroviral transduction efficiencies of *PML-RARA* into CMP, GMP and MEP were 6.0% to 15.2% (median: 6.6%, n = 9), 3.3% to 8.8% (median: 7.1%, n = 8), and 7.8% to 24.6% (median: 8.5%, n = 7) (**Figure 6G**), and the presumed absolute numbers of *PML-RARA* transduced cells in CMP, GMP and MEP utilized for the transplantation were 5,850 to 15,200, 830 to 4,250, and 1,150 to 2,550 cells per mouse, respectively, which were deduced to directly reflect their proportion in the human cord blood. The frequency of induced APL cells in whole bone marrow cells from transplanted NOG mice was higher when using CMP (median, 25.2%) than GMP and MEP (median, 0.15% and 0.01%, respectively) (**Figure 6H**).

Taken together, these findings obtained using our humanized *in vivo* APL model demonstrate that CMP are a target fraction for *PML-RARA* in the development of APL.

Discussion

Our present study revealed that a humanized APL model was successfully established by transplantation of human CD34$^+$ cord blood transduced with *PML-RARA* into immunodeficient mice. Using this model, we demonstrated that the CMP develop into APL by transducing *PML-RARA* whereas the resultant CD34$^-$ APL cells had the ability to maintain the tumor. Our system improves in the following points: The induced APL cells were detected in all of the mice within 150 days if more than 3,000 human CD34$^+$ cells infected with *PML-RARA* were transplanted into NOG mice. The resultant leukemia well recapitulated the human disease phenotypically, genetically and functionally, including the presence of Auer rods and Faggot cells, and the expression pattern of cellular surface markers and transcripts, as well as ATRA sensitivity and low leukemia transplantability. These findings demonstrated that this humanized *in vivo* model is suitable for prospectively analyzing the process of APL development in humans.

The cellular subset from which the APL originates is still controversial. Several lines of evidence using *in vivo* experiments have suggested that APL arises in the committed myeloid progenitors, whereas several clinical observations using FISH and RT-PCR analyses suggest that APL arises in earlier progenitors [4]. A recent report using conditional knock-in mice showed that the induction of *PML-RARA* led to dominant proliferation in a stem cell compartment with multilineage potential, but did not result in myeloproliferation, as if the stem cell compartment would not support leukemogenesis in this model [34,35]. Our *in vitro* and *in vivo* findings are compatible with the previous findings which showed that the generation of *PML-RARA* transgenic mice was only possible by expressing *PML-RARA* in early myeloid cells using the human cathepsin G (hCG) and MRP8 promoters, not the promoters of β-actin, a housekeeping gene, and CD11b which is expressed at a later stage of myeloid differentiation [36].

The leukemogenic function of PML-RARα may require subtle myeloid differentiation, as seen in CMP in the present study; PML-RARα has been reported to possess the inhibitory or toxic effects on the cellular survival, senescence or apoptosis [18,37,38]. CMP are still immature enough to easily acquire stemness and are already committed to the myeloid lineage, which may allow *PML-RARA* to dysregulate RARα-dependent myelopoiesis, rather than hematopoietic stem cells, in agreement with the fact that *RARA* is implicated in the regulation of myelopoiesis, including both early stage and terminal differentiation. In this scenario, the expression of *PML-RARA* would induce differentiation of CMP to promyelocytes, but inhibit their terminal differentiation at the same time [19,39,40]. Therefore, if the CMP expressing *PML-RARA* acquires stemness, this can result in the development of APL. Our findings showed no engraftment of CD34$^+$/CD38$^-$ cells with *PML-RARA* transduction *in vivo*, although their leukemogenic activity cannot be denied, as fewer cells were transplanted in comparison to the CD34$^+$/CD38$^+$ cells. Further analyses are required to evaluate whether CD34$^+$/CD38$^-$ cells possess the ability to cause APL.

Xenograft models using immunodeficient mice are at present the only method for evaluating the maintenance of human leukemia as LIC. The induced APL generated in the NOG mice had a low engraftment efficiency; however, this biological feature well-reproduced the properties of APL cells found in human patients [3,12]. It is possible that the difficulty associated with engrafting APL cells, both primary samples and induced APL cells obtained from cord blood, into NOG mice may depend on the different preferences of human hematopoietic cells between humans and mice. The reconstitution of the human hematopoietic system in NOG mice is achieved with the dominant engraftment of B-cells, in comparison to the myeloid lineage cells [10]. This technical feature may affect the engraftment of each of the transplanted cellular subsets in our study. The slow progressive myeloid tumor cells, such as those involved in myelodysplastic syndromes and chronic myeloid leukemia in the chronic phase, were shown to be difficult to engraft in NOD/SCID-β2-

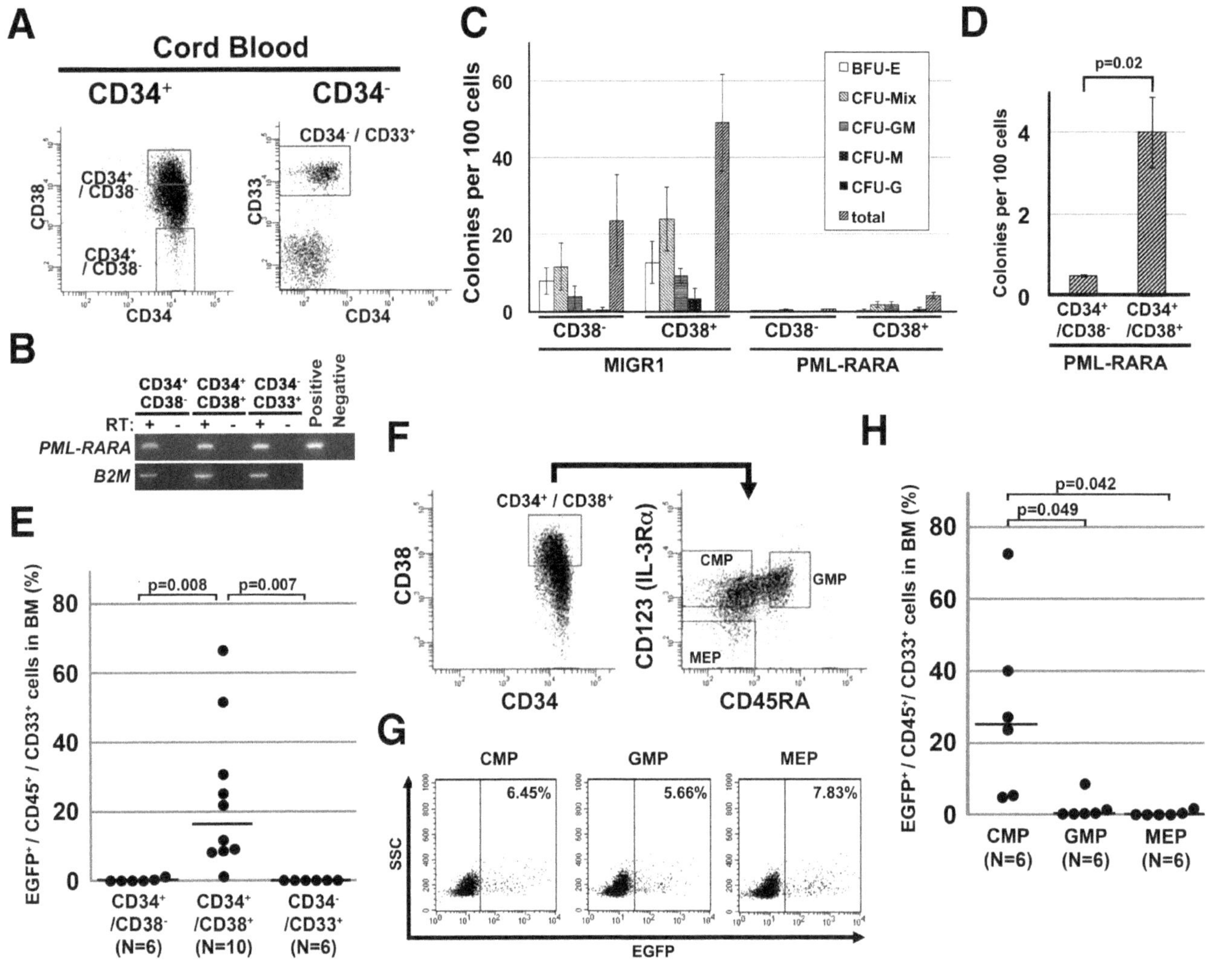

Figure 6. ***PML-RARA*** **targeted human common myeloid progenitors for APL leukemogenesis.** (**A**) The sorting strategy for CD34$^+$/CD38$^-$, CD34$^+$/CD38$^+$ and CD34$^-$/CD33$^+$ cells. Human cord blood was first separated into CD34$^+$ and CD34$^-$ cells by magnetic beads, and then sorted into three fractions by a FACS vantage instrument. (**B**) The expression of *PML-RARA* mRNA in each of the fractions after retroviral transfection. *B2M, beta 2 microglobulin.* The *PML-RARA* expression vector was used as a positive control for the *PML-RARA* analysis. (**C**) A colony-forming assay using *PML-RARA*-transduced CD34$^+$/CD38$^+$ and CD34$^+$/CD38$^-$ cells. The average of three independent experiments is shown. The data represent the means ± SD. (**D**) The total numbers of colonies of *PML-RARA*-transduced CD34$^+$/CD38$^+$ and CD34$^+$/CD38$^-$ cells shown in (C) are highlighted. The data represent the means ± SD (n = 3). (**E**) The development of the induced APL from CD34$^+$/CD38$^+$ cells in NOG mice. Each sorted fraction from human cord blood, as seen in (A), was retrovirally transduced with *PML-RARA* and transplanted into irradiated NOG mice. The percentages were determined by the frequency of EGFP$^+$/CD45$^+$/CD33$^+$ cells at 16 to 20 weeks after transplantation. Each dot represents a single mouse. The horizontal line represents the median value. (**F**) The sorting strategy for common myeloid progenitors (CMP), granulocyte-monocytic progenitors (GMP), and megakaryocyte-erythrocyte progenitors (MEP). Human cord blood was separated into CD34$^+$ cells by magnetic beads, CD34$^+$/CD38$^+$ cells were sorted out, and were finally divided into CMP, GMP and MEP by the FACS vantage instrument. (**G**) The transduction efficiency of *PML-RARA* in CMP, GMP and MEP. Representative data are shown. (**H**) The development of the induced APL from the human hematopoietic progenitors in NOG mice. Each sorted progenitor fraction from human cord blood, as seen in (F), was retrovirally transduced with *PML-RARA* and transplanted into irradiated NOG mice. The percentages were determined by the frequency of EGFP$^+$/CD45$^+$/CD33$^+$ cells at 16 to 20 weeks after transplantation. Each dot represents a single mouse. The horizontal line represents the median value.

microglobulin-deficient or NOG mice (the previous reports [41–43] and our unpublished data), suggesting that the engraftment failure did not always indicate a lack of leukemogenecity of the transplanted cells. Therefore, our study confirmed the leukemogenic activity of the CD34$^-$ induced APL fraction, although it was not strong. These results are consistent with the previous *in vivo* reports which described the some primary CD34$^+$/CD38$^+$ and CD34$^-$ AML cells could function as LIC *in vivo* [44,45].

In conclusion, we demonstrated that the induction of *PML-RARA* targeted human CD34$^+$ cells, including CMP, and led to their ability to cause APL, and that CD34$^-$ APL cells have the capability of maintaining the disease. These findings suggest that it is not necessary that LIC are always consistent with a cellular fraction where leukemia-inducing events occur. Tumor-specific oncogenes, such as *PML-RARA*, effectively function to form tumors with specific characteristics in specific hierarchal stages of myelopoiesis. This model differs from the conventional hierarchal system of AML, in which LIC possess an immature phenotype as seen in hematopoietic stem cells. Since AML is a group of heterogeneous diseases with various causal genetic abnormalities, the present findings will be helpful for the analysis of leukemogenesis in other types of AML which display differentiated leukemic blasts.

Supporting Information

Figure S1 The detection of *PML-RARA* expression in CD34$^+$ cells transduced with *PML-RARA* and their descendent colonies by qualitative RT-PCR. RT, reverse transcription.

Figure S2 Fluorescent images of the colonies derived from the EGFP$^+$ and EGFP$^-$ fractions of the CD34$^+$ cells transduced with *PML-RARA*.

Figure S3 The results of a quantitative analysis of the *PML-RARA* expression in the CD34$^+$ cells 48 hours after *PML-RARA* transduction, the differentiated cells from the resultant colonies and the induced APL cells. There were significant differences in the comparison of the expression level of *PML-RARA*. * indicates p values <0.05.

Figure S4 The heat map of the microarray analysis using the 3,439 probes (3,278 genes) that were differentially expressed in the induced APL (n = 3) and the AML other than APL (n = 62). The gene set separated the induced and human primary APL from the cases of AML other than APL. Red triangles (n = 2 from the total of 16 APL cases) show the clinical APL samples whose microarray data were obtained in this study.

Figure S5 The heat map of the microarray analysis performed using the gene set composed of 573 probes (547 genes), which were specifically expressed in the induced APL in comparison to cases of AML other than APL and normal promyelocytes. The gene set clearly clustered the malignant promyelocytes, such as the induced and human primary APL, apart from the normal promyelocytes. Red triangles (n = 2 of a total 16 APL cases) show the clinical APL samples whose microarray data were obtained in this study.

Table S1 The sequences of the PCR primers and probes.

Table S2 KEGG pathway analysis with the gene sets aberrantly expressed in the induced APL.

Table S3 The gene set apllied in Figure S5 (573 probes).

Table S4 The integration sites of PML-RARA in the induced APL cells.

Acknowledgments

We thank Dr. Warren S. Pear (University of Pennsylvania) for providing the MIGR1 retroviral vector, Dr. Toshio Kitamura (The University of Tokyo) for providing the PLAT-gp packaging cells, Dr. Guilherme Santos (Beth Israel Deaconess Medical Center, Harvard Medical School) for his valuable suggestions and comments, and Tomoko Uno and Tomomi Takanashi (Tokai University School of Medicine) for their expert technical assistance.

Author Contributions

Conceived and designed the experiments: H. Matsushita KA. Performed the experiments: H. Matsushita TY YS YN YM H. Matsuzawa TS AD H. Miyachi. Analyzed the data: H. Matsushita TY MT HH. Contributed reagents/materials/analysis tools: MO MI PPP. Wrote the paper: H. Matsushita TY KA.

References

1. Lowenberg B (2008) Acute myeloid leukemia: the challenge of capturing disease variety. Hematology Am Soc Hematol Educ Program: 1–11.
2. Lapidot T, Sirard C, Vormoor J, Murdoch B, Hoang T, et al. (1994) A cell initiating human acute myeloid leukaemia after transplantation into SCID mice. Nature 367: 645–648.
3. Bonnet D, Dick JE (1997) Human acute myeloid leukemia is organized as a hierarchy that originates from a primitive hematopoietic cell. Nat Med 3: 730–737.
4. Grimwade D, Enver T (2004) Acute promyelocytic leukemia: where does it stem from? Leukemia 18: 375–384.
5. Hope KJ, Jin L, Dick JE (2004) Acute myeloid leukemia originates from a hierarchy of leukemic stem cell classes that differ in self-renewal capacity. Nat Immunol 5: 738–743.
6. Dick JE (2008) Stem cell concepts renew cancer research. Blood 112: 4793–4807.
7. Becker MW, Jordan CT (2011) Leukemia stem cells in 2010: current understanding and future directions. Blood Rev 25: 75–81.
8. de The H, Chen Z (2010) Acute promyelocytic leukaemia: novel insights into the mechanisms of cure. Nat Rev Cancer 10: 775–783.
9. Paietta E (2003) Expression of cell-surface antigens in acute promyelocytic leukaemia. Best Pract Res Clin Haematol 16: 369–385.
10. Ito M, Hiramatsu H, Kobayashi K, Suzue K, Kawahata M, et al. (2002) NOD/SCID/gamma(c)(null) mouse: an excellent recipient mouse model for engraftment of human cells. Blood 100: 3175–3182.
11. Yahata T, Ando K, Nakamura Y, Ueyama Y, Shimamura K, et al. (2002) Functional human T lymphocyte development from cord blood CD34+ cells in nonobese diabetic/Shi-scid, IL-2 receptor gamma null mice. J Immunol 169: 204–209.
12. Patel S, Zhang Y, Cassinat B, Zassadowski F, Ferre N, et al. (2012) Successful xenografts of AML3 samples in immunodeficient NOD/shi-SCID IL2Rgamma(-/-) mice. Leukemia 26: 2432–2435.
13. Guibal FC, Alberich-Jorda M, Hirai H, Ebralidze A, Levantini E, et al. (2009) Identification of a myeloid committed progenitor as the cancer-initiating cell in acute promyelocytic leukemia. Blood 114: 5415–5425.
14. Wojiski S, Guibal FC, Kindler T, Lee BH, Jesneck JL, et al. (2009) PML-RARalpha initiates leukemia by conferring properties of self-renewal to committed promyelocytic progenitors. Leukemia 23: 1462–1471.
15. Brown D, Kogan S, Lagasse E, Weissman I, Alcalay M, et al. (1997) A PMLRARalpha transgene initiates murine acute promyelocytic leukemia. Proc Natl Acad Sci U S A 94: 2551–2556.
16. Grisolano JL, Wesselschmidt RL, Pelicci PG, Ley TJ (1997) Altered myeloid development and acute leukemia in transgenic mice expressing PML-RAR alpha under control of cathepsin G regulatory sequences. Blood 89: 376–387.
17. He LZ, Tribioli C, Rivi R, Peruzzi D, Pelicci PG, et al. (1997) Acute leukemia with promyelocytic features in PML/RARalpha transgenic mice. Proc Natl Acad Sci U S A 94: 5302–5307.
18. Westervelt P, Lane AA, Pollock JL, Oldfather K, Holt MS, et al. (2003) High-penetrance mouse model of acute promyelocytic leukemia with very low levels of PML-RARalpha expression. Blood 102: 1857–1865.
19. Grignani F, Valtieri M, Gabbianelli M, Gelmetti V, Botta R, et al. (2000) PML/RAR alpha fusion protein expression in normal human hematopoietic progenitors dictates myeloid commitment and the promyelocytic phenotype. Blood 96: 1531–1537.
20. Manz MG, Miyamoto T, Akashi K, Weissman IL (2002) Prospective isolation of human clonogenic common myeloid progenitors. Proc Natl Acad Sci U S A 99: 11872–11877.
21. Pear WS, Miller JP, Xu L, Pui JC, Soffer B, et al. (1998) Efficient and rapid induction of a chronic myelogenous leukemia-like myeloproliferative disease in mice receiving P210 bcr/abl-transduced bone marrow. Blood 92: 3780–3792.
22. Matsushita H, Scaglioni PP, Bhaumik M, Rego EM, Cai LF, et al. (2006) In vivo analysis of the role of aberrant histone deacetylase recruitment and RAR alpha blockade in the pathogenesis of acute promyelocytic leukemia. J Exp Med 203: 821–828.
23. Kawada H, Ando K, Tsuji T, Shimakura Y, Nakamura Y, et al. (1999) Rapid ex vivo expansion of human umbilical cord hematopoietic progenitors using a novel culture system. Exp Hematol 27: 904–915.
24. Yahata T, Takanashi T, Muguruma Y, Ibrahim AA, Matsuzawa H, et al. (2011) Accumulation of oxidative DNA damage restricts the self-renewal capacity of human hematopoietic stem cells. Blood 118: 2941–2950.

25. Rego EM, He LZ, Warrell RP Jr, Wang ZG, Pandolfi PP (2000) Retinoic acid (RA) and As2O3 treatment in transgenic models of acute promyelocytic leukemia (APL) unravel the distinct nature of the leukemogenic process induced by the PML-RARalpha and PLZF-RARalpha oncoproteins. Proc Natl Acad Sci U S A 97: 10173–10178.
26. Payton JE, Grieselhuber NR, Chang LW, Murakami M, Geiss GK, et al. (2009) High throughput digital quantification of mRNA abundance in primary human acute myeloid leukemia samples. J Clin Invest 119: 1714–1726.
27. Ando K, Yahata T, Sato T, Miyatake H, Matsuzawa H, et al. (2006) Direct evidence for ex vivo expansion of human hematopoietic stem cells. Blood 107: 3371–3377.
28. Schmidt M, Hoffmann G, Wissler M, Lemke N, Mussig A, et al. (2001) Detection and direct genomic sequencing of multiple rare unknown flanking DNA in highly complex samples. Hum Gene Ther 12: 743–749.
29. Dyck JA, Maul GG, Miller WH Jr, Chen JD, Kakizuka A, et al. (1994) A novel macromolecular structure is a target of the promyelocyte-retinoic acid receptor oncoprotein. Cell 76: 333–343.
30. Weis K, Rambaud S, Lavau C, Jansen J, Carvalho T, et al. (1994) Retinoic acid regulates aberrant nuclear localization of PML-RAR alpha in acute promyelocytic leukemia cells. Cell 76: 345–356.
31. Grignani F, Testa U, Rogaia D, Ferrucci PF, Samoggia P, et al. (1996) Effects on differentiation by the promyelocytic leukemia PML/RARalpha protein depend on the fusion of the PML protein dimerization and RARalpha DNA binding domains. EMBO J 15: 4949–4958.
32. Paietta E, Goloubeva O, Neuberg D, Bennett JM, Gallagher R, et al. (2004) A surrogate marker profile for PML/RAR alpha expressing acute promyelocytic leukemia and the association of immunophenotypic markers with morphologic and molecular subtypes. Cytometry B Clin Cytom 59: 1–9.
33. Welch JS, Ley TJ, Link DC, Miller CA, Larson DE, et al. (2012) The origin and evolution of mutations in acute myeloid leukemia. Cell 150: 264–278.
34. Welch JS, Yuan W, Ley TJ (2011) PML-RARA can increase hematopoietic self-renewal without causing a myeloproliferative disease in mice. J Clin Invest 121: 1636–1645.
35. Wartman LD, Welch JS, Uy GL, Klco JM, Lamprecht T, et al. (2012) Expression and function of PML-RARA in the hematopoietic progenitor cells of Ctsg-PML-RARA mice. PLoS One 7: e46529.
36. Puccetti E, Ruthardt M (2004) Acute promyelocytic leukemia: PML/RARalpha and the leukemic stem cell. Leukemia 18: 1169–1175.
37. Ferrucci PF, Grignani F, Pearson M, Fagioli M, Nicoletti I, et al. (1997) Cell death induction by the acute promyelocytic leukemia-specific PML/RARalpha fusion protein. Proc Natl Acad Sci U S A 94: 10901–10906.
38. Grignani F, Ferrucci PF, Testa U, Talamo G, Fagioli M, et al. (1993) The acute promyelocytic leukemia-specific PML-RAR alpha fusion protein inhibits differentiation and promotes survival of myeloid precursor cells. Cell 74: 423–431.
39. Collins SJ (2002) The role of retinoids and retinoic acid receptors in normal hematopoiesis. Leukemia 16: 1896–1905.
40. Du C, Redner RL, Cooke MP, Lavau C (1999) Overexpression of wild-type retinoic acid receptor alpha (RARalpha) recapitulates retinoic acid-sensitive transformation of primary myeloid progenitors by acute promyelocytic leukemia RARalpha-fusion genes. Blood 94: 793–802.
41. Thanopoulou E, Cashman J, Kakagianne T, Eaves A, Zoumbos N, et al. (2004) Engraftment of NOD/SCID-beta2 microglobulin null mice with multilineage neoplastic cells from patients with myelodysplastic syndrome. Blood 103: 4285–4293.
42. Kerbauy DM, Lesnikov V, Torok-Storb B, Bryant E, Deeg HJ (2004) Engraftment of distinct clonal MDS-derived hematopoietic precursors in NOD/SCID-beta2-microglobulin-deficient mice after intramedullary transplantation of hematopoietic and stromal cells. Blood 104: 2202–2203.
43. Muguruma Y, Matsushita H, Yahata T, Yumino S, Tanaka Y, et al. (2011) Establishment of a xenograft model of human myelodysplastic syndromes. Haematologica 96: 543–551.
44. Taussig DC, Vargaftig J, Miraki-Moud F, Griessinger E, Sharrock K, et al. (2010) Leukemia-initiating cells from some acute myeloid leukemia patients with mutated nucleophosmin reside in the CD34(-) fraction. Blood 115: 1976–1984.
45. Eppert K, Takenaka K, Lechman ER, Waldron L, Nilsson B, et al. (2011) Stem cell gene expression programs influence clinical outcome in human leukemia. Nat Med 17: 1086–1093.

3

Effects of Danshensu on Platelet Aggregation and Thrombosis: *In Vivo* Arteriovenous Shunt and Venous Thrombosis Models in Rats

Chen Yu[1*¶], Dong Qi[2¶], Wei Lian[3], Qing-Zhong Li[1], Hong-Juan Li[1], Hua-Ying Fan[4*]

1 School of Pharmacy, Binzhou Medical University, Yantai, Shandong, China, **2** Department of Nephrology, Yantai Yu-Huang-Ding/Qingdao University Hospital, Yantai, Shandong, China, **3** Yantai Yan-Tai-Shan Hospital, Yantai, Shandong, China, **4** School of Pharmacy, Yantai University, Yantai, Shandong, China

Abstract

Danshensu, a type of dihydroxyphenyl lactic acid, is one of the most abundant active phenolic acids in the dried root of *Salvia miltiorrhizae* (Lamiaceae)—widely used traditional Chinese medicine. The effects of danshensu on platelet aggregation and thrombus formation in rats were examined using various methods. It was found that danshensu significantly reduced thrombus weight in 2 experimental thrombosis models; dose-dependent inhibition of adenosine diphosphate (ADP) and arachidonic acid (AA)-induced platelet aggregation occurred in normal and blood stasis-induced rats; Danshensu also significantly mitigated blood viscosity, plasma viscosity and hematocrit levels. Moreover, danshensu significantly inhibited venous thrombosis-induced expression of cyclooxygenases-2 (COX-2) rather than cyclooxygenases-1(COX-1) in the venous walls, down regulated thromboxane B_2 (TXB_2) and up regulated 6-keto prostaglandin $F_{1\alpha}$ (6-keto-$PGF_{1\alpha}$), normalizing the TXB_2/6-keto-$PGF_{1\alpha}$ ratio. In addition, danshensu did not induce gastric lesions and even had protective effects on aspirin-induced ulcer formation at doses as high as 60 mg/kg. These findings suggest that the antithrombotic and antiplatelet aggregation effects of danshensu are attributed to its highly selective inhibition of COX-2 and ability to normalize the thromboxane A_2(TXA_2)/prostacyclin(PGI_2) balance. These findings suggest that danshensu have great prospects in antithrombotic and antiplatelet therapy.

Editor: Pablo Garcia de Frutos, IIBB-CSIC-IDIBAPS, Spain

Funding: This study was supported by the Project of National Natural Science Foundation of China (Grant No. 81303259), URL: http://www.nsfc.gov.cn/, Shandong Province Natural Science Foundation (No. ZR2010HL065), URL: http://www.sdnsf.gov.cn/portal/, Research Award Fund for Outstanding Young and Middle-aged Scientists of Shandong Province of China (project No. BS2013YY046), URL: http://www.sdstc.gov.cn/, and the Programs for Science and Technology Development and Plan of Yanta (No. 2013WS262), URL: http://www.ytstc.gov.cn/. The funders had no role in study design, data collection and analysis, decision to publish, or preparation of the manuscript.

Competing Interests: The authors have declared that no competing interests exist.

* Email: yuchen810624@163.com (CY); katiefhydong@sina.com (HYF)

¶ These authors contributed equally to this work.

Introduction

Thrombus formation accelerates the progression of various cardiovascular and cerebrovascular disorders. Thromboembolic complications of arteriosclerosis, heart attack, stroke and peripheral vascular disease are the principal causes of death in developed countries. Arterial and venous thrombi comprises primarily platelet aggregates.

Platelets mediate the initiation of thrombosis through platelet adhesion, activation and aggregation [1]. A collaborative meta-analysis of randomized trials has demonstrated that antiplatelet therapy is beneficial in treating thromboembolic diseases and preventing serious vascular events, arterial occlusion and venous thromboembolism in a wide range of patients who are at high risk for occlusive vascular events [2]. Thus, the inhibition of platelet function has the potential to treat circulatory diseases, spurring the development of many antiplatelet and antithrombotic agents and prompting an examination of their effects in preventing thrombosis.

Danshen, the dried root of *Salvia miltiorrhizae* (Lamiaceae), is one of the most widely used traditional herbal medicines against various cardiovascular and cerebrovascular diseases, including coronary heart disease, myocardial infarction, stroke and hypertension. Danshen contains hydrophilic phenolics and lipophilic quinones, which have many pharmacological and therapeutic properties [3].

Increasing data have demonstrated that danshensu is an abundant and representative phenolic acid in danshen [4]. Danshensu (chemical structure shown in Fig. 1)—known as β-3,4-dihydroxyphenyl-lactic acid—has several mechanisms by which it elicits its therapeutic effects. Danshensu can mitigate cardiovascular and cerebrovascular disturbances [5] by improving microcirculation, increasing blood flow, relaxing the coronary arteries and promoting anticoagulation [6].

However, the antithrombotic and antiplatelet effects and mechanisms of danshensu are unknown. The purpose of this study was to determine the effects and mechanisms of danshensu with regard to platelet aggregation, thrombus formation and blood circulation so as to provide pharmacological evidence that supports its clinical application.

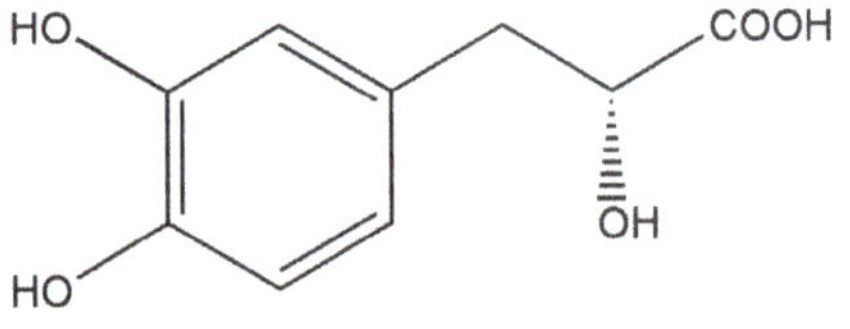

Figure 1. Chemical structure of danshensu ($C_9H_{10}O_5$, molecular weight = 198.17).

Results

Effects on platelet aggregation *in vivo*

To assess the effect of danshensu on platelet aggregation, we measured the inhibition of platelet aggregation on danshensu induced by ADP and AA in normal rats.As shown in Fig. 2, compared with the control group, ADP and AA-induced platelet aggregation was altered by pretreatment with danshensu and aspirin. Danshensu dose-dependently inhibited AA-induced platelet aggregation by approximately 13.9% at 15 mg/kg, 17.9% at 30 mg/kg and 21.5% at 60 mg/kg, respectively. This result showed that similar inhibition in the ADP-induced platelet aggregation.The inhibition of platelet aggregation induced by ADP was 10.5%, 14.6% and 23.5% at doses of 15, 30, and 60 mg/kg, respectively.

Further, we determined effect of danshensu on platelet aggregation in blood stasis rats induced by AA. Blood stasis increased platelet aggregation compared with the control group as shown in Fig. 3, which was also modified by pretreatment with danshensu in a dose-dependent manner. This inhibitory effect of danshensu at dose of 60 mg/kg was comparable with that of aspirin at 20 mg/kg in blood stasis rats.

Effect on thrombus formation

Two rat models of thrombosis were developed by installing an arteriovenous shunt and ligating the inferior vena cava to study the antithrombotic activity and mechanism of danshensu *in vivo*. Pretreatment with danshensu (15 to 60 mg/kg) decreased thrombus formation dose-dependently in the arteriovenous shunt model.The inhibition of thrombus formation was about 12.6%, 18.2% and 29.6% respectively (Fig. 4).

As shown in Fig. 5, this result was confirmed by inferior vena cava model. Residual thrombi from the occlusive vessels of all rats were measured. Compared with the thrombotic control group, aspirin at 20 mg/kg decreased the thrombus weight from 35.37±3.03 mg to 24.14±4.23 mg versus 29.65±5.62 mg with 15 mg/kg, 25.78±3.95 mg with 30 mg/kg and 23.84±2.26 mg with 60 mg/kg of danshensu, respectively. Antithrombotic activity of danshensu at dose of 60 mg/kg is comparable with that of aspirin at 20 mg/kg.

Effects on COX and possible mechanisms

Inhibitory effects of danshensu and aspirin against 2 cyclooxygenases (COX) isoforms were first examined *in vitro* using enzymatic assays. While danshensu had little inhibitory effect on COX-1, danshensu decreased COX-2 activity at 20 to 200 μM even at 200 μM yielding an IC_{50} value of approximately 44 μM (Fig. 6 A vs B).

In contrast, aspirin inhibited COX-1 and COX-2, with geometric mean IC_{50} values of 39.8 and 60.7 μM, respectively. The IC_{50} ratios of COX-1 to COX-2 for danshensu and aspirin exceeded 10 and 0.67 respectively, it is demonstrated that danshensu selectively inhibits COX-2 over COX-1 by approximately 20-fold.

The effects of danshensu on COX-1 and COX-2 levels were examined using western blot technique. As shown in Fig. 7, the expression of COX-1 and COX-2 induced by inferior vena cava ligation was significantly elevated when compared with control group. It is clear that aspirin significantly inhibited both COX-1 and COX-2 expression while danshenu only significantly inhibited COX-2 but not COX-1 expression (Fig. 7B vs D). This observation indicates that danshensu exerts its antiplatelet effect by selectively targeting on COX-2.

Next, we measured the serum concentrations of TXB_2 and 6-keto-PGF1α in the rats. TXB_2 and 6-keto-$PGF_{1\alpha}$ levels increased significantly, accompanying a rise in the TXB_2/6-keto-$PGF_{1\alpha}$

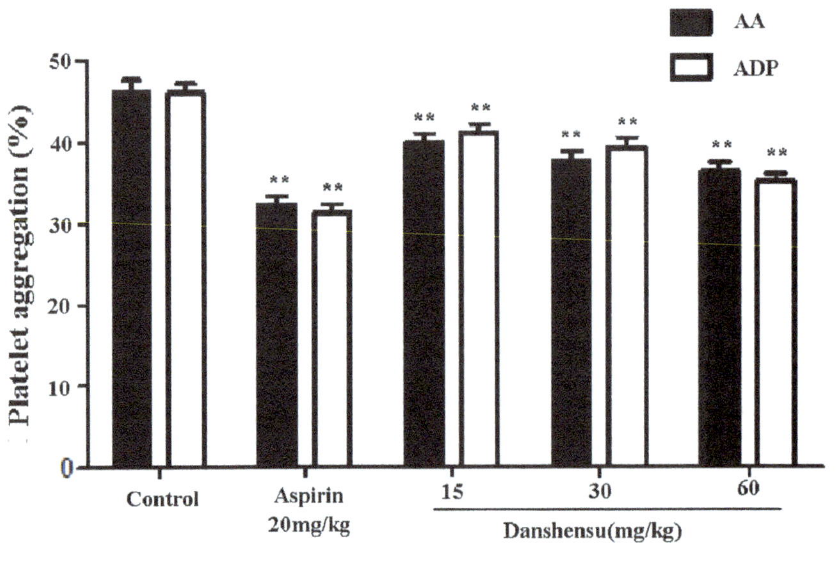

Figure 2. Effect of danshensu on platelet aggregation in normal rats. Blood was drawn 60 min after intragastric danshensu administration. Platelet aggregation was induced by diphosphate (ADP) and arachidonic acid (AA). Data are expressed as mean ± SEM (each group, n = 10). $^{**}P<0.01$ with control group.

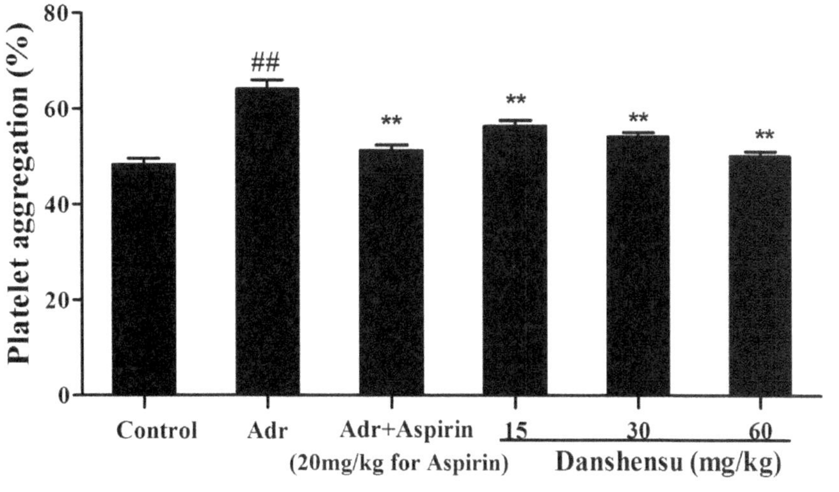

Figure 3. Effect of danshensu on platelet aggregation in blood stasis rats. Blood was drawn 60 min after intragastric danshensu administration. Platelet aggregation was induced by arachidonic acid (AA). Data are expressed as mean ± SEM (each group, n = 10). The blood stasis model was built during the interval between when 2 injections of adrenaline hydrochloride (Adr) were given to rats placed in ice-cold water. ##$P<$ 0.01 compared with normal control. *$P<0.05$ **$P<0.01$ compared with Adr control.

ratio in the 2 thrombosis models. Aspirin significantly reduced TXB_2 and 6-keto-$PGF_{1\alpha}$ levels, decreasing the TXB_2/6-keto-$PGF_{1\alpha}$ ratio. Danshensu downregulated TXB_2 and increased 6-keto-$PGF_{1\alpha}$ levels, especially at 30 and 60 mg/kg, normalizing the TXB_2/6-keto-$PGF_{1\alpha}$ ratio better than aspirin (Tables 1 and 2).

Effect on hemorheology

whole blood viscosity (WBV) at all shear rates, plasma viscosity (PV) and hematocrit values (Hct) significantly rose in blood stasis rats, but danshensu significantly reduced blood viscosity, plasma viscosity and hematocrit, particularly at 30 and 60 mg/kg (Table 3).

Protective effects of danshensu on gastric mucosa

We examined the gastrointestinal (GI) effects of oral administration of danshensu and aspirin in rats for 7 days. The ulcer index for all groups is summarized in Fig. 8. Aspirin resulted in gastric lesions and the ulcer index was significantly higher than the control group. In contrast, danshensu did not induce gastric lesions, even at as high as 60 mg/kg.

We also investigated the effect of danshensu on aspirin-induced gastric lesions. The macroscopic findings of open stomachs are shown in Fig. 9A, we found that oral administration of aspirin (200 mg/kg body weight) induced severe mucosal damage in the gastric corpus of mice. Danshensu had no damaging effects on the stomach. In addition co-administration of danshensu with aspirin could inhibit aspirin-induced ulcer formation. Fig. 9B shows the ulcer score of gastric hemorrhagic ulcers in each group. These data suggest that danshensu has gastroprotective activities and it also prevents aspirin-induced gastric ulcer formation.

Discussion

Many life-threatening diseases, such as atherosclerosis, cerebrovascular thrombosis, coronary artery disease, stroke and tumor metastasis are related with platelet dysfunctions [7]. Many

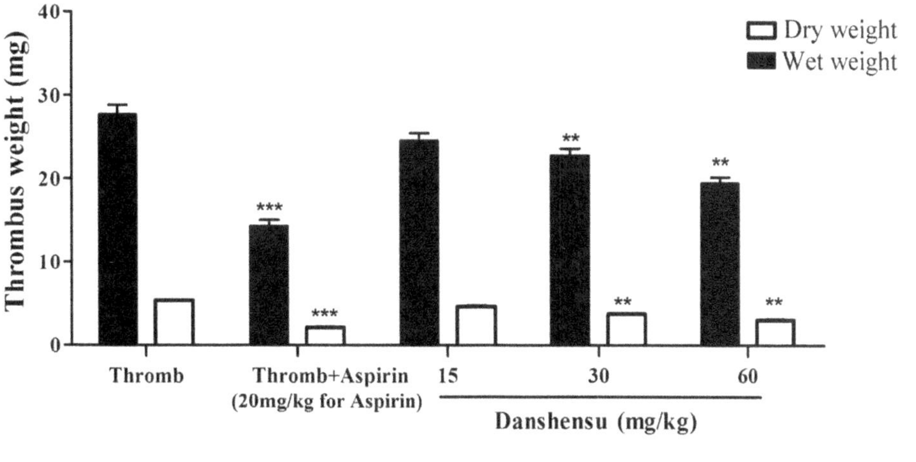

Figure 4. Antithrombotic activity of danshensu in the rat model of arteriovenous shunt. The drug or solvent was administered orally 60 min before thrombogenic challenge. Data are expressed as mean ± SEM (each group, n = 10). Thromb: thrombosis. *$P<0.05$, **$P<0.01$, ***$P<$ 0.001 compared with thrombotic control group.

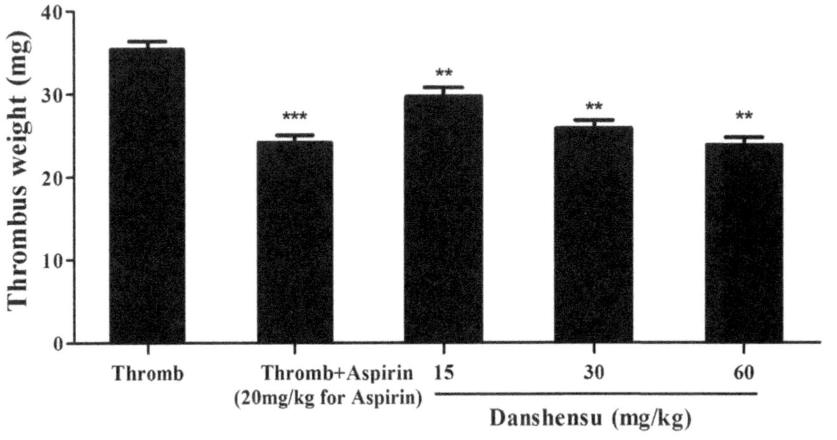

Figure 5. Antithrombotic activity of danshensu in the rat model of ligating inferior vena cava. The drug or solvent was administered orally 60 min before the thrombogenic challenge. Data are expressed as mean ± SEM (each group, n = 10). Thromb: thrombosis. **P*<0.05, ***P*<0.01, ****P*<0.001 compared with thrombotic control group.

available antiplatelet agents interfere with platelet function at various levels of activation, which results in several clinical disadvantages, including gastrointestinal side effects and hemorrhage. For this reason, a search for safer and more effective

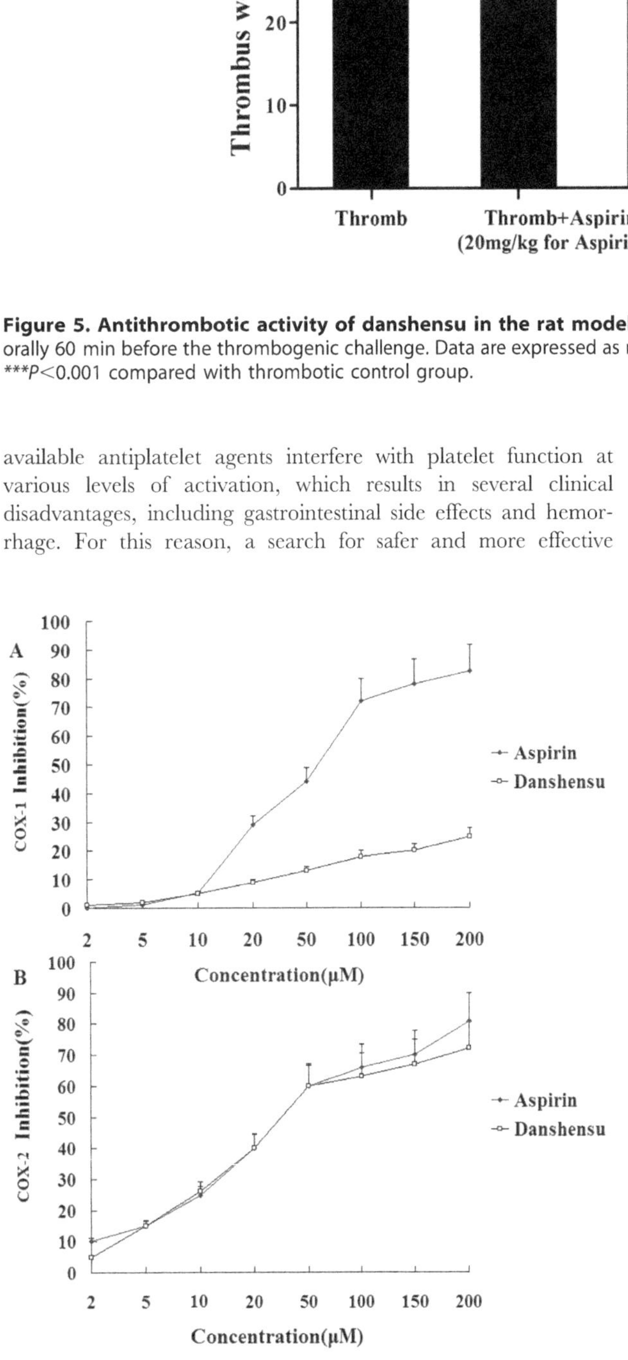

Figure 6. Direct effect of various concentrations of danshensu and aspirin on the enzymatic activities of COX-1 and COX-2. Danshensu and aspirin (water, as a control) were incubated with COX-1 (A) or COX-2 (B) for 10 min and then AA was added. COX enzyme activities are reflected by the amount of PGE_2 produced. PGE_2 production was measured by ELISA. Enzyme activity in the sample without treatment (water alone) served as control and results are expressed as inhibitory rate of COX-1 and COX-2 activity compared with solvent control.

antiplatelet agents without these adverse effects would be highly desirable. In recent years, new therapeutic agents have been derived from Chinese herbs and there is growing interest in this area.

In this study, we examined the antiplatelet and antithrombotic effects of danshensu and the pharmacological mechanisms. We determined effects of danshensu on platelet function by measuring ADP and AA-induced platelet aggregation. Our results showed that danshensu produced marked antiplatelet effect on ADP and AA platelet agonists ex vivo aggregation. This inhibitory effect of danshensu at dose of 60 mg/kg was comparable with aspirin at 20 mg/kg in blood stasis-induced rats.

The effects of danshensu on thrombus formation were studied in arteriovenous shunt model and inferior vena cava model; these models simulate arterial and venous thrombosis observed in humans [8]. Our results demonstrated that danshensu has potent antithrombotic effects against arterial and venous thrombosis.

To assess the effect of danshensu on microcirculation, we evaluated hemorheologic parameters in blood stasis model. Blood stasis can result in platelet aggregation and hemorheological abnormalities. Hemorheological disorders mediate the pathogenesis and development of many cardiovascular and cerebrovascular diseases [9]. In this study, rats were injected subcutaneously with adrenaline hydrochloride (Adr) and treated with cold stress. As a result, blood viscosity, plasma viscosity and hematocrit increased significantly compared with the control group. Our results suggest that Adr combined with exposure to ice-cold water induces blood stasis resulting in hemorheological abnormalities. Platelet aggregation is believed to be a factor that determines blood viscosity [10], consistent with our results that danshensu improves hemorheologic parameters, ameliorates blood stasis and promotes circulation by decreasing whole blood viscosity, secondary to the inhibitory effect on platelet aggregation.

In our study, Danshensu exhibited apparent antiplatelet and antithrombotic activity. In order to explore the further mechanisms of antiplatelet and anti-thrombosis, the activity and expression of COXs were measured. We also evaluated the levels of TXB_2 and 6-keto-$PGF_{1\alpha}$ in both arterial and venous thrombosis models. Our results indicated that danshensu could selectively inhibit COX-2 rather than COX-1 to regulate the balance of TXA_2/PGI_2. Therefore, danshensu exhibited superior antiplatelet and antithrombotic effects compared with aspirin.

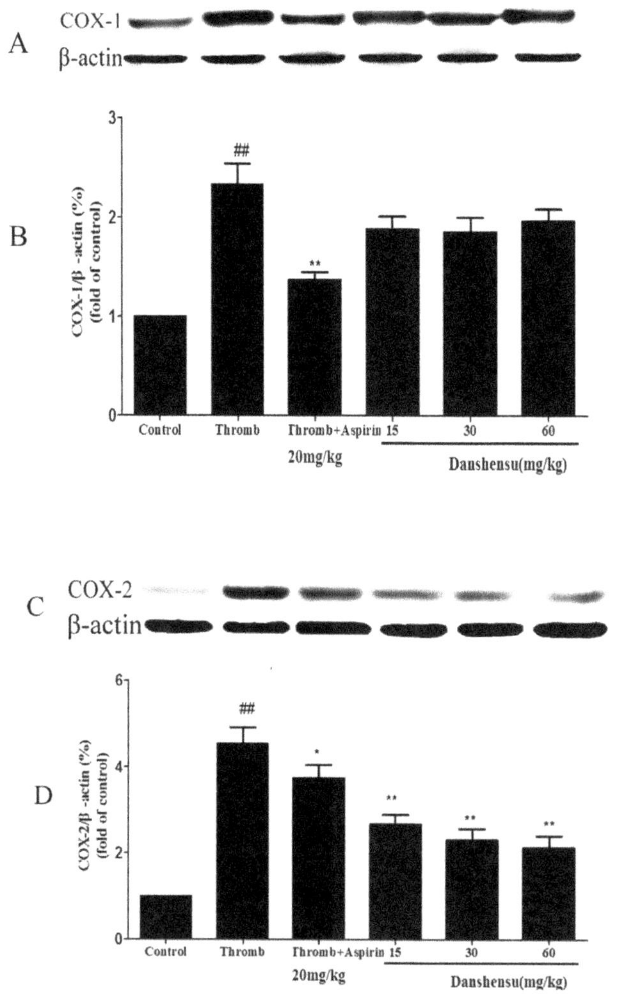

Figure 7. The effects of danshensu on COX expression. Rats were given 15, 30 and 60 mg/kg danshensu intragastrically and 20 mg/kg aspirin for 7 days. Venous thrombus formation was induced by inferior vena cava (IVC) ligation to produce thrombus after last administration.Vein walls were harvested from venous thrombosis and the expression of COX-1 and COX-2 was assessed by western analysis (A and C). β-actin was measured to confirm equal loading of proteins. Densitometric analysis of COX-1 (B) and COX-2 (D) expression is represented by the mean from 3 separate experiments. Data were normalized to β-actin levels. Thromb: thrombosis. ##$P<0.01$ compared with normal control. *$P<0.05$, **$P<0.01$ compared with thrombotic control group.

Disruption of the TXA_2-PGI_2 balance increases the risk of thrombosis [11]. TXA_2 and PGI_2 are metabolites of arachidonic acid, which is hydrolyzed by COXs and transformed into endoperoxides, prostaglandins (PGs) and TXA_2 [12]. COXs exist as 2 distinct isoforms: COX-1 and COX-2. COX-1 which is constitutively expressed in most tissues and has high levels of activity in the the gastrointestinal tract, is thought to exert homeostatic properties that are crucial for gastric physiologic function, including mucosal protectionwhereas COX-2 is absent from most healthy tissues but is induced by proinflammatory and proliferative stimuli after exposure to cytokines, immunological stimuli and growth factors [13,14]. TXA_2 is a potent inducer of platelet aggregation and vasoconstriction and its levels rise in thrombus models. In contrast, PGI_2 is a potent platelet inhibitor. An increase in TXA_2 results in the adhesion, aggregation and release of platelets. However, PGI_2 inhibits platelet aggregation [15,16]. In our study, aspirin significantly decreased both TXB_2 and 6-keto-$PGF_{1\alpha}$ levels due to its non-selective and irreversible COX inhibition. Aspirin exerts its antiplatelet activity through inhibition of both COX-1 and COX-2, therefore inhibits not only the production of TXA_2 in platelets, but also the production of anti-aggregatory PGI_2 in vessel walls. This phenomenon is referred to as the "aspirin dilemma"[17] and is considered to be a reason underlying the insufficient efficacy and unclear dose–response effects of aspirin [18,19]. Compared with aspirin, danshensu with higher selectivity for COX-2 is able to normalize the TXA_2/PGI_2 balance better, by upregulating 6-keto-$PGF_{1\alpha}$ and downregulating TXB_2 simultaneously.

Finally, we evaluated the protective effects of danshensu on gastric mucosa. We compared the ulcerogenic effects of danshensu and aspirin on gastric mucosa and demonstrated that danshensu did not cause any apparent ulceration of the gastric mucosa in rats, even at a dose of 60 mg/kg. In contrast, aspirin had a potent ulcerogenic effect at the antithrombotic dose(20 mg/kg) and produced severe hemorrhagic necrotic lesions in the gastric mucosa even at a dose of 200 mg/kg Aspirin-induced gastric lesion was completely inhibited by the coadministration of danshensu. The observed differences in gastric ulcerogenic properties between danshensu and aspirin may be related with the difference in COX-1 selectivity. COX-1-derived PGs are thought to play a dominant role in gastric mucosal defense and cytoprotection and it has been confirmed that selective inhibition of COX-1 alone may not cause ulcers, but inhibition of both COX-1 and COX-2 is required for the development of gastric lesions [20,21]. Thus, danshensu by selectively inhibit COX-2 only, is considered to be potentially less damaging to the gastrointestinal tract than aspirin that also block COX-1.

In conclusion, our findings suggest that danshensu has potent antithrombotic effects and antiplatelet aggregation activity without inducing GI adverse events. This might be attributed to danshensu's mechanism of its functions as a highly selective COX-2 inhibitor with an ability to normalize TXA_2/PGI_2 balance superior to aspirin. Thus, Danshensu may have good prospects in antithrombotic and antiplatelet therapy.

Materials and Methods

Chemicals and reagents

Danshensu (purity 98%) was provided by Nanjing Zelang Medical Biological Technology Co. Ltd (Nanjing, China). Aspirin (purity 98%) was produced by Anhui Fengyuan Pharmaceutical Co. Ltd (Anhui, China). Arachidonic acid (AA) was purchased from Sigma-Aldrich Chemical Co. (USA). Heparin sodium was purchased from Jiangsu Wanbang Biochemical Medicine Co. Ltd. (Jiangsu, China). Adrenaline hydrochloride was purchased from Tianjin Jinyao Amino Acids Co. Ltd. (Tianjin, China). COX inhibitor screening assay kits were purchased from Cayman Chemical Company (Ann Arbor, MI, USA). Primary antibodies against COX-1, COX-2, β-actin and horseradish peroxidase (HRP)-conjugated secondary antibody were purchased from Santa Cruz Biotechnology, Inc. The thromboxane B_2 (TXB_2) and 6-keto prostaglandin $F_{1\alpha}$ (6-keto-$PGF_{1\alpha}$) radioimmunoassay kits were produced by Tianjin Jiuding Engineering of Medicine and Biology Co. Ltd. (Tianjin, China).

Animals and treatments

Male Sprague-Dawley rats (weight approximately 300 g, 3–4 months each) were purchased from Shandong Lvye Pharmaceu-

Table 1. Effects of danshensu on plasma TXB_2 and 6-keto-$PGF_{1\alpha}$ levels and TXB_2-6-keto-$PGF_{1\alpha}$ ratio in rats in the arteriovenous shunt model.

Group	Dose(mg/kg)	TXB_2 (pg/mL)	6-keto-$PGF_{1\alpha}$ (pg/mL)	TXB_2/6-keto-$PGF_{1\alpha}$
Normal		180.0±8.3	487.3±16.6	0.38±0.01
Thromb		552.2±18.9##	602.5±20.4##	0.93±0.03##
Thromb+Aspirin	20	56.5±1.9***	190.5±7.5***	0.30±0.01***
Thromb +Danshensu	15	258.1±10.2**	621.7±19.8*	0.40±0.01**
	30	228.7±11.5**	638.3±22.1**	0.37±0.02**
	60	206.4±8.9**	649.2±15.8**	0.35±0.02**

Blood was drawn from the abdominal aorta at the end of arteriovenous shunt test period and anticoagulated with indomethacin-EDTA-Na_2. Plasma samples were prepared by centrifugation and analyzed by radioimmunoassay. Data are expressed as mean±SEM (each group, n = 10). #$P<0.05$, ##$P<0.01$ compared with normal group, *$P<0.05$, **$P<0.01$, ***$P<0.001$ compared with thrombotic control group.

tical Co. Ltd., China (certificate No. SCXK (Lu) 20030008). Male ICR mice (weight approximately 25 g, 8–9 weeks each) were purchased from the Animal Department of the College of Medicine, Beijing University (certificate no. SCXK (Jing) 2006–0008).

Animals were acclimated for at least 1 week to a temperature of 24±1°C and humidity of 55±5%. The animals were maintained with free access to standard diet and tap water. The experimental procedures were approved by the Office of Experimental Animal Management.

Committee of Shandong Province, China (certificate No. SYXK (Lu) 20090015). Rats were given 15, 30 and 60 mg/kg danshensu and 20 mg/kg aspirin intragastrically (i.g.). All drugs were dissolved in 0.9% normal saline as vehicle. The control rats were given 0.9% normal saline. All drugs and saline were administered orally to rats once daily at 9 AM for 7 days. All *in vivo* experiments were conducted 60 min after the treatment.

Assay of *ex vivo* Platelet Aggregation in Rats

Blood was collected after the last administration of danshensu and saline. All rats were anesthetized with 10% chloral hydrate and blood was collected from the abdominal aorta and anticoagulated with citrate (3.8%; 1 vol anticoagulant: 9 vol blood). Platelet-rich plasma (PRP) was prepared by centrifuging the blood at 1000 rpm for 8 min and at 3000 rpm for 15 min to prepare platelet-poor plasma (PPP). The platelet concentration was adjusted to $1.8-2\times10^9$/mL with PPP. Then, 0.3 mL of PRP was placed in a cuvette and stirred with a rotor at 37°C for 5 min, after which 6 μM ADP and 100 μM AA was added. Aggregation was measured with a platelet aggregometer (LBY-NJ4, Pulisheng Instrument Co. Ltd. China). Results were recorded as light transmission at maximal aggregation after the addition of an aggregating agent. Data are expressed as percentage of maximal aggregation.

In vivo arteriovenous shunt thrombosis

Rat arterial-venous shunts (silk thread model) were prepared with 2 2-cm-long polyethylene tubes (1 mm i.d.), linked by a central section (8 cm long; 2 mm i.d.) that contained a 5-cm piece of silk thread and was filled with saline solution that contained heparin 50 U/kg. Rats were anesthetized with chloral hydrate (350 mg/kg, i.p.) and an arterial-venous shunt was placed between the right carotid artery and left jugular vein [22,23]. After blood was circulated through the shunt for 15 minutes, both ends of the tube were pinched, the silk thread was removed from the shunt tube and the wet and dry weights were measured by subtracting the pre-experiment weight of the 5-cm silk thread.The rate of inhibition of thrombosis formation was calculated as inhibition (%) = $(A-A_1)/A\times100\%$, where A is the thrombus weight of the thrombosis control group and A_1 is the weight after treatment with the agents. The sham group did not undergo the surgery. All rats fasted overnight before the operation.

Venous thrombosis model

Venous thrombus formation was induced by inferior vena cava (IVC) ligation to produce a stasis thrombus as described [24,25].

Table 2. Effects of danshensu on plasma TXB_2 and 6-keto-$PGF_{1\alpha}$ levels and TXB_2-6-keto-$PGF_{1\alpha}$ ratio in rats the venous thrombosis model.

Group	Dose(mg/kg)	TXB_2 (pg/mL)	6-keto-$PGF_{1\alpha}$ (pg/mL)	TXB_2/6-keto-$PGF_{1\alpha}$
Normal		197.0±8.2	528.3±16.8	0.37±0.03
Thromb		605.2±21.9##	652.5±24.6##	0.95±0.03##
Thromb+Aspirin	20	106.5±4.2***	395.0±14.5***	0.29±0.01***
Thromb +Danshensu	15	358.1±12.8**	663.7±24.2*	0.50±0.02**
	30	328.7±10.6**	684.3±25.1**	0.45±0.02**
	60	306.4±8.2***	719.2±20.9**	0.40±0.02**

Blood was drawn from the abdominal aorta at the end of venous thrombus formation period and anticoagulated with indomethacin-EDTA-Na_2. Plasma samples were prepared by centrifugation and analzyed by radioimmunoassay. Data are expressed as mean±SEM (each group, n = 10). #$P<0.05$, ##$P<0.01$ compared with normal group, *$P<0.05$, **$P<0.01$, ***$P<0.001$ compared with thrombotic control group.

Table 3. The effect of danshensu on the hemorheological parameters in rats.

Group	WBV(mPa.s)			PV(mPa.s)	Hct(%)
	Low shear rate	Medium shear rate	High shear rate		
Normal Control	22.72±1.21	5.88±0.25	4.44±0.11	1.41±0.08	0.41±0.02
Adr Control	39.55±1.35##	9.01±0.32##	6.52±0.23##	2.06±0.06##	0.45±0.02##
Adr Aspirin 20 mg/kg	26.59±0.87**	6.82±0.21**	5.02±0.19**	1.66±0.06*	0.44±0.04
Adr Danshensu 15 mg/kg	35.36±2.25*	8.64±0.51*	6.28±0.31*	1.89±0.08*	0.45±0.02*
Adr Danshensu 30 mg/kg	31.24±1.08**	7.74±0.23**	5.65±0.18**	1.67±0.09*	0.44±0.02*
Adr Danshensu 60 mg/kg	27.12±1.05**	6.65±0.19**	4.78±0.12**	1.45±0.42**	0.43±0.02*

Rats were treated by subcutaneous injection of adrenaline hydrochloride and cold stress. The normal control rats received only saline. Next, blood was collected 30 min after drug administration. Hemorheologic parameters were analyzed by routine laboratory assays. Data are expressed as mean±SEM (each group, n = 10). #P<0.05, ##P<0.01 compared with normal control. *P<0.05 **P<0.01 compared with Adr control. Adr: adrenaline hydrochloride, WBV: whole blood viscosity, PV: plasma viscosity, Hct: hematocrit.

Rats were anesthetized with chloral hydrate (350 mg/kg, i.p.). After the rats were fixed on a temperature-controlled heating pad (38°C) to maintain body temperature, the abdomen was opened surgically. The intestines were moved gently to one side and covered with saline-moistened gauze and the vena cava was exposed by blunt dissection. One millimeter above the bifurcation of the vena iliaca and vena cava, the free vein was ligated by tightening the proximal and distal segments using 4-0 suture (Shinva Medical, China) to induce blood stasis. The abdominal cavity was closed provisionally and blood stasis was maintained for 4 h. After the abdomen was reopened, the ligated venous segment was excised and opened longitudinally to remove the thrombus. The vein wall and thrombus were divided by blunt or sharp dissection. The isolated thrombus was blotted of excess blood and weighed immediately. Harvested vein samples were homogenized for subsequent biochemical analysis. Sham operation was performed in the control group.

Measurement of plasma TXB_2 and 6-keto-$PGF_{1\alpha}$

Blood was drawn from the abdominal aorta at the end of the arteriovenous shunt test period or venous thrombosis model. Plasma was prepared by centrifuging blood at 4000 rpm for 5 min. TXA_2 and PGI_2 levels were estimated by measuring their stable hydrolysis products—TXB_2 and 6-keto-$PGF_{1\alpha}$, respectively—per standard procedures using EIA kits (Cayman Chemical) and expressed as pg/mL.

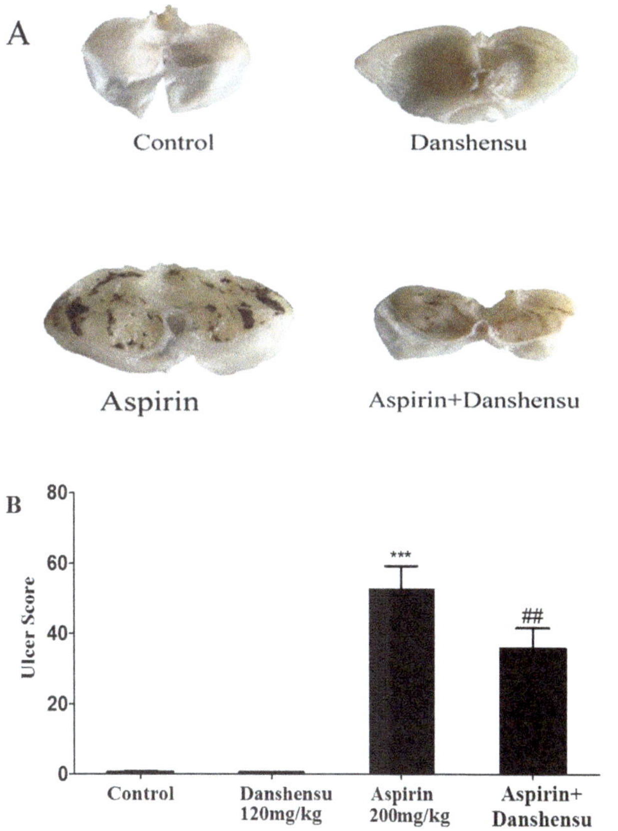

Figure 9. Effects of danshensu on aspirin-induced gastric lesions in mice. A: Photographs of gastric mucosa in the control group and danshensu, aspirin and aspirin + danshensu treatment groups are shown. B: The hemorrhagic ulcer index (mm^2) for each condition. Values are shown as the mean ± SEM(each group, n = 10). **P<0.01 compared with the control rats. ##P<0.01 compared with the aspirin-treated rats.

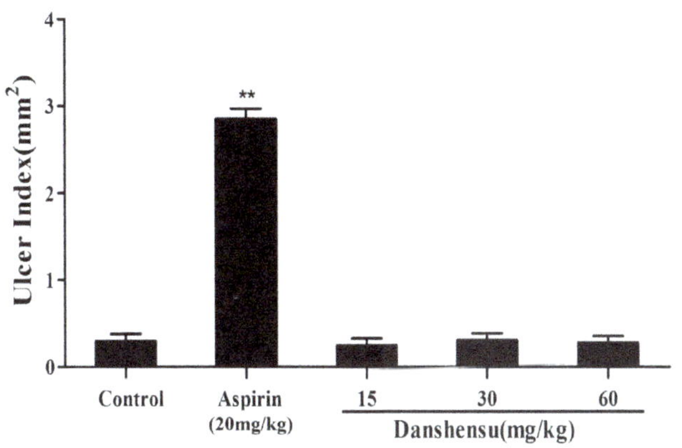

Figure 8. Gastric ulcerogenic response induced by danshensu and aspirin in rats. The test compounds were administered orally at the indicated dose (mg/kg) to rats for 7 days. The animals were sacrificed after the last drug administration and the total length of mucosal lesions in each stomach was used to create an ulcer index. Data are presented as the mean ± SEM (each group, n = 10). **P<0.01 versus the control group.

Effects of Danshensu on COX activity and expression

The inhibition of COX-1 and COX-2 by danshensu and aspirin was determined using COX inhibitor screening assay kits per the manufacturer's instructions. Danshensu and aspirin (with the same volume of water serving as control) were incubated directly with COX-1 or COX-2 in reaction buffer for 10 min. Then, AA was added as substrate and the reaction continued for another 2 min. Then, 0.1 N HCl and saturated stannous fluoride solution were added immediately to stop the enzymatic reaction. The amount of prostaglandin E_2 (PGE_2) that was generated by COX was measured using Cayman ELISA kits. The effects of danshensu and aspirin on COX activity were evaluated by comparing the amounts of PGE_2 production between reactions with and without the drugs. Inhibitory rates were calculated, based on PGE_2 production, as follows: Inhibitory rate (%) = (PGE_2 in Control groups-PGE_2 in drug-treated groups) ×100/PGE_2 in Control groups.

To measure COX-1 and COX-2 expression, venous walls from the venous thrombosis were analyzed by western blot. Venous samples were homogenized mechanically on ice and centrifuged at 4500 g for 10 minutes at 4°C; total proteins were then collected from the supernatants and the protein content was measured using a BCA protein assay kit.

Samples were separated by SDS-PAGE for immunoblot analysis. After the electrophoresis running for 60 min, proteins were transferred onto polyvinylidenedifluoride (PVDF) membranes. The membranes were blocked with 3% skim milk and saturated in Tris-buffered saline with 1% Tween 20 for 1 h at room temperature. Then, the membrane was incubated with primary anti-COX-1 and anti-COX-2 (1:300; Cayman Chemical) overnight at 4°C. The membranes were washed 3 times for 5 min each and incubated in horseradish peroxidase (HRP)-conjugated secondary antibody solution for 1 h at room temperature. The blots were washed again and visualized by using an enhanced chemiluminescence (ECL) detection kit (Beyotime Institute of Biotechnology) and exposure to photographic film. Images were collected and the respective bands were quantitated by densitometric analysis using the DigDoc100 program.

Effects of danshensu on blood stasis

The blood stasis model was established per previous reports [26]. The rats were divided randomly into 6 groups of 10 rats each: normal control, model group given 0.9% normal saline, aspirin (20 mg/kg) and Danshensu (15, 30 and 60 mg/kg). All drugs and saline were administered orally to the rats once per day at 9 AM for 7 days. After the sixth administration, blood stasis was induced by placing the rats in ice-cold water between 2 injections of adrenaline hydrochloride (Adr). All other rats were injected subcutaneously with Adr (0.8 mg/kg), except the control rats, which were injected with 0.9% (w/v) NaCl saline solution. Two hours after the first injection, all rats except the control group were soaked in ice water (0–2°C) for 5 min and reinjected with Adr (0.8 mg/kg) subcutaneously 2 h later to effect blood stasis. Afterward, the rats were placed into cages and fed freely.

Blood samples were collected and anticoagulated with heparin 30 min after the last administration of drugs or saline on the following day. Hemorheologic parameters, including WBV at various shear rates, PV and Hct, were measured by routine laboratory assays. Another aliquot of blood was collected into plastic tubes that contained 3.8% citrate and prepared PRP and PPP as described in *Assay of ex Vivo Platelet Aggregation in Rats*. Platelet aggregation was measured by arachidonic acid-induced.

Ulcerogenic Effects of Danshensu on Gastric Mucosa

Rats were sacrificed by cervical dislocation and the stomachs were removed immediately to determine the gastric ulcer index after the platelet aggregation assayas described with modifications [27,28]. The stomach tissues were split longitudinally and opened along the greater curvature. The total length (mm) of visible mucosal lesions in each stomach sample was measured and used to establish an ulcer index. An independent observer scored the macroscopic appearance of the gastric mucosa. The ulcer area was calculated as $\pi/4 \times a \times b$ mm^2, where a is the long axis and b is the short axis. The ulcer area was expressed as an ulcer index.

Effects of danshensu on aspirin-induced gastric lesion in mice

To investigate the effect of danshensu on aspirin-induced gastric lesions, male ICR mice were randomly divided into 4 groups. Group 1 received 1% carboxymethylcellulose in water as vehicle, Group 2 received danshensu treatment (120 mg/kg body weight), Group 3 received aspirin treatment (200 mg/kg body weight, suspended in 1% carboxymethylcellulose in water) and Group 4 received treatment of aspirin and danshensu. All drugs were administered orally once per day at 9 AM for 7 days. The mice were anesthetized with ether and sacrificed. One hour after the last administration, the isolated stomach was ligated at pylorus and cardia ends, filled with 1.5 mL of 2% formalin and immersed in 2% formalin for 15 min. Then, the stomach was cut along the greater curvature and the lengths of lesions on the stomach wall were measured as described [29].

Statistical analysis

Data were analyzed using SigmaStat 3.1 (SPSS Inc.; Chicago, IL) and expressed as mean±standerd error of means (SEM). $P < 0.05$ was considered to be statistically significant.

Acknowledgments

Chen Yu and Dong Qi contributed equally to this work.

Author Contributions

Conceived and designed the experiments: CY DQ. Performed the experiments: CY DQ. Analyzed the data: WL QZL HJL. Contributed reagents/materials/analysis tools: HJL HYF. Wrote the paper: CY DQ.

References

1. Ruggeri ZM, Loredana Mendolicchio G (2007) Adhesion Mechanisms in Platelet Function Circulation Research. 100: 1673–1685.
2. Antithrombotic Trialists' Collaboration. (2002) Collaborative meta-analysis of randomisedtrials of antiplatelet therapy for prevention of death, myocardial infarction and stroke in high risk patients. BMJ; 324: 71–86.
3. Kang DG, Oh H, Sohn EJ, Hur TY, Lee KC, et al. (2004) Lithospermic acid B isolated from Salviae miltiorrhiza ameliorates ischaemia/reperfusion-induced renal injury in rats. Life Sci. 75: 1801–1816.
4. Chan K, Chui SH, Wong DY, Ha WY, Chan CL, et al (2004) Protective effects of Danshensu from the aqueous extract of Salvia miltiorrhiza (danshen) against homocysteine-induced endothelial dysfunction, Life Sci. 75: 3157–3171.
5. Zhao GR, Zhang HM, Ye TX, Xiang ZJ, Yuan YJ, et al (2008) Characterization of the radical scavenging and antioxidant activities of Danshensu and salvianolic acid B. Food and Chemical Toxicology. 46: 73–81.
6. Chan K, Chui SH, Wong DY, Ha WY, Chan CL, et al (2004) Protective effects of Danshensu from the aqueous extract of Salvia miltiorrhiza (Danshen) against homocysteine-induced endothelial dysfunction. Life Sciences; 75: 3157–3171.

7. Tran H, Anand SS (2004) Oral antiplatelet therapy in cerebrovascular disease, coronary artery disease and peripheral arterial disease. J Am Med Assoc. 292: 1867–1874.
8. Damiano BP, Mitchell JA, Giardino E, Corcoran T, Haertlein BJ, et al (2001) Antiplatelet and Antithrombotic Activity of RWJ-53308, A Novel Orally Active Glycoprotein IIb/IIIa Antagonist. Thromb Res. 104: 113–126.
9. Nosal' R, Jancinova V (2002) Cationic amphiphilic drugs and platelet phospholipase A2 (cPLA2). Thromb Res. 105: 339–345.
10. Ryu KH, Han HY, Lee SY, Jeon SD, Im GJ, et al (2009) Ginkgo biloba extract enhances antiplatelet and antithrombotic effects of cilostazol without prolongation of bleeding time. Thrombosis Research. 124: 328–334.
11. Baskurt OK, Meiselman HJ (2003) Blood Rheology and Hemodynamics. Semin Thromb Hemost. 29: 435–450.
12. Takeuchi K (2012) Pathogenesis of NSAID-induced gastric damage: importance of cyclooxygenase inhibition and gastric hypermotility. World J Gastroenterol18(18).: 2147–2160.
13. Halter F, Tarnawski AS, Schmassmann A (2001) Cyclooxygenase 2-implications on maintenance of gastric mucosal integrity and ulcer healing: controversial issues and perspectives. Gut. 49: 443–453.
14. Masferrer JL, Zweifel BS, Seibert K (1990) Selective regulation of cellular cyclooxygenase by dexamethasone and endotoxin in mice. J Clin Invest. 86: 1375–1379
15. Lechi C, Andrioli G, Gaino S, Tommasoli R, Zuliani V, et al (1996). The antiplatelet effects of a new nitroderivative of acetylsalicylic acid–an in vitro study of inhibition on the early phase of platelet activation and on TXA2 production. Thrombosis and Haemostasis. 76(5): 791–798.
16. Weiss HJ, Turitto VT (1979) Prostacyclin (prostaglandin I2, PGI2) inhibits platelet adhesion and thrombus formation on subendothelium. Blood. 53(2): 244–250
17. Patrono C, Garcia Rodriguez LA, Landolfi R, Baigent C (1979) Low-dose aspirin for the prevention of atherothrombosis. N Engl J Med. 353(22): 2373–83.
18. Collaboration AT (2002). Collaborative meta-analysis of randomised trials of antiplatelet therapy for prevention of death, myocardial infarction and stroke in high risk patients. BMJ. 324 (7329): 71–86.
19. Sakata C, Kawasaki T, Kato Y, Abe M, Suzuki K, et al (2013) ASP6537, a novel highlcy selective cyclooxygenase-1 inhibitor, exerts potent antithrombotic effect without "aspirin dilemma". Thrombosis Research 132: 56–62.
20. Wooten JG, Blikslager AT, Ryan KA, Marks SL, Law JM, et al (2008) Cyclooxygenase expression and prostanoid production in pyloric and duodenal mucosae in dogs after administration of nonsteroidal anti-inflammatory drugs. Am J Vet Res. 69(4): 457–64.
21. Wallace JL, McKnight W, Reuter BK, Vergnolle N (2000) NSAID-induced gastric damage in rats: Requirement for inhibition of bothe cyclooxygenase 1 and 2. Gastroenterology. 119: 706–14.
22. Umar A, Boisseau M, Yusup Az, Upur H, Bégaud B, et al (2004). Interactions between aspirin and COX-2 inhibitors or NSAIDs in a rat thrombosis model. Fundam Clin Pharmacol. 18(5): 559–563.
23. Umoisseau M, Garreau C, Begaud B, Molimard M, Moore N (2003) Effects of armagnac extracts on human platelet function *in vitro* and on rat arteriovenous shunt thrombosis *in vivo*. Thromb Res. 110, 135–140.
24. Henke PK, Varga A, De S, Deatrick CB, Eliason J, et al (2004). Deep vein thrombosis resolution is modulated by monocyte CXCR2-mediated activity in a mouse model. Arterioscler Thromb Vasc Biol. 24: 1130–1137.
25. Henke PK Varma MR, Deatrick KB, Dewyer NA, Lynch EM, et al (2006) Neutrophils modulate post-thrombotic vein wall remodeling but not thrombus neovascularization. Thromb Haemost 2006; 95: 272–281.
26. Chen XP, Wang XW, Zhang YY, Xu XF, Ke WB, et al (2007) Effect of ethanol extract of terminalia chebula on microrheological characteristics in acute blood stasis model rat. Chin J Hemorh. 17(4): 525–528.
27. Sakata C, Kawasaki T, Kato Y, Abe M, Suzuki K, et al (2013) ASP6537, a novel highly selective cyclooxygenase-1 inhibitor, exerts potent antithrombotic effect without"aspirin dilemma" Thrombosis Research. 132: 56–62
28. Mei XT, Xu DH, Xu SK, Zheng YP, Xu SB (2013) Zinc(II)-curcumin accelerates the healing of acetic acid-induced chronicgastric ulcers in rats by decreasing oxidative stress and downregulationof matrix metalloproteinase-9, Food and Chemical Toxicology. 60: 448–454
29. Guth PH, Aures D, Paulsen G (1989) Topical aspirin plus HCl gastric lesion in the rat. Gastroen-terology. 76–88.

4

Increased Bone Marrow (BM) Plasma Level of Soluble CD30 and Correlations with BM Plasma Level of Interferon (IFN)-γ, CD4/CD8 T-Cell Ratio and Disease Severity in Aplastic Anemia

Qingqing Wu[9¶], Jizhou Zhang[9¶], Jun Shi, Meili Ge, Xingxin Li, Yingqi Shao, Jianfeng Yao, Yizhou Zheng*

Severe Aplastic Anemia Studying Program, State Key Laboratory of Experimental Hematology, Institute of Hematology & Blood Diseases Hospital, Chinese Academy of Medical Sciences & Peking Union Medical College, 288 Nanjing Road, Tianjin, 300020, P.R.CHINA

Abstract

Idiopathic aplastic anemia (AA) is an immune-mediated bone marrow failure syndrome. Immune abnormalities such as decreased lymphocyte counts, inverted CD4/CD8 T-cell ratio and increased IFN-γ-producing T cells have been found in AA. CD30, a surface protein belonging to the tumor necrosis factor receptor family and releasing from cell surface as a soluble form (sCD30) after activation, marks a subset of activated T cells secreting IFN-γ when exposed to allogeneic antigens. Our study found elevated BM plasma levels of sCD30 in patients with SAA, which were closely correlated with disease severity, including absolute lymphocyte count (ALC) and absolute netrophil count (ANC). We also noted that sCD30 levels were positively correlated with plasma IFN-γ levels and CD4/CD8 T-cell ratio in patients with SAA. In order to explain these phenomena, we stimulated T cells with alloantigen in vitro and found that $CD30^+$ T cells were the major source of IFN-γ, and induced $CD30^+$ T cells from patients with SAA produced significantly more IFN-γ than that from healthy individuals. In addition, increased proportion of $CD8^+$ T cells in AA showed enhanced allogeneic response by the fact that they expressed more CD30 during allogeneic stimulation. sCD30 levels decreased in patients responded to immunosuppressive therapy. In conclusion, elevated BM plasma levels of sCD30 reflected the enhanced $CD30^+$ T cell-mediated immune response in SAA. CD30 as a molecular marker that transiently expresses on IFN-γ-producing T cells, may participate in mediating bone marrow failure in AA, which also can facilitate our understanding of AA pathogenesis to identify new therapeutic targets.

Editor: Vassiliki A. Boussiotis, Beth Israel Deaconess Medical Center, Harvard Medical School, United States of America

Funding: This study was supported by the National Public Health Grant Research Foundation of China (no. 201202017) to Y.Z., http://www.nhfpc.gov.cn/zhuzhan/index.shtml; the Fundamental Research Funds for the Central Universities of China (no. 2012N05) to Y.Z., http://www.moe.gov.cn/; the National Basic Research Program (2010CB945204) to Y.Z., http://www.nsfc.gov.cn/; the National Natural Science Foundation of China (NNSFC, no. 81330015) to Z.H., http://www.nsfc.gov.cn/; and the NNSFC (no. 81300388) to M.G., http://www.nsfc.gov.cn/. The funders had no role in study design, data collection and analysis, decision to publish, or preparation of the manuscript.

Competing Interests: The authors have declared that no competing interests exist.

* Email: zheng_yizhou@hotmail.com

9 These authors contributed equally to this work.

¶ QW and JZ are co-first authors on this work.

Introduction

Acquired aplastic anemia (AA) is an immune-mediated bone marrow (BM) failure syndrome characterized by persistent peripheral blood (PB) pancytopenia and BM hypoplasia [1]. Immune abnormalities such as decreased lymphocyte counts, inverted CD4/CD8 T-cell ratio and increased IFN-γ-producing T cells have been found in AA [2–4]. Autoreactive T cells activated by specific antigen(s) attacking $CD34^+$ multipotential hematopoietic cells directly [5], and producing type I cytokines such as IFN-γ [6], are thought to be the major villain responsible for destruction of BM hematopoiesis in AA. Effectiveness of immunosuppressive agents further supports the immune-mediated pathogenesis of AA.

Although accumulating laboratory and clinical data suggest that AA is an immune-mediated disorder, the T cell-mediated immunopathology in AA remains to be poorly understood. Recent evidence indicates that oligoclonal expanded cytoxic T cells which are suggestive of an antigen-driven clonal response exist in AA [5,7]. Furthermore, these oligoclones recognize and induce apoptosis of autologous myeloid cells [8]. However, the triggering autoantigens expressed by hematopoietic stem cells (HSC) in AA remain unknown. Only few reports identify autoantibodies in AA, and their pathological significance is unclear [9–12]. In a mouse model the single minor histocompatibility antigen H60 mismatch can trigger immune response and lead to massive BM destruction [13]. Other direct evidence to prove the existence of autoantigen in AA is still limited.

CD30, a cell-surface molecule belonging to the tumor necrosis factor receptor superfamily, is mainly expressed by activated T cells in the physiological condition [14]. CD30 is up-regulated on T cells exposed to allogeneic antigens, and these $CD30^+$ T cells are

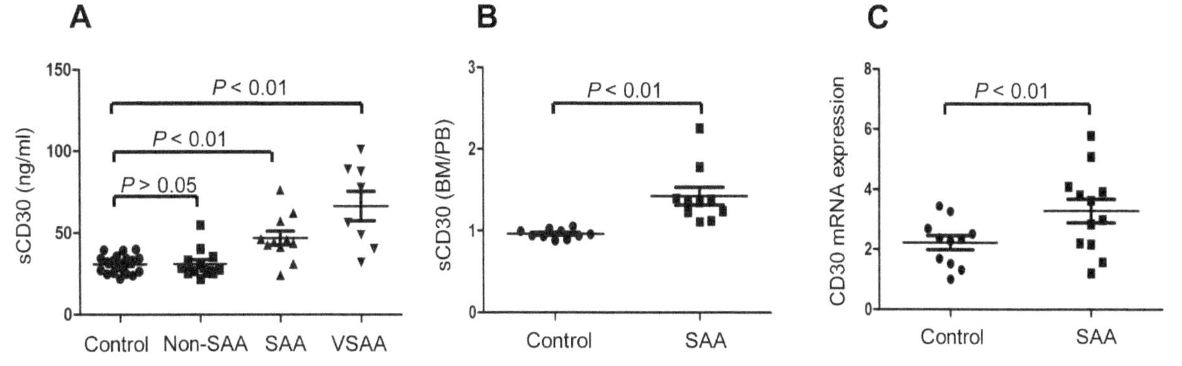

Figure 1. Plasma sCD30 levels and CD30 mRNA expressions in BMMCs from AA patients (n = 42) and healthy individuals (n = 20). (A) BM plasma sCD30 concentrations in healthy individuals (n = 20), Non-SAA patients (n = 13), SAA patients (n = 11) and VSAA patients (n = 8) were measured by ELSIA. (B) The ratios of BM plasma sCD30 level/PB plasma sCD30 level in SAA and VSAA patients (n = 11) and in healthy individuals (n = 11). (C) Relative expressions of CD30 in BMMNCs were measured by real-time PCR in *de novo* SAA patients (n = 12) and healthy individuals (n = 11).

a major source of IFN-γ [15–17]. Quickly after stimulation, surface CD30 is proteolytically cleaved by metalloproteinases and released into bloodstream as soluble CD30 (sCD30) [18]. Therefore, circulating sCD30 is thought to be reflective activation of the immune system.

Low serum levels of sCD30 are detected in healthy individuals [19]. In several classical autoimmune diseases, such as rheumatoid arthritis, atopic dermatitis and systemic lupus erythematosus, high levels of sCD30 have been found to represent the loss of tolerance to self-antigens [20–22]. More interestingly, sCD30 increases significantly in patients who developed acute graft versus host disease (GvHD) after allogeneic hematopoietic cell transplantation (HCT), which implies that elevated levels of sCD30 might be a potential biomarker of allograft rejection in HCT [23–24]. Brentuximab vedotin (SNG35), made by attaching the antitublin agent monomethyl auristatin E (MMAE) to the CD30-specific monoclonal antibody cAC10, has been proved to be efficient in inducing durable objective responses and resulting in tumor regression for CD30-positive lymphomas with only mild-to-moderate toxic effects [25–26]. The US Food and Drug Administration (FDA) has approved Brentuximab vedotin to be used in patients with relapsed/refractory Hodgkin lymphoma and anaplastic large cell lymphoma [27–28].

Thus, it's intriguing to probe whether CD30 is involved in over-production of IFN-γ by T cells given CD30$^+$ T cells are the predominant proliferating and IFN-γ-producing cells in response to alloantigen. So, we carefully evaluated the role of CD30 in the pathogenesis of AA. Our findings suggested that CD30 as a cell surface marker that transiently expressed on activated T cells, might be associated with T cell-mediated bone marrow failure in AA, which could facilitate our understanding of AA pathogenesis to identify new therapeutic targets.

Materials and Methods

Patients and healthy individuals

We analysed samples of PB and BM from 56 patients with AA (median age 28 years, 29 male and 27 female), and 20 BM donors as healthy individuals (median age 27 years, 10 male and 10 female) after written informed consent in accordance with the Declaration of Helsinki, which was approved by the Ethics Committee of the Chinese Academy of Medical Sciences and Peking Union Medical College. The diagnosis and severity classifications of the cohort of patients with AA were established according to the international criteria [29–30], including 13 patients with non-severe AA (Non-SAA), 30 patients SAA and 13 patients very SAA (VSAA). Inherited bone marrow failures and clonal hematologic disorders were excluded from our study. Of 56 patients, 32 patients were analyzed at diagnosis, and 24 patients in complete response (CR) after immunosuppressive therapy (IST) of the combination of antithymocyte globulin (ATG) plus cyclosporine A (CSA). Serial samples pre- and post-ATG/CSA therapy were obtained from 6 patients with SAA. All patients were free from active infection at the time of sampling.

Cell culture

BM mononuclear cells (BMMCs) isolated by Ficoll-Hypaque (1.077 g/mL) density gradient centrifugation were used for the measurements of CD30 mRNA expression. In some experiments, CD3$^+$ T cells were enriched from BMMCs using a commercial CD3$^+$ human T cell isolation kit (Mitenyi Biotec) according to the manufacturer's instructions. CD3$^+$ T cells were mixed at a ratio of 1:1 with autologous or allogenetic PB mononuclear cells pretreated with mitomycin C and seeded at 5×10^5 cells/mL. Cells were cultured for 7 days at 37°C with 5% CO_2 atmosphere, in an optimized serum-free cell culture medium (TexMACS Medium, Miltenyi Biotec) developed for the cultivation and expansion of human T cells, supplemented with 2 mmol/L penicillin/streptomycin. Every 24 h, cells and culture supernatants were collected and analysed by flow cytometry (FCM) and enzyme-linked immune sorbent assay (ELISA), respectively.

Quantitative real-time PCR

Total RNA was isolated from cells with Trizol reagent (Invitrogen) following the manufacturer's instructions. cDNA was synthesized from the purified RNA using a reverse transcription system (Promega) with random primers. Real-time PCR was performed using SYBR green PCR kit (Invitrogen). β-actin was used to normalize gene expression levels. PCR primer sequences were as follows: CD30 forward 5′-GACAAGGCTGTCAGGAGGTG-3′, reverse 5′-ACTGGAGGTTGCTGGGGACA-3′; β-actin forward 5′- CTCTTCCAGCCTTCCTTCCT-3′, reverse 5′- AGCACTGTGTGTTGGCGTACAG-3′.

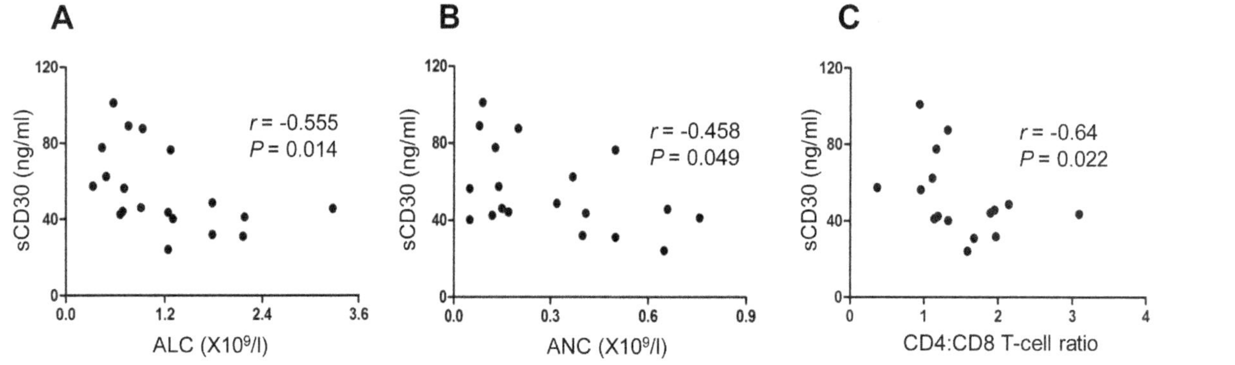

Figure 2. Correlations of BM plasma sCD30 levels with baseline ALC (A), ANC (B), or CD4/CD8 ratio (C) in AA patients (n = 19).

Flow cytometry and cell sorting

In the total 7 days mixed lymphocyte culture system, surface antigen of T cells were analysed by FCM every 24 h. Cultured cells were harvested and washed twice in PBS by centrifugation at 300 g for 5 min. Cells were then stained with the following antibodies: CD3-FITC (Biolegend), CD8-APC (Biolegend), CD30-PE (eBioscience), and the appropriate isotypic control according to the manufacturer's instructions. After incubation, cells were resuspended with 1% paraformaldehyde for FCM analysis. Cell sorting was performed by using BD FACS Canto II (BD Biosciences).

Cytokine ELISA

The plasma and culture supernatants were stored at −80°C until ELISA was performed. The concentrations of sCD30 and IFN-γ were measured by Human sCD30 Instant ELISA kit (eBioscience) and Human IFN-γ ELISA kit (Boshide Biotech, China), respectively.

Statistics

Data were shown as mean ± SEM. The statistical differences were evaluated by the nonparametric Mann–Whitney U-test between unpaired data and by Wilcoxon matched pairs test for two paired variables. The Spearman's rank correlation test was used for correlation analysis. All analyses were performed using SPSS 16.0 software (SPSS Science). *P* values <0.05 were considered statistically significant.

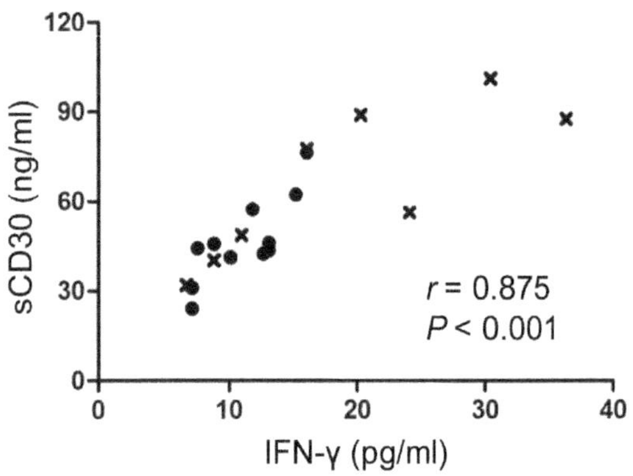

Figure 3. Correlation of BM IFN-γ levels with BM sCD30 levels in SAA patients (•, n = 11) and VSAA patients (×, n = 8).

Ethics Statement

We analysed samples of PB and BM from 56 patients with AA, and 20 BM donors as healthy individuals after written informed consent in accordance with the Declaration of Helsinki to the protocol obtained, which was approved by the Ethics Committee of the Chinese Academy of Medical Sciences and Peking Union Medical College.

Results

Quantitative measurement of sCD30 in AA patients

The comparisons of BM plasma sCD30 levels between *de novo* AA patients (including 13 Non-SAA, 15 SAA and 14 VSAA) and healthy individuals measured by ELISA were shown in Figure 1A. Plasma sCD30 levels were found to be positively correlated with the severity of AA, the median plasma sCD30 levels in healthy individuals, Non-SAA, SAA and VSAA patients were as of 30 ng/mL, 32 ng/mL, 46 ng/mL and 62 ng/mL, respectively.

Because CD30 was suggested to highly express in the target organs of certain autoimmune diseases, we compared sCD30 levels between PB and BM (the latter as the target organ in AA) from 12 SAA and VSAA patients and 11 healthy individuals. Data shown that sCD30 level in BM plasma was higher than its corresponding PB level in each patient with SAA, but healthy individuals had comparable levels of sCD30 between BM and PB, as shown by the significantly higher ratio of BM sCD30/PB sCD30 in patients with SAA in comparison with healthy individuals (Figure 1B). To further confirm CD30 expression in BM, we analysed the mRNA levels of CD30 in BMMCs by real-time PCR, which revealed significantly increased CD30 expression in patients with SAA (Figure 1C).

Correlations between BM plasma sCD30 levels and baseline PB counts

In consideration of alloactivated T cells are the major source of sCD30, we analysed the correlation between BM plasma sCD30 levels and baseline absolute lymphocyte count (ALC), absolute netrophil count (ANC) and absolute reticulocyte count (ARC) in patients with SAA (including VSAA). Our results showed specific inverse correlations between sCD30 levels and ALC (Figure 2A) or ANC (Figure 2B), although no correlation were found between sCD30 levels and ARC (Figure S4).

Interestingly, we also found an inverse correlation between sCD30 levels and CD4/CD8 T-cell ratio (Figure 2C), which suggested patient with a higher $CD8^+$ T cell proportion tended to have a higher plasma level of sCD30.

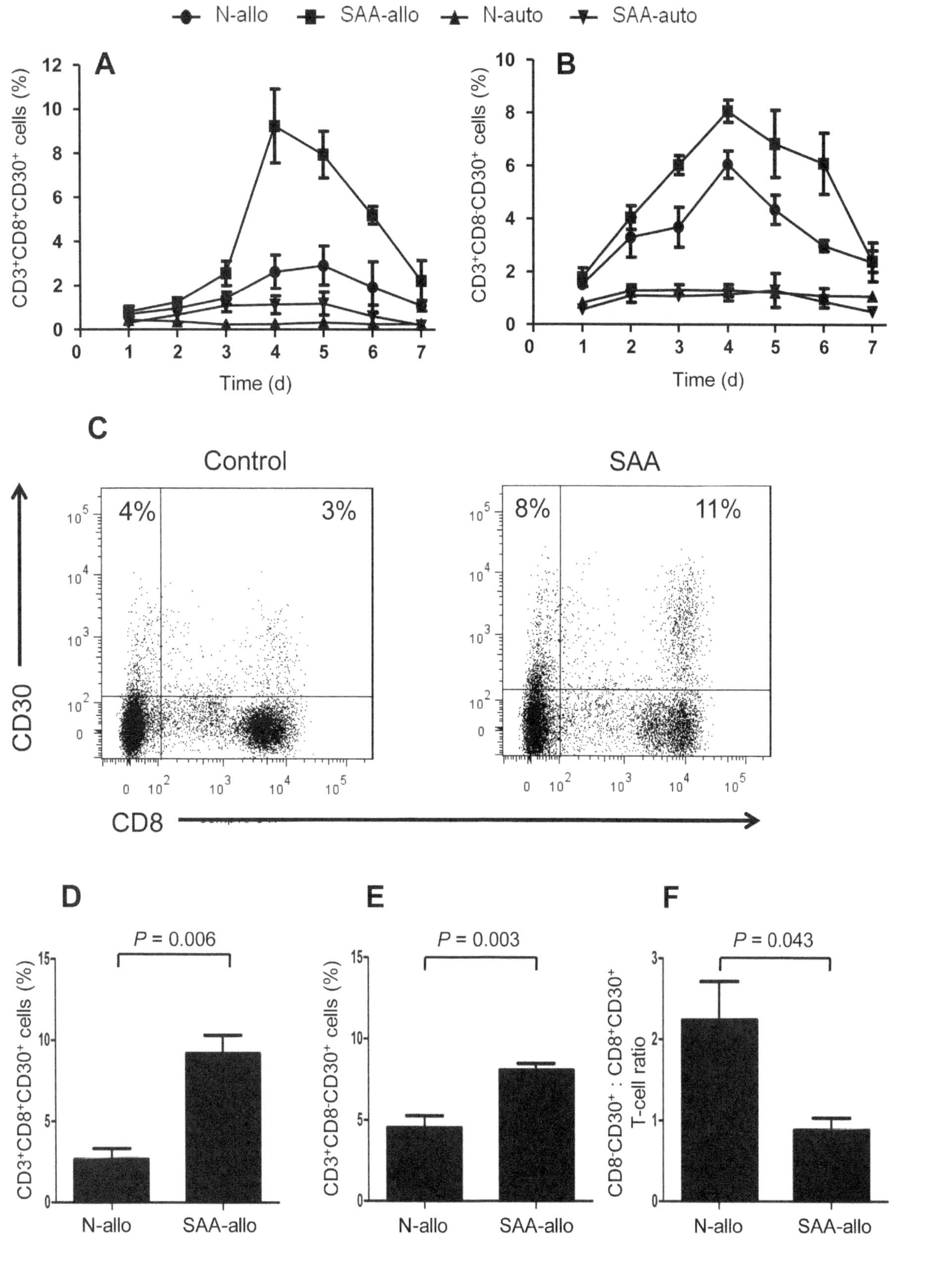

Figure 4. Allogeneic stimulation-induced surface expression of CD30 on T cells. BM $CD3^+$ T cells from healthy individuals and SAA patients were co-cultured with mitomycin C treated autologous or allogenetic mononuclear cells for a total of 7 days, kinetics of cell surface expression of CD30 by $CD3^+CD8^+$ T cells (A) and $CD3^+CD8^-$ T cells (B) were determined by FCM. Data represent mean ± SE of three independent experiments. (C) Representative FCM analyses of cell surface expression of CD30 by T cells from healthy individuals and SAA patients after allogeneic stimulation. Results at day 4 when the maximum CD30 expression reached were shown. (D) and (E) Cells surface expression of CD30 by allogeneic stimulated T-

cell subsets at day 4 were determined in 5 healthy individuals and 6 SAA patients. (F) $CD3^+CD8^-CD30^+$: $CD3^+CD8^+CD30^+$ T-cell ratios in healthy individuals and in SAA patients

Correlation between BM plasma sCD30 levels and BM plasma IFN-γ levels

CD30 was identified as a marker of IFN-γ-producing T cells, so we further determined BM plasma IFN-γ levels in patients with SAA (including VSAA), and found a positive correlation between sCD30 levels and IFN-γ levels (Figure 3), which indicated enhanced CD30 signaling might lead to increased production of IFN-γ in patients with SAA.

Cell surface expression of CD30 by SAA $CD3^+$ T cells during allogeneic stimulation

We had found elevated BM sCD30 levels in SAA, so next we wanted to explore whether T cells from SAA patients expressed more CD30 when exposed to alloantigen compared to those from healthy individuals. To answer this issue, we determined the induction kinetics of CD30 expression on T-cell subsets from SAA patients and healthy individuals after autologous and allogeneic stimulations. The significantly increased percentages of CD30-expressing $CD3^+CD8^+$ (Figure 4A) and $CD3^+CD8^-$ (Figure 4B) T cells in SAA patients as well as in healthy individuals after allogeneic stimulation instead of autologous stimulation were observed. In both SAA patients and healthy individuals, cell surface expression of CD30 by T cells reached peak at day 4 or day 5 during allogeneic stimulation, then quickly decreased to a very low level. Importantly, the significantly higher percentages of CD30-expressing $CD3^+CD8^+$ and $CD3^+CD8^-$ T cells in SAA patients than those in healthy individuals, especially at day 4 were also observed (Figures 4C-E). Furthermore, we found that $CD3^+CD8^-$ T cells expressed more CD30 than $CD3^+CD8^+$ T cells in healthy individuals, whereas the expression levels of CD30 were comparable between $CD3^+CD8^-$ T cells and $CD3^+CD8^+$ T cells in patients with SAA, as shown by the significantly higher $CD3^+CD8^-CD30^+$: $CD3^+CD8^+CD30^+$ T-cell ratios in healthy individuals in comparison with patients with SAA (Figure 4F).

Release of sCD30 and IFN-γ by SAA $CD3^+$ T cells during allogeneic stimulation

Surface CD30 can be cleaved as soluble form, so we measured the kinetics of sCD30 and IFN-γ released into the culture supernatants by autologous and allogeneic stimulated $CD3^+$ T cells. In line with CD30 expression on T cells, significantly

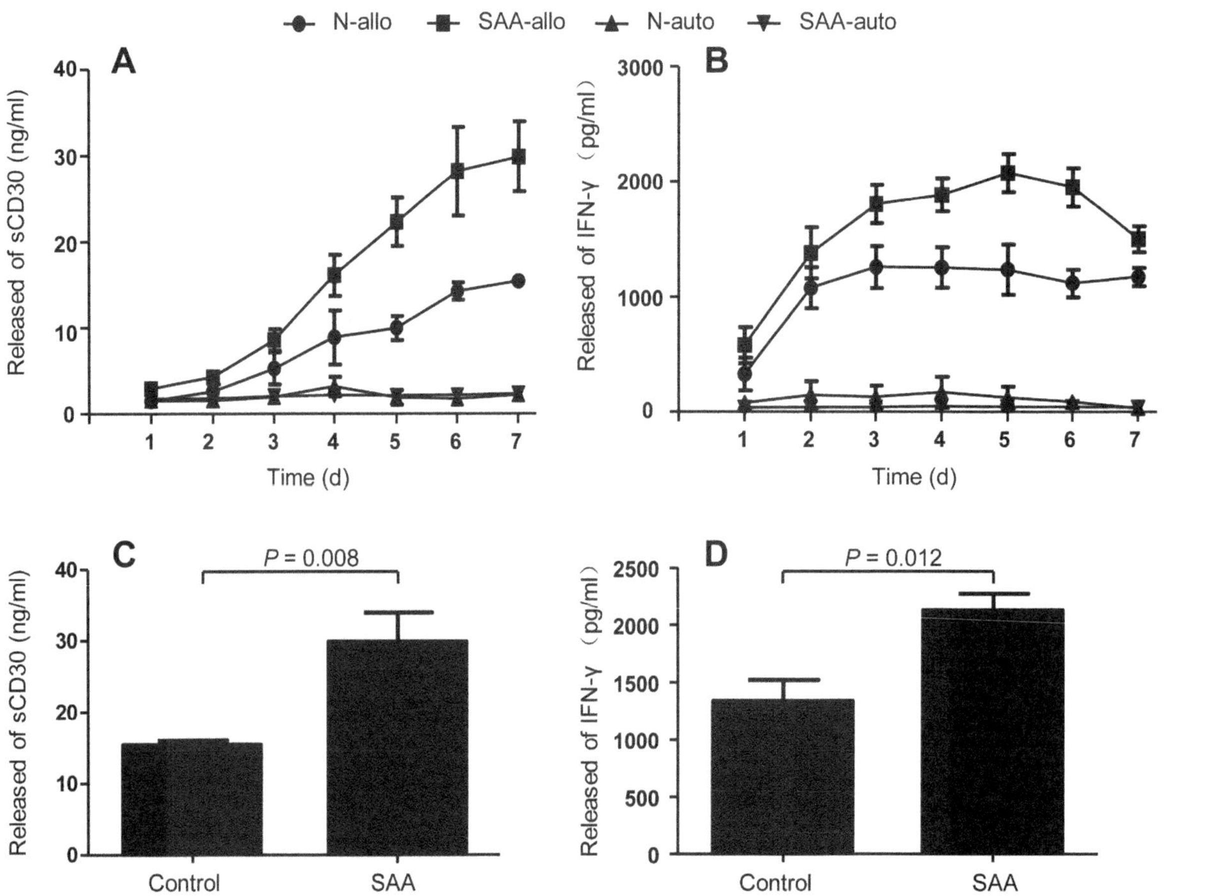

Figure 5. Allogeneic stimulation-induced release of sCD30 and IFN-γ by T cells. BM $CD3^+$ T cells from healthy individuals and SAA patients were co-cultured with mitomycin C treated autologous or allogenetic mononuclear cells for a total of 7 days, kinetics of sCD30 (A) and IFN-γ (B) released into culture supernatants were analysed by ELISA. Data represent mean ± SE of three independent experiments. (C) and (D) Released sCD30 and IFN-γ by allogeneic stimulated T cells at day 4 were determined in 5 healthy individuals and 6 SAA patients.

Table 1. Maximum sCD30 level or IFN-γ level positively correlates with the percentage of $CD30^+$ T cells at day 4 but not day 7 after allogeneic stimulation.

	$CD30^+$ T (%)			
	d4		d7	
	r	p	r	p
sCD30	0.886	0.019	0.23	0.661
IFN-γ 0.018	0.889	0.018	0.126	0.812

Spearman's rank correlation test.

increased levels of sCD30 were detected in culture supernatants from allogeneic stimulated T cells but not from autologous stimulated T cells (Figure 5A). After allogeneic stimulation, sCD30 levels were significant higher in patients with SAA than in healthy individuals (Figure 5C). Distinct correlation was observed between maximum sCD30 level (reached at day 7) and CD30 expression on T cells at day 4 instead of at day 7 (Table 1), when most CD30 had been cleaved from T cells surface.

Significantly elevated levels of IFN-γ were detected in allogeneic cultures but not in autologous cultures (Figure 5B). After allogeneic stimulation, IFN-γ levels were significantly higher in SAA patients than those in healthy individuals (Figure 5D). Once again, specific correlation between maximum IFN-γ levels (reached at day 4 or day 5) and CD30 expression on T cells was observed at day 4 instead of day 7 (Table 1).

Production of IFN-γ by allogeneic sitmulated $CD30^+$ T cells

To assess IFN-γ-producing capacity of induced $CD30^+$ T cells from SAA patients, allogeneic stimulated T cells were separated by FACS day 4 after culture. $CD30^+$ and $CD30^-$ T cells were separately cultured for additional 2 days, followed by determining the levels of IFN-γ in the culture supernatants by ELISA. $CD30^+$ T cells produced significant more IFN-γ than did $CD30^-$ cells in SAA patients as well as in healthy individuals (Figure 6). Importantly, induced $CD30^+$ T cells from SAA patients produced more IFN-γ than healthy individuals.

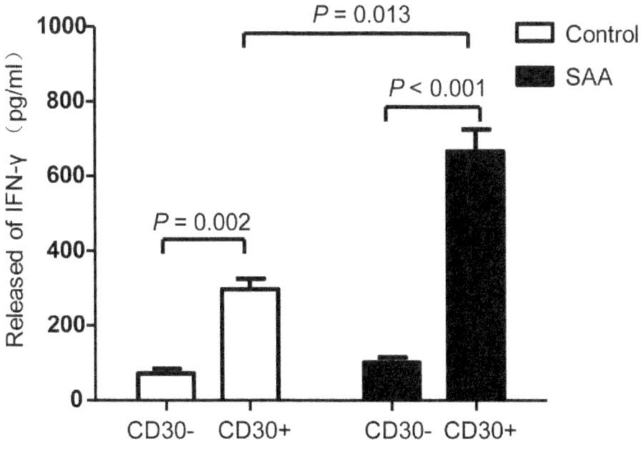

Figure 6. Relationship between CD30 and IFN-γ. After 4 days of culture, allogeneic stimulated T cells were sorted by FACS, $CD30^+$ and $CD30^-$ T cells were separately cultured for additional 2 days, then IFN-γ levels in the culture supernatants were determined by ELISA. Data represent mean ± SE of three independent experiments.

Association between IST and sCD30

In order to investigate the association between sCD30 and disease activity, we detected the sCD30 levels in patients with SAA (including VSAA) at diagnosis (n = 29) and in CR (n = 24). Patients in CR had significantly lower levels of sCD30 than patients at diagnosis (Figure 7A). BM samples pre- and post-IST were collected from 6 SAA patients who had responded to IST, all patients had significant decrease in sCD30 levels after successful IST (Figure 7B).

To test the direct effect of CsA on CD30 expression, we added CsA at 200 ng/mL to the allogeneic cultures. Surface CD30 expression on T cells, and levels of sCD30 and IFN-γ in culture supernatants were analysed at day 4. CsA significantly inhibited CD30 expression on $CD3^+CD8^-$ (Figure 7C) and $CD3^+CD8^+$ T cells (Figure 7D) of both SAA patients and healthy individuals. CsA also reduced sCD30 (Figure 7E) and IFN-γ (Figure 7F) in the culture supernatants from T cells of both SAA patients and healthy individuals.

Discussion

Elevated amounts of sCD30 in blood have been reported in many autoimmune diseases. This is the first study to investigate the role of CD30 in the pathogenesis of AA. We found increased BM plasma levels of sCD30 correlated well with disease severity, CD4/CD8 T-cell ratio and BM plasma levels of IFN-γ in SAA. More interestingly, higher plasma level of sCD30 in BM than in PB was observed in each SAA patient, but not in healthy individual. We also revealed an elevated CD30 expression at mRNA levels in BMMCs of patients with SAA compared with healthy individuals. These data suggested that CD30-associated T cell activation did exist, especially in BM as the target organ of immune attack in patients with SAA. In addition, T cells and in particular $CD8^+$ T cells from patients with SAA showed enhanced allogeneic response by the fact that immune cells from these patients could be induced by alloantigen to express more CD30 than that from healthy controls.

Though the physiological function of CD30 remains unclear, it is unambiguous that CD30 is not a general marker of activated T cells but plays a critical role in alloimmune response. CD30 was suggested to participate in eliminating autoreactive T cells in thymus and inducing T cell apoptosis in periphery *in vivo* [31–34]. Compared with anti-CD3 plus anti-CD28 antibodies and autologous antigen presenting cell (APC), allogeneic APC induced a greater proportion of $CD30^+$ cells which not only were the predominant proliferating T cells in response to alloantigen, but also represented a subset of T cells that were the primary source of IFN-γ *in vitro* [17]. These findings also agreed with the observation that BM plasma levels of sCD30 positively correlated with the levels of IFN-γ in patients with SAA.

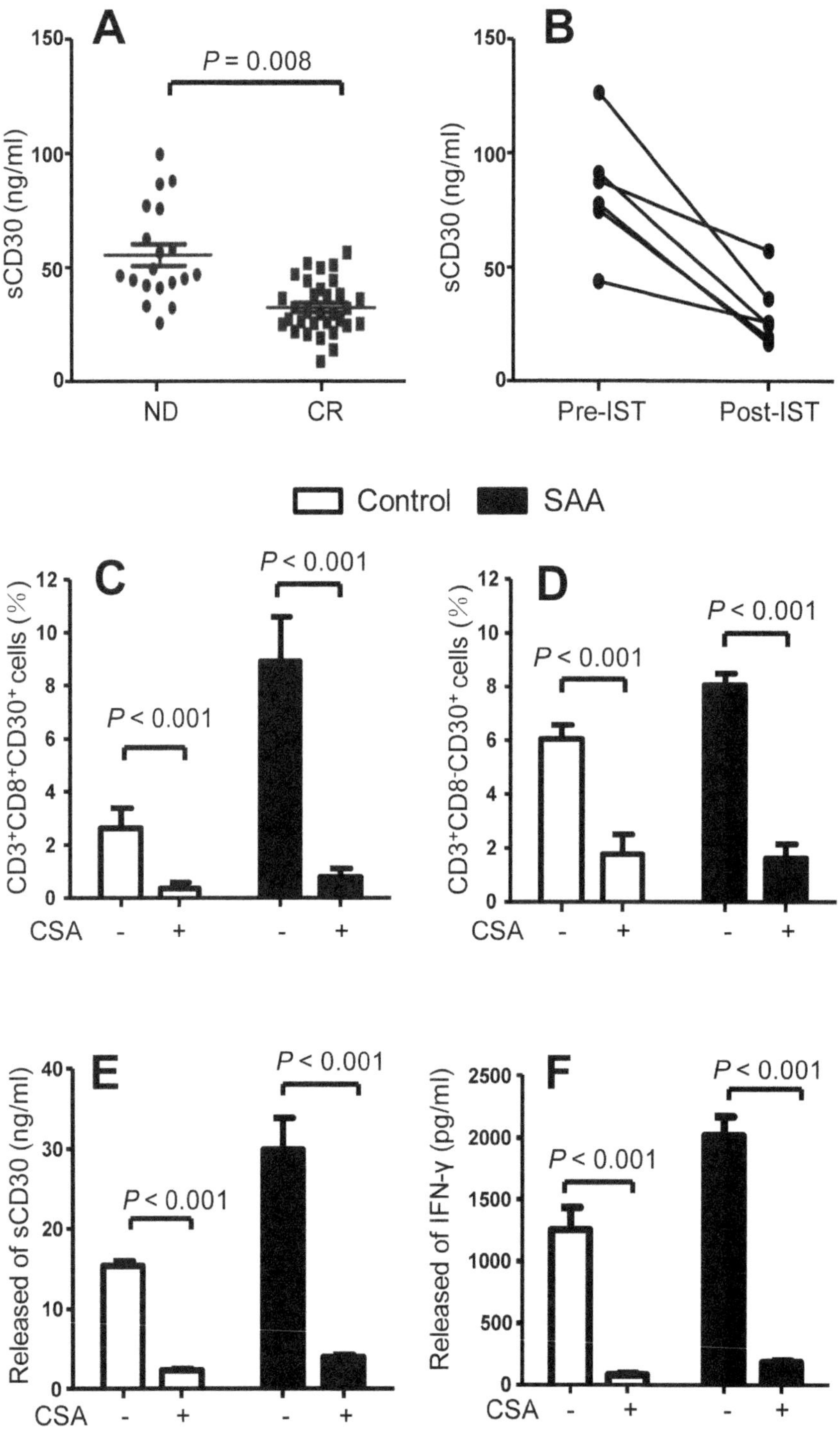

Figure 7. Relationship between BM plasma sCD30 levels and IST. (A) BM plasma sCD30 levels in SAA patients at diagnosis (n = 19) and in CR (n = 24). (B) BM samples pre- and post-IST were collected from 6 SAA patients, BM plasma sCD30 levels were determined by ELISA. CsA was added at 200 ng/mL to the allogeneic stimulated cultures, cells surface CD30 expressions (C and D) and released sCD30 (E) and IFN-γ (F) into culture supernatants were analysed at day 4 by FCM and ELISA, respectively. Data represent mean $\pm$ SE of three independent experiments.

Our *in vitro* stimulation experiments unveiled that the proportion of $CD30^+$ cells increased and peaked at day 4, then decreased quickly, but the sCD30 levels increased in a time-dependent manner paralleled with high production of IFN-γ. Significant correlation of maximum sCD30 level or maximum IFN-γ level with CD30 expression on T cells was observed at day 4, but no at day 7 when most surface CD30 had been cleaved and released as soluble CD30. This observation, consistent with previous studies [35], implied that surface CD30 was transiently expressed by activated T cells, but sCD30 could exist for a relatively longer period, and was easily quantified to reflect the maximum cell surface CD30 expression. It is intriguing to speculate that potent proliferating of $CD30^+$ T cells caused by autoantigens exist abundantly in the early phase of SAA, when the disease still hardly been aware because of lacking obvious clinical symptoms. These $CD30^+$ T cells may have a powerful ability to inhibit hematopoiesis because of enhanced production of IFN-γ. During the aggressive stage of SAA, drastic immune attack eliminates most hematopoietic cells baring autoantigens, leads to few new born $CD30^+$ T cells which only have a transient existence, but sCD30 cleaved from activated $CD30^+$ T cells can circulate in the bloodstream for a relative long time and reflect the degree of T cell activation. This may explain why we can't detect abundant expression of CD30 on T cell surface but elevated sCD30 levels in SAA.

Another interesting observation was the inverse correlation between plasma sCD30 levels and ALC. As we know most SAA patients show activated immune responses and decreased T cell counts. In addition, the baseline ALC is predictive of response at 6 months following IST [2]. The inverse correlation between sCD30 levels and ALC implied that CD30 participated in regulating apoptosis of T cells in SAA patients. However, the role of CD30 in human peripheral T cell apoptosis is still unclear. Only a few studies reported that CD30 regulated apoptosis in human blood eosinophils, anaplastic large cell lymphoma cells and murine $CD8^+$ T cells [34,36,37]. So If CD30 signaling affects the apoptosis of human T cells needs further study, especially in patients with SAA.

Disturbed T-cell subset balance with low CD4/CD8 T-cell ratio is present in many AA patients. We found the inverted CD4/CD8 T-cell ratio correlated with sCD30 levels in patients with SAA. This association was also reported in patients with common variable immunodeficiency [38]. We tried to explain this observation and found that while CD30 was predominantly expressed on $CD3^+CD8^-$ T cells in healthy individuals after allogeneic stimulation, the expression level of CD30 was comparable between $CD3^+8^-$ T cells and $CD3^+CD8^+$ T cells in AA. $CD8^+$ T cells from AA patients expressed more CD30 than that from healthy individuals. Although very preliminary, these findings suggested that activated $CD8^+$ T cells with increased proportion and enhanced allogeneic response might partly contribute to the elevated sCD30 in AA. In addition, we found that the release of IFN-γ reached plateau sooner than the release of sCD30 in allogeneic cultures. This could be explained by a very recent report that IFN-γ was able to trigger the release of sCD30 from allogeneic stimulated T lymphocytes [35]. So, while the CD30 pathway regulate the production of IFN-γ by T cells, IFN-γ may also function as a negative feedback modulator of T cell function by promoting CD30 release from T cells.

Correlations of sCD30 levels with disease activity/severity were reported in patients with systemic lupus erythematosus [22]. Increased levels of sCD30 in serum and synovial fluid were also observed in patients with rheumatoid arthritis [20]. So, sCD30 may be an indicator of immune activation in autoimmune diseases, including AA. Recently, CD30 has been investigated in acute GvHD after HCT [23–24]. The well-known pathophysiology of acute GvHD is clear that donor-derived T cells driven by antigen-present cell participated in the genesis of aGVHD, and minor histocomatibility antigens play a critical role [39]. As a marker of alloimmune responses, the elevated amounts of sCD30 in blood decreased after successful IST in SAA, which was similar with aGvHD. Brentuximab vedotin, an antibody-drug conjugates targeting CD30, has been approved by FDA for treatment of relapsed/refractory Hodgkin lymphoma and anaplastic large cell lymphoma [27–28]. Besides in hematopoietic cancers, Brentuximab vedotin is now being tested in prevention of GvHD after mismatched unrelated allogeneic HCT and treatment of refractory chronic GvHD. So, considering the increased expression of CD30 in many autoimmune diseases, and the treatment effect of CD30 antibody in type-I sensitized mice [40], this drug may have an application prospect in these diseases with elevated levels of sCD30.

Conclusion

In summary, we found that sCD30 plasma levels were increased in AA and correlated with disease severity, IFN-γ levels and CD4/CD8 T-cell ratio. T cells and in particular $CD8^+$ T cells which had increased proportion and enhanced allogeneic response partly contributed to the elevated levels of sCD30 and IFN-γ in AA. CD30 as a molecular marker that transiently express on IFN-γ-producing T cells, may participate in mediating bone marrow failure in AA. Our results shed more insight into the immune pathology involved in SAA. And in light of the importance of IFN-γ in the pathogenesis of SAA, CD30 may be a potent therapeutic target for SAA. CD30-directed drugs, for example, Brentuximab vedotin, should be tested *in vitro* and in AA mouse model for its ability to suppress activation of T cells by alloantigen.

Supporting Information

Figure S1 Expression of CD30 on T cells after allogeneic stimulation. Representative FCM analyses showed the kinetics of cell surface expression of CD30 by $CD3^+CD8^+$ T cells and $CD3^+CD8^-$ T cells after allogeneic stimulation. BM $CD3^+$ T cells from healthy individuals and SAA patients were co-cultured with mitomycin C treated allogenetic mononuclear cells for a total of 7 days.

Figure S2 CD30 positive T cells were mainly contained in the cell population with larger FSC and SSC. Representative FCM analyses showed the cell surface expression of CD30 on T cells at day 4 after allogeneic stimulation.

Figure S3 CsA inhibited the expression of CD30 on T cells after allogeneic stimulation. Representative FCM analyses showed the cell surface expression of CD30 on T cells at day 4 after allogeneic stimulation.

Figure S4 Correlation of BM plasma sCD30 levels with baseline RET in AA patients (n = 19).

Table S1 Characteristics of patients.

Author Contributions

Conceived and designed the experiments: JZ QW YZ. Performed the experiments: JZ QW JS MG XL. Analyzed the data: JZ QW JS MG XL. Contributed reagents/materials/analysis tools: MG XL YS JY. Wrote the paper: JZ QW YZ.

References

1. Brodsky RA, Jones RJ (2005) Aplastic anaemia. Lancet 365: 1647–1656.
2. Scheinberg P, Wu CO, Nunez O, Young NS (2009) Predicting response to immunosuppressive therapy and survival in severe aplastic anaemia. Br J Haematol 144: 206–216.
3. Zoumbos NC, Ferris WO, Hsu SM, Goodman S, Griffith P, et al. (1984) Analysis of lymphocyte subsets in patients with aplastic anaemia. Br J Haematol 58: 95–105.
4. Sloand E, Kim S, Maciejewski JP, Tisdale J, Follmann D, et al. (2002) Intracellular interferon-gamma in circulating and marrow T cells detected by flow cytometry and the response to immunosuppressive therapy in patients with aplastic anemia. Blood 100: 1185–1191
5. Risitano AM, Kook H, Zeng W, Chen G, Young NS, et al. (2002) Oligoclonal and polyclonal CD4 and CD8 lymphocytes in aplastic anemia and paroxysmal nocturnal hemoglobinuria measured by V beta CDR3 spectratyping and flow cytometry. Blood 100: 178–183.
6. Young NS, Scheinberg P, Calado RT (2008) Aplastic anemia. Curr Opin Hematol 15: 162–168.
7. Zeng W, Maciejewski JP, Chen G, Young NS (2001) Limited heterogeneity of T cell receptor BV usage in aplastic anemia. J Clin Invest 108: 765–773.
8. Risitano AM, Maciejewski JP, Green S, Plasilova M, Zeng W, et al. (2004) In-vivo dominant immune responses in aplastic anaemia: molecular tracking of putatively pathogenetic T-cell clones by TCR beta-CDR3 sequencing. Lancet 364: 355–364.
9. Hirano N, Butler MO, Von Bergwelt-Baildon MS, Maecker B, Schultze JL, et al. (2003) Autoantibodies frequently detected in patients with aplastic anemia. Blood 102: 4567–4575.
10. Hirano N, Butler MO, Guinan EC, Nadler LM, Kojima S (2005) Presence of anti-kinectin and anti-PMS1 antibodies in Japanese aplastic anaemia patients. Br J Haematol 128: 221–223.
11. Takamatsu H, Espinoza JL, Lu X, Qi Z, Okawa K, et al. (2009) Anti-moesin antibodies in the serum of patients with aplastic anemia stimulate peripheral blood mononuclear cells to secrete TNF-alpha and IFN-gamma. J Immunol 182: 703–710.
12. Goto M, Kuribayashi K, Takahashi Y, Kondoh T, Tanaka M, et al. (2013) Identification of autoantibodies expressed in acquired aplastic anaemia. Br J Haematol 160: 359–362.
13. Chen J, Ellison FM, Eckhaus MA, Smith AL, Keyvanfar K, et al. (2007) Minor antigen h60-mediated aplastic anemia is ameliorated by immunosuppression and the infusion of regulatory T cells. J Immunol 178: 4159–4168.
14. Ellis TM, Simms PE, Slivnick DJ, Jack HM, Fisher RI (1993) CD30 is a signal-transducing molecule that defines a subset of human activated CD45RO+ T cells. J Immunol 151: 2380–2389.
15. Alzona M, Jack HM, Fisher RI, Ellis TM (1994) CD30 defines a subset of activated human T cells that produce IFN-gamma and IL-5 and exhibit enhanced B cell helper activity. J Immunol 153: 2861–2867.
16. Martinez OM, Villanueva J, Abtahi S, Beatty PR, Esquivel CO, et al. (1998) CD30 expression identifies a functional alloreactive human T-lymphocyte subset. Transplantation 65: 1240–1247.
17. Chan KW, Hopke CD, Krams SM, Martinez OM (2002) CD30 expression identifies the predominant proliferating T lymphocyte population in human alloimmune responses. J Immunol 169: 1784–1791.
18. Hansen HP, Dietrich S, Kisseleva T, Mokros T, Mentlein R, et al. (2000) CD30 shedding from Karpas 299 lymphoma cells is mediated by TNF-alpha-converting enzyme. J Immunol 165: 6703–6709.
19. Schlaf G, Altermann WW, Rothhoff A, Seliger B (2007) Soluble CD30 serum level–an adequate marker for allograft rejection of solid organs? Histol Histopathol 22: 1269–1279.
20. Gerli R, Muscat C, Bistoni O, Falini B, Tomassini C, et al. (1995) High levels of the soluble form of CD30 molecule in rheumatoid arthritis (RA) are expression of CD30+ T cell involvement in the inflamed joints. Clin Exp Immunol 102: 547–550.
21. Dummer W, Brocker EB, Bastian BC (1997) Elevated serum levels of soluble CD30 are associated with atopic dermatitis, but not with respiratory atopic disorders and allergic contact dermatitis. Br J Dermatol 137: 185–187.
22. Caligaris-Cappio F, Bertero MT, Converso M, Stacchini A, Vinante F, et al. (1995) Circulating levels of soluble CD30, a marker of cells producing Th2-type cytokines, are increased in patients with systemic lupus erythematosus and correlate with disease activity. Clin Exp Rheumatol 13: 339–343.
23. Hubel K, Cremer B, Heuser E, von Strandmann EP, Hallek M, et al. (2010) A prospective study of serum soluble CD30 in allogeneic hematopoietic stem cell transplantation. Transpl Immunol 23: 215–219.
24. Chen YB, McDonough S, Hasserjian R, Chen H, Coughlin E, et al. (2012) Expression of CD30 in patients with acute graft-versus-host disease. Blood 120: 691–696.
25. Fanale MA, Forero-Torres A, Rosenblatt JD, Advani RH, Franklin AR, et al. (2012) A phase I weekly dosing study of brentuximab vedotin in patients with relapsed/refractory CD30-positive hematologic malignancies. Clin Cancer Res. 18: 248–255.
26. Younes A, Bartlett NL, Leonard JP, Kennedy DA, Lynch CM, et al. (2010) Brentuximab vedotin (SGN-35) for relapsed CD30-positive lymphomas. N Engl J Med 363: 1812–1821.
27. Sasse S, Rothe A, Goergen H, Eichenauer DA, Lohri A, et al. (2013) Brentuximab vedotin (SGN-35) in patients with transplant-naive relapsed/refractory Hodgkin lymphoma. Leuk Lymphoma 54: 2144–2148.
28. Pro B, Advani R, Brice P, Bartlett NL, Rosenblatt JD, et al. (2012) Brentuximab vedotin (SGN-35) in patients with relapsed or refractory systemic anaplastic large-cell lymphoma: results of a phase II study. J Clin Oncol 30: 2190–2196.
29. Camitta BM, Thomas ED, Nathan DG, Gale RP, Kopecky KJ, et al. (1979) A prospective study of androgens and bone marrow transplantation for treatment of severe aplastic anemia. Blood 53: 504–514.
30. Marsh JC, Ball SE, Cavenagh J, Darbyshire P, Dokal I, et al. (2009) Guidelines for the diagnosis and management of aplastic anaemia. Br J Haematol 147: 43–70.
31. Amakawa R, Hakem A, Kundig TM, Matsuyama T, Simard JJ, et al. (1996) Impaired negative selection of T cells in Hodgkin's disease antigen CD30-deficient mice. Cell 84: 551–562.
32. Chiarle R, Podda A, Prolla G, Podack ER, Thorbecke GJ, et al. (1999) CD30 overexpression enhances negative selection in the thymus and mediates programmed cell death via a Bcl-2-sensitive pathway. J Immunol 163: 194–205.
33. Zeiser R, Nguyen VH, Hou JZ, Beilhack A, Zambricki E, et al. (2007) Early CD30 signaling is critical for adoptively transferred CD4+CD25+ regulatory T cells in prevention of acute graft-versus-host disease. Blood 109: 2225–2233.
34. Telford WG, Nam SY, Podack ER, Miller RA (1997) CD30-regulated apoptosis in murine CD8+ T cells after cessation of TCR signals. Cell Immunol 182: 125–136.
35. Velasquez SY, Garcia LF, Opelz G, Alvarez CM, Susal C (2013) Release of soluble CD30 after allogeneic stimulation is mediated by memory T cells and regulated by IFN-gamma and IL-2. Transplantation 96: 154–161.
36. Berro AI, Perry GA, Agrawal DK (2004) Increased expression and activation of CD30 induce apoptosis in human blood eosinophils. J Immunol 173: 2174–2183.
37. Mir SS, Richter BW, Duckett CS (2000) Differential effects of CD30 activation in anaplastic large cell lymphoma and Hodgkin disease cells. Blood 96: 4307–4312.
38. Rezaei N, Haji-Molla-Hoseini M, Aghamohammadi A, Pourfathollah AA, Moghtadaie M, et al. (2008) Increased serum levels of soluble CD30 in patients with common variable immunodeficiency and its clinical implications. J Clin Immunol 28: 78–84.
39. Couriel D, Caldera H, Champlin R, Komanduri K (2004) Acute graft-versus-host disease: pathophysiology, clinical manifestations, and management. Cancer 101: 1936–1946.
40. Saraiva M, Smith P, Fallon PG, Alcami A (2002) Inhibition of type 1 cytokine-mediated inflammation by a soluble CD30 homologue encoded by ectromelia (mousepox) virus. J Exp Med 196: 829–839.

5

Apolipoprotein E Gene Polymorphisms Are Associated with Primary Hyperuricemia in a Chinese Population

Jie Wu[1]☯, Ling Qiu[1*]☯, Xiu-zhi Guo[1]☯, Tao Xu[2], Xin-qi Cheng[1], Lin Zhang[1], Peng-chang Li[1], Qian Di[1], Qing Wang[3], Lan Ni[3], Guang-jin Zhu[4]

1 Department of Clinical Laboratory, Peking Union Medical College Hospital, Peking Union Medical College & Chinese Academy of Medical Science, Beijing, China, **2** Department of Epidemiology and Statistics, Institute of Basic Medical Sciences, Chinese Academy of Medical Sciences & Peking Union Medical College, Beijing, China, **3** Medical Experimental Center, General Hospital of Ningxia Medical University, Yinchuan, China, **4** Department of Pathophysiology, Institute of Basic Medical Sciences, Chinese Academy of Medical Sciences & Peking Union Medical College, Beijing, China

Abstract

Objective: Primary hyperuricemia, an excess of uric acid in the blood, is a major public health problem. In addition to the morbidity that is attributable to gout, hyperuricemia is also associated with metabolic syndrome, hypertension, and cardiovascular disease. This study aims to assess the genetic associations between Apolipoprotein E (APOE) polymorphisms and hyperuricemia in a Chinese population.

Methods: A total of 770 subjects (356 hyperuricemic cases and 414 normouricemic controls) were recruited from the Ningxia Hui Autonomous Region, China. A physical examination was performed and fasting blood was collected for biochemical tests, including determination of the levels of serum lipid, creatinine, and uric acid. Multi-ARMS PCR was applied to determine the APOE genotypes, followed by an investigation of the distribution of APOE genotypes and alleles frequencies in the controls and cases.

Results: The frequencies of the APOE-ε2ε3 genotype (17.70% vs. 10.39%, $P = 0.003$) and the APOE-ε2 allele (10.53% vs. 5.80%, $P = 0.001$) were significantly higher in the hyperuricemic group than in the normouricemic group. Furthermore, male cases were more likely to have the APOE-ε2ε3 genotype and APOE-ε2 allele, compared with male controls. In both Han and Hui subjects, cases were more likely to have the APOE-ε2ε3 genotype and the APOE-ε2 allele compared with controls. Furthermore, multivariate logistic regression showed that carriers of the APOE-ε2ε3 genotype ($P = 0.001$, OR = 2.194) and the ε2 allele ($P = 0.001$, OR = 2.099) were significantly more likely to experience hyperuricemia than carriers of the ε3/ε3 genotype and the ε3 allele after adjustment for sex, body mass index (BMI), diastolic blood pressure (DBP), triglyceride (TG), low density lipoprotein cholesterol (LDL-C), creatinine (Cr) and fasting blood glucose(FBG).

Conclusions: The APOE-ε2ε3 genotype and the APOE-ε2 allele are associated with serum uric acid levels in Chinese subjects, indicating that individuals carrying the APOE-ε2 allele have a higher risk of hyperuricemia than non-carriers.

Editor: Masaru Katoh, National Cancer Center, Japan

Funding: This work was supported by the Special funding for Key Basic Research Project of the Ministry of Science and Technology of China (2006FY110300), the National Natural Science funding of China (grants 81301508). The funders had no role in study design, data collection and analysis, decision to publish, or preparation of the manuscript.

Competing Interests: The authors have declared that no competing interests exist.

* Email: lingqiubj@aliyun.com

☯ These authors contributed equally to this work.

Introduction

Serum uric acid (SUA) is the final product of purine metabolism in humans. Hyperuricemia(HUA), which is caused by the overproduction of urate or, more commonly, by the reduced renal excretion of urate, contributes to the development of gout [1]. It was reported that 18.8% of patients with HUA developed gout in a 5-year follow-up [2]. Elevation of the SUA level has been identified as a potential risk factor for developing hypertension, insulin resistance, dyslipidemia and obesity, which are hallmarks of metabolic syndrome [3–6]. In addition, multiple epidemiologic studies have confirmed an association between hyperuricemia and cardiovascular disease (CVD) [7–9]. The increasing occurrence of hyperuricemia was observed not only in western populations but also in Asia, including China. Our previous study has shown that the prevalence of HUA is 13.7% in northern China [10]. Recently a meta-analysis demonstrated that in China, the prevalence of hyperuricemia was 21.6% in males and 8.6% in females [11].

The apolipoprotein E (APOE) gene, located in the 19q13 chromosomal region, encodes the ApoE protein, which plays an important role in transporting cholesterol and other lipoproteins. The APOE gene has three common alleles, designated as ε2, ε3, ε4, and six different genotypes, ε2/2, ε2/3, ε2/4, ε3/3, ε3/4, ε4/

4. These three common alleles result from two single-base polymorphisms within exon 4, at codons 112 and 158[12]. APOE-ε3 has a cysteine at residue 112 and an arginine at 158, which are required for normal ApoE functioning. APOE-ε2 (Arg158→Cys) has been shown to be associated with decreased levels of total and low density lipoprotein (LDL) cholesterol, whereas APOE-ε4 (Cys112→Arg) is associated with increased cholesterol levels [13,14].

In addition to the impact on the serum lipid profile, blood pressure levels [15], the occurrence and development of type 2 diabetes mellitus [16] and neurodegenerative disorders [17], polymorphisms of the APOE gene are also associated with the risk of cardiovascular diseases [18]. An association between APOE polymorphisms and SUA was also demonstrated in several studies. However, other studies have reported inconsistent results. Some studies suggest that the ε2 allele is independently associated with increased SUA levels [19,20] and that ε4 is associated with decreased SUA levels [21,22], but others show that the ε4 allele is associated with a higher risk of hyperuricemia [23]. Possible causes include racial and ethnic differences. At present, the correlation between APOE polymorphisms and hyperuricemia remains elusive in China, especially among individuals in an area inhabited by ethnic minorities.

Therefore, the objective of this study was to assess the genetic associations of APOE polymorphisms and hyperuricemia in a Chinese population.

Methods

Subjects

The subjects were selected from a population-based cross-sectional survey, the Chinese Physiological Constant and Health Condition (CPCHC), in the Ningxia Hui Autonomous Region (2011). Briefly, this survey included 6056 participants, aged 10 to 80 years, who underwent physical examination and assays of serum biochemical indicators, including the serum urate levels. Of these 6056 subjects, 356 participants were initially screened as hyperuricemic cases in the present study. One or two region-, gender- and age-matched (the age difference did not exceed 2 years) normouricemic controls for each case were randomly selected at the time of the case diagnosis. Hyperuricemia was defined as SUA≥7 mg/dl (416 μmol/L, male) or SUA≥6 mg/dl (357 μmol/L, female), which is a widely accepted diagnostic criteria [24–26]. Finally, a total of 356 hyperuricemic subjects (243 male and 113 female) and 414 normouricemic individuals (218 male and 196 female) were recruited for genetic analysis. Participants with known systemic diseases, including diabetes mellitus, hypertension, cardiovascular disease, renal or liver disease, gastrointestinal disease, pulmonary disease, or cancer were excluded. Moreover, participants taking any medication known to affect carbohydrate and lipid metabolism were also excluded. The study was conducted in accordance with the Helsinki Declaration and was approved by the Ethics Committee of the Institute of Basic Medical Sciences at the Chinese Academy of Medical Sciences. Written informed consent was obtained from each adult participant before data collection. For minors/children, we sent the parents/guardians an information sheet about the

Table 1. Demographic information and blood chemistry parameters of study subjects.

	Male(n = 461)		Female(n = 309)	
	Normouricemic group	**Hyperuricemic group**	**Normouricemic group**	**Hyperuricemic group**
N(%)	218(47.3%)	243(52.7%)	196(63.4%)	113(36.6%)
Age (years)	24.3(13.9–48.6)	24.0(15.8–45.5)	17.3(15.2–39.1)	18.0(13.2–57.2)
Ethnicity (%)				
Han	103(47.2%)	143(58.8%)	108(55.1%)	63(55.8%)
Hui	112(51.4%)	97(39.9)	88(44.9%)	48(42.5%)
BMI (kg/m^2)	23.0±4.8	24.6±4.5*	21.6±3.5	23.5±5.1*
WC (cm)	76.8±14.2	80.1±12.5*	71.3±10.1	74.3±12.8*
SBP (mmHg)	126.7±21.0	133.3±18.8*	121.3±17.8	127.6±24.2*
DBP (mmHg)	77.4±13.9	82.5±14.7*	76.2±11.6	79.3±14.3
TC (mmol/L)	3.95±0.86	4.11±0.99	3.95±0.84	4.35±1.17*
TG (mmol/L)	1.08(0.65–1.72)	1.33(0.76–2.39)*	0.94(0.58–1.30)	1.20(0.81–1.96)*
HDL-C (mmol/L)	1.13±0.25	1.08±0.28*	1.27±0.27	1.20±0.27*
LDL-C (mmol/L)	2.20(1.76–2.69)	2.34(1.84–2.92)	2.18(1.73–2.61)	2.51(2.03–3.06)*
FBG (mmol/L)	4.96(4.68–5.33)	5.13(4.90–5.51)*	4.87(4.61–5.18)	5.09(4.87–5.52)*
HbA_{1C} (%)	5.10(4.90–5.40)	5.20(5.00–5.50)*	5.10(4.90–5.30)	5.20(5.00–5.60)*
UA (μmmol/L)	297.6±63.0	460.4±45.4*	239.3±55.6	398.4±40.0*
Cr (mmol/L)	80.37±15.4	88.99±18.6*	66.93±8.8	73.03±13.4*
BUN (mmol/L)	4.57±1.29	4.92±1.47*	3.96±1.16	4.47±1.27*

Abbreviations: BMI, Body mass index; WC, Waist circumference; SBP, Systolic blood pressure; DBP, Diastolic blood pressure; TC, Total cholesterol; TG, Triglyceride; HDL-C, High density lipoprotein cholesterol; LDL-C, Low density lipoprotein cholesterol; FBG, Fasting blood glucose; HbA_{1C}, Glycated hemoglobin; UA, Uric acid; Cr, Creatinine; BUN, Blood urea nitrogen.
Data are presented as n (%), mean ± standard deviation (SD); Age, TG, LDL-C, FBG and HbA_{1C} were reported as the medians (interquartile range).
*P<0.05 for Hyperuricemic group vs. Normouricemic group within the same sex.

Table 2. Genotype and allele frequencies of APOE polymorphisms among the study subjects.

	Normouricemic group (%)	Hyperuricemic group (%)	*P value*
	(n=414)	(n=356)	
Genotypes			
ε2ε2	1(0.24%)	3(0.84%)	
ε2ε3	43(10.39%)	63(17.70%)	0.003
ε2ε4	3(0.72%)	6(1.69%)	
ε3ε3	304(73.43%)	230(64.61%)	0.008
ε3ε4	60(14.49%)	52(14.61%)	0.522
ε4ε4	3(0.72%)	2(0.56%)	
Alleles			
ε2	48(5.80%)	75(10.53%)	0.001
ε3	711(85.87%)	575(80.76%)	0.007
ε4	69(8.33%)	62(8.71%)	0.431

The allelic and genotypic frequencies are indicated in absolute values and percentage. *P* value for the overall comparison between the hyperuricemic and normouricemic groups by the chi-square test.
The extremely rare genotypes-ε2ε2, ε2ε4 and ε4ε4 subjects were described but excluded from the statistical analysis.

study and obtained their written informed consent on behalf of the minors/children enrolled in our study.

Clinical Laboratory Tests

All procedures were performed following a 9–12 hour overnight fast and all subjects were told to consume a bland diet before blood testing. Blood pressure (BP) was measured using an OMRON HEM-7000 electronic sphygmomanometer (OMRON Health-Care, Kyoto, Japan) after the participant had rested for ≥10 min. Blood was drawn from the antecubital vein of the arm. Total cholesterol (TC), triglycerides (TG), high-density lipoprotein cholesterol (HDL-C) and low-density lipoprotein cholesterol (LDL-C) were measured with a Beckman AU Series Automatic Biochemical Analyzer (Japan), using Sekisui Medical (Japan) reagents. Fasting blood glucose (FBG), uric acid (UA), creatine (Cr), and blood urea nitrogen (BUN) were measured with the same instrument, using Beckman AU reagents. HbA1c was examined by high-performance liquid chromatography (HPLC) on a Bio-Rad Diamat automated glycosylated hemoglobin analyzer (USA).

APOE Genotyping

Genomic DNA for APOE genotyping was extracted from peripheral blood mononuclear cells with the Genomic DNA Purification System (Promega, Madison, WI, USA). The DNA samples were then analyzed using the amplification refractory mutation system (ARMS)-polymerase chain reaction (PCR) assay

Table 3. The APOE genotype and allele frequencies among the study subjects stratified by gender.

	Male		Female		*P-value*[a]	*P-value*[b]
	Normouricemic group	Hyperuricemic group	Normouricemic group	Hyperuricemic group		
Genotypes						
ε2ε2	1(0.5%)	2(0.8%)	0(0%)	1(0.9%)		
ε2ε3	26(11.9%)	46 (18.9%)	17(8.7%)	17(15.0%)	0.039	0.064
ε2ε4	1(0.5%)	5(2.1%)	2(1.0%)	1(0.9%)		
ε3ε3	160(73.4%)	154(63.4%)	144(73.5%)	76(67.3%)	0.021	0.245
ε3ε4	28(12.8%)	34(14.0%)	32(16.3%)	18(15.9%)	0.718	0.927
ε4ε4	2(0.9%)	2(0.8%)	1(0.5%)	0(0%)		
Total	218	243	196	113		
Alleles						
ε2	29(6.7%)	55(11.3%)	19(4.8%)	20(8.8%)	0.014	0.049
ε3	374(85.8%)	388(79.8%)	337(86.0%)	187(82.7%)	0.017	0.282
ε4	33(7.6%)	43(8.8%)	36(9.2%)	19(8.4%)	0.481	0.744
Total	436	486	392	226		

Subjects with the extremely rare genotypes -ε2ε2, ε2ε4 and ε4ε4 were described but excluded from the statistical analysis.
[a]Hyperuricemic group *vs.* Normouricemic group in males.
[b]Hyperuricemic group *vs.* Normouricemic group in females.

Table 4. The APOE genotype and allele frequencies among the study subjects stratified by ethnic group.

	Han		Hui		*P-value*[a]	*P-value*[b]
	Normouricemic group	**Hyperuricemic group**	**Normouricemic group**	**Hyperuricemic group**		
Genotypes						
ε2ε2	1(0.5%)	1(0.5%)	0(0%)	2(1.4%)		
ε2ε3	20(9.5%)	36(17.5%)	23(11.5%)	27(18.6%)	0.017	0.064
ε2ε4	3(1.4%)	3(1.5%)	0(0%)	3(2.1%)		
ε3ε3	158(74.9%)	131(63.6%)	143(71.5%)	95(65.5%)	0.012	0.236
ε3ε4	28(13.3%)	34(16.5%)	32(16%)	17(11.7%)	0.353	0.261
ε4ε4	1(0.5%)	1(0.5%)	2(1%)	1(0.7%)		
Total	211	206	200	145		
Alleles						
ε2	25(5.9%)	41(10.0%)	23(5.8%)	34(11.7%)	0.021	0.005
ε3	364(86.3%)	332(80.6%)	341(85.3%)	234(80.7%)	0.027	0.113
ε4	33(7.8%)	39(9.5%)	36(9%)	22(7.6%)	0.397	0.509
Total	422	412	400	290		

Subjects with the extremely rare genotypes -ε2ε2, ε2ε4 and ε4ε4 were described but excluded from the statistical analysis.
[a]Hyperuricemic group *vs.* Normouricemic group in Han.
[b]Hyperuricemic group *vs.* Normouricemic group in Hui.

[27]. Briefly, the PCR was conducted with the following primers: Cys158/Arg158 (5′-ATGCCGATGACCTGCAGAATT-3′)/(5′ATGCCGATGACCTGCAGAATC-3′), Cys112/Arg112(5′-CGCGGACATGGAGGACGTTT-3′)/(5′-CGCGGACATG-GAGGACGTTC-3′), and a common reverse primer (5′-GTTCAGTGATTGTCGCTGGGCA-3′). The common primer was paired with Cys158/Arg158 or Cys112/Arg112 and produced an amplicon of 451 and 588 base pairs (bp), respectively. A 218-bp fragment of the LDLR gene was co-amplified to function as an internal positive control, and the PCR primer sequences were 5′- GTGGCACCGAGACCAAACTC-3′ and 5′- AGTG-CAAGGAGACCACGGGA-3′. The PCR conditions were denaturation at 95°C for 5 min, followed by 35 cycles of 95°C for 30 sec, 63°C for 30 sec and 72°C for 30 sec, and a final extension at 72°C for 5 min. At the end of the PCR cycles, the products were resolved by electrophoresis on 2% agarose gels to validate the amplification of the specific PCR product expected.

Statistical Analysis

Continuous variables with a normal distribution are given as the mean ± standard deviation (SD) and were analyzed by t-test. Variables with a non-normal distribution are given as the median (interquartile range) and were compared by the Wilcoxon rank sum test. Categorical variables (such as ethnicity, genotype distribution and allele frequency) were analyzed as percentages using the Chi-squared test. The extremely rare genotype groups (ε2/ε2, ε4/ε4 and ε2/ε4) were excluded from the genotype analyses, but they were included in the allele analyses. ANOVA or the Wilcoxon rank sum test were used to compare the data related to the clinical parameters among the different APOE genotypes. Genotype and alleles frequencies for APOE were calculated and compared between the hyperuricemia cases and the control subjects using the Chi-squared and Fisher's exact test. The associations between the ApoE genotypes and alleles and hyperuricemia were measured by calculating odd ratios (ORs) and 95% confidence intervals (CIs) using logistic regression. Univariate logistic analysis was applied to examine association between each potential risk factor and HUA. In multivariate analyses, all factors that were statistically significant were adjusted as potential confounding variables and the adjusted ORs and 95% CIs were calculated. Hardy-Weinberg equilibrium was assessed using the chi-squared test. In each model, the homozygous ε3/ε3 genotypes formed the reference group. Statistical significance was assumed at $P<0.05$, and all statistical analyses were conducted using SPSS.

Results

Clinical characteristics of the normouricemic and hyperuricemic groups stratified by gender

As shown in Table 1, there was no significant difference in mean age between the normouricemic group and the hyperuricemic group for either men or women. Regardless of gender, the hyperuricemic group had significantly higher values for body mass index (BMI), waist circumference (WC), systolic blood pressure (SBP), total cholesterol (TG), fasting blood glucose FBG, Glycated hemoglobin (HbA_{1C}), uric acid (UA), creatine (Cr) and blood urea nitrogen (BUN), but they had lower high-density lipoprotein cholesterol (HDL-C) levels compared with the normouricemic group ($P<0.05$). The levels of Total cholesterol (TC) and low-density lipoprotein cholesterol (LDL-C) were significantly higher among women in the hyperuricemic group than in the normouricemic group, while the diastolic blood pressure (DBP) was significantly higher for men in the hyperuricemic group than in the normouricemic group.

Distribution of APOE genotypes and alleles among the study subjects

A total of 356 hyperuricemic cases and 414 normouricemic subjects were evaluated, and the frequencies of the APOE genotypes and alleles are shown in Table 2. The allele frequencies were within Hardy-Weinberg equilibrium ($P>0.05$). The frequencies of the ε2ε3 genotype and the ε2 allele in the hyperuricemic group were significantly higher than those in the normouricemic

Table 5. The effects of APOE genotypes on clinical and metabolic parameters.

	Normouricemic group			Hyperuricemic group			*P-value**	*P-value*#
	ε2/3(n = 43)	ε3/3(n = 304)	ε3/4(n = 60)	ε2/3(n = 63)	ε3/3(n = 230)	ε3/4(n = 52)		
Age (years)	22.6(15.0–44.2)	22.1(14.9–45.4)	19.7(13.0–43.7)	19.0(14.0–47.1)	21.0(15.7–51.4)	19.1(13.2–43.4)	0.916	0.225
BMI(kg/m^2)	22.4±3.86	22.3±4.31	22.0±4.21	24.5±5.12	24.1±4.68	24.2±4.44	0.879	0.898
WC(cm)	74.6±11.3	74.2±12.7	73.1±13.6	79.1±13.1	77.8±12.9	78.7±11.3	0.808	0.749
SBP	122.9±20.1	124.3±19.3	124.3±22.0	133.8±21.3	132.2±21.3	135.9±17.4	0.920	0.801
DBP	75.1±12.9	76.9±12.9	77.3±12.6	83.2±15.4	80.9±14.9	81.8±13.3	0.666	0.547
TC(mmol/L)	3.68±0.75[ab]	3.98±0.87	4.01±0.80	3.81±1.09[ab]	4.27±1.04	4.35±1.00	0.049	0.005
TG(mmol/L)	0.84(0.53–1.28)	0.99(0.62–1.51)	1.05(0.62–1.52)	1.35(0.88–2.68)	1.21(0.73–2.13)	1.53(0.97–2.58)[C]	0.327	0.054
HDL-C(mmol/L)	1.27±0.28	1.20±0.27	1.19±0.27	1.11±0.27	1.13±0.29	1.05±0.20	0.219	0.105
LDL-C(mmol/L)	1.89(1.45–2.38)[ab]	2.21(1.76–2.71)	2.18(1.87–2.57)	1.83(1.53–2.35)[ab]	2.45(2.01–3.06)	2.68(2.22–3.16)	0.005	<0.001
FBG(mmol/L)	4.85(4.59–5.22)	4.93(4.65–5.25)	4.92(4.60–5.22)	5.14(4.97–5.58)	5.12(4.89–5.49)	5.13(4.67–5.59)	0.536	0.349
HbA_{1C} (%)	5.10(5.00–5.30)	5.10(4.90–5.30)	5.10(4.80–5.40)	5.20(5.10–5.50)	5.20(5.00–5.50)	5.20(5.00–5.60)	0.932	0.922
UA(μmol/L)	283.7±57.3[a]	264.9±57.4	273.2±52.8	448.4±54.4[a]	432.4±52.1	437.2±52.4	0.039	0.024
Cr (mmol/L)	75.1±13.6	74.2±14.9	72.2±12.4	83.2±17.6	84.6±18.9	81.0±18.5	0.540	0.430
BUN (mmol/L)	4.25±1.31	4.32±1.22	4.18±1.31	4.52±1.44	4.87±1.44	4.61±1.36	0.741	0.168

Abbreviations: BMI, Body mass index; WC, Waist circumference; SBP, Systolic blood pressure; DBP, Diastolic blood pressure; TC, Total cholesterol; TG, Triglyceride; HDL-C, High density lipoprotein cholesterol; LDL-C, Low density lipoprotein cholesterol; FBG, Fasting blood glucose; HbA_{1C}, Glycated hemoglobin; UA, Uric acid; Cr, Creatinine; BUN, Blood urea nitrogen.

LSD and SNK test were applied to analyze the differences between each pair of groups.

[a]ε2/3 vs. ε3/3, $p<0.05$;

[b]ε2/3 vs. ε3/4, $p<0.05$;

[C]ε3/4 vs. ε3/3, $p<0.05$.

*Comparison of genotypes in Normouricemic group.

#Comparison of genotypes in Hyperuricemic group.

Table 6. Univariate analysis of the association between APOE polymorphism, metabolic parameters and hyperuricemia.

	OR (95%CI)	*P value*
Genotypes		
ε3ε3	1(Reference)	
ε2ε3	1.937(1.267–2.959)	0.002
ε3ε4	1.146(0.761–1.724)	0.515
Alleles		
ε3	1(Reference)	
ε2	1.932(1.323–2.821)	0.001
ε4	1.111(0.775–1.593)	0.567
Sex		
Female	1(Reference)	
Male	1.933(1.439–2.597)	<0.001
Age(years)	1.006(0.998–1.013)	0.129
BMI(kg/m^2)	1.097(1.061–1.133)	<0.001
WC(cm)	1.025(1.014–1.037)	<0.001
SBP	1.018(1.010–1.025)	<0.001
DBP	1.025(1.014–1.036)	<0.001
TC(mmol/L)	1.299(1.116–1.512)	0.001
TG(mmol/L)	1.534(1.325–1.776)	<0.001
HDL-C(mmol/L)	0.342(0.200–0.585)	<0.001
LDL-C(mmol/L)	1.419(1.167–1.726)	<0.001
FBG(mmol/L)	1.648(1.303–2.084)	<0.001
HbA_{1C} (%)	2.052(1.447–2.910)	<0.001
Cr(mmol/L)	1.040(1.029–1.050)	<0.001
BUN(mmol/L)	1.316(1.179–1.469)	<0.001

Abbreviations: BMI, Body mass index; WC, Waist circumference; SBP, Systolic blood pressure; DBP, Diastolic blood pressure; TC, Total cholesterol; TG, Triglyceride; HDL-C, High density lipoprotein cholesterol; LDL-C, Low density lipoprotein cholesterol; FBG, Fasting blood glucose; HbA_{1C}, Glycated hemoglobin; Cr, Creatinine; BUN, Blood urea nitrogen.

P-values and their ORs for the genotypes and clinical parameters were calculated by univariate logistic regression analysis.

group ($P = 0.003$ and $P = 0.001$, respectively). However, the distributions of the ε3ε3 genotype and the ε3 allele were significantly lower in the hyperuricemic individuals ($P = 0.008$ and $P = 0.007$, respectively).

Distribution of APOE genotypes and alleles based on gender and ethnicity

Table 3 and 4 present the APOE genotype and allele frequencies distributed by gender and ethnic group, respectively. The ε2ε3 genotype frequency in the hyperuricemic group was significantly higher than that in the normouricemic group for males ($P = 0.039$). Furthermore, the APOE ε2 allele frequency was significantly higher in the hyperuricemic group compared with the normouricemic group both in males ($P = 0.014$) and females ($P = 0.049$). In addition, the frequencies of the APOE-ε3ε3 genotype and the ε3 allele in the hyperuricemic group were significantly lower than those in the normouricemic group in males but not in females. Meanwhile, we observed that the prevalence of the APOE ε2 allele in males was higher than that in females in both the hyperuricemic (11.3% vs. 8.8%) and the normouricemic (6.7% vs. 4.8%) groups, although the difference was not statistically significant. Similar results were obtained from different ethnic groups (Table 4). The frequencies of the ε2ε3 genotype and the ε2 allele were significantly higher, but those of the ε3ε3 genotype and the ε3 allele were significantly lower in the hyperuricemic group compared with the normouricemic group in the Han population. Moreover, in the Hui population, a significant difference in the distribution of the ε2 allele between the control and hyperuricemic groups was identified.

Effect of APOE gene polymorphism on metabolic parameters and serum uric acid concentrations

We further analyzed the effects of the APOE genotypes on the clinical and metabolic parameters and serum uric acid levels in both the normouricemic group and hyperuricemic group. As shown in Table 5, the levels of TC, LCL-C and UA were significantly different among the APOE genotype groups in both the normouricemic group and hyperuricemic group. The ε2/3 group had significantly higher levels of serum uric acid compared with the ε3/3 group ($P<0.05$).

Table 6 presents the association between the presence of APOE gene polymorphism, clinical metabolic parameters and hyperuricemia. The results of univariate logistic regression revealed that carriers of the ε2ε3 genotype ($P = 0.002$, OR = 1.937, 95% CI 1.267–2.959) and ε2 allele ($P = 0.001$, OR = 1.932, 95% CI 1.323–2.821) were significantly more likely to present hyperuricemia when the ε3/ε3 genotypes was set as the reference group. Furthermore, sex, BMI, WC, SBP, DBP, TC, TG, HDL-C, LDL-C, BUN, Cr, FBG and HbA_{1C} were found significantly associated with hyperuricemia. Considering the high degree of correlation

Table 7. Multivariate analysis of the independent association between APOE polymorphism and hyperuricemia.

	OR (95%CI)	*P value*
Genotypes		
ε3ε3	1(Reference)	
ε2ε3	2.194(1.362–3.537)	0.001
ε3ε4	1.175(0.755–1.828)	0.475
Alleles		
ε3	1(Reference)	
ε2	2.099(1.379–3.195)	0.001
ε4	1.076(0.730–1.588)	0.710
Sex		
Female	1(Reference)	
Male	1.093(0.757–1.579)	0.635
BMI(kg/m^2)	0.988(0.940–1.037)	0.621
DBP	1.000(0.986–1.014)	0.957
TG(mmol/L)	1.227(1.034–1.455)	0.019
LDL-C(mmol/L)	1.149(0.891–1.481)	0.285
FBG(mmol/L)	1.378(1.060–1.792)	0.017
Cr(mmol/L)	1.033(1.018–1.047)	<0.001

Abbreviations: BMI, Body mass index; DBP, Diastolic blood pressure; TG, Triglyceride; LDL-C, Low density lipoprotein cholesterol; FBG, Fasting blood glucose; Cr, Creatinine.
P -values and adjusted ORs for the multivariate logistic regression analyses were adjusted for sex, BMI, DBP, TG, LDL-C, FBG and Cr.

between some variables (for example, SBP and DBP), in the next multivariate logistic regression model, only key factors sex, BMI, DBP, TG, LDL-C, Cr and FBG were included and adjusted as potential confounding variables. As shown in Table 7, the ε2ε3 genotype ($P = 0.001$, OR = 2.194, 95% CI 1.362–3.537) and ε2 allele ($P = 0.001$, OR = 2.099, 95% CI 1.379–3.195) were also significantly associated with hyperuricemia after adjusting for sex, BMI, DBP, TG, LDL-C, Cr and FBG.

Discussion

In the present study we observed that APOE gene polymorphism is associated with hyperuricemia in Chinese subjects. The frequencies of both the APOE-ε2ε3 genotype and ε2 allele were higher in the hyperuricemic group than in the normouricemic group (p<0.01), and individuals with the ε2ε3 genotype or ε2 allele had significantly higher SUA levels than ε3ε3 genotype or ε3 allele carriers. To the best of our knowledge, this is the first study to examine the possible associations between APOE polymorphism and hyperuricemia in China.

APOE gene polymorphism is known to be closely related to cardiovascular disease, hypertension, dyslipidemia, diabetes, and metabolic syndrome [28]. Hyperuricemia is an independent risk factor for coronary artery disease(CAD), hypertension, and obesity-related metabolic syndrome [29]. Therefore, it is reasonable to explore the connections between APOE gene polymorphism and hyperuricemia. Cardona et al. reported that the prevalence of the ε2 allele was greater in the patients with gout than in the healthy subjects and proposed that the reduced renal excretion of uric acid in patients with gout is mediated by the high prevalence of the ε2 allele of the APOE gene [19]. Another study in Caucasians also suggested that the APOE-ε2 allele is independently associated with increased SUA levels in healthy individuals [20]. In addition, according to various studies, the association between the ε4 allele and serum uric acid levels is controversial. Different studies have shown that APOE-ε4 allele carriers have lower [21,22] or higher [23] SUA levels compared with APOE-ε3 allele carriers.

In this Chinese population study, the frequencies of the ε2ε3 genotype and the ε2 allele in hyperuricemic individuals were significantly higher than those in normouricemic subjects, but no difference in the frequency of the ε4 allele was found between the two groups. We further analyzed the associations of gender and ethnicity with APOE polymorphism, and we found that the APOE ε2 allele frequency was also significantly higher in the hyperuricemic group compared with the normouricemic group, not only in males and females but also in the Han and Hui populations(Table 3 and Table 4). Interestingly, we observed that the prevalence of the APOE ε2 allele in males was higher than that in females in both the hyperuricemic (11.3% vs. 8.8%) and normouricemic (6.7% vs. 4.8%) groups (Table 3), which may be another reason besides differences in sex hormones for the reduced renal excretion of uric acid and the high incidence of hyperuricemia in males. Denzer et al. reported a significantly positive association between plasma testosterone and uric acid concentrations in obese children and adolescents [30]. In addition, animal studies have demonstrated gender differences in uric acid transporters and showed that male mice have a higher reabsorption of uric acid than female mice [31]. The higher APOE ε2 allele frequency in men and its possible impact requires further confirmation and clarification. The frequencies of the APOE alleles are highly variable among different ethnic populations; for example, the ε4 allele frequency is significantly higher in African-American than in Asians [32]. Therefore, in this study, we explored the difference in the frequencies of APOE gene polymorphisms between Han and Hui populations, but we did not find any significant difference between the two groups.

A logistic regression model demonstrated that the ε2ε3 genotype and the ε2 allele were significantly positively associated with hyperuricemia, and the association remained significant after adjustment for gender, BMI, DBP, TG, LDL-C, FBG and Cr. The ε2ε3 genotype or ε2 allele could be considered as independent risk factors of hyperuricemia. The underlying mechanisms for the increased risk of hyperuricemia in individuals with the ε2ε3 genotype or the ε2 allele are largely unknown, but they are most likely related to increased purine metabolism and uric acid production or decreased renal clearance of uric acid. The presence of the APOE-ε2 allele in patients with gout is associated with reduced renal excretion of urates [19]. In fact, in this study, the positive association between the ε2 allele and hyperuricemia persists after excluding the impact of serum creatinine (SCr), suggesting that the main reason is not reduced renal clearance of uric acid, but more likely increased production of uric acid. The presence of APOE gene polymorphism has been demonstrated to influence serum levels of C-reactive protein (CRP) [33]. Moreover, epidemiological studies have confirmed that children with high concentrations of CRP are more susceptible to hyperuricemia, and the serum uric acid concentration increased with rising CRP levels [34]. Whether the APOE-ε2 allele could stimulate uric acid production and the underlying mechanisms require further experimental exploration. In this study, we did not find that BMI and DBP were independently associated with hyperuricemia (Table 7), probably because of the special nature of the study population. Patients included in this study are patients with primary hyperuricemia, among whom hypertension, diabetes and other diseases have been ruled out. In addition, teenagers are the main body of the study population. Therefore, in this population, it is possible that ApoE genotype, but not BMI and DBP, is independently associated with hyperuricemia.

Dietary habits, the intensity of physical activity, drinking and smoking may also be associated with the serum uric acid level. However, we did not include these factors in the multivariable analysis, which is a limitation of our study. In addition, due to the small sample size for subjects with the ε2ε2, ε2ε4 and ε4ε4 genotypes, these genotypes were not included in the logistic regression analysis.

In conclusion, this study is the first to report that the APOE ε2 allele is positively associated with SUA and could be an independent risk factor for hyperuricemia in a Chinese population. Larger studies in the future will further clarify the correlation between APOE polymorphisms and uric acid metabolism.

Acknowledgments

We thank Dr. Li-quan Zhou for his kind assistance with the language editing. We are grateful to the participants, primary care doctors and nurses who took part in the survey.

Author Contributions

Conceived and designed the experiments: JW LQ GJZ. Performed the experiments: JW XZG LZ PCL QW LN. Analyzed the data: JW TX XQC QD. Contributed reagents/materials/analysis tools: JW LQ XZG TX GJZ. Contributed to the writing of the manuscript: JW LQ LZ TX.

References

1. Neogi T (2011) Clinical practice. Gout. N Engl J Med 364: 443–452.
2. Lin KC, Lin HY, Chou P (2000) The interaction between uric acid level and other risk factors on the development of gout among asymptomatic hyperuricemic men in a prospective study. J Rheumatol 27: 1501–1505.
3. Masuo K, Kawaguchi H, Mikami H, Ogihara T, Tuck ML (2003) Serum uric acid and plasma norepinephrine concentrations predict subsequent weight gain and blood pressure elevation. Hypertension 42: 474–480.
4. Sundstrom J, Sullivan L, D'Agostino RB, Levy D, Kannel WB, et al. (2005) Relations of serum uric acid to longitudinal blood pressure tracking and hypertension incidence. Hypertension 45: 28–33.
5. Borges RL, Ribeiro AB, Zanella MT, Batista MC (2010) Uric acid as a factor in the metabolic syndrome. Curr Hypertens Rep 12: 113–119.
6. Yoo TW, Sung KC, Shin HS, Kim BJ, Kim BS, et al. (2005) Relationship between serum uric acid concentration and insulin resistance and metabolic syndrome. Circ J 69: 928–933.
7. Gagliardi AC, Miname MH, Santos RD (2009) Uric acid: A marker of increased cardiovascular risk. Atherosclerosis 202: 11–17.
8. Johnson RJ, Kang DH, Feig D, Kivlighn S, Kanellis J, et al. (2003) Is there a pathogenetic role for uric acid in hypertension and cardiovascular and renal disease? Hypertension 41: 1183–1190.
9. Edwards NL (2009) The role of hyperuricemia in vascular disorders. Curr Opin Rheumatol 21: 132–137.
10. Qiu L, Cheng XQ, Wu J, Liu JT, Xu T, et al. (2013) Prevalence of hyperuricemia and its related risk factors in healthy adults from Northern and Northeastern Chinese provinces. BMC Public Health 13: 664.
11. B L, T W, Hn Z, Ww Y, Hp Y, et al. (2011) The prevalence of hyperuricemia in China: a meta-analysis. BMC Public Health 11: 832.
12. Rall SC, Jr., Weisgraber KH, Mahley RW (1982) Human apolipoprotein E. The complete amino acid sequence. J Biol Chem 257: 4171–4178.
13. Mahley RW, Rall SC, Jr. (2000) Apolipoprotein E: far more than a lipid transport protein. Annu Rev Genomics Hum Genet 1: 507–537.
14. Liberopoulos EN, Miltiadous GA, Cariolou M, Tselepis AD, Siamopoulos KC, et al. (2004) The influence of serum apolipoprotein E concentration and polymorphism on serum lipid parameters in hemodialysis patients. Am J Kidney Dis 44: 300–308.
15. Lea Correa Leite M, Lima-Costa MF, Moriguchi EH (2013) Age-related trends of blood pressure levels by apolipoprotein E genotype: the Bambui Cohort Study of Ageing (1997–2008). Hypertens Res 36: 270–276.
16. Yin YW, Qiao L, Sun QQ, Hu AM, Liu HL, et al. (2013) Influence of apolipoprotein E gene polymorphism on development of type 2 diabetes mellitus in Chinese Han population: A meta-analysis of 29 studies. Metabolism.
17. Crunkhorn S (2013) Neurodegenerative disorders: Linking apolipoprotein E to LOAD. Nat Rev Drug Discov 12: 664.
18. Song Y, Stampfer MJ, Liu S (2004) Meta-analysis: apolipoprotein E genotypes and risk for coronary heart disease. Ann Intern Med 141: 137–147.
19. Cardona F, Tinahones FJ, Collantes E, Escudero A, Garcia-Fuentes E, et al. (2003) The elevated prevalence of apolipoprotein E2 in patients with gout is associated with reduced renal excretion of urates. Rheumatology (Oxford) 42: 468–472.
20. Liberopoulos EN, Miltiadous GA, Athyros VG, Ganotakis M, Cariolou M, et al. (2005) Effect of apolipoprotein E polymorphism on serum uric acid levels in healthy subjects. J Investig Med 53: 116–122.
21. Fernandes MA, Proenca MT, Nogueira AJ, Grazina MM, Oliveira LM, et al. (1999) Influence of apolipoprotein E genotype on blood redox status of Alzheimer's disease patients. Int J Mol Med 4: 179–186.
22. Bazrgar M, Karimi M (2012) Is the apolipoprotein E4 allele always hazardous? Serum uric acid level as a conflict. Genet Test Mol Biomarkers 16: 920–923.
23. Alvim RO, Freitas SR, Ferreira NE, Santos PC, Cunha RS, et al. (2010) APOE polymorphism is associated with lipid profile, but not with arterial stiffness in the general population. Lipids Health Dis 9: 128.
24. Becker MA, Schumacher HR, Jr., Wortmann RL, MacDonald PA, Eustace D, et al. (2005) Febuxostat compared with allopurinol in patients with hyperuricemia and gout. N Engl J Med 353: 2450–2461.
25. Nagahama K, Inoue T, Iseki K, Touma T, Kinjo K, et al. (2004) Hyperuricemia as a predictor of hypertension in a screened cohort in Okinawa, Japan. Hypertens Res 27: 835–841.
26. Zhang W, Doherty M, Bardin T, Pascual E, Barskova V, et al. (2006) EULAR evidence based recommendations for gout. Part II: Management. Report of a task force of the EULAR Standing Committee for International Clinical Studies Including Therapeutics (ESCISIT). Ann Rheum Dis 65: 1312–1324.
27. Donohoe GG, Salomaki A, Lehtimaki T, Pulkki K, Kairisto V (1999) Rapid identification of apolipoprotein E genotypes by multiplex amplification refractory mutation system PCR and capillary gel electrophoresis. Clin Chem 45: 143–146.
28. Ang LS, Cruz RP, Hendel A, Granville DJ (2008) Apolipoprotein E, an important player in longevity and age-related diseases. Exp Gerontol 43: 615–622.
29. Soltani Z, Rasheed K, Kapusta DR, Reisin E (2013) Potential role of uric acid in metabolic syndrome, hypertension, kidney injury, and cardiovascular diseases: is it time for reappraisal? Curr Hypertens Rep 15: 175–181.
30. Denzer C, Muche R, Mayer H, Heinze E, Debatin KM, et al. (2003) Serum uric acid levels in obese children and adolescents: linkage to testosterone levels and pre-metabolic syndrome. J Pediatr Endocrinol Metab 16: 1225–1232.
31. Sekine T, Miyazaki H, Endou H (2006) Molecular physiology of renal organic anion transporters. Am J Physiol Renal Physiol 290: F251–261.

32. Liang S, Pan M, Geng HH, Chen H, Gu LQ, et al. (2009) Apolipoprotein E polymorphism in normal Han Chinese population: frequency and effect on lipid parameters. Mol Biol Rep 36: 1251–1256.
33. Austin MA, Zhang C, Humphries SE, Chandler WL, Talmud PJ, et al. (2004) Heritability of C-reactive protein and association with apolipoprotein E genotypes in Japanese Americans. Ann Hum Genet 68: 179–188.
34. Yoshida T, Kaneshi T, Shimabukuro T, Sunagawa M, Ohta T (2006) Serum C-reactive protein and its relation to cardiovascular risk factors and adipocytokines in Japanese children. J Clin Endocrinol Metab 91: 2133–2137.

6

Orp8 Deficiency in Bone Marrow-Derived Cells Reduces Atherosclerotic Lesion Progression in LDL Receptor Knockout Mice

Erik van Kampen[1]*, Olivier Beaslas[2], Reeni B. Hildebrand[1], Bart Lammers[1], Theo J. C. Van Berkel[1], Vesa M. Olkkonen[2], Miranda Van Eck[1]

1 Div. of Biopharmaceutics, Cluster of BioTherapeutics, Leiden Academic Centre for Drug Research, Leiden, The Netherlands, **2** Dept. of Lipid Signalling and Homeostasis, Minerva Foundation Institute for Medical Research, Helsinki, Finland

Abstract

Introduction: Oxysterol binding protein Related Proteins (ORPs) mediate intracellular lipid transport and homeostatic regulation. ORP8 downregulates ABCA1 expression in macrophages and cellular cholesterol efflux to apolipoprotein A-I. In line, ORP8 knockout mice display increased amounts of HDL cholesterol in blood. However, the role of macrophage ORP8 in atherosclerotic lesion development is unknown.

Methods and Results: LDL receptor knockout (KO) mice were transplanted with bone marrow (BM) from ORP8 KO mice and C57Bl/6 wild type mice. Subsequently, the animals were challenged with a high fat/high cholesterol Western-type diet to induce atherosclerosis. After 9 weeks of Western-Type diet feeding, serum levels of VLDL cholesterol were increased by 50% in ORP8 KO BM recipients compared to the wild-type recipients. However, no differences were observed in HDL cholesterol. Despite the increase in VLDL cholesterol, lesions in mice transplanted with ORP8 KO bone marrow were 20% smaller compared to WT transplanted controls. In addition, ORP8 KO transplanted mice displayed a modest increase in the percentage of macrophages in the lesion as compared to the wild-type transplanted group. ORP8 deficient macrophages displayed decreased production of pro-inflammatory factors IL-6 and TNFα, decreased expression of differentiation markers and showed a reduced capacity to form foam cells in the peritoneal cavity.

Conclusions: Deletion of ORP8 in bone marrow-derived cells, including macrophages, reduces lesion progression after 9 weeks of WTD challenge, despite increased amounts of circulating pro-atherogenic VLDL. Reduced macrophage foam cell formation and lower macrophage inflammatory potential are plausible mechanisms contributing to the observed reduction in atherosclerosis.

Editor: Olivier Kocher, Harvard Medical School, United States of America

Funding: This work was supported by The Netherlands Heart Foundation (Grant 2009B075 (EvK)), www.hartstichting.nl; The Netherlands Organization for Scientific Research (VICI Grant 91813603 (MVE)), www.nwo.nl/; the Sigrid Juselius Foundation, the Finnish Foundation for Cardiovascular Research, the Magnus Ehrnrooth Foundation, and the Academy of Finland (grant 121457 to VMO), www.sigridjuselius.fi/foundation, www.sydantutkimussaatio.fi, pro.tsv.fi/magnusehrnrooth, www.aka.fi. MVE is an Established Investigator of the Netherlands Heart Foundation (Grant 2007T056), www.hartstichting.nl. The funders had no role in study design, data collection and analysis, decision to publish, or preparation of the manuscript.

Competing Interests: The authors have declared that no competing interests exist.

* Email: e.van.kampen.3@lacdr.leidenuniv.nl

Introduction

ORPs are Oxysterol binding protein Related Proteins and comprise an evolutionary conserved family of 12 members. Although the family as a whole has a range of functions, a unifying theme is that ORPs can act as sterol sensors communicating with different signaling pathways [1]. Sterol signaling mediates several processes important to macrophage function in atherosclerosis, such as macrophage cholesterol efflux, pro-inflammatory signaling and the ability of macrophages to differentiate to functionally diverse subtypes [2,3,4]. Previous studies have demonstrated that altering the expression of ORPs in macrophages results in changes in cellular function and atherosclerosis susceptibility. Silencing of ORP1L reduced cholesterol efflux from macrophages, while overexpression of ORP1L led to increased atherosclerosis development in Low-Density Lipoprotein receptor knockout (LDLr KO) mice [5,6]. ORP3 overexpression inhibits phagocytosis by macrophages, and macrophage intracellular cholesterol transport is disrupted in cells deficient in ORP5 [7,8]. Furthermore, mutations in the ORP7 gene are associated with increased LDL and total cholesterol, risk factors for atherosclerosis [9]. Additionally, ORP8 is a potentially interesting target for atherosclerosis research.

In humans, mutations in the ORP8 gene are associated with changes in High-Density Lipoprotein (HDL) cholesterol levels in blood [10]. Furthermore, ORP8 is expressed by macrophages in human atherosclerotic lesions [11]. THP-1 macrophages in which ORP8 has been knocked down display an increased ability to efflux cholesterol to nascent HDL particles due to increased expression of ATP-Binding Cassette transporter A1 (ABCA1), which is essential for cholesterol transport to lipid-poor apoAI, the primary apolipoprotein of HDL [11]. Similarly, female ORP8 KO mice display a markedly increased expression of ABCA1 in the liver, as well as increased levels of HDL cholesterol and ApoAI particles in blood [12,13]. This indicates a role for ORP8 as a regulator of cellular cholesterol metabolism and efflux.

The aim of the current study is to investigate the effects of ORP8 deletion in macrophages on atherosclerotic lesion development. Hereto irradiated LDLr KO mice were transplanted with ORP8 KO bone marrow (BM) and fed a high fat/high cholesterol Western-Type Diet (WTD) for periods of 6 and 9 weeks. We show that mice receiving ORP8 KO BM developed smaller atherosclerotic plaques despite increased levels of pro-atherogenic lipoproteins and propose a possible mechanism for the observed decrease in atherosclerosis.

Materials and Methods

Perivascular Collar Placement

LDL receptor knockout (LDLr KO) mice were obtained from the Jackson Laboratory and bred at the Gorlaeus Laboratories in Leiden, the Netherlands.

To assess gene expression during atherosclerotic plaque development, mice were fed a high-fat/high-cholesterol Western-Type Diet (WTD), containing 15% cacao butter and 0.25% cholesterol (WTD; Special Diet Services) for 2, 4, 6, 8, 10 and 12 weeks. At two weeks a baseline group was sacrificed and atherosclerotic carotid artery lesions were induced by perivascular collar placement as described previously [14]. At the end of the WTD feeding period the mice were anaesthetized using a mix of rompun, ketamine and atropine at a lethal dose. Mice were then exsanguinated and perfused with PBS.

Animal experiments were approved by the Ethics Committee for Animal Experiments of Leiden University (permit number 08015) and performed at the Gorlaeus Laboratories of the Leiden Academic Center for Drug Research in accordance with the National Laws and the Directive 2010/63/EU of the European Parliament.

Bone Marrow-Derived Macrophage Generation and Culturing

Bone Marrow was isolated from ORP8 KO male mice (age 10 weeks). Bone marrow cells were plated in DMEM/20% FCS/1% penicillin/1% streptomycin and differentiated into macrophages by addition of 30% L929 cell-conditioned media (as a source of M-CSF) for 7 days according to Van Eck et al. [15] Macrophages were incubated for 24 h in cell culture plates (Greiner Bio-One) the absence or presence of 100 ng/mL LPS (Salmonella Typhosa, Sigma) or 20 ng/mL IL-4 (Sigma) and subsequently lysed for mRNA extraction or analyzed by FACS.

Flow Cytometry Analysis

BMDMs were stained using antibodies against CD40 and CD80 (eBioscience) and analyzed on a FACS Canto II (BD Biosciences, Mountain View, CA).

Cytokine Quantification

Concentrations of murine TNFα and IL-6 in the supernatant of BMDMs were assayed using an ELISA kit according to the manufacturer's protocol (BD Bioscience). Absorbance was detected at 450 nm.

mRNA Expression Analysis by Microarray and Real Time PCR

Carotid arteries with collar-induced plaques of female LDLr KO mice which were fed WTD for 2, 4, 6, 8, 10 and 12 weeks were isolated. Samples were digested with proteinase K and mechanically homogenized. Total RNA from samples was isolated using the guanidinium thiocyanate (GTC) method [16] and a microarray was performed by Service XS (Leiden, The Netherlands).

Furthermore, total RNA from Bone Marrow-Derived Macrophages (BMDMs) was isolated using the same GTC method and reverse transcribed using a RevertAid M-MuLV enzyme (Fermentas, Burlington, Canada). The mRNA expression levels were assessed by real time PCR (ABI PRISM 7500; Applied Biosystems, Foster City, CA) using SYBR Green technology (Applied Biosystems). The average of GAPDH and 36B4 or ß-actin expression was used as a housekeeping control.

Bone Marrow Transplantation

To study the effect of ORP8 deletion in hematopoietic cells, bone marrow (BM) of male ORP8 KO mice and WT controls (age 12 weeks) was obtained from the laboratory of Dr. Olkkonen (Minerva Foundation Institute for Medical Research, Helsinki, Finland) for transplantation to female LDLr KO mice (age 12 weeks) at the Leiden Academic Centre for Drug Research. In short, 5×10^6 bone marrow cells were injected into the tail vein of lethally irradiated recipients [15].

After 8 weeks recovery, recipient mice were fed WTD for 6 and for 9 weeks. At the end of the WTD feeding period the mice were anaesthetized using a mix of rompun, ketamine and atropine at a lethal dose, after which peritoneal cells were isolated by peritoneal lavage with PBS. Mice were then exsanguinated, perfused with PBS, and organs were harvested.

Serum cholesterol, triglycerides and cytokines

Serum concentrations of free cholesterol were determined by enzymatic colorimetric assays with 0.048 U/mL cholesterol oxidase (228250, Calbiochem) and 0.065 U/mL peroxidase (P8375, Sigma) in reaction buffer (1.0 KPi buffer, pH = 7.7 containing 0.01 M phenol, 1 mM 4-amino-antipyrine, 1% polyoxyethylene-9-laurylether, and 7.5% methanol). For the determination of total cholesterol, 0.03 U/mL cholesteryl esterase (228180, Calbiochem) was added to the reaction solution. Absorbance was read at 490 nm. Serum triglycerides were measured using a colorimetric assay (Roche Diagnostics, Mannheim Germany) according to the manufacturer's instructions. The distribution of cholesterol and triglycerides over the different lipoproteins in serum was determined by fractionation of 25 µL of serum of each mouse using a Superose 6 column (3.2×300 mm, Smart-System; Pharmacia, Uppsala, Sweden). Total cholesterol content of the effluent was determined as described above. Concentrations of murine TNFα and IL-6 in the plasma were assayed using an ELISA kit according to the manufacturer's protocol (BD Bioscience). Absorbance was detected at 450 nm.

Blood Cell Analysis

An automated Sysmex XT-2000iV Veterinary Haematology analyzer (Sysmex Corporation) was used to analyze leukocyte numbers and composition in blood and peritoneal leukocyte samples.

Macrophage cholesterol efflux studies

Bone marrow-derived macrophages were incubated with 0.5 μCi/mL ^{3}H-cholesterol in DMEM/0.2% free fatty acid free BSA for 24 hours at 37°C. To determine cholesterol loading, cells were washed three times with washing buffer (50 mmol/L Tris, containing 0.9% NaCl, 1 mmol/L EDTA, 5 mmol/L $CaCl_2$, pH 7.4), lysed in 0.1 mol/L NaOH, and the radioactivity was determined by liquid scintillation counting. Cholesterol efflux was studied by incubating the cells with DMEM/0.2% BSA alone, or with DMEM/0.2% BSA supplemented with either 10 μg/mL apolipoprotein AI (Calbiochem) or 50 μg/mL human HDL (isolated according to Redgrave, as described previously [17]). Radioactivity in the medium was determined by scintillation counting after 24 hours of incubation. Cholesterol efflux was defined as $(dpm_{medium}/dpm_{cell}+dpm_{medium})\times 100\%$.

Histological Analysis of the Aortic Root

Serial sections (7 μm) of the aortic root were cut using a Leica CM3050S cryostat and stained for lipids using oil red-O. The atherosclerotic lesion areas in oil red-O stained cryostat sections of the aortic root were quantified using the Leica image analysis system, consisting of a Leica DMRE microscope coupled to a video camera and Leica Qwin Imaging software (Leica Ltd, Cambridge, UK). Mean lesion area (in μm^2) was calculated from 10 consecutive oil red-O stained sections, starting at the appearance of the tricuspid valves. For the assessment of the macrophage area, sections were immunolabeled with MOMA-2 (Research Diagnostics Inc; dilution 1:50). The MOMA-2-positive lesion area was subsequently quantified using the Leica image analysis system and expressed as a fraction of total lesion area. Apoptosis in the plaque was visualized using an *In-Situ* Cell Death Detection Kit (POD) (11 684 817 910, Roche) as per manufacturer's instructions. The tissue was counter stained using 0.3% Methyl Green for 2 minutes. Methyl Green positive nuclei and TUNEL positive nuclei in the plaque were counted and the fraction of TUNEL positive nuclei of total Methyl Green positive nuclei was calculated. Furthermore, presence of CD3$^+$ T cells in aortic root sections was visualized using an anti-CD3 antibody (RM-9107, Thermo Scientific; dilution 1:150). Leica Qwin software was used to quantify adventitia size in the stained sections. CD3$^+$ T cells were quantified and normalized for adventitia size. A Masson Trichrome kit consisting of Biebrich Scarlet Acid Fuchsin, Phosphotungstic Acid, Phosphomolybdic Acid and Aniline Blue was used according to manufacturer's instructions (Procedure HT15) to visualize plaque collagen.

Statistical Analysis

Statistically significant differences were tested with the appropriate tests as indicated using Graphpad Prism software. The probability level (alpha) for statistical significance was set at 0.05. Results are expressed as an average ± SEM.

Results

Expression of ORP8 is detectable in the atherosclerotic plaque and correlates with expression of macrophage marker CD68

Atherosclerotic plaques were induced in the carotid artery of LDLr KO mice by surgically placing a collar around the carotid artery and subjecting the animals to an atherogenic Western-Type Diet (WTD) for up to 12 weeks. Animals were sacrificed every two weeks starting at two weeks after collar placement. RNA was isolated from the carotid arteries with atherosclerotic lesions and analyzed by microarray. RNA expression of ORP8 was increased during atherosclerosis progression up to 66% after 12 weeks of WTD feeding ($P<0.05$, figure 1A). Expression of CD68, indicative of macrophage infiltration, in the collar-induced plaques followed a strikingly similar pattern to the expression pattern of ORP8. At 12 weeks of WTD feeding expression of CD68 was increased 17-fold ($P<0.01$, figure 1A). Relative expression of ORP8 and CD68 were plotted against each other, and linear regression analysis showed a correlation between ORP8 and CD68 expression in the atherosclerotic carotid arteries, indicating that ORP8 is primarily expressed by macrophages in the murine lesions ($P<0.001$, figure 1B).

Decreased expression of macrophage differentiation markers, pro-inflammatory cytokines and co-stimulatory molecules by ORP8 KO BMDMs

Next, the effects of ORP8 deficiency on macrophage gene expression were investigated. Macrophages are capable of

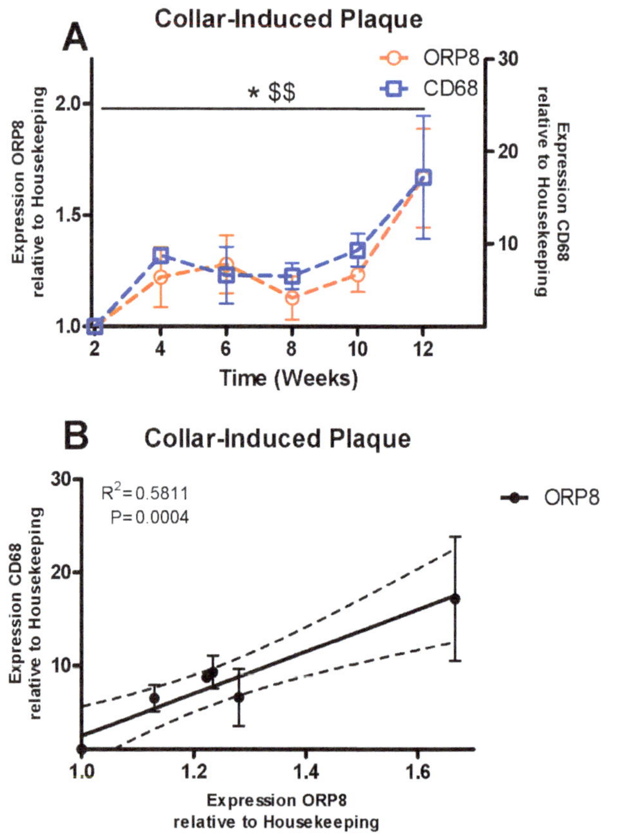

Figure 1. ORP8 expression detected in murine atherosclerotic plaques correlates with expression of CD68. mRNA was isolated from collar-induced plaques located in the carotid artery of LDLr KO mice. Samples were taken at 2 week intervals from week 2 baseline until week 12. Expression of ORP8 and the monocyte/macrophage marker CD68 was measured at each timepoint by microarray analysis and normalized for expression at baseline. A) ORP8 was found to be upregulated during plaque progression, as was CD68 (* $P<0.05$; $$< 0.01, respectively). N = 3, values are expressed as mean ± SEM. Significance was assessed by ANOVA with Dunnetts post-test. B) Expression of ORP8 in murine atherosclerotic plaques correlated with expression of CD68 ($P<0.001$). Significance was assessed by linear regression.

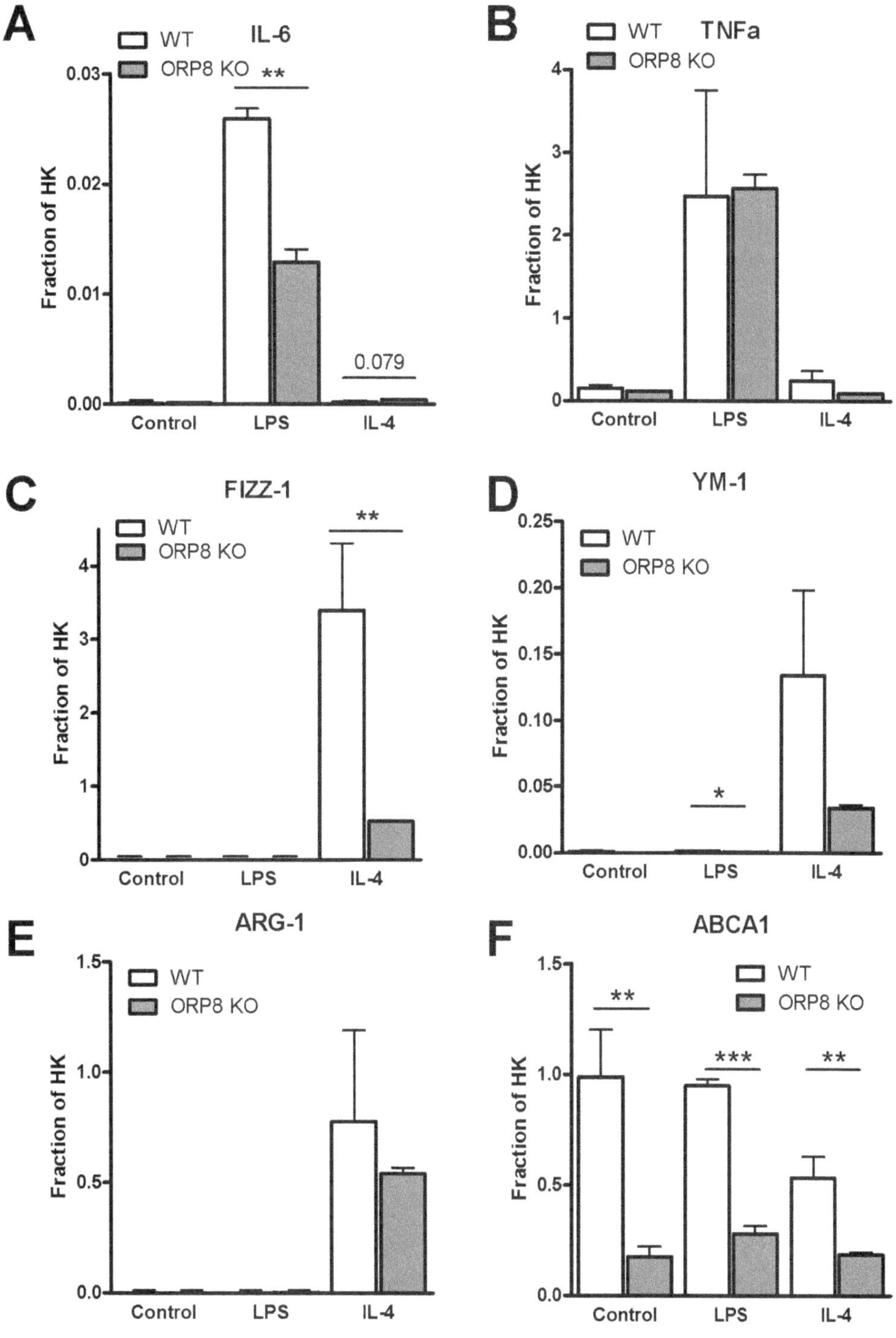

Figure 2. ORP8 KO BMDMs display reduced expression of macrophage differentiation factors and excrete less of pro-inflammatory cytokines. Bone Marrow-Derived Macrophages (BMDM) were generated from bone marrow of ORP8 KO mice or WT controls and incubated with LPS (100 ng/mL), IL-4 (20 ng/ml) or PBS. Expression of macrophage differentiation markers was measured by QPCR and calculated as relative to housekeeping (HK) for the M1 markers IL-6 (A) and TNFα (B), the M2 markers FIZZ-1 (C), YM-1 (D), Arg1 (E), and ABCA1 (F) (N = 3). Significance was determined by Student T-test, data are expressed as mean ±SEM. Statistical significant difference * $P<0.05$, ** $P<0.01$, *** $P<0.001$ as compared to controls.

differentiating into a range of subtypes which vary widely in inflammatory potential and wound healing ability, the extreme ends of the subtype distribution being the pro-inflammatory M1 and the anti-inflammatory M2 macrophages [18,19,20]. BMDMs were cultured from bone marrow of male ORP8 KO mice and stimulated with LPS, IL-4 or left unstimulated to generate M1, M2 or naïve macrophages, respectively. At 24 hours after stimulation RNA was isolated and expression of macrophage differentiation markers was measured. As anticipated, stimulation with LPS induced the expression of the M1 markers IL-6 and TNFα, while

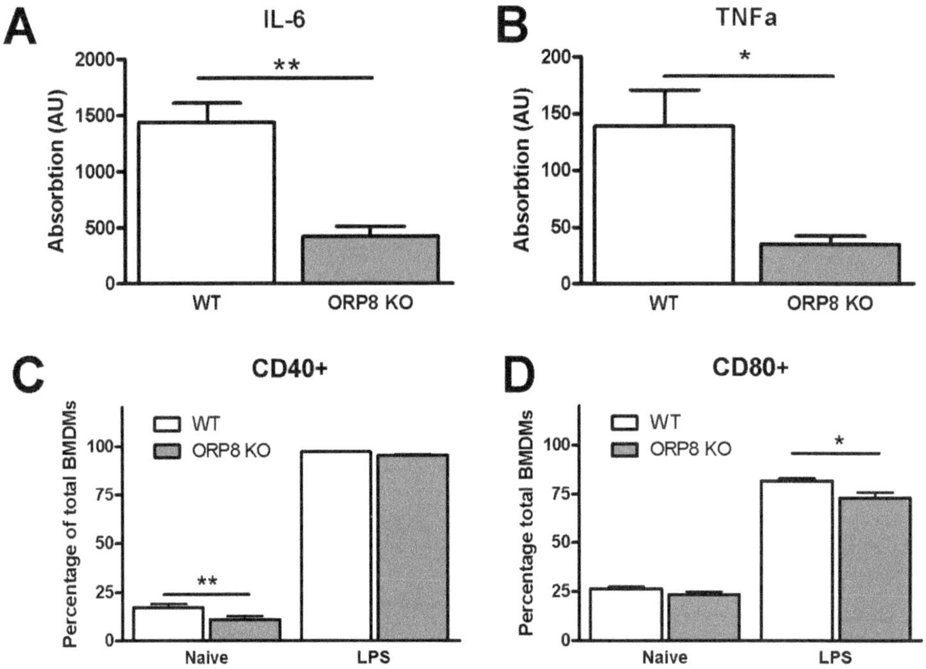

Figure 3. ORP8 KO BMDMs have reduced excretion of pro-inflammatory cytokines and reduced expression of co-stimulatory factors. Bone Marrow-Derived Macrophages (BMDMs) were generated from bone marrow of ORP8 KO mice or WT controls and stimulated with LPS (100 ng/mL). A) A decrease in secretion of IL-6 by LPS stimulated ORP8 KO BMDMs was measured using ELISA. (** $P<0.01$, N = 4) B) Similarly, TNFα secretion was also decreased in LPS-stimulated ORP8 KO BMDMs. (* $P<0.05$, N = 4). Expression of co-stimulatory factors CD40 and CD80 on BMDMs from ORP8 BM and WT BM was measured using FACS C) The percentage of unstimulated BMDMs expressing CD40 was decreased in the ORP8 KO group. (** $P<0.01$, N = 5) D) After stimulation with LPS, the percentage of BMDMs expressing CD80 was decreased in the ORP8 KO group (* $P<0.05$, N = 5). Significance of ELISA results was determined by Student T-test. Significance of FACS results was assessed by two-way ANOVA with Bonferroni post-tests. Data are expressed as mean ± SEM.

IL-4 stimulation led to augmented expression of the M2 markers FIZZ-1, YM-1, and Arginase 1 (Arg1) (figure 2A–E). In LPS-stimulated ORP8 KO BMDMs, a significant 2-fold decrease in expression of the M1 marker IL-6 was found ($P<0.01$, figure 2A), while no differences in expression of TNFα could be found (figure 2B). Expression of the M2 marker FIZZ-1 was decreased 6-fold in IL-4 stimulated ORP8 KO BMDMs ($P<0.01$, figure 2C). There was also a trend towards a decrease in expression of YM-1 in ORP8 KO BMDMs in all treatment groups. However, this only reached significance in the LPS-stimulated cells ($P<0.05$, figure 2D), but expression of YM-1 under these conditions is extremely low. No significant difference was found in the expression of Arg1 (figure 2E). Expression of ABCA1 was measured, as ORP8 has previously been shown to regulate expression of ABCA1 [11]. There was a strong decrease in expression of ABCA1 in naïve macrophages and macrophages stimulated with LPS and IL-4 (5-fold $P<0.01$, 3.4-fold $P<0.001$ and 2.9-fold $P<0.01$, respectively, figure 2F).

In addition to mRNA expression analysis, cytokine concentrations in supernatant of LPS stimulated BMDMs were measured by ELISA, showing decreased production of the pro-inflammatory cytokines IL-6 (3.5-fold, $P<0.01$) and TNFα (4-fold, $P<0.05$) by the ORP8 KO cells (figure 3A–B). Furthermore, the percentage of unstimulated BMDMs expressing CD40 was decreased in the ORP8 deficient group (0.6-fold, $P<0.01$), while there was also a small, but significant decrease (0.9-fold, $P<0.05$) in the amount of CD80 expressing ORP8 KO BMDMs after stimulation with LPS, compared to WT BMDMs (figure 3C–D).

Increased Cholesterol and Triglycerides in the VLDL fraction of blood from ORP8 KO BM recipient mice

To study the effect of macrophage ORP8 deletion on atherosclerosis, bone marrow from ORP8 KO mice and WT mice was transplanted into recipient LDLr KO animals. The recipients were then fed a chow diet for 8 weeks and consecutively WTD for a maximum of 9 weeks. No difference in body weight was observed between the groups throughout the experiment. At the end of both periods of dietary feeding blood was taken for lipid analysis (table 1). Although there was a small increase in free cholesterol in ORP8 KO BM recipients on chow diet at 18 weeks after transplantation, no difference between the groups was found after 6 and 9 weeks of WTD feeding. However, at 9 weeks of WTD feeding a 1.4-fold increase in plasma triglycerides was found in the ORP8 KO BM recipient mice ($P<0.05$, table 1). Serum from animals after 9 weeks of WTD feeding was fractionated by FPLC and analyzed for cholesterol and triglyceride content. VLDL cholesterol was increased 1.2-fold in the ORP8 KO BM recipients ($P<0.05$, figure 4A). While there was also a 1.2-fold increase in total cholesterol, this failed to reach statistical significance. Additionally, a 1.6-fold increase in VLDL triglycerides was found ($P<0.05$, figure 4B). Following the observation that IL-6 and TNFα secretion were decreased in ORP8 KO BMDMs, IL6 and TNFα were measured in blood samples of the BM recipients. However, the concentration of these cytokines was below the threshold of detection (data not shown).

Table 1. After 6 and 9 weeks of WTD feeding no difference in blood cholesterol levels was found between LDLr KO mice receiving ORP8 KO BM or WT BM.

	0 weeks		6 weeks		9 weeks	
	WT BM	ORP8 KO BM	WT BM	ORP8 KO BM	WT BM	ORP8 KO BM
Body Weight (gr)	25.7 (±0.4)	26.8 (±1.0)	29.3 (±1.3)	27.2 (±0.7)	27.1 (±0.9)	27.2 (±0.6)
Triglycerides (μg/ml)	-	-	-	-	1263 (±95)	1794 (±166)*
Free Cholesterol (μg/ml)	678 (±20)	745 (±19)	3966 (±259)	4151 (±203)	3665 (±194)	3749 (±229)
Esterified Cholesterol (μg/ml)	4467 (±175)	4468 (±138)	9336 (±1003)	11577 (±1552)	12901 (±759)	14185 (±1129)
Total Cholesterol (μg/ml)	5148 (±189)	5213 (±139)	13302 (±1273)	15727 (±1723)	16566 (±939)	17934 (±1351)

Body weight was measured during the chow feeding and the WTD feeding period, but no difference between the groups was found. At the end of the 9 weeks WTD feeding period ORP8 KO BM recipients had increased blood triglycerides (TG) (N = 15, *P<0.05). Furthermore, free cholesterol (FC), cholesteryl esters (CE) and total cholesterol (TC) were measured in WT BM and ORP8 KO BM recipients on chow diet and after 6 and 9 weeks on WTD. A small increase in FC was observed in the ORP8 KO BM recipients on chow diet, but no differences could be found after WTD feeding (N = 11, * P<0.05, significance was assessed by Student T-test with Welsh correction if required). Results are expressed as mean ± SEM.

No change in circulating leukocytes, but increased amounts of foam cells in the peritoneal cavity

After 9 weeks of WTD feeding, blood samples and peritoneal lavage from LDLr KO mice transplanted with ORP8 KO BM or WT BM were analyzed for leukocyte content. The number of circulating leukocytes was not changed between the WT BM recipients and the ORP8 KO BM recipients (figure 5A). Furthermore, there was no detectable difference in leukocyte composition, as the proportion of lymphocytes, monocytes and neutrophils in blood were all unchanged (figure 5B–D).

Similarly, no difference in the total amount of leukocytes and the proportion of lymphocytes and neutrophils was found in the peritoneal cavity (figure 6A–C). However, there was a significant 35% increase in the proportion of peritoneal monocytes, but not macrophages (P<0.05, figure 6D).

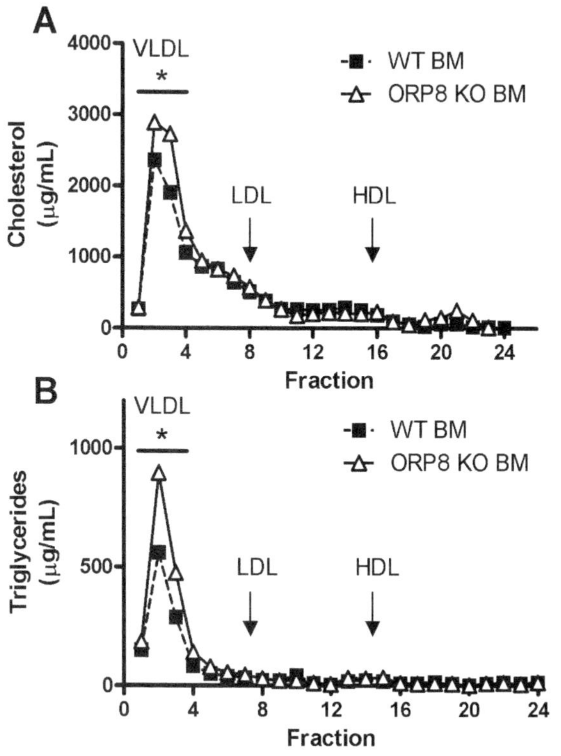

Figure 4. Increased VLDL cholesterol and triglycerides in LDLr KO mice receiving ORP8 KO bone marrow. Blood was isolated from LDLr KO mice after transplantation with ORP8 KO bone marrow (BM) or Wild Type (WT) BM. Lipoproteins were fractioned by size using FPLC and cholesterol and triglyceride contents were measured in each fraction. A) 17 weeks after transplantation and after 9 weeks of WTD feeding ORP8 KO BM recipients exhibit increased VLDL cholesterol (* P<0.05) B) Similarly, an increase in triglycerides in the VLDL fraction in blood of ORP8 KO BM recipients on WTD was found (* P<0.05). Significance was determined by Student t-test. N = 7, data are expressed as mean ±SEM.

Decreased foam cell formation in the presence of reduced ABCA1 expression in peritoneal cells of ORP8 KO BM recipients, but unaffected macrophage cholesterol efflux

Interestingly, although no difference in the amount of peritoneal macrophages was found, the amount of foam cells in the peritoneal cavity was strongly decreased (2.5-fold P<0.05, figure 7A). Additionally, in line with the reduced expression of ABCA1 in ORP8 KO BMDMs (figure 2F), ABCA1 expression in *ex-vivo* peritoneal leukocytes from ORP8 KO BM recipients was reduced 8-fold (P<0.01, figure 7B). However, no difference in cholesterol efflux from ^{3}H-cholesterol labeled BMDMs to ApoA1 or to HDL was observed (figure 7C), indicating that the level of ABCA1 expression remained sufficiently high to maintain proper macrophage cholesterol efflux.

Reduced atherosclerotic plaque size after 9 weeks Western-type diet challenge, together with increased macrophage area in plaques of ORP8 KO BM recipients

Despite the observed increased VLDL cholesterol and triglycerides in the blood of the ORP8 KO BM recipients, Oil Red-O staining of atherosclerotic plaques revealed a 20% reduction in plaque size after 9 weeks of WTD feeding (P<0.05, figure 8A, F). No significant difference in plaque size was found after 6 weeks of WTD feeding, indicating that macrophage ORP8 deficiency did not significantly affect development of early atherosclerotic plaques of less than 200.000 μm^{2}. Further morphological analysis by MOMA-2 staining of atherosclerotic plaques after 9 weeks of WTD challenge revealed that a 20% larger fraction of the plaques in the ORP8 KO BM recipients was made up of macrophages (P<0.05, figure 8B, F). Sections were stained with a Masson's

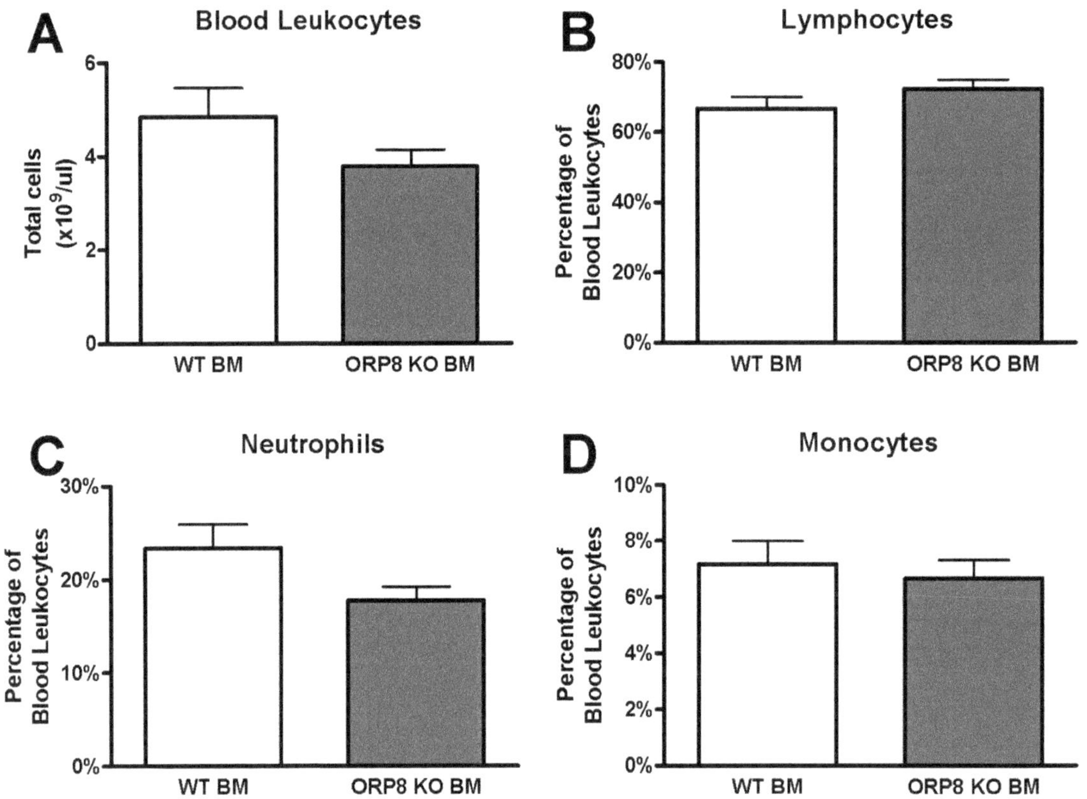

Figure 5. No effect on blood leukocyte counts in LDLr KO mice receiving ORP8 KO bone marrow. At 17 weeks after transplantation and after 9 weeks of WTD feeding, blood was isolated from bone marrow recipient animals. Blood leukocytes were counted using a hematology analyzer, and different subpopulations were quantified as percentage of total leukocytes. A) No difference between the ORP8 KO BM recipients and the wildtype (WT) BM recipients in the amount of circulating leukocytes. B–D) Similarly, there was no difference in the percentage of lymphocytes, neutrophils and monocytes of total leukocytes. N = 15, results are expressed as mean ±SEM and significance was assessed by Student T-test.

Trichrome kit to visualize collagen deposition in the plaques. However, no difference was found (figure 8C, F). Moreover, TUNEL staining revealed no difference in the amount of apoptotic cells in the plaque, indicating that deficiency of ORP8 in macrophages did not result in differences in cell death by apoptosis. (figure 8D, F). *In vitro* studies using BMDMs indicated decreased inflammatory potential of macrophages lacking ORP8, as evidenced by a reduced secretion of cytokines IL-6 and TNFα (figure 2G–H). Therefore also a CD3 staining was carried out to quantify the T cells in the adventitia underlying the atherosclerotic plaque, but no difference was found between the groups (figure 8E, F).

Discussion

In the current study we showed that ORP8 expression is increased during atherosclerotic lesion development, a process which coincides with macrophage infiltration. This corresponds with the finding that ORP8 is present in human atherosclerotic plaques as opposed to healthy arteries, and is produced there by macrophages [21]. To investigate the role of macrophage ORP8 in atherosclerotic lesion development we transplanted ORP8 knockout (KO) bone marrow into atherosclerosis susceptible LDLr KO mice. Deletion of ORP8 in bone marrow-derived cells resulted in increased levels of VLDL cholesterol and triglycerides in the blood, but also a decrease in atherosclerotic plaque size.

ORP8 KO animals on a C57Bl/6 background exhibit increased levels of HDL cholesterol in the blood, and increased ApoAI production by hepatocytes [13]. Upon transplantation of ORP8 KO bone marrow into LDLr KO mice, we did not find any differences in HDL cholesterol in the blood of the BM recipients. This is not surprising, as the contribution of macrophages to HDL formation is minor [22]. It is thus likely that the HDL phenotype observed previously in the total body ORP8 KO animals is primarily hepatocyte driven. In contrast, we did observe a marked increase in VLDL cholesterol and triglycerides in ORP8 KO BM recipient mice on WTD. Interestingly, also in total body ORP8 KO mice a strong tendency towards an increase in blood triglycerides was observed, which in the female mice could be ascribed to an increase in the VLDL fraction [13]. This change was attributed to reduced lipoprotein lipase activity and possible changes in SREBP signaling [13,23]. Hence, it is tempting to speculate that the increase in VLDL triglycerides in the total body ORP8 KO mice is the consequence of alterations induced by deletion on ORP8 in bone marrow cells. Indeed, ORP8 mRNA expression in liver samples of ORP8 KO BM recipients was decreased. No differences in liver CD68 mRNA or Kupffer cell numbers were observed, suggesting that ORP8 deletion likely resulted in altered macrophage function but not viability (figure S1). Whether the increased VLDL cholesterol and triglycerides in our model, as opposed to the increase in HDL cholesterol described previously is a consequence of the more pro-atherogenic phenotype of the LDLr KO recipient mice requires further study.

VLDL cholesterol is a strong inducer of atherosclerosis development, which makes the decrease in plaque development after 9 weeks of WTD feeding in our model a striking finding [24].

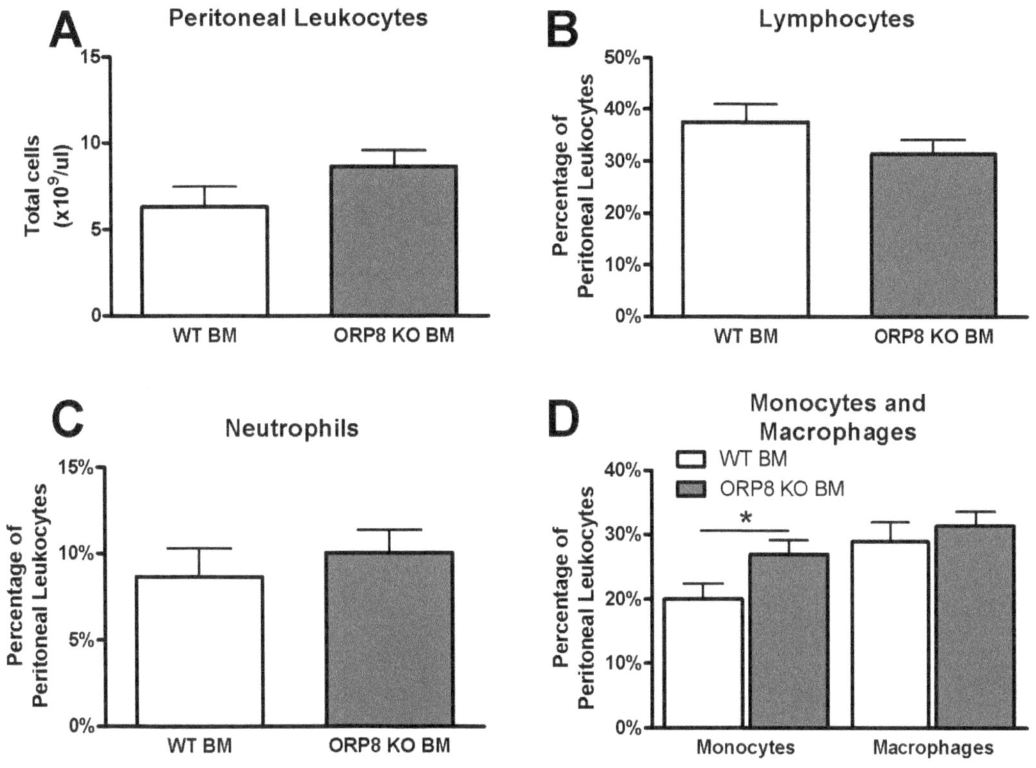

Figure 6. Increase in peritoneal monocytes in LDLr KO mice receiving ORP8 KO BM, but decrease in peritoneal foam cells. Peritoneal leukocytes were isolated from ORP8 KO BM recipients and wild type BM recipients and counted using a hematology analyzer at 17 weeks after BMT and 9 weeks WTD feeding. A) No difference between treatment groups was found in the total number of peritoneal leukocytes. B) The amount of peritoneal lymphocytes did not differ between the groups. C) Similarly, there was no difference between the groups in the amount of neutrophils in the peritoneum. D) However, there was an increase in the percentage of peritoneal monocytes out of total leukocytes in the ORP8 KO BM recipients, but no difference in macrophage content (* $P<0.05$). N = 15, significance was assessed by Student T-test. Results are expressed as mean ±SEM.

In line with the decreased atherosclerosis, we also found reduced foam cell formation in the peritoneal cavity of ORP8 KO BM recipients. Macrophage foam cell formation is determined by a disruption of the balance of cholesterol synthesis, cholesterol influx and cholesterol efflux. Considering the observed increased levels of VLDL cholesterol, it is unlikely that the decreased foam cell formation is due to decreased influx. Moreover, the reduced foam cell formation could not be explained by enhanced cholesterol efflux as *ex vivo* cholesterol efflux experiments failed to show significant differences. Notably ABCA1 mRNA expression was reduced both *ex vivo* in peritoneal macrophages and *in vitro* in bone marrow-derived macrophages.

Previous publications have reported an increase in ABCA1 expression when expression of ORP8 was ablated, both in THP-1 cells and in female mouse liver samples [11,13]. In THP-1 cells, the increase in ABCA1 expression after siRNA mediated silencing

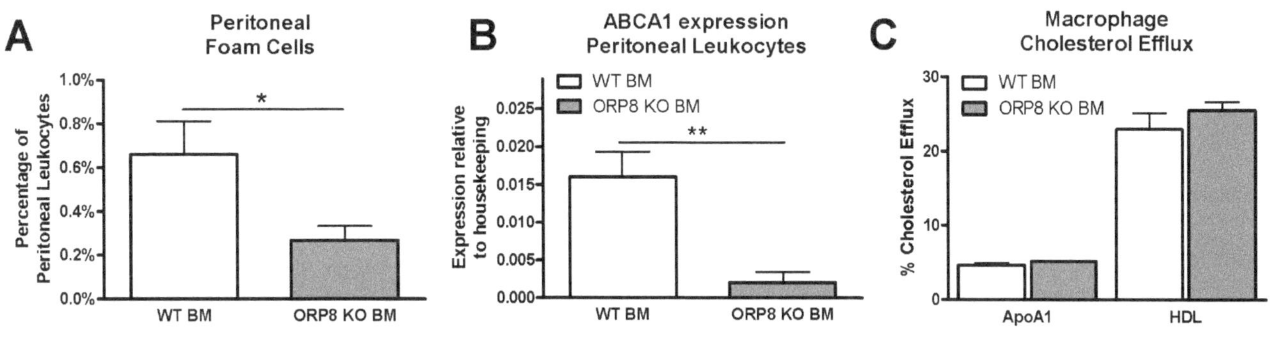

Figure 7. Reduced peritoneal foam cell formation and lower expression of ABCA1 in ORP8 KO macrophages, but no change in cellular cholesterol efflux. Expression of ABCA1 was measured by QPCR in Peritoneal Leukocytes isolated from LDLr KO mice at 17 weeks after transplantation with WT BM or ORP8 KO BM and 9 weeks WTD feeding. A) The ORP8 KO transplanted group displays a reduced amount of foam cells when expressed as a percentage of total peritoneal leukocytes. B) In line, expression of ABCA1 in peritoneal leukocytes of ORP8 KO BM recipients is reduced. (** $P<0.01$, N = 4) C) However, no change in cholesterol efflux of BMDMs to ApoA1 or HDL was found (N = 5). Results are expressed as mean ± SEM after subtraction of baseline efflux to BSA. Significance was determined by Student t-test.

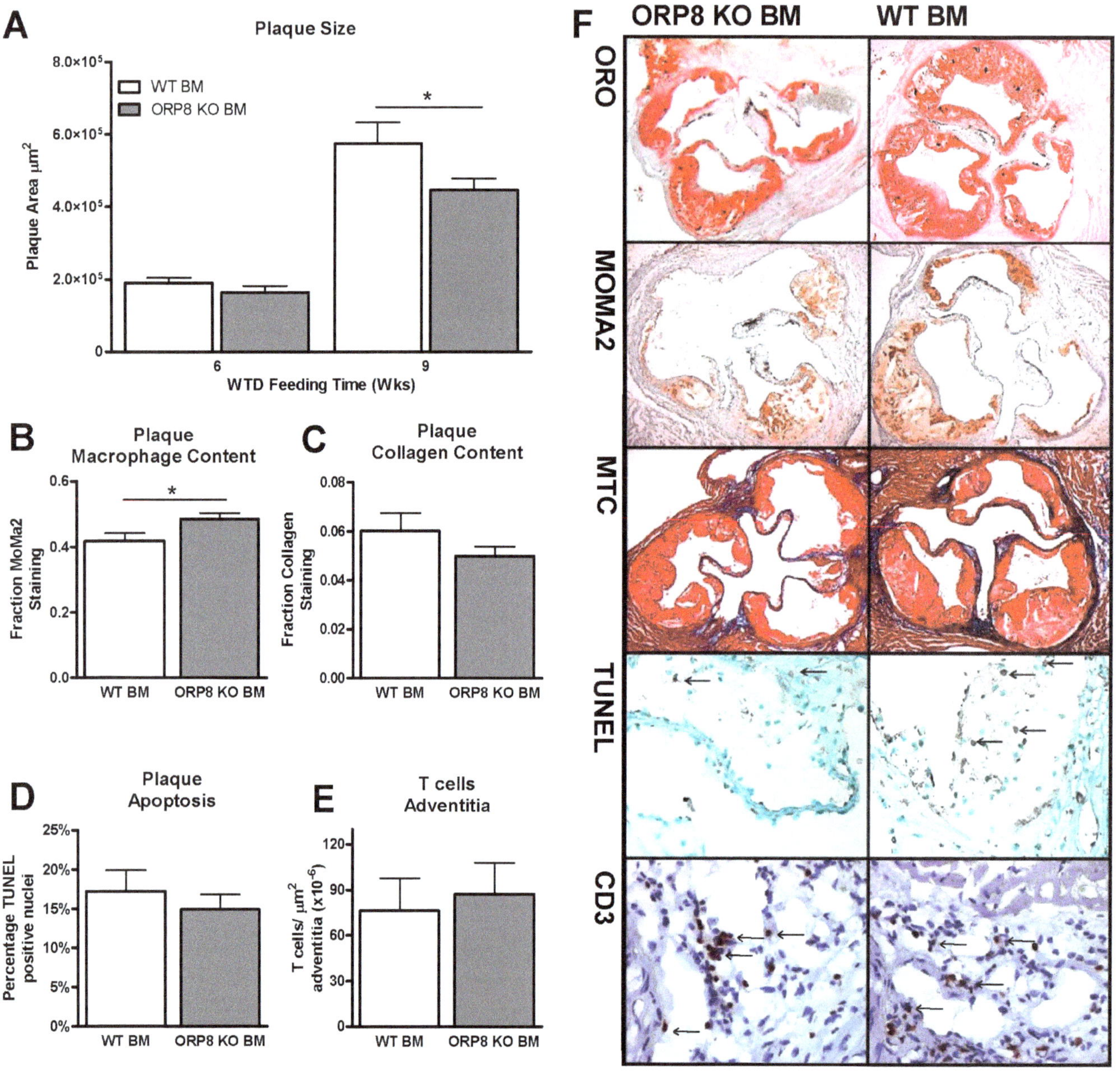

Figure 8. Decreased plaque size in ORP8 KO BM recipients and increased plaque macrophage content after 9 weeks WTD feeding. A) Plaque size was quantified in Oil Red O stained sections. After 9 weeks of WTD feeding following BMT, a decrease in plaque size could be measured. No difference was observed after 6 weeks of dietary challenge. (N = 13 * P<0.05, data was analyzed by two-way ANOVA with Bonferroni post-tests) B) Plaque macrophages were visualized using MoMa2 staining and quantified as a percentage of total plaque area. After 9 weeks of WTD feeding, an increase in the MoMa2 positive fraction was detected in the ORP8 KO BM recipients. (N = 13 * P<0.05, data was analyzed by two-way ANOVA with Bonferroni post-tests) C) Collagen was visualized by staining plaques from ORP8 BM and WT BM recipients with a Masson's Trichrome (MTC) kit, but no difference was found between the groups (N = 15, significance was assessed by Student T test). D) Apoptotic cells in atherosclerotic plaques of ORP8 KO BM recipients and WT BM controls were visualized by TUNEL staining. No difference in the amount of apoptotic cells was detected between treatment groups (N = 8, significance was assessed by Student T test). E) Aortic root sections from ORP8 KO BM recipients and WT BM controls were stained for CD3 to detect T cells. No difference between the groups was detected (N = 8, significance was assessed by Student T test). F) Representative images of Oil-Red O (ORO), MoMa2, TUNEL, CD3 and MTC stainings performed on atherosclerotic plaques of mice receiving ORP8 KO BM or WT BM. Images of ORO, Moma2 and MTC stainings, original magnification 5×. Images of TUNEL and CD3 stainings, original magnification 20×.

of ORP8 was accompanied with increased cholesterol efflux to apoA-I [11]. In livers of female ORP8 KO mice expression of ABCA1 was also strongly increased, but this did not translate into a difference in protein expression. In contrast, in male ORP8 KO mice hepatic expression of ABCA1 showed a trend towards a decrease in expression on both RNA and on protein levels. In line, in our study the bone marrow donors were male and we observed a decrease in ABCA1 expression both in peritoneal leukocytes and in BMDMs. Lentiviral silencing of ORP8 in RAW 264.7 cells results in a modest increase in SREBP1 and SREBP2 expression, and ORP8 silencing in HuH7 cells leads to increased expression of SREBP target genes, including HMG-CoA reductase and LDLr

[23,25]. ORP8 likely affects ABCA1 expression by interfering with LXR signaling and SREBP activity [21,23,24]. The reduction in ABCA1 expression did not translate into differences in macrophage cholesterol efflux. ABCA1 mRNA expression is not always an accurate reflection for ABCA1 protein abundance, and previous studies on ORP8 KO liver have demonstrated changes in ABCA1 mRNA expression without corresponding changes in protein levels [13,21]. Alternatively, the level of ABCA1 expression was still sufficient for maintaining a proper cholesterol efflux capacity under the studied conditions. In the current study the reduction in ABCA1 expression could also simply be a result of the observed reduction in lipid loading in the peritoneal cells. Previous studies in male ORP8 KO mice showed decreased expression of HMG-CoA reductase [13]. The down-regulation of HMG-CoA reductase, which is the rate limiting enzyme for cholesterol production, could result in reduced cholesterol loading. This might explain that ORP8 deletion resulted in reduced *in vivo* macrophage foam cell formation. Importantly, the reduced foam cell formation upon deletion of ORP8 in bone marrow-derived cells could have contributed to the observed reduction in lesion development. This however does not explain why macrophage ORP8 deletion primarily affects the progression of early atherosclerotic lesions, rich in macrophage foam cells, to more advance atherosclerotic lesions. *In vitro* studies using bone marrow-derived macrophages also point towards a role for ORP8 in regulation of macrophage differentiation toward different subtypes.

A study by Beaslas et al. has demonstrated that silencing of ORP8 expression in the murine RAW 264.7 macrophage cell line results in down regulation of gene pathways associated with lysosomal function, growth-factor activity and immunity Major Histocompatibility Complex type I (MCH-I) function and increased macrophage migration [25]. This could result in a reduced capacity to present antigens to immune cells such as T-cells [26]. In line, the observed decrease in CD40 and CD80 expression in ORP8 KO BMDMs indicates a reduced co-stimulatory potential and a decreased capacity to activate T-cells [26]. In the current study we also demonstrated a decrease in mRNA expression of IL-6 and excretion of TNFα and IL-6 by LPS-stimulated M1 BMDMs lacking ORP8. Furthermore, mRNA expression of the M2 markers YM-1 and FIZZ-1 was decreased. Upon deletion of ORP8, macrophages thus show a reduced polarization towards both M1 and M2 subtypes [27]. The effects of ORP8 deficiency on macrophage inflammatory signaling could provide a mechanistic explanation for the increase in VLDL levels in mice lacking macrophage ORP8. However, decreased excretion of TNFα and IL-6 would lead to decreased synthesis of cholesterol, triglycerides and VLDL particles [28]. Therefore it is unlikely that the observed increase in VLDL levels in ORP8 KO BM recipients can be attributed to a decrease in production of pro-inflammatory cytokines by Kupffer cells lacking ORP8.

Importantly, macrophage differentiation plays a crucial role in the advanced stages of atherosclerotic plaque development. "Wound healing" M2 macrophages promote plaque stability, whereas "classically activated" M1 macrophages contribute to the thinning of the fibrous cap [29]. Both types of macrophages can be found in advanced plaques, creating a complex dynamic equilibrium that determines the structure of the plaque and its likelihood to rupture [18,29,30,31]. In human plaques, expression of ORP8 is localized in the shoulder region [11]. Research on human carotid artery sections has shown that macrophages in the shoulder region of the plaque strongly exhibit markers of M1 macrophages such as iNOS and HLA [29]. Moreover, an increase in TNFα and IL-6 mRNA is observed in ruptured plaque segments [29]. By producing pro-inflammatory factors such as TNFα and IL-6, M1 macrophages are able to drive the inflammatory reaction and thereby enhance the development of atherosclerosis [32,33,34,35]. The observed decrease in the production of TNFα and IL-6 and reduced expression of co-stimulatory molecules by macrophages lacking ORP8 is thus expected to lead to reduced inflammatory activity in the plaque.

In summary, ORP8 KO macrophages have a decreased ability to drive atherosclerosis due to lowered production of pro-inflammatory cytokines and a reduced formation of foam cells. In concert, these two effects may result in a reduced size of atherosclerotic plaques in ORP8 KO BM recipients after 9 weeks of WTD feeding, despite the observed increase in VLDL cholesterol and triglycerides.

Supporting Information

Figure S1 Transplantation of LDLr KO mice with ORP8 KO bone marrow (BM) results in decreased expression of ORP8 in the liver, but no changes in Kupffer cell content. Livers were isolated at 17 weeks after transplantation and after 9 weeks of WTD feeding. A) A reduction in RNA expression of ORP8 as a fraction of housekeeping (HK) in liver lysates was measured by QPCR (* $P<0.05$). B) No difference in expression of the macrophage marker CD68 could be detected using QPCR. C) Liver sections were stained for F4/80 and F4/80 positive cells were quantified as percentage of total cells counted. No difference in liver F4/80 positive cells could be found. D) Representative images of F4/80 stained liver sections. Original magnification 40×. Significance was determined by Student T-test.

Author Contributions

Conceived and designed the experiments: EvK OB TJCvB VMO MvE. Performed the experiments: EvK OB RBH BL. Analyzed the data: EvK OB RBH. Contributed reagents/materials/analysis tools: EvK VMO MvE. Wrote the paper: EvK TJCvB VMO MvE.

References

1. Olkkonen VM, Johansson M, Suchanek M, Yan D, Hynynen R, et al. (2006) The OSBP-related proteins (ORPs): global sterol sensors for co-ordination of cellular lipid metabolism, membrane trafficking and signalling processes? Biochemical Society transactions 34: 389–391.
2. Shibata N, Glass CK (2010) Macrophages, oxysterols and atherosclerosis. Circulation journal: official journal of the Japanese Circulation Society 74: 2045–2051.
3. Im SS, Osborne TF (2011) Liver x receptors in atherosclerosis and inflammation. Circulation research 108: 996–1001.
4. Lemaire-Ewing S, Prunet C, Montange T, Vejux A, Berthier A, et al. (2005) Comparison of the cytotoxic, pro-oxidant and pro-inflammatory characteristics of different oxysterols. Cell biology and toxicology 21: 97–114.
5. Vihervaara T, Uronen RL, Wohlfahrt G, Bjorkhem I, Ikonen E, et al. (2011) Sterol binding by OSBP-related protein 1L regulates late endosome motility and function. Cellular and molecular life sciences: CMLS 68: 537–551.
6. Yan D, Jauhiainen M, Hildebrand RB, Willems van Dijk K, Van Berkel TJ, et al. (2007) Expression of human OSBP-related protein 1L in macrophages enhances atherosclerotic lesion development in LDL receptor-deficient mice. Arteriosclerosis, thrombosis, and vascular biology 27: 1618–1624.
7. Lehto M, Mayranpaa MI, Pellinen T, Ihalmo P, Lehtonen S, et al. (2008) The R-Ras interaction partner ORP3 regulates cell adhesion. Journal of cell science 121: 695–705.
8. Du X, Kumar J, Ferguson C, Schulz TA, Ong YS, et al. (2011) A role for oxysterol-binding protein-related protein 5 in endosomal cholesterol trafficking. The Journal of cell biology 192: 121–135.

9. Teslovich TM, Musunuru K, Smith AV, Edmondson AC, Stylianou IM, et al. (2010) Biological, clinical and population relevance of 95 loci for blood lipids. Nature 466: 707–713.
10. Ma L, Yang J, Runesha HB, Tanaka T, Ferrucci L, et al. (2010) Genome-wide association analysis of total cholesterol and high-density lipoprotein cholesterol levels using the Framingham heart study data. BMC medical genetics 11: 55.
11. Yan D, Mayranpaa MI, Wong J, Perttila J, Lehto M, et al. (2008) OSBP-related protein 8 (ORP8) suppresses ABCA1 expression and cholesterol efflux from macrophages. The Journal of biological chemistry 283: 332–340.
12. Tall AR (2003) Role of ABCA1 in cellular cholesterol efflux and reverse cholesterol transport. Arteriosclerosis, thrombosis, and vascular biology 23: 710–711.
13. Beaslas O, Metso J, Nissila E, Laurila PP, Kaiharju E, et al. (2013) Osbpl8 deficiency in mouse causes an elevation of high-density lipoproteins and gender-specific alterations of lipid metabolism. PloS one 8: e58856.
14. von der Thusen JH, van Berkel TJ, Biessen EA (2001) Induction of rapid atherogenesis by perivascular carotid collar placement in apolipoprotein E-deficient and low-density lipoprotein receptor-deficient mice. Circulation 103: 1164–1170.
15. Van Eck M, Bos IS, Hildebrand RB, Van Rij BT, Van Berkel TJ (2004) Dual role for scavenger receptor class B, type I on bone marrow-derived cells in atherosclerotic lesion development. The American journal of pathology 165: 785–794.
16. Chomczynski P, Sacchi N (1987) Single-step method of RNA isolation by acid guanidinium thiocyanate-phenol-chloroform extraction. Analytical biochemistry 162: 156–159.
17. Redgrave TG, Roberts DC, West CE (1975) Separation of plasma lipoproteins by density-gradient ultracentrifugation. Analytical biochemistry 65: 42–49.
18. Feig JE, Rong JX, Shamir R, Sanson M, Vengrenyuk Y, et al. (2011) HDL promotes rapid atherosclerosis regression in mice and alters inflammatory properties of plaque monocyte-derived cells. Proceedings of the National Academy of Sciences of the United States of America 108: 7166–7171.
19. Patel PJ, Khera AV, Wilensky RL, Rader DJ (2013) Anti-oxidative and cholesterol efflux capacities of high-density lipoprotein are reduced in ischaemic cardiomyopathy. European journal of heart failure.
20. Nagy L, Tontonoz P, Alvarez JG, Chen H, Evans RM (1998) Oxidized LDL regulates macrophage gene expression through ligand activation of PPAR-gamma. Cell 93: 229–240.
21. Wellington CL, Walker EK, Suarez A, Kwok A, Bissada N, et al. (2002) ABCA1 mRNA and protein distribution patterns predict multiple different roles and levels of regulation. Laboratory investigation; a journal of technical methods and pathology 82: 273–283.
22. Haghpassand M, Bourassa PA, Francone OL, Aiello RJ (2001) Monocyte/macrophage expression of ABCA1 has minimal contribution to plasma HDL levels. The Journal of clinical investigation 108: 1315–1320.
23. Zhou T, Li S, Zhong W, Vihervaara T, Beaslas O, et al. (2011) OSBP-related protein 8 (ORP8) regulates plasma and liver tissue lipid levels and interacts with the nucleoporin Nup62. PloS one 6: e21078.
24. Mahley RW, Innerarity TL, Rall SC, Jr., Weisgraber KH (1985) Lipoproteins of special significance in atherosclerosis. Insights provided by studies of type III hyperlipoproteinemia. Annals of the New York Academy of Sciences 454: 209–221.
25. Beaslas O, Vihervaara T, Li J, Laurila PP, Yan D, et al. (2012) Silencing of OSBP-related protein 8 (ORP8) modifies the macrophage transcriptome, nucleoporin p62 distribution, and migration capacity. Experimental cell research 318: 1933–1945.
26. Dion S, Germon S, Guiton R, Ducournau C, Dimier-Poisson I (2011) Functional activation of T cells by dendritic cells and macrophages exposed to the intracellular parasite Neospora caninum. International journal for parasitology 41: 685–695.
27. Nair MG, Cochrane DW, Allen JE (2003) Macrophages in chronic type 2 inflammation have a novel phenotype characterized by the abundant expression of Ym1 and Fizz1 that can be partly replicated in vitro. Immunology letters 85: 173–180.
28. Khovidhunkit W, Kim MS, Memon RA, Shigenaga JK, Moser AH, et al. (2004) Effects of infection and inflammation on lipid and lipoprotein metabolism: mechanisms and consequences to the host. Journal of lipid research 45: 1169–1196.
29. Stoger JL, Gijbels MJ, van der Velden S, Manca M, van der Loos CM, et al. (2012) Distribution of macrophage polarization markers in human atherosclerosis. Atherosclerosis 225: 461–468.
30. Cho KY, Miyoshi H, Kuroda S, Yasuda H, Kamiyama K, et al. (2013) The phenotype of infiltrating macrophages influences arteriosclerotic plaque vulnerability in the carotid artery. Journal of stroke and cerebrovascular diseases: the official journal of National Stroke Association 22: 910–918.
31. Oh J, Riek AE, Weng S, Petty M, Kim D, et al. (2012) Endoplasmic reticulum stress controls M2 macrophage differentiation and foam cell formation. The Journal of biological chemistry 287: 11629–11641.
32. Mantovani A, Sica A, Sozzani S, Allavena P, Vecchi A, et al. (2004) The chemokine system in diverse forms of macrophage activation and polarization. Trends in immunology 25: 677–686.
33. Ridker PM, Rifai N, Pfeffer M, Sacks F, Lepage S, et al. (2000) Elevation of tumor necrosis factor-alpha and increased risk of recurrent coronary events after myocardial infarction. Circulation 101: 2149–2153.
34. Ridker PM, Rifai N, Stampfer MJ, Hennekens CH (2000) Plasma concentration of interleukin-6 and the risk of future myocardial infarction among apparently healthy men. Circulation 101: 1767–1772.
35. Naugler WE, Karin M (2008) The wolf in sheep's clothing: the role of interleukin-6 in immunity, inflammation and cancer. Trends in molecular medicine 14: 109–119.

7

Assessment of Toxic Effects of the Methanol Extract of *Citrus macroptera* Montr. Fruit via Biochemical and Hematological Evaluation in Female Sprague-Dawley Rats

Nizam Uddin*, Md. Rakib Hasan, Md. Mahadi Hasan, Md. Monir Hossain, Md. Robiul Alam, Mohammad Raquibul Hasan, A. F. M. Mahmudul Islam, Tasmina Rahman, Md. Sohel Rana

Department of Pharmacy, Jahangirnagar University, Savar, Dhaka, 1342, Bangladesh

Abstract

Citrus macroptera Montr. (*C. macroptera*) is locally known as Satkara. The fruit of this plant is used as appetite stimulant and in the treatment of fever. This study therefore aimed to evaluate the toxic effects of the fruit extract using some biochemical and hematological parameters in rat model. The effects of methanol extract of *Citrus macroptera* Montr. fruit administered at 250, 500 and 1000 mg/kg body weight were investigated on hematological and biochemical parameters in Sprague-Dawley female rats. Moreover, histopathological study was performed to observe the presence of pathological lesions in primary body organs. The extract presented no significant effect on body weight, percent water content, relative organ weight and hematological parameters in rat. Significant decrease from control group was observed in the levels of triglyceride, total cholesterol, low density lipoprotein and very low density lipoprotein; thus leading to significant decrease of cardiac risk ratio, castelli's risk index-2, atherogenic coefficient and atherogenic index of plasma at all doses. 500 mg/kg dose significantly decreased alkaline phosphatase ($P<0.05$), 1000 mg/kg dose significantly increased high density lipoprotein cholesterol ($P<0.05$) and 250 mg/kg dose significantly decreased the level of glycated hemoglobin ($P<0.05$) from the control group. There were no significant alterations observed with other serum biochemical parameters. Histopathological study confirmed the absence of inflammatory and necrotic features in the primary body organs. Study results indicate that methanolic fruit extract is unlikely to have significant toxicity. Moreover, these findings justified the cardio-protective, moderate hepato-protective and glucose controlling activities of the fruit extract.

Editor: Michael Bader, Max-Delbrück Center for Molecular Medicine (MDC), Germany

Funding: This study was supported with funding from Jahangirnagar University Annual Research Grant (Grant no: JU-ARG-2012-005). The funder had no role in study design, data collection and analysis, decision to publish, or preparation of the manuscript.

Competing Interests: The authors have declared that no competing interests exist.

* Email: sami.pharm22@gmail.com

Introduction

Medicinal plants were and are still one of the major sources of modern medicine. Interest in medicinal plant's pharmacognosy has increased due to using trend of phytotherapy as alternative medicine [1,2]. Plants produce bioactive compounds that act as defense mechanism against predators and at the same time may be toxic in nature for our health. With the increased interest in the pharmacological activities of the medicinal plants, there is a surge for thorough scientific investigations of these medicinal plants for efficacy and potential toxicity. Proper scientific evidence is necessary to establish the use of plants for medicinal purposes as safe, non-toxic and pharmacologically active.

Citrus macroptera Montr., a semi wild species of citrus genus, is known as 'Satkara' in Bangladesh. It may be mentioned here that the English meaning of Satkara is 'Wild orange'. The maximum height of the tree of this fruit is 5 meter. The diameter of the fruit is 6–7 cm. The fruit becomes yellow when it ripens and its rind is thick. As the pulp of this fruit is somewhat dry, it does not have enough juice, which is very sour and a bit bitter [3]. Chowdhury et al. (2008) reported the antioxidant activities of crude extracts of the stem bark of ***Citrus macroptera* and isolated** lupeol and stigmasterol [4]. Waikedre et al. (2010) reported the anti-microbial activity of essential oil of ***Citrus macroptera* a**gainst five bacteria and five fungi strains. Besides, the author found the presence of beta-pinene as major component [5]. Rana et al. (2012) reported that essential oils obtained by hydro-distillation from the fresh peels of *Citrus macroptera* contained limonene, beta-caryophyllene and geranial as main compounds [6]. Gaillard et al. (1995) isolated edulinine, ribalinine and isoplatydesmine and five aromatic compounds [7]. The people of Bangladesh eat this fruit as a vegetable. The fruit is used as ingredient in cooking different kinds of meat and chicken. Nowadays many Bangladeshi and Indian restaurants offer meat and chicken curries cooked with Satkara. Traditionally, this fruit is used as appetite stimulant and in treatment of fever [8]. In spite of the diverse uses of this fruit, there seems to be a dearth of information about the toxicity of this fruit. Therefore, we have designed our study protocol to evaluate the possible toxicity of the methanolic fruit extract via biochemical and hematological assessment as well as histopathological study in rat model. In addition, the results of the study can provide researchers with the safe levels of the doses of methanolic fruit extract. In this study we used methanol solvent for extraction because this solvent can dissolve various polar bioactive compounds as well as lipophilic compounds. Moreover, it is easy to evaporate this solvent and we get maximum bioactive compounds of the extract by minimizing the loss of compounds due to excessive heat [9].

Materials and Methods

Chemicals and reagents

Methanol was bought from SIGMA (Sigma-Aldrich, St Louis, USA). Ketamine inj. was obtained from ACI Pharmaceuticals Ltd., Bangladesh. All clinical diagnostic kits were purchased from Human Laboratories, Germany. All other chemicals and reagents used were of analytical grade.

Plant material

Fruits of *Citrus macroptera* were collected from Sylhet, Bangladesh and authenticated by an expert Taxonomist. A voucher specimen (Acc. No. 38619) was deposited in Bangladesh National Herbarium for future reference. No field studies were carried out in this study as the fruits were purchased from some local markets of Sylhet, Bangladesh. No specific permissions were required.

Preparation of plant extract

At first peels were removed. Then the pulp were cut into pieces and then dried in a hot air oven (Size 1, Gallen kamp) at reduced temperature (not more than 50°C) to make suitable for extraction process. Then the dried fruit materials (500 gm) were treated with sufficient amount of pure methanol (1000 ml) for one week at room temperature with occasional shaking (solvent to fruit ratio was 2:1). The extract was filtered through a cotton plug followed by Whatman No. 1 filter paper. The filtrate was then evaporated under reduced pressure to give a dark green viscous mass and stored at 4°C until it was used. The yield value for the methanol extract was 29.02%.

Animals and experimental set-up

Sprague-Dawley female rats weighing between 170–230 g were collected from Pharmacology Laboratory, Department of Pharmacy, Jahangirnagar University and were acclimatized to normal laboratory conditions for one week prior to study and were assessed to pellet diet and water *ad libitum*. Temperature of facility was (22±3) °C and light/darkness alternated 12 h apart. The research activities were conducted in accordance with the internationally accepted principles of the US guidelines (NIH publication #85–23, revised in 1985) and following the approval by the Biosafety, Biosecurity and Ethical Committee [Approval Number: BBECJU/N2013(21)] of Faculty of Biological Sciences of Jahangirnagar University, Savar, Dhaka, Bangladesh. The study was carried out in the Department of Pharmacy, Jahangirnagar University.

Experimental procedure

The animals were assigned to four groups of five animals each. Group-1 was treated as control and group-2, 3 and 4 were treated with 250 mg/kg, 500 mg/kg and 1000 mg/kg doses of methanol extract of *C. macroptera* fruit respectively for 21 days. Different doses of the extract of *C. macroptera* were administered orally by stomach tube. Rats were weighed weekly and observed for behavioral changes, feeding and drinking habits, and general morphological changes. At the end of the 21-day treatment period, after 18 hours fasting, rats from each group were anaesthetized by administration (i.p) of ketamine (500 mg/kg body weight) [10]. Blood samples were collected from post vena cava of rats into EDTA (Ethylene diamine tetra acetic acid) sample tubes for hematological analysis and plain sample tubes for serum generation for biochemical analysis. Serum was obtained after allowing blood to coagulate for 30 minutes and centrifuged at 4000 g for 10 min using bench top centrifuge (MSE Minor, England). The supernatant serum samples were collected using dry Pasteur pipette and stored in the refrigerator for further analysis. All analyses were completed within 24 hours of sample collection [11].

Hematological analysis

Blood samples were analyzed using established procedures and automated Sysmex KX-21 hematology analyzer. Parameters that were recorded included Hemoglobin (Hb), Red blood cells (RBC), White blood cells (WBC), Platelets, Erythrocyte Sedimentation Rate (ESR), Packed cell Volume (PCV), Mean corpuscular volume (MCV), Mean corpuscular hemoglobin (MCH), Mean corpuscular hemoglobin concentration (MCHC), Pro-calcitonin (PCT), Packed cell volume (PCV), Red cell distribution width - standard deviation (RDW–SD), Red cell distribution width - coefficient of variation (RDW-CV), Platelet larger cell ratio (P-LCR), Platelet distribution width (PDW), Mean platelet volume (MPV), Neutrophils, Basophils, Lymphocytes, Monocytes and Eosinophils.

Biochemical analysis

Serum samples were analyzed for urea, albumin, total protein, total cholesterol (TC), high density lipoprotein (HDL) cholesterol, triglycerides (TG), uric acid, alkaline phosphatase (ALP), aspartate transaminase (AST) and alanine transaminase (ALT) using Human commercial kits and Humalyzer 3500. Moreover, glycated hemoglobin (HbA1c) test was performed to find out the amount of glycated hemoglobin (HbA1c) using Bio Rad D-10 analyzer. Very low density lipoprotein (VLDL) cholesterol and Low density lipoprotein (LDL) cholesterol concentrations were calculated using the following Friedewald equations [12]:

$$\text{i. LDL cholesterol (mg/dL)} = (\text{Total cholesterol} - \text{HDL cholesterol} - \text{Triglyceride} / 5)$$

$$\text{ii. VLDL cholesterol (mg/dL)} = \text{Triglyceride} / 5.$$

The atherogenic indices were calculated as follows:

Cardiac Risk Ratio (CRR) $= TC/HDL-C$ [13]

Atherogenic Coefficient (AC) $= (TC-HDL-C)/HDL-C$ [14]

Atherogenic Index of Plasma (AIP) $= \log(TG/HDL-C)$ [15]

Castelli's Risk Index−2 (CRI−2) $= LDL-C/HDL-C$ [16]

Histopathology

After the collection of blood, all the animals were euthanized for gross pathological examinations of the major organs. The organs such as: hearts, kidneys, lungs, livers, spleens, fallopian tubes, thymuses and ovaries were collected from all the animals for histopathology. The weights of the organs were determined. The relative organ weights were calculated by dividing the individual weight of each organ with the final body weight of each rat. The percent water content was determined by subtracting the dry weight of each organ from the respective weight of each wet organ. Then it was planned to perform histo-pathological examination for the control and high dose group initially. If any histopatholgical findings were observed with high dose group, the mid and low dose groups were to be studied. The selected organs were fixed in 10% neutral buffered formalin, trimmed and a 4–5 μm thickness of tissue sections were stained with hematoxylin and eosin for histopathological investigation using established protocols [17]. The photomicrographs were taken with Olympus DP 72 microscope.

Data analysis

Data were expressed as mean ± SEM (Standard Error of Mean). Repeated measures ANOVA and One-way ANOVA followed by Dunnett's multiple comparison was performed to analyze data sets. $P<0.05$ was considered significant. Statistical programs used were SPSS (version 16, IBM software Inc, USA) and GRAPHPAD PRISM (version 6.02; GraphPad Software Inc., San Diego, CA, USA).

Result

Effect of the extract on the body weight, % water content and relative organ weight of rats

There were no signs and symptoms of toxicity and death recorded after three week treatment period. From the figure 1 it is ascertained that body weight did not gradually increase at all doses in comparison with control. There was no significant deviation in weight gain from control at any doses in this three- week treatment period. Table-1 and 2 present effects of different doses of methanol extract on % water content and relative weight of different body organs of rats. No significant difference was noticed in % water content and relative organ weight of primary body organs (Table 1 and 2).

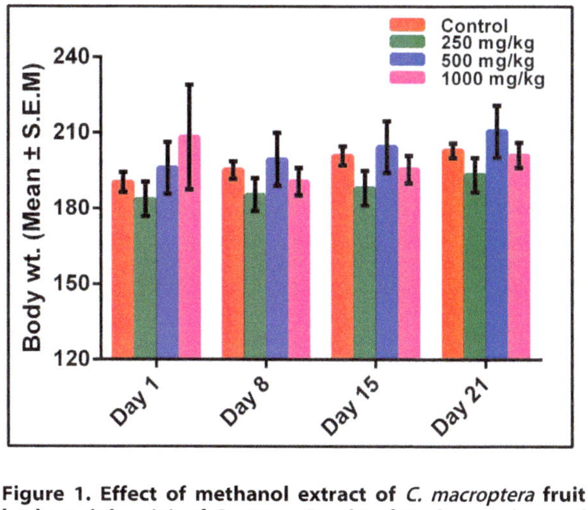

Figure 1. Effect of methanol extract of *C. macroptera* fruit on body weights (g) of Sprague-Dawley female rats in 21 days treatment period. RM ANOVA with Dunnett's multiple comparison was performed to analyze this weight variation in different days. No significant different was found when compared to control group. Time effect was found not significant ($P>0.05$).

Effect of extract on the hematological parameters

The effects of different doses of the extract on the hematological parameters are tabulated in table 3. No significant difference was found with all hematological parameters.

Effect of extract on the biochemical parameters

Treatment with different doses of methanol extract did not have any significant adverse effect on hepatic biomarker enzymes ALT and AST while 500 mg/kg dose significantly decreased the activity of ALP enzyme. Moreover, three different doses of the extract did not alter the level of total protein and albumin which are major tests to assess liver damage (Table 4). Besides, methanol extract significantly reduced the level of LDL, VLDL, TG, TC, CRR, CRI-2, AC and AIP which are the imperative assays for cardiovascular diseases. Furthermore, 1000 mg/kg dose significantly ($P<0.05$) increased the level of HDL. The determination of uric acid and urea is the biomarker of the normal function of kidney. Insignificant ($P>0.05$) changes were found in the level of these two renal biomarkers. Moreover, 250 mg/kg dose significantly reduced HbA1c ($P<0.05$) whereas in high doses the fruit extract failed to show positive response (Table 4).

Histopathological observations

There were no overt pathological lesions observed both at high and low doses of the methanol extract in histopathological study. In the figure 2 photomicrograph of histopathological study of 1000 mg/kg dose and control were presented. No abnormal signs of toxicity were found in the high dose. Histopathological observations confirmed the normal cellular architecture of the tested organs.

Discussion

Daily oral doses of the methanol extract up to 1000 mg/kg did not cause any physical abnormalities or death after three week treatment period. In a previous study Uddin et al (2014) performed the acute toxicity of this fruit extract. Administration of doses up to 4000 mg/kg (the highest dose) produced no mortality which was accompanied by normal physical activity of the tested animals [18]. This study strengthens the safety of the extract.

The body of a human being manages a large number of complicated interactions with a view to maintaining balance within a usual range. These interactions make compensatory changes easier which support normal physical and psychological functions. This process is indispensable to the survival of humans and other species. This process is essential to the survival of the person and to our species [19]. 75% weight of the body of an infant and 55% weight of the body of an elderly person are water. It is vital for maintaining cellular homeostasis. Dehydration can cause several physiological disorders [20]. In our study we found no significant alteration in % water content of primary organs from control group which buttresses the claim that the fruit extract does not have toxic effects on normal fluid content and role of body fluid in maintaining homeostasis system. Alteration in the normal weight of the body indicates impairment of normal function of different body organs. Methanol extract did not show any significant alteration on the body weight of the rats compared to control group in 3-week treatment period (Figure 1). It can be

Table 1. % Water content of different organs treated with different doses of methanol extract of *C. macroptera* fruit.

Organ	Control	250 mg/kg	500 mg/kg	1000 mg/kg
Heart	34.04±1.867	36.121±1.523	34.973±3.011	36.262±2.262
Kidney	47.008±1.458	48.565±1.043	48.403±1.011	48.276±2.007
Lung	42.271±4.066	51.637±0.481	49.128±2.862	42.75±4.877
Liver	58.263±1.185	62.147±1.817	60.882±1.688	61.082±2.068
Spleen	38.909±0.820	43.386±2.043	34.971±1.291	34.202±0.887

Values are presented as mean±S.E.M (n = 5). No significant result was found when compared against control. One way ANOVA followed by Dunnett's multiple comparison was performed to analyze this data set.

suggested that this extract has no negative impact on the body weight of rats treated with three different doses. Relative organ weight may serve as indication of pathological and physiological status in man and animals. Toxic substances induce abnormal metabolic reactions that affect primary organs such as heart, liver, spleen, kidney and lung [21]. Our findings suggest that three doses of the methanol extract of fruit are non-toxic on all vital organs tested in this study. Furthermore, three doses of the fruit extract showed no toxicity on reproductive organs such as fallopian tube and ovary. Therefore, this fruit extract is considered safe for maintaining the normal function of the organs.

Hematological assessment is useful to determine the extent of toxic effects of plant extracts on the blood constituents of an animal [22]. The analysis of blood parameters is closely related to risk evaluation because when tests involve rodents, the hematological system has a higher predictive value of any abnormal toxicity signs and symbols in humans [23]. We found no noticeable hemolytic changes on RBC, Hb, PCV, MCH, MCV, MCHC, RDW-SD and RDW-CV. These findings exclude the possibility of occurrence of anemic condition and other erythrocyte cells related disorders (thalassemia, polycythemia, liver disease, hypothyroidism etc.). Increase in the production of WBC and it's differentials is generally considered to be a marker of stress and a defence mechanism triggered by immune system against various inflammatory conditions (Polymyalgia rheumatica, bacterial infections, hemorrhage, leukemia etc.). The non-significant changes in the level of WBC and differentials including platelet and its indices, neutrophils, lymphocytes, monocytes and eosinophils observed in this study at three doses level suggest the non-toxicity of the fruit extract. Platelet indices are important biomarkers for the early diagnosis of thromboembolic diseases. MPV and PDW are simple platelet indices which are increased during platelet activation [24]. Besides, P-LCR is also considered as an indicator of risk factor associated with thromboembolic ischemic events [25]. A high ESR and PCT indicates that inflammation (Bacterial infections, sepsis, arthritis, etc.) occurs somewhere in the body. Therefore, non-significant impact on the ESR, PCT, WBC and differential counts posits that the fruit extract has no contribution to the induction of infectious diseases and thromboembolic disorders. Moreover, it is safe for hematopoietic system of the body.

Urea and uric acid are the biomarkers of kidney function and retention of these products in the body indicates renal damage [26–28]. In this present study, there was no significant increase ($P>0.05$) in the amount of urea and uric acid when compared with the control group. Hence this fruit extract is considered safe and has no destructive effect on normal kidney functions. Elevation in the level of serum transaminase enzymes activities is highly indicative of hepatic impairment in animals [29]. The insignificant change in plasma ALT activity with AST at the doses of 250, 500 and 1000 mg/kg indicates that the extract caused no changes in the liver. ALT is a kind of cytoplasmic enzyme that increases in plasma which is an indication of injuries caused by toxic agents to the liver. Liver injury is characterized by predominant elevation of the ALT and increased activity of mitochondrial enzyme AST in plasma reflects severe tissue injuries [30]. However, 500 mg/kg dose significantly ($P<0.05$) reduced ALP level (table 4) which may account for protective effect on liver disorders. But in 1000 mg/kg the extract did not present significant result. It would indicate selective activity in the median dose and non-selective activity in the highest dose. That is why further research work should be conducted to verify this reason.

Table 2. Relative Organ weight profile of rats treated with different doses of methanol extract of *C. macroptera*.

Organ	Control	250 mg/kg	500 mg/kg	1000 mg/kg
Heart	0.2245±0.002	0.2428±0.007	0.227±0.003	0.243±0.009
Kidney	0.2246±0.004	0.2484±0.016	0.231±0.009	0.215±0.020
Lung	0.5019±0.067	0.457±0.009	0.4±0.024	0.481±0.041
Liver	2.025±0.100	2.387±0.121	2.04±0.08	2.3±0.078
Spleen	0.2749±0.008	0.313±0.005	0.314±0.02	0.304±0.013
Ovary	0.0235±0.002	0.026±0.001	0.024±0.001	0.025±0.001
Fallopian tube	0.2122±0.016	0.2127±0.016	0.204±0.03	0.2±0.026
Thymus	0.127±0.007	0.1078±0.011	0.120±0.004	0.110±0.004

Values are presented as mean±S.E.M (n = 5). No significant result was found when compared against control. One way ANOVA followed by Dunnett's multiple comparison was performed to analyze this data set.

Table 3. Effect of different doses of methanol extract of *C. macroptera* fruit on the hematological parameters of rats.

Hematological parameters	Control	250 mg/kg	500 mg/kg	1000 mg/kg
ESR(mm)	5.4±0.748	8±0.836	5.2±1.012	6.6±1.077
RBC($\times$ 10^{12}/L)	7.016±0.192	6.532±0.245	7.402±0.241	7.388±0.088
WBC ($\times 10^9$/L	5.32±0.5	4.95±0.76	4.944±0.421	3.538±0.530
PLT($\times$ 10^9/L)	417.2±43.787	412.8±11.425	468.2±51.361	417±40.707
Hb(g/dl)	13.4±0.448	14.125±0.125	13.74±0.430	14.04±0.252
HCT/PCV(%)	48.04±1.403	47.56±1.307	47.18±1.383	47.78±1.012
MCV(fL)	67.84±1.525	73.62±3.103	63.76±0.78	64.66±0.951
MCHC (g/dl)	27.86±0.235	25.72±1.437	29.1±0.23	29.42±0.284
MCH (pg)	19.12±0.385	18.86±1.084	18.58±0.162	19.02±0.172
RDW-SD (fL)	43.72±1.184	49.275±4.636	38.76±0.62	40.52±1.66
RDW-CV (%)	19.66±0.250	21.5±1.662	19.36±0.097	19.46±0.764
PDW (μm)	13.56±0.892	14.55±1.12	12.44±0.242	13.04±0.654
MPV (fL)	10.3±0.3	11.175±0.45	10.22±0.156	10.24±0.273
P-LCR	28.62±2.383	34.275±3.456	27.92±1.151	28.46±1.92
PCT (μg/L)	0.432±0.050	0.67±0.106	0.506±0.064	0.428±0.042
N (%)	39.48±4.233	39.92±3.222	34.92±0.421	31.725±3.164
L (%)	57.84±4.212	53.84±4.84	58.16±2.13	60.06±3.504
M (%)	1.66±0.13	4.86±2.345	2.94±0.271	2.94±0.842
E (%)	1.02±0.351	1.38±0.871	1.32±0.554	3.675±1.575
N/L	0.7218±0.137	0.7892±0.134	0.603±0.017	0.416±0.061

Here N= Neutrophils, L = Lymphocyte, M=Monocyte, E = Eosinophils, PLT= Platelet and N/L=Neutrophil/Lymphocyte ratio. Values are presented as mean±S.E.M (n=5). No significant result was found when compared against control. One way ANOVA followed by Dunnett's multiple comparison was performed to analyze this data set.

Table 4. Effect of different doses of methanol extract of *C. macroptera* fruit on biochemical safety parameters in rats.

Biochemical parameters	Control	250 mg/kg	500 mg/kg	1000 mg/kg
TP(g/dl)	5.096±0.077	4.544±0.214	5.194±0.156	5.188±0.21
ALB(g/dl)	3.82±0.216	3.4±0.124	3.5234±0.090	3.7142±0.186
GLB(g/dl)	1.276±0.251	1.1442±0.27	1.671±.150	1.4744±0.144
A/G	3.620±0.907	3.9837±1.20	2.1732±0.181	2.6292±0.308
TG (mg/dl)	67.222±1.195	46.854±2.928*	36.84±1.501*	34.22±4.94*
TC (mg/dl)	75.946±1.964	69.326±0.267*	68.608±0.515*	66.102±0.896*
HDL (mg/dl)	56.9498±1.802	59.674±0.6	60.609±0.34	62.17±0.636*
LDL (mg/dl)	5.5518±1.097	0.2812±0.134*	0.631±0.301*	0.388±0.061*
VLDL (mg/dl)	13.4444±0.241	9.3708±0.585*	7.368±0.3*	6.844±0.987*
ALT(IU/L)	49.136±1.634	45.95±0.735	49.48±1.43	46.42±0.852
AST(IU/L)	94.54±1.740	90.8±1.870	90.058±0.48	90.248±0.472
ALP(IU/L)	361.62±7.891	353.86±15.523	314.63±2.826*	363.5±4.193
U (mg/dl)	34.684±2.316	34.716±1.258	38.528±2.647	39.83±2.342
UA (mg/dl)	2.0824±0.283	3.0162±0.331	1.7098±0.236	1.4068±0.143
HbA1c (%)	2.74±0.16	1.92±0.115*	2.92±0.243	2.72±0.213
CRR	1.3353±0.022	1.1622±0.011*	1.132±0.008*	1.0638±0.02*
CRI-2	0.097±0.012	0.004±0.002*	0.010±0.005*	0.006±0.001*
AC	0.3353±0.022	0.1622±0.011*	0.132±0.007*	0.0638±0.02*
AIP	1.042±0.012	0.941±0.017*	0.878±0.009*	0.845±0.033*

TP = Total protein, ALB = Albumin, GLB= Globulin, U= Urea and UA= Uric Acid. Values are presented as mean±S.E.M (n=5). One way ANOVA followed by Dunnett's multiple comparison was performed to analyze this data set. * $P<0.05$ when compared against control.

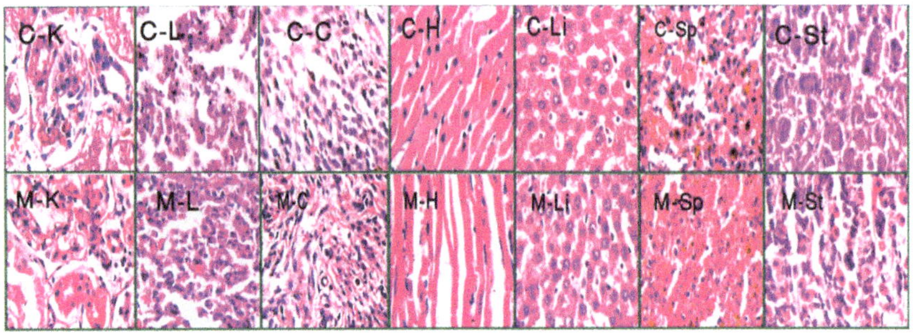

Figure 2. Histopathological photomicrographs of control group and 1000 mg/kg dose group of *C. macroptera* (×100 magnification). No presence of discernible lesions including inflammation and necrosis were observed. Here, C-K = Control-Kidney, C-L = Control-Lung, C-C = Control-Cecum, C-H = Control-Heart, C-Li = Control-Liver, C-Sp = Control-Spleen, C-St = Control-Stomach, M-K = 1000 mg/kg dose-Kidney, M-L = 1000 mg/kg dose-Lung, M-C = 1000 mg/kg dose-Cecum, M-H = 1000 mg/kg dose-Heart, M-Li = 1000 mg/kg dose-Liver, M-Sp = 1000 mg/kg dose-Spleen and M-St = 1000 mg/kg dose-Stomach.

The level of plasma albumin decreases in response to inflammation [31]. Recent studies have shown that not only albumin concentration but also albumin function are reduced in liver disorders such as liver cirrhosis [32]. The non-significant variation in the level of TP, albumin, globulin and albumin-globulin ratio provides logistic support behind the non-toxic effect of this fruit extract on liver and no link with liver dysfunction.

A high plasma triglyceride level is both an independent and synergistic risk factor for cardiovascular diseases [33] and is often related to hypertension [34], obesity and diabetes mellitus [35]. Elevated total cholesterol level is a familiar and well-known risk factor for developing atherosclerosis and other cardiovascular diseases [36]. High levels of plasma LDL and VLDL cholesterol are responsible for cardiovascular diseases [37] which are accompanied with hypertension and obesity [38]. In this study a very significant decrease was observed in the levels of TC, TG, LDL and VLDL cholesterol which strengthen the lipid lowering activity and represents cardio-protective effect of the fruit extract. Low plasma HDL cholesterol is also a major predictor for cardiovascular diseases [37]. High plasma HDL cholesterol exerts a protective effect by enhancing reverse cholesterol transport through scavenging excess cholesterol from peripheral tissues in our body. 1000 mg/kg dose exhibited very good activity ($P<0.05$) by increasing the level of HDL. This finding further gives strong support for cardio-protective effect of the extract. With these findings (discussed above) in hand we evaluated atherogenic indices which are powerful indicators of the risk of cardiovascular diseases. The higher the values of atherogenic indices the higher the risk of developing cardiovascular disease and vice versa [36]. Methanolic fruit extract reduced three atherogenic indices with significant value $P<0.05$. Moreover. three doses of the fruit extract significantly lowered the value of AIP ($P<0.05$). Hematological parameters MPV and P-LCR are also related to cardiovascular disorders. Higher levels of these parameters coupled with neutrophil/lymphocyte ratio can serve as indication of coronary heart disease [25,39,40]. In this study non-significant variation of these parameters from control group provides vital evidences in favor of reduced atherogenic indices and protective effect of the methanolic fruit extract against cardiovascular disorders. Moreover, at low dose fruit extract prevented significant increase in HbA1c in blood. In diabetic condition the level of HbA1c is enhanced due to the production of excessive glucose in blood which further react with blood hemoglobin and creates glycated hemoglobin [41]. Uddin et al (2014) found hypoglycemic activity of the same fruit extract via both *in-vivo* OGTT (Oral Glucose Tolerance Test) model and *in-vitro* α- amylase inhibitory assay, which further substantiated blood glucose level controlling activity [18]. In high doses we did not find any significant HbA1c reduction activity. This may have happened due to the loss of selective activity. That is why further study is required to find out the exact reason. Lipid metabolism abnormality in diabetes is characterized by increase in TC, TG, LDL cholesterol and fall in HDL cholesterol [34]. We recorded significant decrease in the serum levels of these biomarkers which is discussed previously. Moderate activity in decreasing glycated hemoglobin coupled with the reduction of lipid profile proved the efficacy of the fruit extract as moderate hypoglycemic agent and it can control blood glucose level.

Furthermore, up to 1000 mg/kg no discernible lesions including inflammation and necrosis were found. That is why it is logical to infer that methanol extract has no toxic effect on primary body organs when administered at 250, 500 and 1000 mg/kg doses for 3 weeks in rats. Uddin et al, (2014) detected the presence of saponins, steroids and terpenoids in the fruit extract. Therefore, these phytochemicals may exert the non-toxic effect as well as afore-mentioned therapeutic potentials [18].

Conclusions

In a nutshell, the non-toxic effect evaluated by biochemical and hematological assessment suggests a wide margin of safety for therapeutic doses. The extract has no significant toxic effect on biological parameters. Besides the medicinal uses, we recorded significant cardio-protective effect with moderate hepato-protective and hypoglycemic activities exerted by this fruit extract. These findings justify the therapeutic potential of the fruit. Further research projects should be launched to isolate and characterize active principles and elucidate molecular structures with precise pharmacology.

Acknowledgments

The authors are greatly thankful to Wazed Miah Science Research Center (WMSRC), Jahangirnagar University for taking photomicrographs of histopathological slides to complete this research work.

Author Contributions

Conceived and designed the experiments: NU M. Rakib Hasan. Performed the experiments: NU M. Rakib Hasan M. M. Hasan M. M. Hossain MRA M. Raquibul Hasan. Analyzed the data: NU M. Rakib Hasan. Contributed reagents/materials/analysis tools: TR MSR. Wrote the paper: NU MSR. Managed Literature search: AFMMI.

References

1. Gupta SS (1994) Propects and perpectives of normal plants products in medicine. Indian J Pharmacol 26: 1–12.
2. Das SS, Das S, Pal S, Mujib A, Dey S (1999) Biotechnology of medicinal plants-Recent advances and potential. UK 992 Publications: Hyderabad. pp.126–139.
3. Elevitch CR (2006) Traditional Trees of Pacific Islands: Their Culture, Environment, and Use. Hawaii: Permanent Agriculture Resources. pp.243–276.
4. Chowdhury SA, Sohrab MH, Datta BK, Hasan CM (2008) Chemical and Antioxidant Studies of *Citrus macroptera*. Bang J Sci Ind Res 43: 449–454.
5. Waikedre J, Dugay A, Barrachina I, Herrenknecht C, Cabalion P, et al. (2010) Chemical composition and antimicrobial activity of the essential oils from New Caledonian *Citrus macroptera* and *Citrus hystrix*. Chem Biodivers 7: 871–877.
6. Rana VS, Blazquez MA (2012) Compositions of the volatile oils of *Citrus macroptera* and *C. maxima*. Nat Prod Commun 7: 1371–1372.
7. Gaillard E, Muyard F, Bevalot F, Regnier A, Vaquette J (1995) [Rutacea from New Caledonia. Chemical composition of stem bark of *Citrus macroptera* Montr]. Ann Pharm Fr 53: 75–78.
8. Rahmatullah M, Afsana K, Morshed N, Prashanta KN, Sadar UK, et al. (2010) A Randomized Survey of Medicinal Plants used by Folk Medicinal Healers of Sylhet Division, Bangladesh. Adv in Nat App Sci 4: 52–62.
9. Jaroszynska J (2003) The Influence of Solvent Choice on the Recovery of Phytogenic Phenolic Compounds Extracted from Plant Material. Pol J Environ Stud 12: 481–484.
10. Ringer DH, Dabich L (1979) Hematology and clinical biochemistry. In: Baker HJ, Lindsey JR, Weisbroth SH, editors. The laboratory Rat, volume 1, Biology and diseases. San Diego: Academic Press. pp.105–121.
11. Wolford ST, Schroer RA, Gohs FX, Gallo PP, Brodeck M, et al. (1986) Reference range data base for serum chemistry and hematology values in laboratory animals. J Toxicol Environ Health 18: 161–188.
12. Friedewald WT, Levy RI, Fredrickson DS (1972) Estimation of the concentration of low-density lipoprotein cholesterol in plasma, without use of the preparative ultracentrifuge. Clin Chem 18: 499–502.
13. Martirosyan DM, Miroshnichenko LA, Kulakova SN, Pogojeva AV, Zoloedov VI (2007) Amaranth oil application for coronary heart disease and hypertension. Lipids Health Dis 6: 1.
14. Brehm A, Pfeiler G, Pacini G, Vierhapper H, Roden M (2004) Relationship between serum lipoprotein ratios and insulin resistance in obesity. Clin Chem 50: 2316–2322.
15. Dobiasova M (2004) Atherogenic index of plasma [log(triglycerides/HDL-cholesterol)]: theoretical and practical implications. Clin Chem 50: 1113–1115.
16. Castelli WP, Abbott RD, McNamara PM (1983) Summary estimates of cholesterol used to predict coronary heart disease. Circulation 67: 730–734.
17. Carleton H (1980) Carleton's Histological techniques. London: Oxford University Press.
18. Uddin N, Hasan MR, Hossain MM, Sarker A, Hasan AH, et al. (2014) *In vitro* alpha-amylase inhibitory activity and *in vivo* hypoglycemic effect of methanol extract of Citrus macroptera Montr. fruit. Asian Pac J Trop Biomed 4: 473–479.
19. Guyton CA (1986) Textbook of Medical Physiology. Philadelphia: W.B Saunders Company. pp.2–7.
20. Popkin BM, D'Anci KE, Rosenberg IH (2010) Water, hydration, and health. Nutr Rev 68: 439–458.
21. Dybing E, Doe J, Groten J, Kleiner J, O'Brien J, et al. (2002) Hazard characterisation of chemicals in food and diet. dose response, mechanisms and extrapolation issues. Food Chem Toxicol 40: 237–282.
22. Ashafa AOT, Yakubu MT, Grierson DS, Afolayan AJ (2009) Effects of aqueous leaf extract from the leaves of *Chrysocoma ciliate* L. on some biochemical parameters of Wistar rats. Afr J Biotechnol 8: 1425–1430.
23. Olson H, Betton G, Robinson D, Thomas K, Monro A, et al. (2000) Concordance of the toxicity of pharmaceuticals in humans and in animals. Regul Toxicol Pharmacol 32: 56–67.
24. Vagdatli E, Gounari E, Lazaridou E, Katsibourlia E, Tsikopoulou F, et al. (2010) Platelet distribution width: a simple, practical and specific marker of activation of coagulation. Hippokratia 14: 28–32.
25. Grotto HZ, Noronha JF (2004) Platelet larger cell ratio (P-LCR) in patients with dyslipidemia. Clin Lab Haematol 26: 347–349.
26. Newman DJ, Price C (1998) Renal function and nitrogen metabolites. In: Burtis CA, Ashwood ER, editors. Tietz Texbook of Clinical Chemistry. Philadelphia: W.B. Saunders; 1998. pp.1204–1270.
27. Odutola AA A, Co Zaria S (1992) Rapid Interpretation of Routine Clinical Laboratory Test. Nigeria: Asekome, S and Company, Zaria. pp.1–30.
28. Johnson RJ, Nakagawa T, Jalal D, Sanchez-Lozada LG, Kang DH, et al. (2013) Uric acid and chronic kidney disease: which is chasing which? Nephrol Dial Transplant 28: 2221–2228.
29. Tennant BC (1997) Hepatic function. In: Kaneko JJ, Harvey JW, Bruss ML, editors. Clinical Biochemistry of Domestic Animals. Singapore: Harcourt Brace and Company Asia PTE. Limited. pp.327–52.
30. Martins AC (2006) Clinical chemistry and metabolic medicine. UK: Edward Arnold Ltd. pp.7–15.
31. Ruot B, Breuille D, Rambourdin F, Bayle G, Capitan P, et al. (2000) Synthesis rate of plasma albumin is a good indicator of liver albumin synthesis in sepsis. Am J Physiol Endocrinol Metab 279: E244–251.
32. Garcia-Martinez R, Caraceni P, Bernardi M, Gines P, Arroyo V, et al. (2013) Albumin: pathophysiologic basis of its role in the treatment of cirrhosis and its complications. Hepatology 58: 1836–1846.
33. McBride P (2008) Triglycerides and risk for coronary artery disease. Curr Atheroscler Rep 10: 386–390.
34. Zicha J, Kunes J, Devynck MA (1999) Abnormalities of membrane function and lipid metabolism in hypertension: a review. Am J Hypertens 12: 315–331.
35. Shen GX (2007) Lipid disorders in diabetes mellitus and current management. Curr Pharm Anal 3: 17–24.
36. Ademuyiwa O, Ugbaja RN, Idumebor F, Adebawo O (2005) Plasma lipid profiles and risk of cardiovascular disease in occupational lead exposure in Abeokuta, Nigeria. Lipids Health Dis 4: 19.
37. Lichtenstein AH, Appel LJ, Brands M, Carnethon M, Daniels S, et al. (2006) Diet and lifestyle recommendations revision 2006: a scientific statement from the American Heart Association Nutrition Committee. Circulation 114: 82–96.
38. Shepherd J (1998) Identifying patients at risk for coronary heart disease: treatment implications. Eur Heart J 19: 1776–1783.
39. Ayhan S, Ozturk S, Erdem A, Ozlu MF, Memioglu T, et al. (2013) Hematological parameters and coronary collateral circulation in patients with stable coronary artery disease. Exp Clin Cardiol 18: e12–15.
40. Endler G, Klimesch A, Sunder-Plassmann H, Schillinger M, Exner M, et al. (2002) Mean platelet volume is an independent risk factor for myocardial infarction but not for coronary artery disease. Br J Haematol 117: 399–404.
41. Pari L, Saravanan R (2004) Antidiabetic effect of diasulin, a herbal drug, on blood glucose, plasma insulin and hepatic enzymes of glucose metabolism in hyperglycaemic rats. Diabetes Obes Metab 6: 286–292.

Whole Grain Rye Intake, Reflected by a Biomarker, Is Associated with Favorable Blood Lipid Outcomes in Subjects with the Metabolic Syndrome

Ola Kally Magnusdottir[1]*, Rikard Landberg[2,3], Ingibjorg Gunnarsdottir[1], Lieselotte Cloetens[4], Björn Åkesson[4,5], Fredrik Rosqvist[6], Ursula Schwab[7,8], Karl-Heinz Herzig[9], Janne Hukkanen[10], Markku J. Savolainen[10], Lea Brader[11], Kjeld Hermansen[11], Marjukka Kolehmainen[7,12], Kaisa Poutanen[7,12], Matti Uusitupa[7,13], Ulf Risérus[6], Inga Thorsdottir[1]

1 Unit for Nutrition Research, Landspitali -The National University Hospital of Iceland and Faculty of Food Science and Nutrition, School of Health Sciences, University of Iceland, Reykjavík, Iceland, **2** Department of Food Science, BioCenter, Swedish University of Agricultural Sciences, Uppsala, Sweden, **3** Division of Nutritional Epidemiology, Institute of Environmental Medicine, Karolinska Institutet, Stockholm, Sweden, **4** Biomedical Nutrition, Pure and Applied Biochemistry, Lund University, Lund, Sweden, **5** Department of Clinical Nutrition, Skåne University Hospital, Lund, Sweden, **6** Department of Public Health and Caring Sciences, Clinical Nutrition and Metabolism, Uppsala University, Uppsala, Sweden, **7** Institute of Public Health and Clinical Nutrition, University of Eastern Finland, Kuopio, Finland, **8** Institute of Clinical Medicine, Internal Medicine, Kuopio University Hospital, Kuopio, Finland, **9** Institute of Biomedicine, Department of Physiology and Biocenter, Oulu University, Oulu, Finland and Department of Psychiatry, Kuopio University Hospital, Kuopio, Finland, **10** Department of Internal Medicine and Biocenter, Institute of Clinical Medicine, University of Oulu, Oulu, Finland and Clinical Research Center, Oulu University Hospital, Oulu, Finland, **11** Department of Endocrinology and Internal Medicine, Aarhus University Hospital, Aarhus, Denmark, **12** VTT Technical Research Centre of Finland, Espoo and Kuopio, Finland, **13** Research Unit, Kuopio University Hospital, Kuopio, Finland

Abstract

Background and Aim: Few studies have explored the possible plasma cholesterol lowering effects of rye consumption. The aim of this secondary analysis in the SYSDIET study was to investigate the association between plasma alkylresorcinols (AR), a biomarker for whole grain wheat and rye intake, and blood lipid concentrations in a population with metabolic syndrome. Furthermore, we analyzed the associations between the AR C17:0/C21:0 ratio, a suggested marker of the relative intake of whole grain/bran rye, and blood lipid concentrations.

Methods: Participants were 30–65 years of age, with body mass index (BMI) 27–40 kg/m^2 and had metabolic syndrome. Individuals were recruited through six centers in the Nordic countries and randomized either to a healthy Nordic diet (ND, n = 93), rich in whole grain rye and wheat, as well as berries, fruits and vegetables, rapeseed oil, three fish meals per week and low-fat dairy products, or a control diet (n = 65) for 18/24 weeks. Associations between total plasma AR concentration and C17:0/C21:0 homologue ratio and blood lipids were investigated in pooled (ND + control group) regression analyses at 18/24 weeks adjusted for baseline value for the dependent variable, age, BMI and statin use.

Results: When adjusted for confounders, total plasma AR at 18/24 weeks was not significantly associated with blood lipids but the AR ratio C17:0/C21:0 was inversely associated with LDL cholesterol concentrations (B (95% CI): −0.41 (−0.80 to −0.02)), log LDL/HDL cholesterol ratio (−0.20 (−0.37 to −0.03)), log non-HDL cholesterol (−0.20 (−0.37 to −0.03)), log apolipoprotein B (−0.12 (−0.24 to 0.00)) and log triglyceride concentrations (−0.35 (−0.59 to −0.12)).

Discussion: Increased proportion of whole grain rye, reflected by a biomarker, in the diet is associated with favorable blood lipid outcomes, a relationship that should be further investigated.

Trial Registration: ClinicalTrials.gov NCT00992641

Editor: Mario D. Cordero, University of Sevilla, Spain

Funding: The study was supported by NordForsk NCoE in Food Nutrition and Health: Project 070014 SYSDIET (Systems biology in controlled dietary interventions and cohort studies. http://www.nordforsk.org/en?set_language = en. This study was also funded by the Academy of Finland, Finnish Diabetes Research Foundation, Finnish Foundation for Cardiovascular Research, The Sigrid Juselius Foundation, and EVO funding from Kuopio University Hospital (Finland: US, KHH, JH, MJS, MK, KP, MU); the Druvan Foundation, ESPEN, Skåne County Council Research and Development Foundation, Swedish Research Council for Health, Working Life and Welfare, EXODIAB (Excellence of Diabetes Research in Sweden), The Heart-Lung Foundation, Diabetesfonden and Foundation Cerealia

(Sweden: RL, LC, BÅ, FR, UR); The Danish Obesity Research Centre (DanORC, www.danorc.dk), The Danish Council for Strategic Research (DairyHealth, BioFunCarb) (Denmark: LB, KH), The Agricultural Productivity Fund (Iceland: IG, OKM, IT) and the Icelandic Research Fund for graduate students (1206880061)http://rannis.is/ (OKM). The following companies provided food products for the study participants: Kesko Food Ltd, Raisio Group, Bunge Finland Ltd (Finland); Belico Food AB, Fazer Bageri Sverige, Lantmännen, Oatly AB, Olle Svensson AB, Procordia Food AB, Pågen AB, Unilever, Wasabröd AB (Sweden); Lantmännen Food R&D, Jan Import A/S, Ardo A/S, Scandic Food A/S, WASA, Glyngøre Limfjord A/S, Royal Greenland A/S, Arla Foods (Denmark); The Mother Earth Farm at Vallanes (Iceland); and Unilever Nordic (Sweden, Denmark, Iceland). The funders had no role in study design, data collection and analysis, decision to publish, or preparation of the manuscript.

Competing Interests: The following companies provided food products for the study participants: Kesko Food Ltd, Raisio Group, Bunge Finland Ltd (Finland); Belico Food AB, Fazer Bageri Sverige, Lantmännen, Oatly AB, Olle Svensson AB, Procordia Food AB, Pågen AB, Unilever, Wasabröd AB (Sweden); Lantmännen Food R & D, Jan Import A/S, Ardo A/S, Scandic Food A/S, WASA, Glyngøre Limfjord A/S, Royal Greenland A/S, Arla Foods (Denmark); The Mother Earth Farm at Vallanes (Iceland); and Unilever Nordic (Sweden, Denmark, Iceland).

* Email: olakally@landspitali.is

Introduction

Epidemiological studies have shown an inverse relationship between diets rich in whole grain and the risk of many diet-related diseases, including cardiovascular diseases [1,2], metabolic syndrome [3] and type 2 diabetes [4]. A number of intervention studies have shown that intake of whole grains lowers serum total and LDL cholesterol concentrations [5–8], blood pressure [9,10] and improves insulin sensitivity [11–13]. Animal studies have shown cholesterol lowering effects of rye consumption [14–16] but few intervention studies have studied the effects of rye on blood lipids in humans, despite the fact that whole grain rye products contain substantial amounts of extractable arabinoxylans and β-glucans [17] that may contribute to cholesterol reduction. One study has shown that rye bread consumption decreased total and LDL cholesterol concentrations in men with moderately elevated serum cholesterol [5] but another study showed an unfavorable shift in serum cholesterol concentrations after rye bread intake in postmenopausal women [18].

In nutritional science it is essential to have accurate dietary information to assess compliance to dietary interventions and to investigate diet-disease associations. Collecting valid data on whole grain intake can, however, be challenging due to the broad selection of foods contributing to these intakes [19]. The use of alkylresorcinols (AR) as dietary biomarkers for whole grain wheat and rye intake could improve the validity of dietary assessment of whole grain in combination with, or as an alternative for, self-reports [19–22]. It may also be used as a tool for secondary analysis, where non-compliant individuals can be excluded on the basis of the biomarker measurements. AR are 3,5-dihydroxyphenolic lipids with an odd-numbered alkyl chain generally ranging from C17 to C25. Among commonly consumed foods, AR are almost exclusively present in the outer parts of wheat and rye grains, and just at trace amounts in refined white flour [23,24]. The ratio of the AR homologues C17:0 and C21:0 differs between cereals but is consistent within cereal species (approximately 0.1 in wheat and 1 in rye) [24] and may be used to differentiate sources of cereals consumed via plasma measurements [25]. We have previously demonstrated that AR are useful biomarkers for whole grain wheat and rye intake as part of a healthy Nordic diet [26]. Furthermore, significant between-group changes in non-HDL cholesterol concentrations and LDL to HDL cholesterol ratio was found in the randomized dietary intervention with a healthy Nordic diet (SYSDIET) [27].

The present study is based on a secondary analysis of the SYSDIET intervention trial and the aim was to investigate the association between plasma AR, a biomarker for whole grain wheat and rye intake, and blood lipid concentrations in a population with metabolic syndrome (MetS) participating in a randomized dietary intervention. Furthermore, the associations between the AR C17:0/C21:0 ratio, a suggested marker of the relative whole grain/bran rye intake, and blood lipids were analyzed.

Methods

The current study was a part of the SYSDIET study, a randomized controlled multicenter parallel group study with balanced randomization (1:1) performed in six intervention centers (Kuopio and Oulu, Finland; Lund and Uppsala, Sweden; Aarhus, Denmark and Reykjavik, Iceland) examining the health effects of a healthy Nordic diet (ND) in a population with MetS. The protocol for this trial and supporting CONSORT checklist are available as supporting information; see Checklist S1 and Protocol S1.

All local ethical committees (Research Ethics Committee of the Hospital District of Northern Savo and Northern Ostrobothnia Hospital District, Oulu, Finland, Regional Ethical Review Board, Lund and The Regional Ethical Review Board in Uppsala, Sweden, Ethical Committee of Aarhus County, Denmark and The Icelandic Bioethics Committee, Iceland) approved the SYSDIET study protocol which followed the Helsinki declaration guidelines and informed written consent was obtained from all participants. The trial was registered at ClinicalTrials.gov (ClinicalTrials identifier: NCT00992641, http://clinicaltrials.gov/ct2/show/NCT00992641?term=NCT00992641&rank=1) in October 2009, once all local ethical committees had given their approval. The authors confirm that all ongoing and related trials for this intervention are registered.

The study design, inclusion and exclusion criteria, study diets, the main measurements and analyses performed at each time point and main results have previously been reported in detail [27]. The present study is a secondary analysis where the association between AR and blood lipids at the end of the intervention was examined.

Study participants

Participants in the study were primarily recruited through advertisements in newspapers, but also from previous clinical or epidemiological trials. In brief, the inclusion criteria were age 30–65 years, body mass index (BMI) 27–40 kg/m^2, and two diagnostic criteria for metabolic syndrome as outlined by the International Diabetes Federation [28], except type 2 diabetes.

Study design

Participants were randomly assigned to either a healthy Nordic diet or an average Nordic (control) diet for 18 or 24 weeks. Due to financial and logistic reasons the study period was 18 weeks at 4 centers (Aarhus, Uppsala, Reykjavik and Oulu) and 24 weeks at 2 centers (Lund and Kuopio) where the intervention was initiated earlier [27]. The major visits to the study clinics were on week 0 (baseline), week 12 and week 18/24. In Kuopio and Lund, the intervention was carried out from October 2009 to June 2010, in Aarhus, from January 2010 to September 2010, in Oulu, from

December 2009 to October 2010, in Reykjavik, from March 2010 to October 2010 and in Uppsala, from June 2010 to November 2010.

The randomization was done by staff in each study center as described elsewhere [26]. The staff in all study centers was trained to perform measurements in a similar way and the quality management protocol was available for all staff members. The allowed weight change during the study was aimed to be less than ±4 kg due to the isocaloric design applied.

Study diets

The study diets were planned to be isocaloric. Nordic nutrition recommendations formed the basis of the diet in the ND group [29] and the mean nutrient intake in the Nordic countries formed the basis for the control diet. Participants in the ND group were advised to consume ≥25% of total energy as whole grain, of which ≥50% was comprised of rye, barley and oat which included ≥6 slices/day of bread with ≥6 g fiber/100 g (one slice equals 30–40 g of bread). Participants in the control group were asked to consume ≥25% of energy as refined grain, of which ≥90% made from wheat. Furthermore, the participants in the ND group were encouraged to consume ≥500 g of fruits, vegetables and berries daily, use rapeseed and/or sunflower and/or soybean oil based margarines, choose low fat milk and dairy products, consume three fish meals a week, choose low fat meat, and to avoid sugar-sweetened beverages while the control group was advised to keep their habitual diet. Key food products were provided to the study participants in both groups. The individuals in the ND group received whole grain products such as oatmeal and barley, crisp breads, whole grain wheat and rye breads. The individuals in the control group received low fiber cereal products, e.g. breads with fiber content less than 6 g/100 g and ordinary pasta. The study diets have previously been described in detail [27].

The participants were instructed by a clinical nutritionist or a dietitian at all study visits. The study participants kept dietary records regarding the intake of cereal products. These records were checked at each visit to the study center, including the visits when the groceries were delivered to the participants, i.e. at 1–2 week intervals and the subjects also returned 4-day weighed food records at baseline, week 2, 12 and 18/24 [27].

Biochemical measurements

Blood samples were collected at week 0, 12 and 18/24. Automated clinical chemistry analyzers and routine clinical chemistry methods were used to measure concentrations of total and HDL cholesterol, triglycerides and apoplipoproteins A1 and B. The equipment and system reagents and CV%'s have been described previously [27]. LDL cholesterol concentrations were calculated using Friedewald's formula.

Determination of AR in plasma samples were made in collaboration with the HELGA-Centre at Department of Food Science, BioCenter at Swedish University of Agricultural Sciences. A gas chromatography mass spectrometry (GC-MS) method was used to quantify AR homologues C17:0–C25:0 in 0.2 ml plasma samples as described previously [30]. Quality control samples (n = 4) was included in each batch to ensure appropriate within- and between batch precision (CV <15%). Samples from each subject were analyzed within the same batch and samples from different centers were allocated randomly between batches.

Data pooling and statistical analysis

All intervention centers entered their data into Microsoft Office Excel 2007 (Windows) data form prior to pooling the data in a joint database maintained at VTT Technical Research Centre of Finland. Data was exported from the database and imported to SPSS (Statistical Package for the Social Sciences) for Windows, version 20.0 (SPSS Inc., Chicago, Illinois, USA) for statistical analysis. Level of significance in all analyses was set at $P<0.05$.

Normality of variables was checked by inspection and by using the Kolmogorov–Smirnov test. Values are described as means and standard deviations (SD) if normally distributed or as medians and interquartile range (IQR) if not normally distributed.

The analyses were performed with data from the ND and control groups combined and associations between total AR and the AR C17:0/C21:0 ratio at 18/24 weeks and various blood lipid outcomes were analyzed. Where distributions were skewed (every variable except total and LDL cholesterol concentrations), log-transformation was performed on dependent variables for linear regression to better approximate normal distribution. The distribution of AR C17:0/C21:0 ratio across total plasma AR was checked by inspection.

Linear regressions for fasting concentrations of total, LDL, HDL, non-HDL cholesterol, apolipoproteins A1 and B, triglycerides and LDL/HDL cholesterol ratio with total plasma AR or AR C17:0/C21:0 ratio (model 1), baseline value for the dependent variable, age, BMI and statin use, as factors were performed. As rye often contains more AR than wheat, total plasma AR was added as a variable, in addition to the variables in model 1 when the associations between AR C17:0/C21:0 ratio was examined, to prevent confounding of high AR content (model 2). To account for multiple testing, we used the Bonferroni correction approach, using a significance level of alpha divided by the number of independent outcomes, that is 0.05/8 = 0.006. Furthermore, we individually adjusted for saturated fat intake calculated from food records and serum phospholipid fatty acids myristic acid, palmitic acid, omega-3 fatty acids and C15:0, to prevent confounding of dietary fat intake.

Results

Altogether 166 participants finished the study and of those 158 subjects had blood samples for AR and blood lipid analyses from all time points and that group was used for analyses in the present study (Figure 1). There was no difference between dropouts and those who completed the study in baseline BMI ($P = 0.797$), waist circumference ($P = 0.228$), age ($P = 0.959$) or triglyceride ($P = 0.055$), total cholesterol ($P = 0.743$), HDL cholesterol ($P = 0.216$) or LDL cholesterol ($P = 0.686$) concentrations.

There was no change in total energy intake during the study and energy intake was not different between the groups, hence, body weight remained constant during the intervention in both groups. The mean age of the participants was 54.5 (8.2) years, body weight 91.2 (13.5) kg, BMI 31.7 (3.2) kg/m^2 and waist circumference 104.3 (9.7) cm as described previously [31]. Baseline lipid concentrations and the number of statin users in by intervention group, are shown in Table 1. The prevalence of MetS was 90%. No differences were observed between the groups at baseline in clinical characteristics.

There were small, but significant, decrease in concentrations of total cholesterol (5.1 (1.2) mmol/L at 18/24 weeks, $P = 0.018$), LDL (3.2 (1.1) mmol/L at 18/24 weeks, $P = 0.006$) and non-HDL cholesterol (3.8 (1.3) mmol/L at 18/24 weeks, $P = 0.006$) and LDL/HDL cholesterol ratio (2.3 (1.3) at 18/24 weeks, $P = 0.003$) within the ND group from week 0 to 18/24 but not within the control group. Results on the effects of the SYSDIET intervention, with ND, on blood lipid concentrations and other health outcomes have been reported previously [27]. Both total plasma AR concentration and the ratio of C17:0/C21:0 were significantly

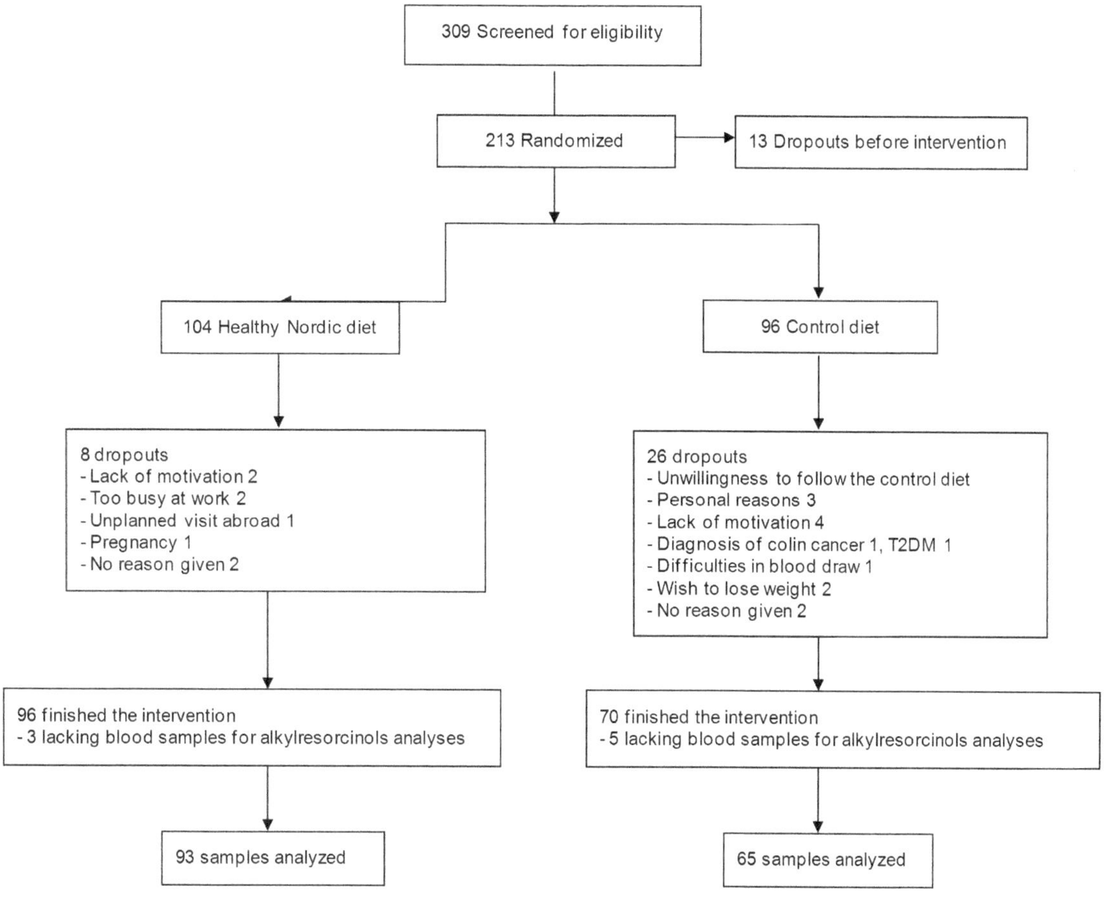

Figure 1. Flow chart of the study.

higher in the ND group than in the control group at 18/24 week (Table 2) and the range of total plasma AR was 14 to 499 nmol/L. There was no skew towards higher AR C17:0/C21:0 ratios for higher total plasma AR concentrations.

All participants (both ND and control groups) were combined for secondary analyses on the associations between AR and blood lipids concentrations at 18/24 weeks. Total plasma AR concentration at 18/24 weeks was not significantly correlated with concentrations of fasting serum total cholesterol ($P = 0.95$), LDL cholesterol ($P = 0.23$), HDL cholesterol ($P = 0.25$), LDL-C/HDL-C ratio ($P = 0.13$), triglycerides ($P = 0.14$), apolipoprotein A1 ($P = 0.09$) or apolipoprotein B ($P = 0.86$) after adjusting for

Table 1. Baseline blood lipid concentrations and statin use of the participants.

	ND group (n = 93)	Control group (n = 65)
Total cholesterol, *mmol/L*	5.3 (1.2)	5.1 (1.5)
HDL cholesterol, *mmol/L*	1.4 (0.5)	1.3 (0.6)
LDL cholesterol, *mmol/L*	3.2 (1.1)	3.1 (1.5)
Non-HDL cholesterol, *mmol/L*	3.9 (1.3)	3.7 (1.6)
LDL-C/HDL-C	2.5 (1.4)	2.4 (1.8)
Triglycerides 0 min, *mmol/L*	1.3 (0.8)	1.4 (0.8)
Apolipoprotein A1, *g/L*	1.4 (0.3)	1.4 (0.3)
Apolipoprotein B, *g/L*	1.0 (0.4)	1.0 (0.4)
Statin use, *n*	19	18

Values are presented as medians (IQR).
Abbreviations: HDL, high-density lipoprotein; LDL, low-density lipoprotein.

Table 2. Dietary fiber intake, total plasma alkylresorcinols (AR) concentration and AR C17:0/C21:0 ratio for the healthy Nordic diet group (ND) and control group at baseline and after the 18/24 week intervention.

	ND group (n = 93)		Control group (n = 65)	
	Week 0	**Week 18/24**	**Week 0**	**Week 18/24**
Dietary fiber intake[1,2], *g/day*	21.1 (8.8)	36.0 (15.1)[#]	20.0 (7.1)	16.0 (6.2)*[#]
Total plasma AR[1], *nmol/L*	73 (88)	106 (108)[#]	71 (70)	61 (40)*[#]
C17:0/C21:0 ratio[1]	0.3±0.2	0.3±0.2	0.3±0.2	0.2±0.2*[#]

Values are medians (IQR).
*significantly different from ND group at that time point.
[#]significantly different from baseline.
[1]Data published previously [31].
[2]n = 140, ND group n = 80 and control group n = 40.
Abbreviations: ND, healthy Nordic diet; AR, alkylresorcinols.

confounders. However, the AR C17:0/C21:0 ratio, which reflects the proportion of whole grain rye of whole grain rye and whole grain wheat combined, was inversely associated with LDL cholesterol concentration when adjusted for baseline LDL cholesterol concentration, BMI, age and statin use (model 1, $P = 0.040$) and also when total plasma AR was added to the regression model (model 2, $P = 0.046$) (Table 3).

Table 3. Regression models for concentrations of serum total, HDL, LDL, non HDL cholesterol and triglycerides and the cholesterol LDL-C/HDL-C ratio.

Dependent variable at 18/24 weeks	Independent variable at 18/24 weeks	B[1] (95% CI)
Total cholesterol		
Model 1	AR C17:0/C21:0	−0.33 (−0.78 to 0.12)
Model 2	AR C17:0/C21:0	−0.33 (−0.78 to 0.12)
LDL cholesterol		
Model 1	AR C17:0/C21:0	−0.41 (−0.80 to −0.02)
Model 2	AR C17:0/C21:0	−0.40 (−0.79 to −0.01)
Log HDL cholesterol		
Model 1	AR C17:0/C21:0	0.11 (0.00 to 0.21)
Model 2	AR C17:0/C21:0	0.11 (0.00 to 0.21)
Log LDL-C/HDL-C cholesterol		
Model 1	AR C17:0/C21:0	−0.20 (−0.37 to −0.03)
Model 2	AR C17:0/C21:0	−0.20 (−0.37 to −0.03)
Log non HDL cholesterol		
Model 1	AR C17:0/C21:0	−0.84 (−1.22 to −0.45)
Model 2	AR C17:0/C21:0	−0.81 (−1.19 to −0.44)
Log triglycerides		
Model 1	AR C17:0/C21:0	−0.35 (−0.59 to −0.12)
Model 2	AR C17:0/C21:0	−0.37 (−0.60 to −0.13)
Log apolipoprotein A1		
Model 1	AR C17:0/C21:0	0.05 (−0.03 to 0.13)
Model 2	AR C17:0/C21:0	0.05 (−0.03 to 0.13)
Log apoliprotein B		
Model 1	AR C17:0/C21:0	−0.12 (−0.24 to 0.00)
Model 2	AR C17:0/C21:0	−0.12 (−0.24 to 0.00)

[1]B reflects the change in the log-transformed outcome variable for each 1-unit changes in the independent variable.
Model 1: adjusted for baseline value of the dependent variable, BMI, age and statin use.
Model 2: adjusted for baseline value of the dependent variable, total AR, BMI, age and statin use.
Abbreviations: ND, healthy Nordic diet; AR, alkylresorcinols; HDL, high-density lipoprotein; LDL, low-density lipoprotein; BMI, body mass index.

Similarly, AR C17:0/C21:0 ratio was inversely associated with LDL/HDL cholesterol ratio ($P = 0.020$ and $P = 0.024$ for model 1 and model 2, respectively), non-HDL cholesterol ($P<0.001$ for both model 1 and model 2), triglyceride ($P = 0.004$ and $P = 0.002$ for model 1 and model 2, respectively) and apolipoprotein B concentrations ($P = 0.047$ for both model 1 and model 2) and positively associated with HDL cholesterol concentration ($P = 0.044$ and $P = 0.049$ for model 1 and model 2, respectively). Including saturated fatty acids calculated from food records to the models did not change the results nor did including the serum phospholipid fatty acids myristic acid, palmitic acid, omega-3 fatty acids and C15:0, except for HDL cholesterol in which the association with C17:0/C21:0 became borderline significant ($P = 0.067$). However, using the Bonferroni correction approach to account for multiple testing the associations for LDL cholesterol, HDL cholesterol, LDL/HDL cholesterol ratio and apolipoprotein B concentrations would not be considered significant while associations for non-HDL cholesterol and triglyceride concentration are robust for this correction ($P<0.006$).

Discussion

Favorable changes in serum LDL cholesterol concentration and LDL to HDL cholesterol ratio were observed in participants consuming a healthy Nordic diet, established with a healthy dietary pattern approach, and thus also rich in whole grain cereals, for either 18 or 24 weeks [27]. In the intervention the participants in the ND group were advised to consume ≥25% of total energy as whole grain, of which ≥50% was comprised of rye, barley and oat, and to make favorable changes in dietary fat intake, and therefore a change in serum cholesterol concentration in the ND group was expected. Some studies have found that whole grain diets lower serum total and LDL cholesterol concentrations [5–8]. The cholesterol lowering effects of β-glucans in oats and barley have been extensively studied [32,33] and the European Food Safety Authority (EFSA) has approved two health claims on the subject: β-glucans contribute to the maintenance of normal blood cholesterol levels [34] and oat β-glucan has been shown to lower/reduce blood cholesterol. Blood cholesterol lowering by increased oats intake may reduce the risk of (coronary) heart disease [35].

In the present study, both ND and control groups were pooled for secondary analysis on the association between plasma AR and blood lipids at 18/24 weeks. Plasma AR has been established as a biomarker for whole grain wheat and rye intake [19,21,26] and has previously been studied regarding associations with BMI and metabolic risk factors [36,37]. We observed no association between total plasma AR concentration and serum lipid concentrations, possibly due to a considerable amount of AR intake originating from whole grain wheat. Whole grain wheat intake does typically not affect blood cholesterol and is thus often used as a control in experimental studies [38]. Interestingly, the AR C17:0/C21:0 ratio, an indicator of relative rye intake, was associated with favorable changes in concentrations of LDL-, HDL-, and non HDL cholesterol, LDL/HDL cholesterol ratio and triglycerides, even after adjustment for fatty acids composition of serum phospholipids, with the exception of HDL cholesterol where the association became borderline significant. The ratio of the AR homologues C17:0 and C21:0 differs between cereal species and can be used to differentiate between the whole grain sources in food products [24]. The ratio of AR C17:0/C21:0 is approximately 0.1 in wheat and 1 in rye and the ratio is to some extent reflected in fasting plasma samples, although it is generally lower, typically around 0.6–0.8 in fasting samples after a whole grain rye intervention for 1–8 weeks, and can be used to differentiate which AR containing cereals have been consumed [25,39,40].

Health effects of rye are far less studied than oats and barley and studies on the effects of rye consumption on cholesterol are scarce. The mechanisms that have been proposed to cause the reduction in plasma cholesterol levels focus on the fiber and phytochemical content of whole grains, particularly water-soluble viscose fiber [41,42], and it has been established that the cholesterol lowering effect of β-glucans is dependent on the molecular weight and subsequent viscosity [43]. Rye is particularly high in dietary fiber, ranging between 18–22%, and it contains substantial amounts of extractable β-glucans and arabinoxylans, which could contribute to cholesterol reduction through a similar mechanism as β-glucans from oats and barley [17,44]. Animal studies have shown that rye could affect blood lipid concentrations by increasing the total concentration of bile acids in the bile [14–15].

Previous studies have shown that rye bread consumption decreases total and LDL cholesterol concentrations in men with moderately elevated serum cholesterol [5], and lower concentrations of plasma free-cholesterol, total cholesterol, triglycerides and phospholipids have been demonstrated after a high fiber rye diet than a low fiber wheat diet [6]. Additionally, animal studies have shown cholesterol lowering effects of rye consumption [14–16]. However, Moazzami et al showed an unfavorable shift in serum cholesterol levels after rye bread intake in postmenopausal women [18]. Processing of rye and other whole grains, such as fermentation, have been reported to influence the molecular weight of cereal dietary fiber, hence it is possible that lower viscosity of the fibers could explain the lack of beneficial effects reported in some studies [17]. Nevertheless, the results of the present study suggest that whole grain rye consumption is associated with favorable outcomes in blood lipids and this association should be further studied.

One of the strengths of the present study is that we used AR as a dietary biomarker for whole grain rye and wheat intake instead of self-reported estimates. As collecting valid data on whole grain intake can be challenging, the use of biomarkers to assess intake and/or compliance to dietary interventions is a way to avoid some of the obstacles associated with self-reporting [19]. Previously, we have demonstrated that AR is a good biomarker for the ND under intervention conditions with moderate to good reliability [26] and our data supports the use of the AR C17:0/C21:0 ratio as an indicator for whole grain rye intake in intervention studies where a diet rich in whole grain rye is being investigated [31]. Although the AR C17:0/C21:0 ratio reflects only the relative whole grain/bran rye consumption of total whole grain wheat and rye intake, and not the total rye intake, the advised whole grain rye intake in the present study was high in relation to other sources of AR and therefore the ratio should reflect the total rye intake reasonably well. However, the present study does not offer any mechanistic explanations behind the possible cholesterol-lowering by whole grain rye, and more needs to be done to explain the association. Nevertheless, the results do motivate further research on this topic. Some confounding effects from oats intake are possible, as participants consuming more rye might also consume more oats, and confounding effects from other food sources cannot be excluded. However, this is probably not explaining the main results. Previous studies suggest that plasma AR may be transported in VLDL and HDL [45], which could affect the results of the present study, as well as numerous dietary and non-dietary factors potentially influencing biomarker concentrations [19]. Nevertheless, since the AR C17:0/C21:0 ratio, but not total plasma AR, was associated with cholesterol concentrations, and the associations did not change when adjusted for total plasma

AR, we believe our findings indicate that the associations we found are related to whole grain rye intake and not by the fact that AR may be transported in certain lipoproteins.

Conclusion

Our findings suggest that a greater proportion of whole grain rye in a Nordic diet is associated with favorable outcomes in blood lipid concentrations, an association that warrants further investigation.

Supporting Information

Checklist S1 Consort 2010 checklist of information to include when reporting a randomized trial.

Protocol S1 SYSDIET study plan.

Acknowledgments

Authors express sincere gratitude to the participants taking part in the study. We also thank all staff involved in the intervention.

Author Contributions

Conceived and designed the experiments: BÅ US KHH MJS KH MK KP MU UR IT. Performed the experiments: OKM IG LC FR US JH LB MK UR. Analyzed the data: OKM RL. Contributed reagents/materials/analysis tools: RL. Contributed to the writing of the manuscript: OKM RL IG BÅ MU UR IT.

References

1. McKeown NM, Meigs JB, Liu S, Wilson PW, Jacques PF (2002) Whole-grain intake is favorably associated with metabolic risk factors for type 2 diabetes and cardiovascular disease in the Framingham Offspring Study. Am J Clin Nutr 76: 390–398.
2. Mellen PB, Walsh TF, Herrington DM (2008) Whole grain intake and cardiovascular disease: a meta-analysis. Nutr Metab Cardiovasc Dis 18: 283–290.
3. Sahyoun NR, Jacques PF, Zhang XL, Juan W, McKeown NM (2006) Whole-grain intake is inversely associated with the metabolic syndrome and mortality in older adults. Am J Clin Nutr 83: 124–131.
4. de Munter JS, Hu FB, Spiegelman D, Franz M, van Dam RM (2007) Whole grain, bran, and germ intake and risk of type 2 diabetes: a prospective cohort study and systematic review. PLoS Med 4: e261.
5. Leinonen KS, Poutanen KS, Mykkanen HM (2000) Rye bread decreases serum total and LDL cholesterol in men with moderately elevated serum cholesterol. J Nutr 130: 164–170.
6. Lundin EA, Zhang JX, Lairon D, Tidehag P, Aman P, et al. (2004) Effects of meal frequency and high-fibre rye-bread diet on glucose and lipid metabolism and ileal excretion of energy and sterols in ileostomy subjects. Eur J Clin Nutr 58: 1410–1419.
7. Giacco R, Clemente G, Cipriano D, Luongo D, Viscovo D, et al. (2010) Effects of the regular consumption of wholemeal wheat foods on cardiovascular risk factors in healthy people. Nutr Metab Cardiovasc Dis 20: 186–194.
8. Ross AB, Bruce SJ, Blondel-Lubrano A, Oguey-Araymon S, Beaumont M, et al. (2011) A whole-grain cereal-rich diet increases plasma betaine, and tends to decrease total and LDL-cholesterol compared with a refined-grain diet in healthy subjects. Br J Nutr 105: 1492–1502.
9. Behall KM, Scholfield DJ, Hallfrisch J (2006) Whole-grain diets reduce blood pressure in mildly hypercholesterolemic men and women. J Am Diet Assoc 106: 1445–1449.
10. Tighe P, Duthie G, Vaughan N, Brittenden J, Simpson WG, et al. (2010) Effect of increased consumption of whole-grain foods on blood pressure and other cardiovascular risk markers in healthy middle-aged persons: a randomized controlled trial. Am J Clin Nutr 92: 733–740.
11. Leinonen K, Liukkonen K, Poutanen K, Uusitupa M, Mykkanen H (1999) Rye bread decreases postprandial insulin response but does not alter glucose response in healthy Finnish subjects. Eur J Clin Nutr 53: 262–267.
12. Juntunen KS, Laaksonen DE, Poutanen KS, Niskanen LK, Mykkanen HM (2003) High-fiber rye bread and insulin secretion and sensitivity in healthy postmenopausal women. Am J Clin Nutr 77: 385–391.
13. Pereira MA, Jacobs DR, Jr., Pins JJ, Raatz SK, Gross MD, et al. (2002) Effect of whole grains on insulin sensitivity in overweight hyperinsulinemic adults. Am J Clin Nutr 75: 848–855.
14. Lund EK, Salf KL, Johnson IT (1993) Baked rye products modify cholesterol metabolism and crypt cell proliferation rates in rats. J Nutr 123: 1834–1843.
15. Zhang JX, Lundin E, Reuterving CO, Hallmans G, Stenling R, et al. (1994) Effects of rye bran, oat bran and soya-bean fibre on bile composition, gallstone formation, gall-bladder morphology and serum cholesterol in Syrian golden hamsters (Mesocricetus auratus). Br J Nutr 71: 861–870.
16. Andersson U, Rosen L, Ostman E, Strom K, Wierup N, et al. (2010) Metabolic effects of whole grain wheat and whole grain rye in the C57BL/6J mouse. Nutrition 26: 230–239.
17. Rakha A, Åman P, Andersson R (2010) Characterisation of dietary fibre components in rye products. Food Chemistry 119: 859–867.
18. Moazzami AA, Bondia-Pons I, Hanhineva K, Juntunen K, Antl N, et al. (2012) Metabolomics reveals the metabolic shifts following an intervention with rye bread in postmenopausal women–a randomized control trial. Nutr J 11: 88.
19. Ross AB, Bourgeois A, Macharia HN, Kochhar S, Jebb SA, et al. (2012) Plasma alkylresorcinols as a biomarker of whole-grain food consumption in a large population: results from the WHOLEheart Intervention Study. Am J Clin Nutr 95: 204–211.
20. Ross AB, Kamal-Eldin A, Aman P (2004) Dietary alkylresorcinols: absorption, bioactivities, and possible use as biomarkers of whole-grain wheat- and rye-rich foods. Nutr Rev 62: 81–95.
21. Landberg R, Kamal-Eldin A, Andersson A, Vessby B, Aman P (2008) Alkylresorcinols as biomarkers of whole-grain wheat and rye intake: plasma concentration and intake estimated from dietary records. Am J Clin Nutr 87: 832–838.
22. Montonen J, Landberg R, Kamal-Eldin A, Aman P, Knueppel S, et al. (2010) Reliability of fasting plasma alkylresorcinol concentrations measured 4 months apart. Eur J Clin Nutr 64: 698–703.
23. Ross AB, Shepherd MJ, Schupphaus M, Sinclair V, Alfaro B, et al. (2003) Alkylresorcinols in cereals and cereal products. J Agric Food Chem 51: 4111–4118.
24. Chen Y, Ross AB, Aman P, Kamal-Eldin A (2004) Alkylresorcinols as markers of whole grain wheat and rye in cereal products. J Agric Food Chem 52: 8242–8246.
25. Linko-Parvinen AM, Landberg R, Tikkanen MJ, Adlercreutz H, Penalvo JL (2007) Alkylresorcinols from whole-grain wheat and rye are transported in human plasma lipoproteins. J Nutr 137: 1137–1142.
26. Magnusdottir OK, Landberg R, Gunnarsdottir I, Cloetens L, Akesson B, et al. (2013) Plasma Alkylresorcinols Reflect Important Whole-Grain Components of a Healthy Nordic Diet. J Nutr.
27. Uusitupa M, Hermansen K, Savolainen MJ, Schwab U, Kolehmainen M, et al. (2013) Effects of an isocaloric healthy Nordic diet on insulin sensitivity, lipid profile and inflammation markers in metabolic syndrome – a randomized study (SYSDIET). J Intern Med 274: 52–66.
28. Alberti KG, Eckel RH, Grundy SM, Zimmet PZ, Cleeman JI, et al. (2009) Harmonizing the metabolic syndrome: a joint interim statement of the International Diabetes Federation Task Force on Epidemiology and Prevention; National Heart, Lung, and Blood Institute; American Heart Association; World Heart Federation; International Atherosclerosis Society; and International Association for the Study of Obesity. Circulation 120: 1640–1645.
29. (2004) Nordic Nutrition Recommendations 2004 Intergrating nutrition and physical activity. Copenhagen: Nordic Council of Ministers.
30. Landberg R, Åman P, Kamal-Eldin A (2009) A rapid gas chromatography-mass spectrometry method for quantification of alkylresorcinols in human plasma. Anal Biochem 385: 7–12.
31. Magnusdottir OK, Landberg R, Gunnarsdottir I, Cloetens L, Akesson B, et al. (2014) Plasma alkylresorcinols C17: 0/C21: 0 ratio, a biomarker of relative whole-grain rye intake, is associated to insulin sensitivity: a randomized study. Eur J Clin Nutr 68: 453–458.
32. Tiwari U, Cummins E (2011) Meta-analysis of the effect of beta-glucan intake on blood cholesterol and glucose levels. Nutrition 27: 1008–1016.
33. Othman RA, Moghadasian MH, Jones PJ (2011) Cholesterol-lowering effects of oat beta-glucan. Nutr Rev 69: 299–309.
34. EFSA Panel on Dietetic Products, Nutrition and Allergies (NDA). *Scientific Opinion on the substantiation of health claims related to beta glucans and maintenance of normal blood cholesterol concentrations (ID 754, 755, 757, 801, 1465, 2934) and maintenance or achievement of a normal body weight (ID 820, 823) pursuant to Article 13(1) of Regulation (EC) No 1924/2006.* EFSA Journal 2009; 7(9): 1254 [18]. 10.2903/j.efsa.2009.1254 Available online: www.efsa.europa.eu/efsajournal. Accessed February 20 2014.
35. EFSA Panel on Dietetic Products, Nutrition and Allergies (NDA). *Scientific Opinion on the substantiation of a health claim related to oat beta glucan and lowering blood cholesterol and reduced risk of (coronary) heart disease pursuant to Article 14 of Regulation (EC) No 1924/2006.* EFSA Journal 2010;8(12): 1885 [15]. 10.2903/j.efsa.2010.1885 Available online:www.efsa.europa.eu/efsajournal. Accessed February 20 2014.

36. Ma J, Ross AB, Shea MK, Bruce SJ, Jacques PF, et al. (2012) Plasma Alkylresorcinols, Biomarkers of Whole-Grain Intake, Are Related to Lower BMI in Older Adults. J Nutr 142: 1859–1864.
37. Magnusdottir OK, Landberg R, Gunnarsdottir I, Cloetens L, Akesson B, et al. (2014) Plasma alkylresorcinols C17: 0/C21: 0 ratio, a biomarker of relative whole-grain rye intake, is associated to insulin sensitivity: a randomized study. Eur J Clin Nutr.
38. Jenkins DJ, Kendall CW, Vuksan V, Augustin LS, Mehling C, et al. (1999) Effect of wheat bran on serum lipids: influence of particle size and wheat protein. J Am Coll Nutr 18: 159–165.
39. Landberg R, Aman P, Friberg LE, Vessby B, Adlercreutz H, et al. (2009) Dose response of whole-grain biomarkers: alkylresorcinols in human plasma and their metabolites in urine in relation to intake. Am J Clin Nutr 89: 290–296.
40. Ross AB (2012) Present status and perspectives on the use of alkylresorcinols as biomarkers of wholegrain wheat and rye intake. J Nutr Metab 2012: 462967.
41. Slavin JL, Jacobs D, Marquart L, Wiemer K (2001) The role of whole grains in disease prevention. J Am Diet Assoc 101: 780–785.
42. Fardet A (2010) New hypotheses for the health-protective mechanisms of whole-grain cereals: what is beyond fibre? Nutr Res Rev 23: 65–134.
43. Wolever TM, Tosh SM, Gibbs AL, Brand-Miller J, Duncan AM, et al. (2010) Physicochemical properties of oat beta-glucan influence its ability to reduce serum LDL cholesterol in humans: a randomized clinical trial. Am J Clin Nutr 92: 723–732.
44. Hansen HB, Rasmussen CV, Bach Knudsen KE, Hansen Å (2003) Effects of genotype and harvest year on content and composition of dietary fibre in rye (Secale cereale L) grain. Journal of the Science of Food and Agriculture 83: 76–85.
45. Linko-Parvinen AM, Landberg R, Tikkarren MJ, Adlercreutz H, Penalvo JL (2007) Alkylresorcinols from whole-grain wheat and rye are transported in human plasma lipoproteins. Journal of Nutrition 137: 1137–1142.

Erythrocytic Mobilization Enhanced by the Granulocyte Colony-Stimulating Factor Is Associated with Reduced Anthrax-Lethal-Toxin-Induced Mortality in Mice

Hsin-Hou Chang[1,2], Ya-Wen Chiang[1], Ting-Kai Lin[1], Guan-Ling Lin[2], You-Yen Lin[2], Jyh-Hwa Kau[3], Hsin-Hsien Huang[4], Hui-Ling Hsu[4], Jen-Hung Wang[5], Der-Shan Sun[1,2]*

1 Department of Molecular Biology and Human Genetics, Tzu-Chi University, Hualien, Taiwan, **2** Institute of Medical Sciences, Tzu-Chi University, Hualien, Taiwan, **3** Department of Microbiology and Immunology, National Defense Medical Center, Taipei, Taiwan, **4** Institute of Preventive Medicine, National Defense Medical Center, Taipei, Taiwan, **5** Department of Medical Research, Tzu Chi General Hospital, Hualien, Taiwan

Abstract

Anthrax lethal toxin (LT), one of the primary virulence factors of *Bacillus anthracis*, causes anthrax-like symptoms and death in animals. Experiments have indicated that levels of erythrocytopenia and hypoxic stress are associated with disease severity after administering LT. In this study, the granulocyte colony-stimulating factor (G-CSF) was used as a therapeutic agent to ameliorate anthrax-LT- and spore-induced mortality in C57BL/6J mice. We demonstrated that G-CSF promoted the mobilization of mature erythrocytes to peripheral blood, resulting in a significantly faster recovery from erythrocytopenia. In addition, combined treatment using G-CSF and erythropoietin tended to ameliorate *B. anthracis*-spore-elicited mortality in mice. Although specific treatments against LT-mediated pathogenesis remain elusive, these results may be useful in developing feasible strategies to treat anthrax.

Editor: Nupur Gangopadhyay, University of Pittsburgh, United States of America

Funding: This work was supported by grants of National Science Council http://web1.nsc.gov.tw/mp.aspx (NSC 96-2311-B-320-005-MY3 and NSC 99-2311-B-320-003-MY3) and Tzu-Chi University http://www.tcu.edu.tw/ (610400130). The funders had no role in study design, data collection and analysis, decision to publish, or preparation of the manuscript.

Competing Interests: The authors have declared that no competing interests exist.

* Email: dssun@mail.tcu.edu.tw

Introduction

Infection with *Bacillus anthracis*, a gram-positive spore-forming bacterium, can lead to life-threatening anthrax [1]. Anthrax lethal toxin (LT) is comprised of a protective antigen (PA, 83 kDa) and lethal factor (LF, 90 kDa) [2–4], and is one of the primary virulence factors of *B. anthracis*. LF is a specific metalloprotease for mitogen-activated protein kinase (MAPK) kinases (MKKs/MEKs) [5], and can thus disrupt MAPK signaling cascades including p38 MAPK, p42/44 extracellular signal-regulated kinase (ERK), and c-Jun N-terminal kinase (JNK) [6,7]. All of these 3 MAPK pathways are critical in maintaining fundamental cellular homeostasis, including cell proliferation, differentiation, and apoptosis [8]. LF can be delivered into cells by PA, a cell-receptor binding component [3,9]. Although experimental LT treatments may not reproduce the full pathogenesis of anthrax, LT studies in cell or animal models have revealed certain pathogenic progressions. Various cell types, which include macrophages [10,11], dendritic cells [12], lymphocytes [13,14], erythrocytes [15], and megakaryocytes [16], cardiomyocytes [17], and smooth muscle [17], are sensitive to LT treatment. LT has been shown to suppress the differentiation and maturation of the progenitors of macrophages, megakaryocytes, and erythrocytes [15,16,18]. In addition, blood cell count analyses have indicated that LT treatment significantly reduced levels of circulating red blood cells (RBCs) and platelets in mice [15,16], suggesting multiple targets of LT in hematopoietic lineage cells. Deficiencies of platelets and RBCs may lead to hemorrhage and lethal hypoxic damage [19,20]. Because high levels of LT accumulate in the body when anthrax enters the bacteremia stage, death is typically inevitable even after aggressive antibiotic treatments. This suggests that a specific treatment to overcome the toxic effect is crucial in controlling the disease [21]. Unfortunately, an effective therapeutic approach against LT remains elusive.

Cytokine treatments, particularly hematopoietic growth factors, have been used in various clinical settings to rescue pathological defects [22]. Our previous demonstration was the first to indicate that thrombopoietin (TPO), a megakaryopoiesis-enhancing cytokine [23], can ameliorate LT-induced thrombopoiesis suppression, thrombocytopenia, and likely reduce the mortality in mice [16]. Our data also revealed that erythropoietin (EPO), a potent erythropoiesis-stimulating cytokine [24], ameliorated LT-induced erythropoiesis suppression (particularly those precursors in early erythropoiesis stages), erythrocytopenia, and reduced mortality rates from 100% to 50% after lethal-dose LT challenges in experimental mice [15]. Bone marrow is the primary stem niche supporting erythropoiesis, displaying technically-divided 4-differentiation stages of erythroblasts based on the expression levels of surface markers CD71 and TER-119 [25]. The transferrin receptor (CD71) is first expressed on early erythroblasts, such as erythroid burst-forming units (BFU-Es) and erythroid colony-forming units (CFU-Es) cells. Erythrocytic CD71 is downregulated by more mature erythroblasts [26]. By contrast, TER-119 is primarily expressed on relatively mature erythroblasts, reticulocytes, and mature erythrocytes [27]. Accordingly, 4 cell populations (CD71^{high}TER-119^{med}, CD71^{high}TER-119^{high}, CD71^{med}-TER-119^{high}, and CD71^{low}TER-119^{high}) can be defined, which are morphologically equivalent to proerythroblasts (flow cytometry-gated region 1; R1), basophilic erythroblasts (R2), late basophilic and polychromatophilic erythroblasts (R3), and orthochromatophilic erythroblasts (R4), from the early to late stages of erythroid differentiation, respectively [25]. Following these approaches, we are thus able to characterize the mechanism to use hematopoietic cytokines/growth factors as ameliorative agents to rescue anthrax LT-induced mortality [15,16].

The granulocyte colony-stimulating factor (G-CSF) has been found to regulate granulopoiesis [28], and is a multifunctional cytokine. For example, it has been found to stimulate cell proliferation, differentiation, enhance hematopoiesis, mobilize hematopoietic stem cells, and induce anti-apoptotic and anti-inflammatory effects [29–31]. Both G-CSF and EPO are U.S. FDA-approved drugs. Although the mechanism remains unclear, combined treatments using G-CSF and EPO were shown to ameliorate aplastic anemia in patients with myelodysplastic syndrome [32–36]. Given that EPO treatments are beneficial for LT-challenged mice [15], we hypothesized that combining G-CSF and EPO may be useful in treating anthrax. Consequently, we used mouse models to discuss the combined treatments of G-CSF and EPO on reduced anthrax LT and spore-induced mortality. In addition, we also discussed the differential erythropoietic regulation in response to G-CSF and EPO treatments.

Materials and Methods

Ethics Statement

Our research approaches involving experimental mice were approved by the Institutional Animal Care and Use Committee of Tzu Chi University (Approval ID: 98104) and the National Defense Medical Center (Approval ID: AN-100-04).

Toxins and spores

B. anthracis-derived LT was purified according to previously described procedures [49]. LT was delivered in a 1:5 ratio of LF and PA [16]. Spores derived from the *B. anthracis*-nonencapsulated mutant strain (pXO1$^+$, pXO2$^-$) were purchased from the American Type Culture Collection (Manassas, VA, USA) (ATCC 14186).

Erythroid colony-forming cell assay

The erythroid colony-forming cell assay was conducted according to the manufacturer's instructions (MethoCult M3334, StemCell Technologies). For the *in vitro* erythroid colony-forming cell assay, bone marrow cells were collected from the femurs and tibiae of C57BL/6J mice. C57BL/6J mice (males, 8–10 wk of age) were obtained from the National Laboratory Animal Center (Taipei, Taiwan) and kept in a specific pathogen-free (SPF) environment in the experimental animal center of Tzu Chi University. For the *ex vivo* erythroid colony-forming cell assay, C57BL/6J mice were retro-orbitally injected with 55 μg/kg/d of recombinant human G-CSF (Filgrastim, Kirin, Tokyo, Japan) in 250 μl saline, once daily for 5 d, initiated 5 d before the challenges of a lethal dose of LT (1.5 mg/kg in 250 μl saline, retro-orbitally injected). Treatments using saline, G-CSF, and LT alone were used as comparison controls. Bone marrow cells were collected at 69 h after LT treatment and flushed with Roswell Park Memorial Institute medium (RPMI)-1640 containing 20% anticoagulant acid citrate dextrose formula A (ACD-A: 38 mM citric acid, 75 mM trisodium citrate, 139 mM D-glucose, 12.5 mM EDTA [15]). After depleting RBCs by adding a hypotonic buffer (153 mM NH_4Cl and 17 mM Tris-HCl) at room temperature for 10 min, 100 μl of remaining cells (9×10^5/ml) were resuspended in Iscove's Modified Dulbecco's Medium (IMDM) (StemCell Technologies) and mixed with 1 ml of semisolid methylcellulose-based medium containing 3 units of EPO. Finally, each 1.1 ml of methylcellulose-cell suspension was mixed with or without a dose of G-CSF (20 ng/ml or 764 ng/ml) and duplicate seeded in 35-mm dishes. A G-CSF dose of 20 ng/ml was used in the colony-forming cell assay for hematopoietic cells [50]. Because the volume of mice blood is 70–80 ml/kg [51], a dose of 764 ng/ml approximated the dose used to ameliorate LT-induced mortality in the experiments. Two doses of G-CSF (20 ng/ml and 764 ng/ml) were added to the medium supplement of the erythroid colony-forming cell assay. The cultures were incubated at 37°C for 14 d. Dynamic changes in colony number were measured on Days 3, 7, and 14 after initiating the colony assay. The erythroid colonies were separated into 3 groups by size: small (8–50 cells), medium (more than 50, but less than 200 cells), and large (more than 200 cells).

Analysis of erythropoiesis in bone marrow

Bone marrow cells were purified and blocked with 5% bovine serum albumin in RPMI medium at 37°C for 1 h and incubated in 500 μl RPMI-1640 medium with 1 μl of fluorescein (FITC)-conjugated rat anti-mouse CD71 antibody (BioLegend) and 3 μl of R-Phycoerythrin (R-PE)-conjugated rat anti-mouse TER-119 antibody (BD Immunocytometry System) at 37°C for 1 h. After washing with phosphate-buffered saline (PBS), the cells were measured and analyzed using a FACSCalibur flow cytometer and the CellQuest^{TM} Pro program (Becton-Dickinson).

Flow cytometry analysis of peripheral blood cells of G-CSF-treated EGFP mice

EGFP mice [C57BL/6J-Tg (Pgk1-EGFP) 03Narl, males, 10–12 wk of age] were obtained from the National Laboratory Animal Center (Taipei, Taiwan) and maintained in the aforementioned SPF environments. EGFP mice were retro-orbitally injected with G-CSF (55 μg/kg/d in 250 μl saline) once daily for 4 d. To detect the erythrocytes' specific surface markers, 50 μl of retro-orbital blood samples were obtained 22, 44, 66, and 94 h after the initial G-CSF injection, and subsequently mixed with 450 μl of anticoagulant ACD-A (1:9). Cells were incubated in 300 μl of RPMI-1640 medium with 3 μl of the R-Phycoerythrin (R-PE)-conjugated rat anti-mouse TER-119 antibody (BD Immunocytometry System) at 37°C for 1 h. After washing with PBS, the cells were analyzed using a FACSCalibur flow cytometer and the CellQuest^{TM} Pro program.

G-CSF treatment to reduce LT-induced mortality

C57BL/6J mice (males, 8–10 wk of age) were retro-orbitally injected with 55 μg/kg/d of recombinant human G-CSF in 250 μl saline, once daily for 5 d, initiated 5 d before or 1 d after the challenges of a lethal dose of LT (1.5 mg/kg in 250 μl saline, retro-orbitally injected). Treatments using saline, G-CSF, and LT alone were used as comparison controls. Because no suitable potential predictor of death/survival exists for LT-challenged mice, we used death as an endpoint for the survival experiment. The survival time and mortality of mice were recorded after the LT challenges. LT treatment in mice did not induce obvious discomfort and body weight loss, except for reducing activities. The experimental mice were continually monitored up to 250 h

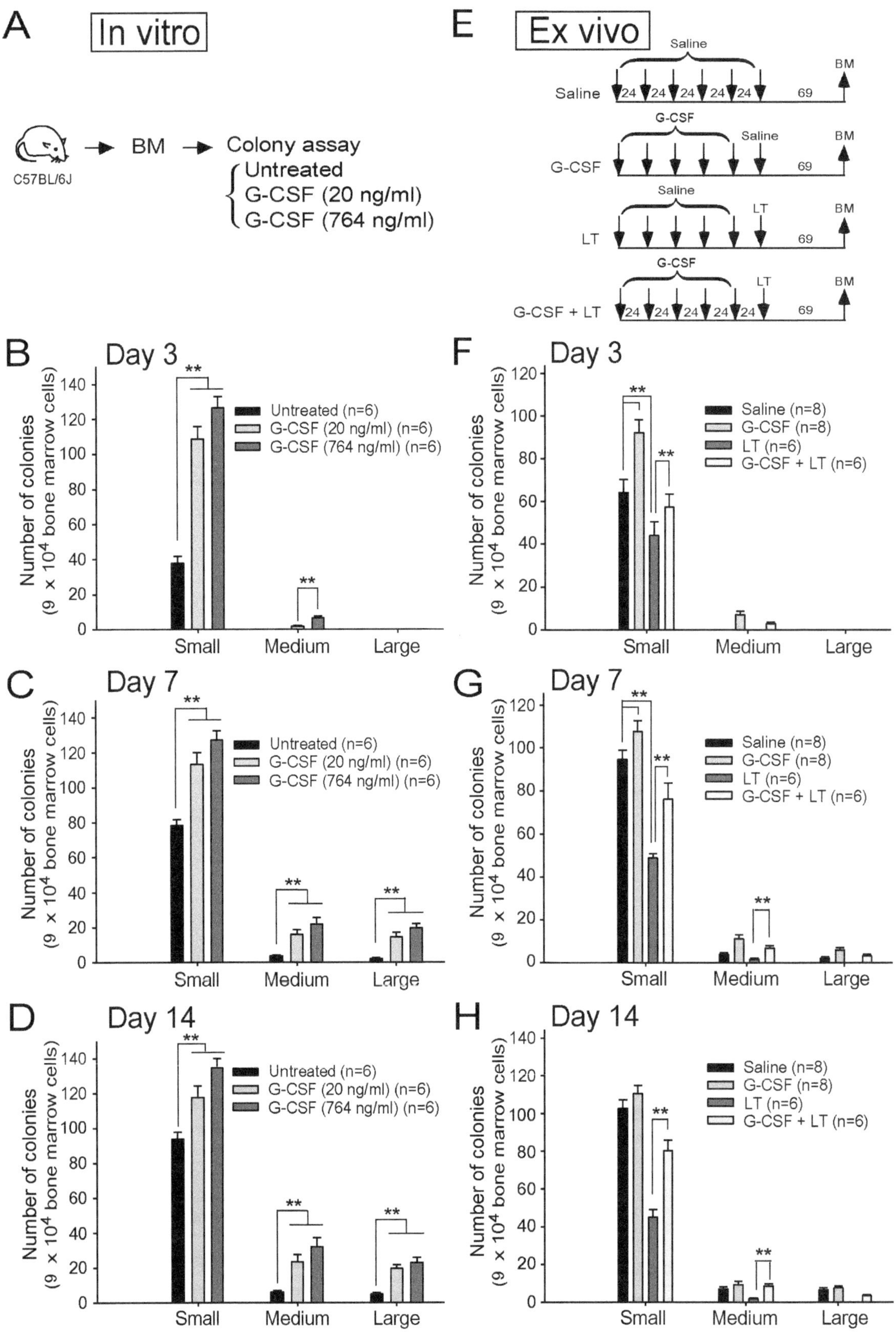

Figure 1. Erythroid colony-forming cell assays to measure the effect of G-CSF on erythropoiesis. The experimental outlines of *in vitro* (A) and *ex vivo* (E) analyses are shown. An *in vitro* assay was performed using murine bone marrow (BM) cells that were incubated with [20 ng/ml (n = 6) or 764 ng/ml (n = 6)], or without G-CSF (n = 6). The colonies were quantified on Days 3 (B), 7 (C), and 14 (D). Untreated bone marrow cells were used

as a control. Colony numbers of bone marrow cells from mice, which were treated with G-CSF (n = 8), LT (n = 6), or G-CSF and LT (n = 6), were measured on Days 3 (F), 7 (G), and 14 (H) following the *ex vivo* colony assay. Bone marrow cells from saline treated mice (n = 8) served as controls. **$P<0.01$ was compared between the indicated groups. Data are shown as mean ± standard deviation (SD) and represent results from 2 independent experiments. The mouse drawing used in this and all following figures was originally published in *Blood*. Huang, H. S., Sun, D. S., Lien, T. S. and Chang, H. H. Dendritic cells modulate platelet activity in IVIg-mediated amelioration of ITP in mice. *Blood*. 2010; 116: 5002–5009. © the American Society of Hematology.

for every 4–6 h. All surviving mice were monitored each day for 2 subsequent mo. For hematopoietic parameters, 50 µl of retro-orbital blood samples were collected at 22, 44, and 66 h after LT challenges and analyzed by an automated hematology analyzer (KX-21, Sysmex Corporation).

Combined treatments with G-CSF and EPO to reduce anthrax-spore-induced mortality

C57BL/6J mice were retro-orbitally injected with G-CSF (55 µg/kg/d in 250 µl saline) daily for 5 consecutive d or injected with a combination of recombinant human EPO (rhEPO, Neorecormon, Roche, Mannheim, Germany) (2 IU/g, in 250 µl saline) twice at 24 and 48 h after injecting spores (1×10^7 in 1 ml saline, intraperitoneal injection). The survival times and mortality of mice were recorded. Because no suitable potential predictor of death/survival exists for spore-challenged mice, we used death as an endpoint for the survival experiment. Spore treatment in mice did not induce obvious discomfort and body weight loss, except for reducing activities. The experimental mice were continually

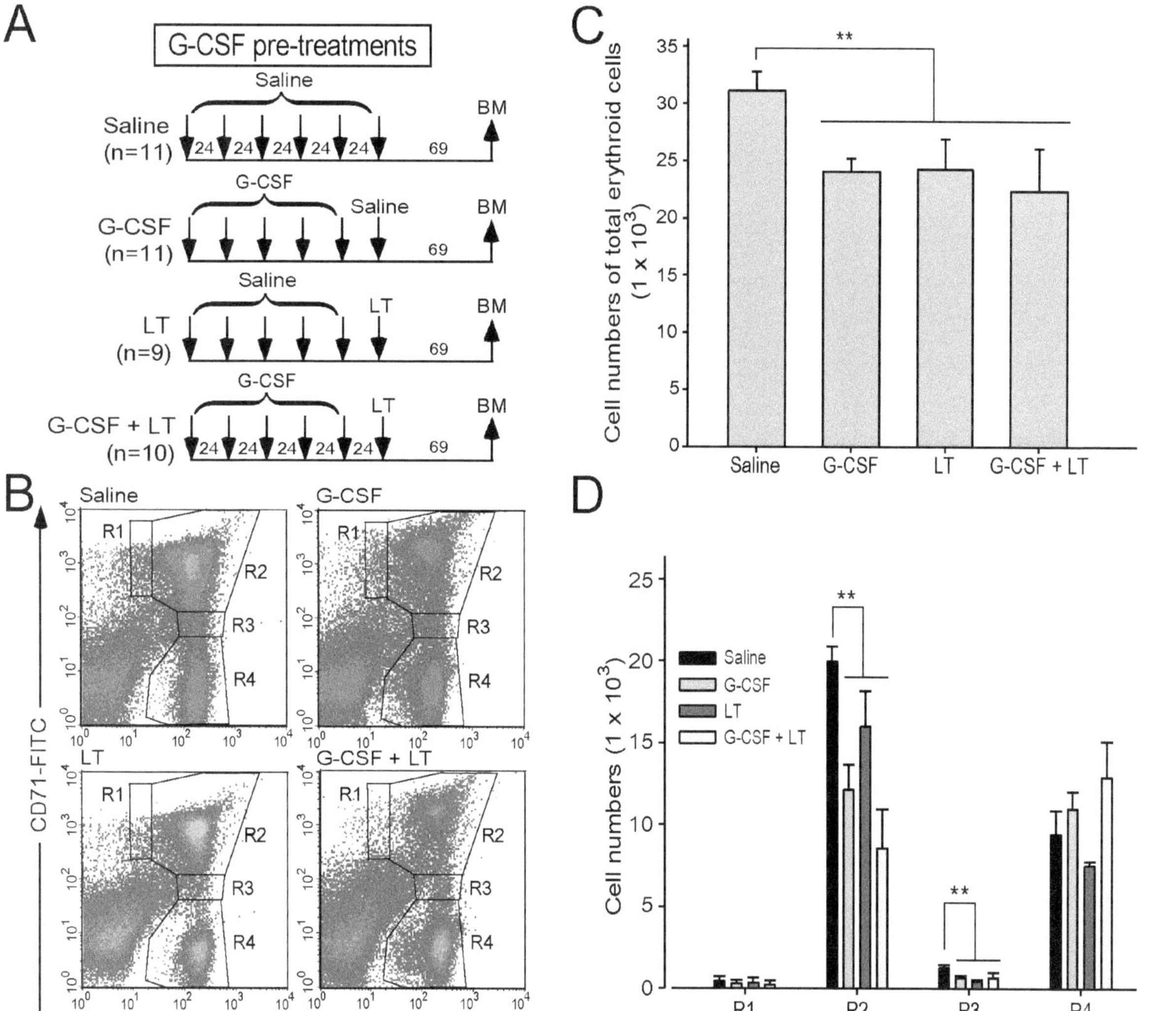

Figure 2. Regulation of G-CSF on bone marrow erythroblast populations. The experimental outlines are illustrated (A). Mice were treated with saline (n = 11), G-CSF (n = 11), LT (n = 9), or G-CSF plus LT (n = 10). Flow cytometry analysis analyzed erythroblast populations of BM cells at 69 h after LT challenges. The erythroblast cells were gated as R1 ($CD71^{high}$, $TER\text{-}119^{med}$), R2 ($CD71^{high}$, $TER\text{-}119^{high}$), R3 ($CD71^{med}$, $TER\text{-}119^{high}$), and R4 ($CD71^{low}$, $TER\text{-}119^{high}$) in all groups (B) as described [25]. The cell numbers of all erythroblast cells (sum of R1 to R4) (C) and individual erythroblast (R1, R2, R3, and R4) (D) in each group were quantified. **$P<0.01$ was compared between indicated groups. Data are showed as mean ± SD and represent the results from 2 independent experiments.

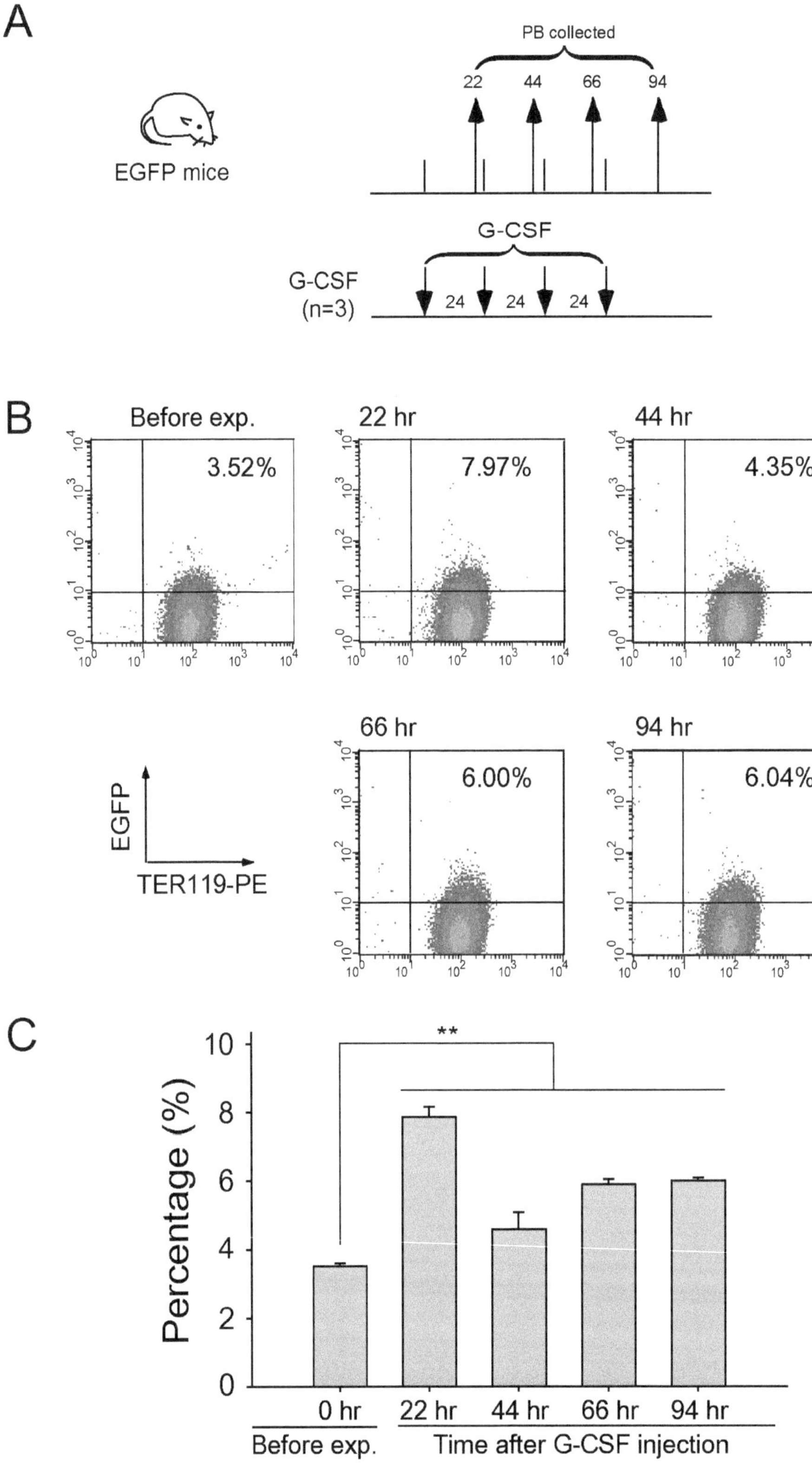

Figure 3. Mobilization of newly synthesized erythrocytes into peripheral blood by G-CSF. The experimental outline is illustrated (A). The EGFP mice were injected with G-CSF (n = 3). The percentage of $EGFP^+/TER119^+$ cells in peripheral blood (PB) was analyzed by flow cytometry (B) and quantified (C) at 22, 44, 66, and 94 h after G-CSF injection. PB collected from mice before G-CSF injection served as the negative control. $^{**}P<0.01$ was compared to the negative control. Data are shown as mean ± SD.

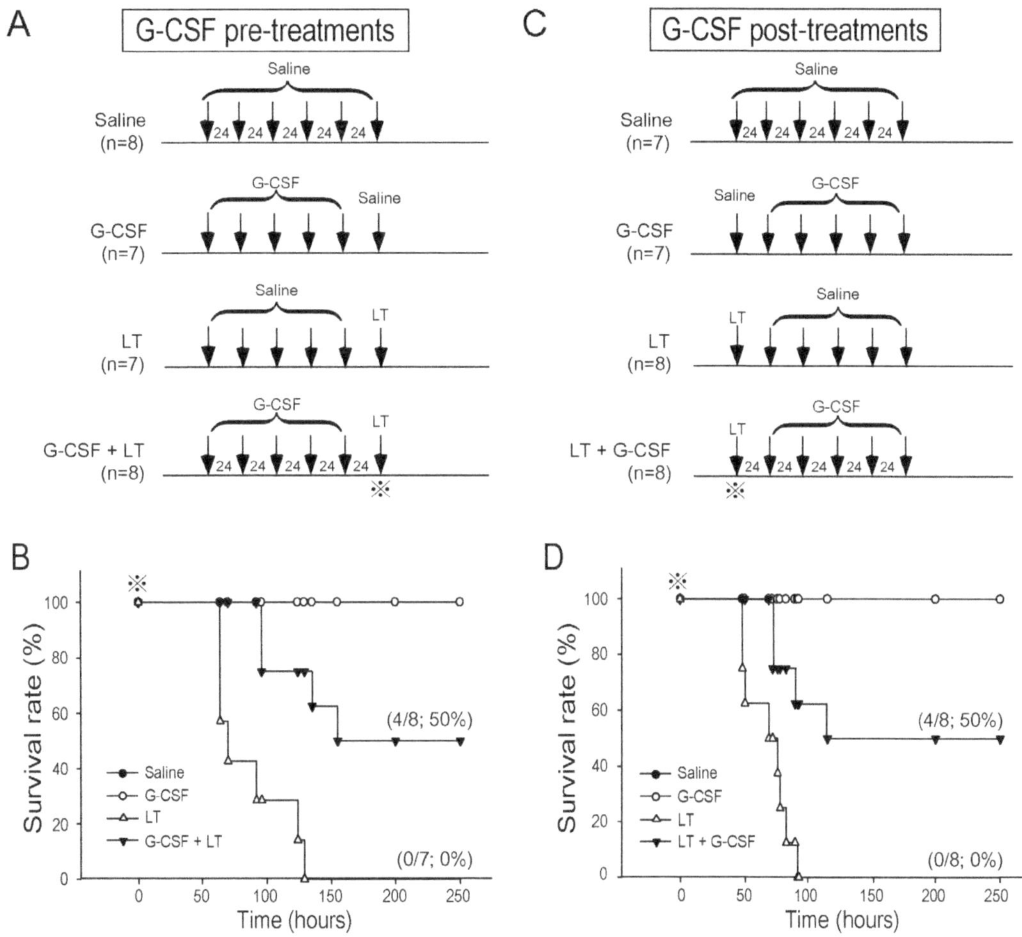

Figure 4. G-CSF treatments ameliorated LT-elicited mortality in mice. The experimental timetable (A), (C), and the survival rates of mice pre-treated (B) and post-treated (D) with G-CSF, LT, or G-CSF and LT are indicated. Saline treated mice served as negative controls. The symbol (※) in (A) to (D) indicates the onset time point for recording survival rates.

monitored up to 15 d for every 4–6 h. All surviving mice were monitored each day for 2 subsequent mo.

Statistics

All results are presented as the mean ± SD (standard deviation) for each group. Data significance was examined by one-way ANOVA followed by the post-hoc Bonferroni-corrected *t*-test. Univariate Kaplan-Meier analysis was used to compare the difference in survival rate between groups with various treatments. *P*-values were calculated and log-rank tests were performed to determine statistical significance. A probability of type 1 error $\alpha = 0.05$ was recognized as the threshold of statistical significance. Statistical analysis was conducted using the statistical software SPSS, version 17.0 (SPSS Inc., Chicago, IL, USA).

Results

G-CSF treatment promoted erythrocytic differentiation and proliferation *in vitro* and *ex vivo*

To elucidate the role of G-CSF on erythrocytic differentiation and proliferation, an *in vitro* erythroid colony-forming cell assay was performed to quantify BFU-Es and CFU-Es. Control groups without using filgrastim G-CSF supplements formed only medium-sized colonies by Day 7 (Figure 1C). By contrast, G-CSF treatments accelerated the formation of medium-sized colonies, which appeared earlier by Day 3 (Figure 1B). Following G-CSF treatment, the numbers of colonies in all colony sizes were greater than those in the untreated control groups (Figure 1B–1D). Based on the traditional concept that G-CSF primarily regulates granulopoiesis [28], those colonies to be affected by G-CSF treatment may not be exclusively erythroid-origin cells. Consequently, 3, 3′-diaminobenzidine tetrahydrochloride (DAB) [37] was used to identify erythroid colonies, and the pseudoperoxidase activity of erythroid cells was stained on Day 14. Compared with the untreated groups, the number of DAB^+ colonies was greater in G-CSF-treated groups (Figure S1). This data indicated that G-CSF treatment enhances the proliferation and differentiation of erythrocytes *in vitro*. Further experiments were performed to investigate the effect of G-CSF and LT treatments *ex vivo* (Figure 1E). The number of erythroid colonies sharply decreased with LT treatment on Days 3, 7 and 14 (Figure 1F–1H). Medium-sized colonies first appeared on Day 3 in G-CSF treated groups (Figure 1F), compared with saline and LT-treated groups, whereas medium-sized colonies only appeared on Day 7 (Figure 1G). In addition, G-CSF treatments ameliorated LT-induced suppression on erythropoiesis in the *ex vivo* erythroid colony-forming cell assay (Figure 1F–1H). These results indicated that G-CSF promoted erythrocytic proliferation and differentiation *in vitro* and *ex vivo*

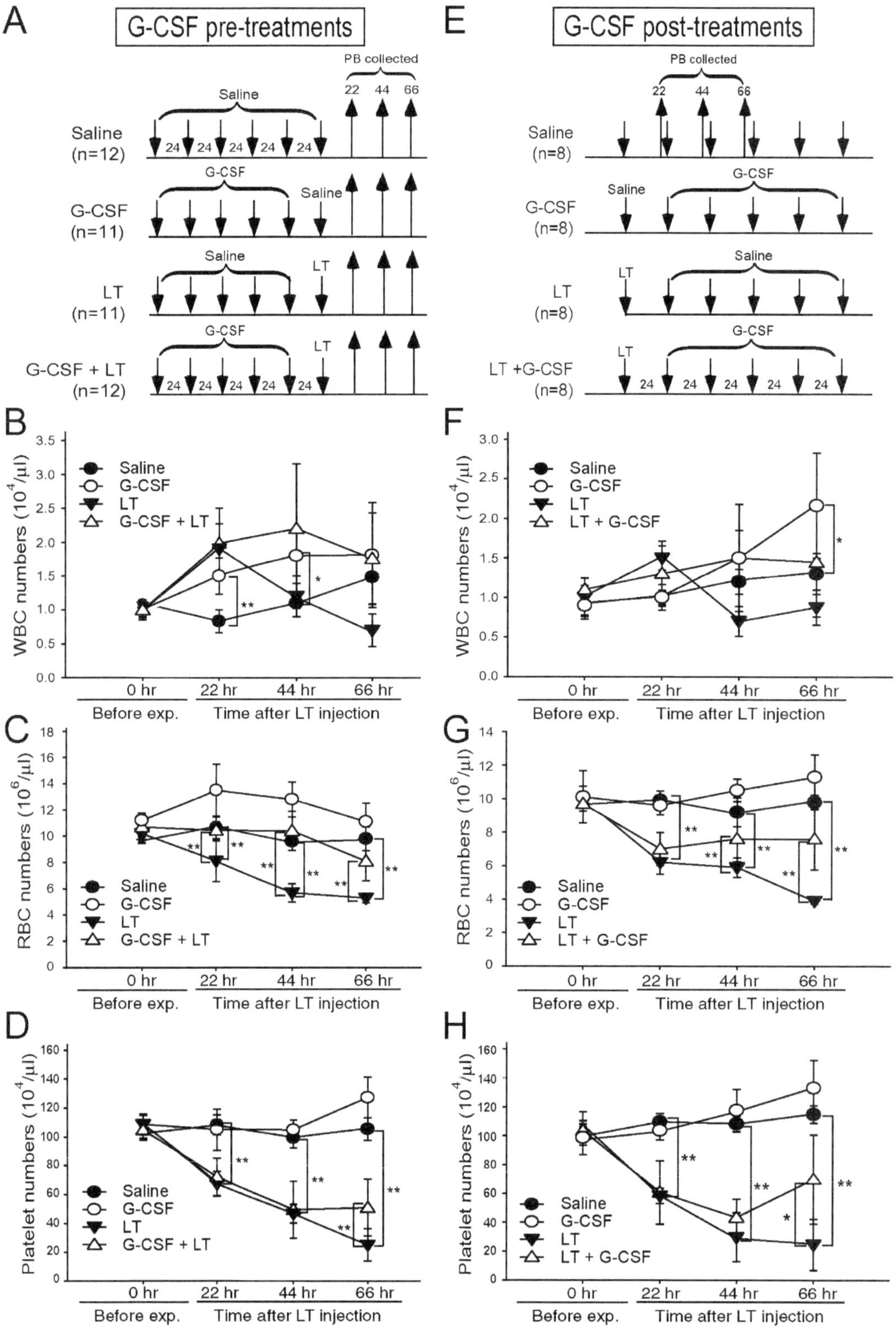

Figure 5. Amelioration of LT-induced erythrocytopenic response by G-CSF. The experimental outlines are indicated (A), (E). Mice were treated with saline (n = 12), G-CSF (n = 11), LT (n = 11), and G-CSF plus LT (n = 12) before (A) or saline (n = 8), G-CSF (n = 8), LT (n = 8), and LT plus G-CSF (n = 8) after (E) the LT challenges; their WBC, RBC, and platelet counts were subsequently analyzed at 22, 44, and 66 h after the LT challenges. Saline-treated mice were used as negative controls. $^{*}P<0.05$, $^{**}P<0.01$ were compared between the indicated groups. Data are shown as mean ± SD and represent the results from 2 independent experiments.

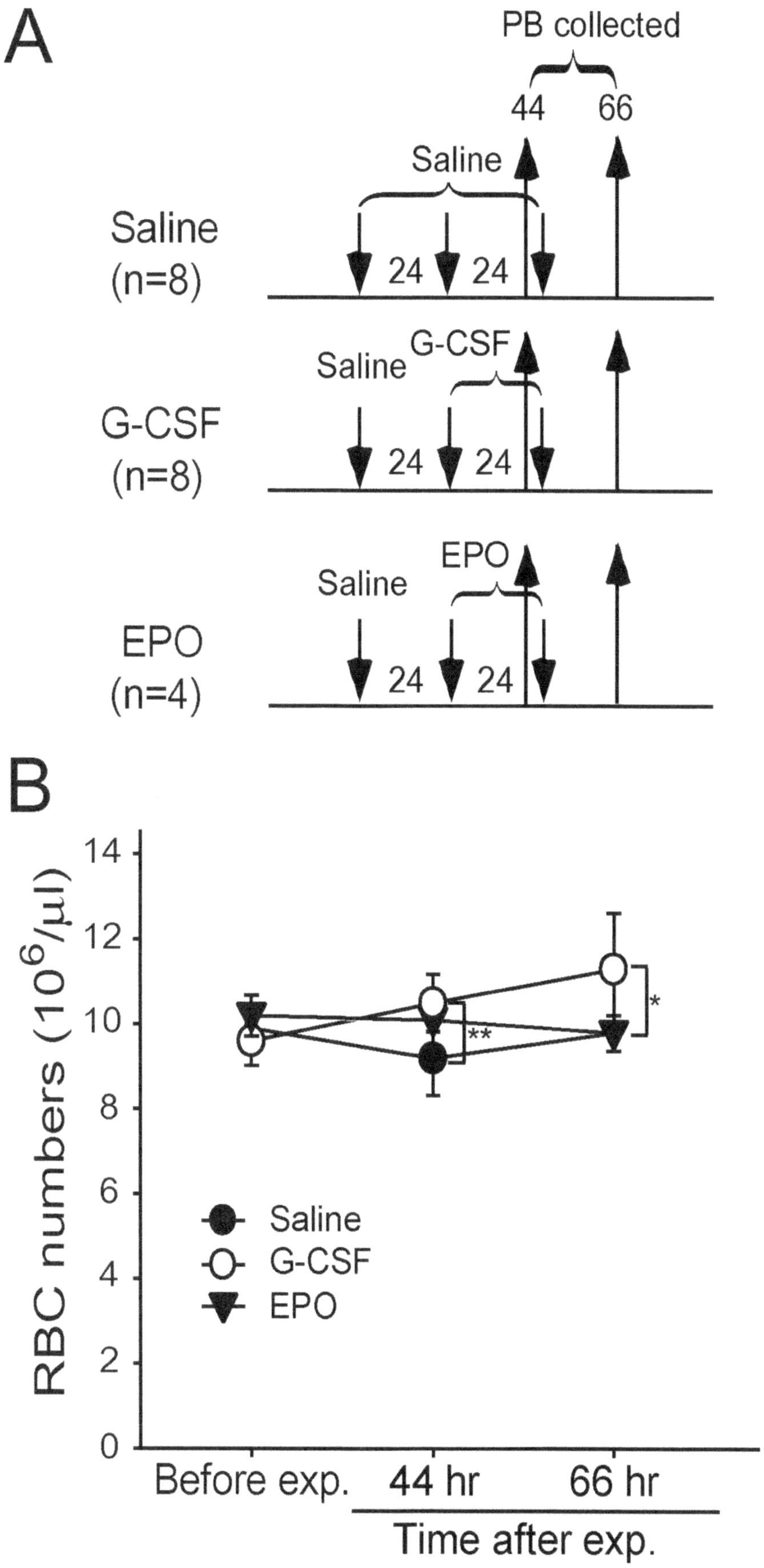
A
PB collected
44
66
Saline
Saline
(n=8)
24
24
G-CSF
Saline
G-CSF
(n=8)
24
24
EPO
Saline
EPO
(n=4)
24
24
B
RBC numbers (10^6/μl)
14
12
10
8
6
4
2
0
**
*
Saline
G-CSF
EPO
Before exp.
44 hr
66 hr
Time after exp.

Figure 6. Fast mobilization of erythrocytes into peripheral blood by G-CSF versus EPO treatments. Experimental outline for measuring the PB-RBC counts of mice treated with G-CSF (n = 8) or EPO (n = 4) for 2 consecutive d (A). The PB RBC counts were measured before the experiments and at 44 and 66 h after the first saline injection (B). Data are shown as mean ± SD and represent the results from 2 independent experiments. Saline treated groups (n = 8) were used as the negative control. *$P<0.05$, **$P<0.01$ were compared to the negative control.

and ameliorated LT-induced erythropoiesis suppression in the *ex vivo* erythroid colony-forming cell assay.

G-CSF treatment promoted mobilization of newly synthesized RBC to peripheral blood

After the promising analyses *in vitro* and *ex vivo*, this study investigated the erythropoietic progression *in vivo*. Our previous report revealed that LT suppressed erythropoiesis in bone marrow [15]. Following similar approaches [15,25], we used surface expression of CD71 and TER-119 to verify the maturation status of various bone marrow erythroblasts under the G-CSF treatments with or without anthrax LT challenges. Although we found that G-CSF treatment rescued LT-induced erythrocytopenia (please see the following section), G-CSF pre-treatments could not overcome LT-mediated suppression on the cell numbers of both total erythroblast and individual subpopulations of erythroblast (R1 to R4 populations) (Figure 2C and 2D). This prompted us to verify whether G-CSF could mobilize mature erythrocytes into peripheral blood; we employed C57BL/6J mice with the whole-body-expressing enhanced-green-fluorescence-protein (EGFP) transgene. Prior to G-CSF analyses, we found that only a small fraction of $EGFP^+$ RBCs was detectable in the peripheral blood of normal control groups (Figure 3, 3.5% cells, before exp. groups). This is likely because mature erythrocytes do not have a nucleus, and that newly differentiated RBCs, rather than aged RBCs, express detectable EGFP. We employed an acute hemorrhage model, in which 35% of total blood was removed, to provoke the natural induction of erythropoiesis to investigate whether newly synthesized erythrocytes contain additional fluorescence. Our data revealed that $EGFP^+$/TER-119^+ erythrocytes increased consistently by Days 2, 4, and 6 after acute anemia (Figure S2). This suggested that $EGFP^+$/TER-119^+ cells are newly synthesized erythrocytes. Using the same strategy, analyses revealed that G-CSF treatment can mobilize newly synthesized erythrocytes to peripheral blood in mice (Figure 3, beginning at 22 h after G-CSF injections).

G-CSF treatment reduced LT-mediated mortality, erythrocytopenia, and thrombocytopenia

To investigate the ameliorative effect of G-CSF on LT, C57BL/6J mice were treated with G-CSF according to the manufacturer's instructions (once daily for 5 d). Treatments of G-CSF were initiated 5 d before (Figure 4A) or 1 d after the challenges of a lethal dose of LT (Figure 4C). LT initiated mortality within 48 to 129 h (Figure 4B and 4D, LT groups). Administration of 5 doses of G-CSF before (Figure 4A) and after (Figure 4C) the LT challenges significantly improved survival rates (Figure 4B and 4D) ($P<0.01$). Treatments using saline, G-CSF, and LT alone served as the controls (Figure 4B and 4D). The peripheral white blood cell (WBC) counts of the G-CSF-treated groups increased approximately 2-fold at 22 and 44 h (Figure 5A and 5B), as well as at 66 h (Figure 5E and 5F) following the implementation of differing G-CSF regimens; this is in consistent with a previous G-CSF report [38]. Notably, both G-CSF treatments significantly ameliorated LT-induced erythrocytopenia (Figure 5C, G-CSF + LT vs. LT; Figure 5G, LT + G-CSF vs. LT). Compared with RBC counts, the ameliorative effect of G-CSF on LT-induced thrombocytopenia was somewhat later and was observed at approximately 66 h after LT treatment (Figure 5D and 5H). These results indicated that G-CSF positively regulated both RBC and platelet counts.

G-CSF treatment induced erythrocytes to mobilize into peripheral blood faster than EPO

Our previous study showed that EPO up-regulated RBC counts in peripheral blood [15]. To compare the EPO and G-CSF treatments in their efficiency at increasing RBC counts, mice were injected with 2 doses of either G-CSF or EPO. The circulating RBC counts were measured (Figure 6). Our data revealed that G-CSF induced a faster increase of RBC counts, within 20 h of the first G-CSF administration, than the EPO treatment, in which no increased RBC counts were observed (Figure 6B, G-CSF vs. EPO). These results suggested that G-CSF induced a faster mobilization of erythrocytes into peripheral blood than that of EPO.

Combined G-CSF and EPO had an ameliorative effect on anthrax-spore-induced mortality in C57BL/6J mice

Our previous report suggested that EPO ameliorates LT-mediated erythrocytopenia by enhancing erythropoiesis [15]. Because G-CSF increases the erythrocyte supply through a diverse mechanism by enhancing the mobilization of erythrocytes into peripheral blood, these results prompted us to investigate whether combined treatments using G-CSF and EPO may be more effective than respective single treatments alone. The analysis indicated that EPO treatment did not exert a protective effect on anthrax-spore-challenged mice (Figure 7B, Spore + EPO vs. Spore only). This is consistent with another line of evidence; the survival rates of anthrax LT-challenged mice increased only 25% following EPO post-treatment (Figure S3, LT + EPO vs. LT, $P = 0.101$). By contrast, G-CSF treatments with or without EPO effectively increased the survival rate of anthrax spore-challenged mice from 18.75% to 37.5% (Figure 7, Spore + G-CSF vs. Spore only). Post-treatments combining G-CSF and EPO prolonged the survival period of anthrax-spore-challenged mice (Figure 7, Spore + G-CSF + EPO vs. Spore + G-CSF). Statistical analysis revealed that the P value is marginally significant (Figure 7, $P = 0.094$, Spore + G-CSF + EPO vs. Spore; $P = 0.088$, Spore + G-CSF + EPO vs. Spore + EPO). These results suggested that combined treatment using G-CSF and EPO tended to ameliorate anthrax-spore-induced mortality in mice.

Discussion

This study demonstrated that G-CSF, a stimulating factor for granulopoiesis, enhanced erythrocytic mobilization, by which it enhanced RBC counts in peripheral blood. This likely therefore rescued anthrax LT-induced anemia and mortality in mice.

Our *in vitro* (Figure 1A–1D) and *ex vivo* (Figure 1E–1H) evidence suggested that G-CSF may promote erythropoiesis. The *in vivo* analyses revealed that G-CSF ameliorated LT-induced erythrocytopenia in peripheral blood (Figure 5C and 5G), but did not increase erythroblast cell numbers in bone marrow (Figure 2). Therefore, the effects of G-CSF on erythropoiesis *in vivo* require clarification. One study demonstrated that G-CSF had a negative effect on bone marrow erythropoiesis in mice [39].

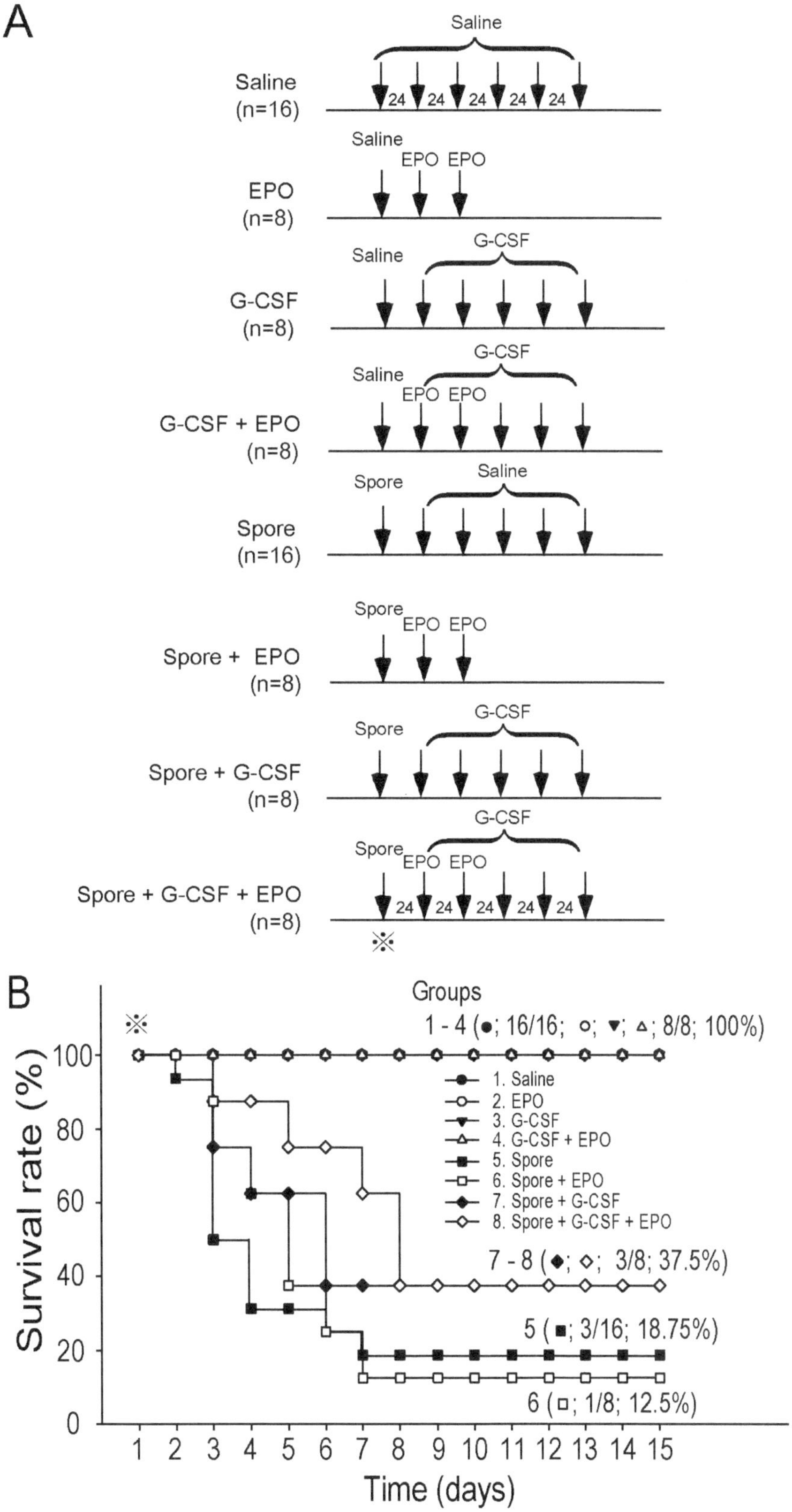

Figure 7. Post-treatments of G-CSF and EPO tended to ameliorate anthrax spore elicited-lethality in mice. Experimental outlines (A) and the survival rates of mice treated with G-CSF (n = 8), EPO (n = 8), and G-CSF combined with EPO (n = 8) after anthrax spore injection (B). Saline (n = 16), EPO (n = 8), G-CSF (n = 8), G-CSF and EPO (n = 8), and anthrax spore (n = 16) injected groups were used for comparisons. The symbol (※) in (A) and (B) indicates the onset time point for recording survival rates. Data represent the results from 2 independent experiments.

However, another study demonstrated that G-CSF treatments in humans increased immature reticulocytes in peripheral blood [40]. Clinical observations also found that the reticulocyte fraction, an assessment of immature erythroid cells in peripheral blood, was an early surrogate marker for the rise of $CD34^+$ hematopoietic stem cells during G-CSF mobilization [41]. This evidence suggests that G-CSF is involved in regulating erythroid precursor cells in humans.

G-CSF induced fast mobilization of RBCs to peripheral blood within 20 h of the first G-CSF administration, compared with the EPO treatment (Figure 6). This data is consistent with the EGFP mice experiment, regarding the time in which G-CSF treatment increased the percentage of newly synthesized erythrocytes in peripheral blood (Figure 3). Thus, a single post-treatment dose of G-CSF was sufficient to save approximately 40% of mice within 24 h (Figure 4D, 100% and 60% survival rates in LT + G-CSF and LT, 48 h groups, respectively). The advantage of fast mobilization of RBCs of G-CSF can also be confirmed by the higher survival rate of G-CSF compared with EPO in LT-induced (Figure 4D vs. Figure S3B) and LT-spore-induced (Figure 7B) mortality in mice.

G-CSF is a multi-function cytokine that stimulates the proliferation and differentiation of myeloid precursors and modulates mature cells [29]. G-CSF is also used to prevent or shorten neutropenia in chemotherapy-induced or primary congenital neutropenia [42], and mobilize hematopoietic stem cells to peripheral blood for transplantation [43]. Probably because of the anti-apoptotic and anti-inflammatory effects, G-CSF has also been used to treat nonhematopoietic targets including cerebral ischemia [44], spinal cord ischemia [45], infarct heart [46], and end stage liver disease [47]. Consequently, the effects of G-CSF on other cell types (e.g., macrophage, lymphocyte, endothelial, dendritic cells, cardiomyocytes, and smooth muscle) may not be completely excluded from the rescue mechanism of G-CSF. Although the mechanism is unclear, combination therapy using G-CSF and EPO has been used to treat myelodysplastic anemia in clinical settings [32–36,48]. This suggests that the medical community has empirically recognized the RBC-enhancing effect of the combination treatment using G-CSF and EPO. One critical aspect of G-CSF is the rapid induction of peripheral RBCs, a property superior to EPO, which may be applied to anthrax or other diseases with urgent RBC and oxygen demands. Further detailed and well-designed clinical studies are required to explore the therapeutic potential of combination treatment using G-CSF and EPO.

In this study, we demonstrated that G-CSF mobilized erythrocytes into peripheral blood. In addition, combined treatments of G-CSF and EPO tended to ameliorate anthrax spore-induced mortality. An optimized rescue protocol may provide new perspectives and assist the development of a feasible therapeutic strategy against anthrax.

Supporting Information

Figure S1 G-CSF treatments enhanced bone marrow erythroid colony numbers. An *in vitro* erythroid colony-forming cell assay was performed using murine bone marrow (BM) cells incubated with [20 ng/ml (n = 6) or 764 ng/ml (n = 6)] or without G-CSF (n = 6). The erythroid colonies were confirmed by 3, 3′-diaminobenzidine tetrahydrochloride (DAB) staining (A) and quantified on Day 14 (B). Untreated BM cells were used as the control. $^{**}P<0.01$ was compared to the untreated groups. Scale bar: 500 μm. Data are shown as mean ± SD.

Figure S2 Mobilization of newly synthesized erythrocytes ($EGFP^+/TER\text{-}119^+$) into peripheral blood by acute anemia in EGFP transgenic mice. Experimental timetable used in acute anima assay (A). During acute anima (after aspirating 35% of total blood), the population of $EGFP^+/TER\text{-}119^+$ cells in peripheral blood (PB) of EGFP mice was gated as R1 and quantified. The total cell number was defined as 100%. The percentage of R1 was analyzed by flow cytometry (B) on Day 2, 4, and 6 after the removal of 35% of total blood. PB samples from mice before acute anemia were used as negative controls. Data were collected from 2 representative EGFP mice.

Figure S3 Post-treatments of EPO increased the survival rates of LT-challenged mice. Experimental timetable (A). The survival rates of mice challenged with EPO (n = 4), LT (n = 4), or LT plus EPO (n = 4) are shown (B). Saline-treated mice were used as controls (n = 4). C57BL/6J mice were retro-orbitally injected with recombinant human EPO (rhEPO, Neorecormon, Roche, Mannheim, Germany) (2 IU/g, in 250 μl saline) twice every 24 h after the challenges of a lethal dose of LT (1.5 mg/kg in 250 μl saline, retro-orbitally injected). The symbol (※) in (A) and (B) indicates the onset time point for recording the survival rates of mice.

Methods S1 Supplemental experimental procedures.

Acknowledgments

We wish to thank Professor Yu MS for providing 3, 3′-diaminobenzidine tetrahydrochloride (DAB) tablets. We also wish to thank Professor Wang MH and his team, the Experimental Animal Center of Tzu-Chi University for animal care.

Author Contributions

Conceived and designed the experiments: HHC DSS. Performed the experiments: YWC TKL GLL YYL JHK HHH HLH. Analyzed the data: HHC JHW DSS. Contributed reagents/materials/analysis tools: JHK HHH HLH JHW. Wrote the paper: HHC DSS.

References

1. Mock M, Fouet A (2001) Anthrax. Annu Rev Microbiol 55: 647–671.
2. Brossier F, Mock M (2001) Toxins of Bacillus anthracis. Toxicon 39: 1747–1755.
3. Collier RJ, Young JA (2003) Anthrax toxin. Annu Rev Cell Dev Biol 19: 45–70.
4. Mourez M (2004) Anthrax toxins. Rev Physiol Biochem Pharmacol 152: 135–164.
5. Bardwell AJ, Abdollahi M, Bardwell L (2004) Anthrax lethal factor-cleavage products of MAPK (mitogen-activated protein kinase) kinases exhibit reduced binding to their cognate MAPKs. Biochem J 378: 569–577.
6. Hagemann C, Blank JL (2001) The ups and downs of MEK kinase interactions. Cell Signal 13: 863–875.
7. Wada T, Penninger JM (2004) Mitogen-activated protein kinases in apoptosis regulation. Oncogene 23: 2838–2849.
8. Raman M, Chen W, Cobb MH (2007) Differential regulation and properties of MAPKs. Oncogene 26: 3100–3112.
9. Moayeri M, Leppla SH (2004) The roles of anthrax toxin in pathogenesis. Curr Opin Microbiol 7: 19–24.
10. Kau JH, Sun DS, Huang HS, Lien TS, Huang HH, et al. (2010) Sublethal doses of anthrax lethal toxin on the suppression of macrophage phagocytosis. PLoS One 5: e14289.
11. Muehlbauer SM, Evering TH, Bonuccelli G, Squires RC, Ashton AW, et al. (2007) Anthrax lethal toxin kills macrophages in a strain-specific manner by apoptosis or caspase-1-mediated necrosis. Cell Cycle 6: 758–766.
12. Alileche A, Serfass ER, Muehlbauer SM, Porcelli SA, Brojatsch J (2005) Anthrax lethal toxin-mediated killing of human and murine dendritic cells impairs the adaptive immune response. PLoS Pathog 1: e19.

13. Comer JE, Chopra AK, Peterson JW, Konig R (2005) Direct inhibition of T-lymphocyte activation by anthrax toxins in vivo. Infect Immun 73: 8275–8281.
14. Fang H, Xu L, Chen TY, Cyr JM, Frucht DM (2006) Anthrax lethal toxin has direct and potent inhibitory effects on B cell proliferation and immunoglobulin production. J Immunol 176: 6155–6161.
15. Chang HH, Wang TP, Chen PK, Lin YY, Liao CH, et al. (2013) Erythropoiesis suppression is associated with anthrax lethal toxin-mediated pathogenic progression. PLoS One 8: e71718.
16. Chen PK, Chang HH, Lin GL, Wang TP, Lai YL, et al. (2013) Suppressive effects of anthrax lethal toxin on megakaryopoiesis. PLoS One 8: e59512.
17. Liu S, Zhang Y, Moayeri M, Liu J, Crown D, et al. (2013) Key tissue targets responsible for anthrax-toxin-induced lethality. Nature 501: 63–68.
18. Kassam A, Der SD, Mogridge J (2005) Differentiation of human monocytic cell lines confers susceptibility to Bacillus anthracis lethal toxin. Cell Microbiol 7: 281–292.
19. Kau JH, Sun DS, Tsai WJ, Shyu HF, Huang HH, et al. (2005) Antiplatelet activities of anthrax lethal toxin are associated with suppressed p42/44 and p38 mitogen-activated protein kinase pathways in the platelets. J Infect Dis 192: 1465–1474.
20. Moayeri M, Haines D, Young HA, Leppla SH (2003) Bacillus anthracis lethal toxin induces TNF-alpha-independent hypoxia-mediated toxicity in mice. J Clin Invest 112: 670–682.
21. Rainey GJ, Young JA (2004) Antitoxins: novel strategies to target agents of bioterrorism. Nat Rev Microbiol 2: 721–726.
22. Wadhwa M, Thorpe R (2008) Haematopoietic growth factors and their therapeutic use. Thromb Haemost 99: 863–873.
23. Debili N, Wendling F, Katz A, Guichard J, Breton-Gorius J, et al. (1995) The Mpl-ligand or thrombopoietin or megakaryocyte growth and differentiative factor has both direct proliferative and differentiative activities on human megakaryocyte progenitors. Blood 86: 2516–2525.
24. Fisher JW (2003) Erythropoietin: physiology and pharmacology update. Exp Biol Med (Maywood) 228: 1–14.
25. Socolovsky M, Nam H, Fleming MD, Haase VH, Brugnara C, et al. (2001) Ineffective erythropoiesis in Stat5a(−/−)5b(−/−) mice due to decreased survival of early erythroblasts. Blood 98: 3261–3273.
26. Trowbridge IS, Lesley J, Schulte R (1982) Murine cell surface transferrin receptor: studies with an anti-receptor monoclonal antibody. J Cell Physiol 112: 403–410.
27. Kina T, Ikuta K, Takayama E, Wada K, Majumdar AS, et al. (2000) The monoclonal antibody TER-119 recognizes a molecule associated with glycophorin A and specifically marks the late stages of murine erythroid lineage. Br J Haematol 109: 280–287.
28. Hubel K, Dale DC, Liles WC (2002) Therapeutic use of cytokines to modulate phagocyte function for the treatment of infectious diseases: current status of granulocyte colony-stimulating factor, granulocyte-macrophage colony-stimulating factor, macrophage colony-stimulating factor, and interferon-gamma. J Infect Dis 185: 1490–1501.
29. Morstyn G, Burgess AW (1988) Hemopoietic growth factors: a review. Cancer Res 48: 5624–5637.
30. Metcalf D (2008) Hematopoietic cytokines. Blood 111: 485–491.
31. Xiao BG, Lu CZ, Link H (2007) Cell biology and clinical promise of G-CSF: immunomodulation and neuroprotection. J Cell Mol Med 11: 1272–1290.
32. Bessho M, Hirashima K, Asano S, Ikeda Y, Ogawa N, et al. (1997) Treatment of the anemia of aplastic anemia patients with recombinant human erythropoietin in combination with granulocyte colony-stimulating factor: a multicenter randomized controlled study. Multicenter Study Group. Eur J Haematol 58: 265–272.
33. Greenberg PL, Sun Z, Miller KB, Bennett JM, Tallman MS, et al. (2009) Treatment of myelodysplastic syndrome patients with erythropoietin with or without granulocyte colony-stimulating factor: results of a prospective randomized phase 3 trial by the Eastern Cooperative Oncology Group (E1996). Blood 114: 2393–2400.
34. Hellstrom-Lindberg E, Gulbrandsen N, Lindberg G, Ahlgren T, Dahl IM, et al. (2003) A validated decision model for treating the anaemia of myelodysplastic syndromes with erythropoietin + granulocyte colony-stimulating factor: significant effects on quality of life. Br J Haematol 120: 1037–1046.
35. Hellstrom-Lindberg E, Negrin R, Stein R, Krantz S, Lindberg G, et al. (1997) Erythroid response to treatment with G-CSF plus erythropoietin for the anaemia of patients with myelodysplastic syndromes: proposal for a predictive model. Br J Haematol 99: 344–351.
36. Negrin RS, Stein R, Doherty K, Cornwell J, Vardiman J, et al. (1996) Maintenance treatment of the anemia of myelodysplastic syndromes with recombinant human granulocyte colony-stimulating factor and erythropoietin: evidence for in vivo synergy. Blood 87: 4076–4081.
37. Ogawa M, Parmley RT, Bank HL, Spicer SS (1976) Human marrow erythropoiesis in culture. I. Characterization of methylcellulose colony assay. Blood 48: 407–417.
38. Kikuta T, Shimazaki C, Ashihara E, Sudo Y, Hirai H, et al. (2000) Mobilization of hematopoietic primitive and committed progenitor cells into blood in mice by anti-vascular adhesion molecule-1 antibody alone or in combination with granulocyte colony-stimulating factor. Exp Hematol 28: 311–317.
39. Nijhof W, De Haan G, Dontje B, Loeffler M (1994) Effects of G-CSF on erythropoiesis. Ann N Y Acad Sci 718: 312–324; discussion 324–315.
40. Park K, Im T, Sasaki A, Yamane T, Nakao Y, et al. (1991) Positive effect of granulocyte-colony stimulating factor on erythropoiesis in humans. Osaka City Med J 37: 123–132.
41. Remacha AF, Martino R, Sureda A, Sarda MP, Sola C, et al. (1996) Changes in reticulocyte fractions during peripheral stem cell harvesting: role in monitoring stem cell collection. Bone Marrow Transplant 17: 163–168.
42. Page AV, Liles WC (2011) Colony-stimulating factors in the prevention and management of infectious diseases. Infect Dis Clin North Am 25: 803–817.
43. Rankin SM (2012) Chemokines and adult bone marrow stem cells. Immunol Lett 145: 47–54.
44. Abe K, Yamashita T, Takizawa S, Kuroda S, Kinouchi H, et al. (2012) Stem cell therapy for cerebral ischemia: from basic science to clinical applications. J Cereb Blood Flow Metab 32: 1317–1331.
45. Chen WF, Jean YH, Sung CS, Wu GJ, Huang SY, et al. (2008) Intrathecally injected granulocyte colony-stimulating factor produced neuroprotective effects in spinal cord ischemia via the mitogen-activated protein kinase and Akt pathways. Neuroscience 153: 31–43.
46. Baldo MP, Davel AP, Damas-Souza DM, Nicoletti-Carvalho JE, Bordin S, et al. (2011) The antiapoptotic effect of granulocyte colony-stimulating factor reduces infarct size and prevents heart failure development in rats. Cell Physiol Biochem 28: 33–40.
47. Gaia S, Smedile A, Omede P, Olivero A, Sanavio F, et al. (2006) Feasibility and safety of G-CSF administration to induce bone marrow-derived cells mobilization in patients with end stage liver disease. J Hepatol 45: 13–19.
48. Jadersten M, Montgomery SM, Dybedal I, Porwit-MacDonald A, Hellstrom-Lindberg E (2005) Long-term outcome of treatment of anemia in MDS with erythropoietin and G-CSF. Blood 106: 803–811.
49. Kau JH, Lin CG, Huang HH, Hsu HL, Chen KC, et al. (2002) Calyculin A sensitive protein phosphatase is required for Bacillus anthracis lethal toxin induced cytotoxicity. Curr Microbiol 44: 106–111.
50. Sarma NJ, Takeda A, Yaseen NR (2010) Colony forming cell (CFC) assay for human hematopoietic cells. J Vis Exp.
51. Harkness JE, Wagner JE (1995) Clinical procedures: Biology and Medicine of Rabbits and Rodents 93.

10

Single Nucleotide Polymorphisms in Noncoding Regions of *Rad51C* Do Not Change the Risk of Unselected Breast Cancer but They Modulate the Level of Oxidative Stress and the DNA Damage Characteristics

Peter Gresner[1]*, Jolanta Gromadzinska[1], Ewa Jablonska[1], Maciej Stepnik[1], Oscar Zambrano Quispe[2], Ewa Twardowska[1], Wojciech Wasowicz[1]

1 Department of Toxicology and Carcinogenesis, Nofer Institute of Occupational Medicine, Lodz, Poland, **2** Department of Oncology, Herlev Hospital, Herlev, Denmark

Abstract

Deleterious and missense mutations of *RAD51C* have recently been suggested to modulate the individual susceptibility to hereditary breast and ovarian cancer and unselected ovarian cancer, but not unselected breast cancer (BrC). We enrolled 132 unselected BrC females and 189 cancer-free female subjects to investigate whether common single nucleotide polymorphisms (SNPs) in non-coding regions of *RAD51C* modulate the risk of BrC, and whether they affect the level of oxidative stress and the extent/characteristics of DNA damage. Neither SNPs nor reconstructed haplotypes were found to significantly affect the unselected BrC risk. Contrary to this, carriers of rs12946522, rs16943176, rs12946397 and rs17222691 rare-alleles were found to present significantly increased level of blood plasma TBARS compared to respective wild-type homozygotes ($p<0.05$). Furthermore, these carriers showed significantly decreased fraction of oxidatively generated DNA damage (34% of total damaged DNA) in favor of DNA strand breakage, with no effect on total DNA damage, unlike respective wild-types, among which more evenly distributed proportions between oxidatively damaged DNA (48% of total DNA damage) and DNA strand breakage was found ($p<0.0005$ for the difference). Such effects were found among both the BrC cases and healthy subjects, indicating that they cannot be assumed as causal factors contributing to BrC development.

Editor: Gayle E. Woloschak, Northwestern University Feinberg School of Medicine, United States of America

Funding: The study was supported by the Nofer Institute of Occupational Medicine fund no. IMP1.5/2011. The funders had no role in study design, data collection and analysis, decision to publish, or preparation of the manuscript.

Competing Interests: The authors have declared that no competing interests exist.

* Email: pgresner@imp.lodz.pl

Introduction

Breast cancer (BrC) is the most common malignancy among women, with nearly 1.4 million new BrC cases causing nearly 460,000 deaths per year worldwide [1]. Although vast majority of BrC cases are sporadic, approximately 5–10% of them are considered familial, occurring at unusually young ages in members of families with strong history of hereditary breast and/or ovarian cancer (HBOC) [2]. Studies have shown that familial BrC is likely a polygenic disease caused by mutations in several high-, moderate- and low-penetrance susceptibility genes. Genes like *BRCA1*, *BRCA2*, *TP53* and *PTEN* are well-known high-penetrance susceptibility genes, although nowadays it is assumed, that they account for roughly some 20% of all hereditary breast cancer cases [3–5]. Therefore, the ongoing quest to identify additional BrC-susceptibility genes resulted in identification of several moderate-penetrance BrC-susceptibilty genes, the majority of which are somewhat related to *Brca1/Brca2*-mediated pathways. These include *CHEK2*, *ATM*, *BRIP1*, *PALB2* and recently also *RAD51C*, all of which are involved in various steps of DNA recombination repair [5–7]. An approximately 2-fold relative risk increase among carriers of heterozygous mutations in these genes has been implied [8].

Members of the *RAD51* gene family are often found among genes tested as possible BrC susceptibility genes. This family consists of *RAD51*, a key player in the homologous recombination (HR) double-strand breaks (DSBs) DNA damage response pathway, and its five paralogs: *RAD51B*, *RAD51C*, *RAD51D*, *XRCC2* and *XRCC3*. Protein products of these five genes interact with each other to create hetero-tetrameric and hetero-dimeric complexes crucial for the HR machinery [9]. Out of all *RAD51* paralogs, protein product of *RAD51C* (*RAD51* homolog C, *S. cervisiae*; 17q25.1) seems to play a prominent role as it is found in both the above mentioned complexes. Indeed, RAD51C localizes to the sites of DNA DSBs in early stage of HR, which is thought to be a prerequisite for RAD51/DNA nucleoprotein filament assembly, a key event in the whole HR reaction [10]. Other identified functions of this protein include facilitating the migration and resolution of Holliday junctions in late stages of HR [11], repair of interstrand cross-links [12], distinct functions related to DNA damage response and checkpoint activation [10] and a function of tumor suppressor and cancer susceptibility gene [5,13–15]. It has also been shown, that HR complexes involving *RAD51C* protein product are engaged in repair of stalled/collapsed replication forks induced by single strand breaks (SSBs) of DNA [16]. Interestingly, a recent study has proposed that RAD51C (together with other RAD51 paralogs) may play a role in protection of mitochondrial genome against oxidative damage as well, as mitochondrial level of this protein was found to increase with oxidative stress and its depletion leads to dramatic decrease of mtDNA copy number [17].

Meindl et al. identified deleterious frame-shift, splice-site and missense mutations in *RAD51C* to associate with HBOC families [13] and this observation was further confirmed by other studies including those on unselected ovarian cancer (OC) cases [14,18–22]. Despite the discussion on possible involvement of *RAD51C* genotyping in the routine clinical testing [18], there is still a considerable amount of studies which failed to find any association between *RAD51C* mutations and HBOC [15,23–27], a fact, which is usually explained by very rare occurrence of these mutations. It is, however, intriguing that while all these mutations were associated with HBOC or OC only families, none of the above cited studies identified *RAD51C* mutations associated with BrC only families. This somehow indicates, that *RAD51C* is a susceptibility gene for HBOC and OC, but not for BrC and other cancers [28].

As all *RAD51* paralogs are generally considered conservative with the frequency of missense mutations being very low, we recently focused on single nucleotide polymorphisms (SNPs) occurring in promoter, 5′ untranslated region (5′UTR) of exon 1 and intron 1 of these genes and found that genetic variability of *XRCC3* and *RAD51* may be of relevance with respect to head and neck cancer (HNC) [29]. In the case of *RAD51C*, its association with BrC is generally sought in terms of its missense mutations in coding regions, while the intronic/promoter variability is rather underestimated. Interestingly, our recent study revealed that non-coding SNPs spanning from *RAD51C* promoter to its intron 1 form a linkage-disequilibrium (LD) block significantly associated with HNC risk [30]. Therefore, here we present a study, in which we employed a case-control setup to find out whether common SNPs occurring in non-coding regions (promoter, 5′UTR of exon 1, intron 1) of *RAD51C* may influence the risk of BrC. To this purpose, both single-site and haplotype analyses were performed. Moreover, in order to inspect the possible role of *RAD51C* in BrC more profoundly, we examined whether such variability of *RAD51C* affects the level of oxidative stress, and the extent of DNA strand breakage and/or oxidatively generated DNA damage, and if so, whether such effect may be associated with the development of BrC. In further we show that even though the variability in noncoding regions of *RAD51C* may not alter the risk of unselected BrC, it may be involved in modulation of the oxidative stress and may determine the characteristics of resulting DNA damage.

Material and Methods

Reagents

Diethylpyrocarbonate-treated water used for genotyping of *Rad51C* was obtained from Promega (Madison, WI, USA). Tetrasodium and disodium salts of ethylenediamine tetraacetic acid (Na_2EDTA, Na_4EDTA), thiobarbituric acid (TBA), acetic acid, 1-butanol, Tris base, type VII and type I agarose, Triton X-100, RPMI-1640 medium and 4′6-diamidino-2-phenylindole dyhydrochloride (DAPI) were purchased from Sigma-Aldrich (St. Louis, MO, USA), Phosphate buffered saline (PBS) and hydrochloric acid were from Polish Chemicals (Gliwice, Poland), while 1,1,3,3-tetraaethoxy-propan was obtained from Fluka (Buchs, Switzerland).

Subjects

All breast cancer subjects enrolled in the study were of European descent and residents of Lodz district in Poland. The study involved 132 female patients aged 36–86 years (median age at the time of diagnosis 57 years; interquartile range (IQR): 15 years) hospitalized at the Department of Oncology, Memorial Copernicus Hospital in Lodz, Poland between February 2007 and May 2008 with diagnosis of BrC confirmed histopathologically by two independent histopathologists. Only female patients with primary breast cancer tumor without metastases and without any history of previous anti-cancer treatment, undergoing curative resection therapy or chemotherapy were eligible for the study. The control group consisted of 189 healthy cancer-free volunteer females of European descent who agreed to undergo examinations, aged 35 – 54 years (median age at the time of examination 43 years; IQR: 6 years). All control subjects were also residents of Lodz district in Poland.

Additional information on tobacco-smoking habits was collected for both controls and BrC cases and the individual's lifetime tobacco consumption was expressed by means of the pack-years (i.e. the number of cigarette packs smoked per day times the number of years as a smoker).

For the purposes of DNA damage assays, a subset of 40 controls randomly selected from the group of all control females enrolled in the study was created. To achieve this goal, a method of age-stratified randomization was employed in order to ensure that age distribution in the control subset match the one in the group of BrC females. Following randomization, the matching of SNP distribution between control subset and the whole control group was also checked.

Prior to experiments, written and informed consent for participation in this study was obtained from each subject enrolled. The study was performed under the guidelines of the Helsinki Declaration for human research and was approved by the Bioethics Committee in the Nofer Institute of Occupational Medicine (resolution no. 5/2007). Characteristics of the breast cancer group, the control group as well as the subset of controls used for DNA damage assays are summarized in Table 1.

Blood collection

A sample of peripheral blood was collected from each subject involved in the study by venipuncture into tubes containing either EDTA or heparin as anticoagulants. Heparinized blood samples were then centrifuged (10 min, 1500×g, 4°C) to obtain plasma and used for assessment of the level of oxidative stress. Whole blood samples collected on EDTA were further used in genotyping and DNA damage assays.

DNA isolation

Genomic DNA was isolated from peripheral blood leukocytes using the QIAamp DNA Blood Mini Kit (Qiagen, Germany) according to the manufacturer's instruction. The RNA contamination was removed by digestion with 1 mg/ml RNase A (Qiagen, Hilden, Germany) and obtained DNA was further quantified and the protein content and DNA purity was checked using an Eppendorf BioPhotometer (Eppendorf, Hamburg, Germany) instrument. Samples were stored at -80°C until further processing.

Table 1. Characteristics of the groups of subjects involved in the study.

Feature	Cancer cases	Control subjects	DNA damage assay control subset [a]
Total number	132	189	40
Age [years]	57 [50–65] [b]	43 [40–46]	43 [40–48]
Smoking status [never/ever]	55/63 (47%/53%) [c]	120/68 (64%/36%)	24/16 (60%/40%)
Pack-years	11.3 [6.0–20.0] [d, e]	2.0 [1.0–4.6]	1.0 [0.8–4.6]
Tumor staging [f]			
T [1/2/3/4/x]	44/45/1/6/1	-	-
N [0/1/2/3/x]	44/24/10/2/20	-	-
Tumor grade			
G [1/2/3/x]	7/37/40/13	-	-

Numerical data for age and pack-years presented as median [interquartile range].
[a] DNA damage assay control subset consisted of 40 subjects randomly selected from the whole control group by means of the age-stratified randomization;
[b] $p << 0.001$ cancer cases vs. controls, Mann-Whitney *U* test;
[c] $p < 0.005$, cancer cases vs. controls; two-sided mid-P test;
[d] $p << 0.0001$, cancer cases vs. controls, Mann-Whitney *U* test;
[e] $p < 0.001$, cancer cases vs. DNA damage assay control subset, Kruskal-Wallis *H* test *post-hoc* analysis;
[f] Tumor staging classification: T – describes the size of the primary tumor and its invasiveness, N – describes the regional lymph nodes involved, *x* –data not available.

Genotyping

In this study, we focused on single nucleotide polymorphisms (SNPs) occurring predominantly in non-coding region of *RAD51C*, as it is assumed that these SNPs may be involved in gene expression regulation. We involved seven SNPs localized in gene's promoter, 5′UTR of exon 1 and intron 1. Only those SNPs the minor allele frequency (MAF) of which in the Caucasian population exceeded 10% (according to data contained in dbSNP database [31]) were selected for the study. Possible involvement of selected SNPs in regulation of *RAD51C* expression was tested by is-rSNP algorithm [32], an *in-silico* method for prediction whether an SNP can be considered as regulatory (i.e. disrupting the transcription factor binding). Exemplary results of such prediction for selected well-known nuclear transcription factors together with other detailed information on SNPs analyzed in this study are provided in Table 2.

All SNPs involved in this study were genotyped in DNA isolated from the whole blood samples by means of the real-time PCR technique using either custom or pre-designed commercially available TaqMan SNP Genotyping Assays (Life Technologies, Carlsbad, CA, USA) according to manufacturer's instructions. Genotyping was performed on BioRad's iQ5 iCycler Multicolor Real Time PCR Detection System (BioRad, Hercules, CA, USA) in 20-μl aliquots containing 16 ng DNA. The cycling conditions, preceded by polymerase activation (95°C, 10 min) consisted of 50 cycles involving DNA denaturation at 95°C for 15 s followed by a combined annealing-elongation step at 61.5°C for 1 min, during which the fluorescence signal was measured. The genotype recognition of analyzed subjects was performed automatically using the BioRad's iQ5 Optical System Software ver. 2.0.

Ten per cent of obtained results were verified by repeated genotyping using the same technique.

Determination of thiobarbituric acid-reactive species in blood plasma

An individual's level of oxidative stress was evaluated based on the amount of thiobarbituric acid-reactive species (TBARS) assayed in the plasma obtained from the heparinized peripheral blood sample. The concentration of TBARS was determined using the method previously described by Wasowicz et al. [33], based on the reaction of 2-thiobarbituric acid (TBA) with malondialdehyde, which is a naturally occurring side-product of lipid peroxidation. Briefly, a 50-μl aliquot of blood plasma was mixed with 1 ml deionized water, 25 μl of 5 M HCl and 1 ml of 12.2% (v/v) acetic acid containing 29 mM TBA. The mixtures were incubated for 1 h at 95–100°C and subsequently cooled on ice. After addition of 3.5 ml of 1-butanol, the samples were vortexed thoroughly for 2 min and centrifuged at 2880×g, room temperature for 10 min. Finally, the concentration of TBARS was assessed by measuring the fluorescence of the butanol extract at wavelength of 547 nm following excitation at 525 nm on using a PerkinElmer LS50-B instrument (PerkinElmer, Shelton, CT, USA). The concentration of TBARS in blood plasma was expressed in μM. A dilution series of 1,1,3,3-tetraaethoxypropane was used for standard curve preparation.

DNA damage assays

DNA damage including the single-strand breaks (SSBs) and alkali-labile sites (ALSs) was assayed in whole blood using alkaline single-cell gel electrophoresis (SCGE; comet assay) method as described by Singh et al. [34] and modified by Mc Kelvey-Martin et al. [35]. One aliquot of whole blood was mixed with nine aliquots of RPMI-1640 medium containing 10% fetal calf serum and ten aliquots of 2% (in PBS) molten agarose type VII (Low gelling temperature). The mixture was then spread on a slide (Sigma-Aldrich) earlier covered with agarose type I (Low EEO) at 1% concentration in water and dried. The cells embedded in the agarose gel were lysed in cold lysing solution (2.5 M NaCl, 100 mM Na_2EDTA, 10 mM Tris base, pH 10, with 1% Triton X-100 added just before use) at 4°C for at least 1 hour. Subsequently, DNA was unwound in alkaline electrophoresis buffer (1 mM Na_2EDTA, 300 mM NaOH, pH >13) for 20 min to produce single stranded DNA and to express SSBs and ALSs and electrophoresed in the same alkaline conditions (30 min, 25 V, 300 mA, 0.93 V/cm). The gels were then neutralized by rinsing three times with 0.4 M Tris buffer (pH 7.5) and the slides were dried for storage.

In parallel analyses, oxidatively generated damage to DNA bases was identified using modified comet assay as described earlier by Collins et al. [36]. After lysis, the slides were washed

Table 2. Resume of *RAD51C* SNPs analyzed in the study.

rs-code	New name	Other names	SNP position	MAF	Disruption of binding of selected nuclear transcription factors (*p-value*)				
					NF-κB	Pax-5	Bcl-6	c-Myb	p53
rs302874	c.-2009C>T	g.3034C>T	5' near gene (promoter)	T: 0.42	-	-	-	-	0.0052
rs12946522	c.-1902T>G	g.3141T>G	5' near gene (promoter)	G: 0.17	0.0023	-	0.0028	-	0.0076
rs302873	c.-524C>G	g.4519C>G	5' near gene (promoter)	G: 0.41	0.0448	0.0698	-	0.0002	-
rs16943176	c.-118G>A	g.4925G>A	5' near gene (promoter)	A: 0.20	0.0133	0.0385	0.0391	0.0281	0.0490
rs12946397	c.-26C>T	g.5017C>T	exon 1 (5'UTR)	T: 0.21	0.0117	0.0642	0.0069	-	0.0196
rs17222691	c.145+947C>T	g.6134C>T	intron 1	T: 0.20	0.0461	0.0051	0.0257	0.0131	0.0034
rs28363302	c.146-706delC	g.6624delC	intron 1	del: 0.18	*NA*	*NA*	*NA*	*NA*	*NA*

SNP nomenclature, localization and minor allele frequencies (MAF) are provided according to data obtained from the dbSNP database [31]. Additionally, the levels of significance (p-values) for observing the change in binding affinity between the *RAD51C* promoter and several well-known transcription factors caused by SNPs investigated in our study, as inferred by the is-rSNP algorithm [32] against the Transfac database [48] are also provided. Dash indicates that the given SNP is unlikely to affect the binding of given transcription factor. *NA* - not applicable.

three times with enzyme buffer (0.1 M KCl, 0.5 mM Na_2EDTA, 40 mM HEPES-KOH, 0.2 mg/ml bovine serum albumin, pH 8) and incubated with formamidopyrimidine glycosylase (FPG) at 1 μg/ml in this buffer (kept at −80°C) for 30 min at 37°C. The slides were then electrophoresed and neutralized as described above. Finally, the slides were stained with 5 μg/ml DAPI and 50 cells from each slide were analyzed using an Olympus fluorescence microscope (a BX40 instrument; Olympus, Tokyo, Japan) equipped with an image analysis system (Comet IV, Perceptive Instruments, UK).

In the case of each individual, four slides were prepared simultaneously - two for assessment of DNA strand breakage and the other two, which included also the FPG treatment, for the assessment of total DNA damage (i.e. DNA strand breakage and oxidatively generated DNA damage). Relative amount of DNA in the comet tail (henceforth referred to as % DNA) obtained based on computer-aided image analysis was used as the marker of respective DNA damage. Oxidatively generated DNA damage was expressed as the difference between the total DNA damage and DNA strand breakage. For the purposes of analysis, the ratio of oxidatively generated DNA damage to DNA strand breakage was used and was calculated as

$$R = \frac{\textit{total DNA damage (in \% DNA)}}{\textit{DNA strand breakage(in \% DNA)}} - 1.$$

Statistical analysis

Both absolute and relative allelic/genotypic frequencies are provided for each analyzed SNP. The Hardy-Weinberg equilibrium (HWE) was tested by a goodness-of-fit chi-square test. Inter-group comparisons of observed allelic/genotypic frequencies were performed using unconditional logistic regression and the strength of association between SNPs and breast cancer was expressed by means of age-adjusted odds ratio (OR). All ORs are provided together with corresponding 95% confidence intervals (95% CI). In the case of genotypic comparisons, both dominant and recessive genetic models were assumed.

To account for possible non-random associations between investigated *Rad51C* SNPs, linkage disequilibrium analysis and haplotype reconstruction were performed using the Haploview package [37]. LD was expressed by means of a normalized measure of allelic association |D'| [38] and LD blocks were inferred using the confidence interval method described by Gabriel et al. [39]. Briefly, a pair of SNPs is said to be in "strong LD", if the upper confidence bound of |D'|>0.98 and the lower one >0.7. Contrary to this, a "strong recombination" between a pair of SNPs is inferred, if the upper confidence bound of |D'|< 0.90. All other possibilities were classified as inconclusive. A block of "strong LD" (or a haplotype block) is defined as a region in which 95% of comparisons among informative SNPs show strong evidence of LD. Haplotypes reconstructed within each block were tested for differences in their frequencies between the control and BrC group and the significance of such differences was assessed using the two-sided exact mid-P test. Possible linkage between haplotypes and BrC was assessed based on OR with corresponding 95% CI.

Normal distribution of numerical data was tested by means of the Shapiro-Wilk *W* test. Data departing from normal distribution are provided as median [interquartile range]. As data for TBARS and relative amount of DNA in comet tails met all relevant criteria for normal distribution but were found to be significantly right-skewed, they were logarithmically transformed prior to any further analyses. Transformed data fulfilling all the criteria for normal distribution are presented as mean ± standard deviation (SD) and expressed in log-units. Analysis of outliers was performed on the basis of estimated Cook's distances. Inter-group comparisons of normally distributed data adjusted for differences in age were performed using the two-way analysis of covariance (ANCOVA) involving the subjects' age as covariate. Post-hoc comparisons were performed using the Scheffé test. In all analyses investigating the effect of *RAD51C* SNPs on markers of DNA damage, only the dominant genetic model was assumed due to limited number of rare homozygotes. In the case of blood plasma TBARS, dominant as well as additive genetic models were used. The recessive genetic model was omitted due to low number of rare homozygotes.

The significance of differences between groups in other non-paired data (such as individuals' age, sex and tobacco consumption) were assessed using the Mann-Whitney *U*, Student's *t*, or two-sided exact mid-P test, depending on the character and distribution of data. The Spearman's rank correlation (R_S) was used to identify possible additional confounders, which were also involved in ANCOVA when appropriate to ensure the robustness of identified effects.

All statistical calculations were performed using the Statistica 8.0 package (StatSoft, Tulsa, USA).

Results

Genetic variability of *RAD51C* SNPs and association with breast cancer

Single-site analyses of all SNPs with respect to their possible association with BrC risk were performed. All analyzed SNPs presented the observed genotype frequencies which were found to be in agreement with the ones predicted by the Hardy-Weinberg law in both the control and breast cancer groups. Nevertheless, comparing the allelic frequencies between the two groups, none of the analyzed SNPs of *RAD51C* was found to present significantly different distributions of its alleles, suggesting that neither allele of any SNP can be assumed to be associated with increased BrC risk. Comparing the genotypic frequencies, neither SNP was found to present significantly different distributions of corresponding genotypes, either under dominant or recessive genetic models (Table 3).

Analysis of LD between *RAD51C* SNPs revealed a "strong LD" block spanning from rs16943176 (c.-118G>A) in 5′near gene region, through rs12946397 (c.-26C>T) in exon 1 to rs17222691 (c.145+947C>T) in intron 1 of *RAD51C* (Figure 1). Within this LD block, three rare and two common haplotypes ($^{-118}$G/$^{-26}$C/$^{145+957}$C and $^{-118}$A/$^{-26}$T/$^{145+957}$T) were reconstructed. Common haplotypes encompassed together 99.7% of all haplotypes (Table 3), nevertheless, they failed to present any significant differences in distribution between controls and BrC subjects, suggesting that haplotypes in non-coding region of *RAD51C* neither are associated with the increased risk of BrC.

Effect of *RAD51C* SNPs on blood plasma levels of TBARS. Interaction with BrC

Overall levels of TBARS in blood plasma from BrC cases and healthy controls are shown in Figure 2, and were found to be significantly higher among BrC cases compared to controls ($p<0.0001$). To investigate how *RAD51C* SNPs interact with BrC in affecting the blood plasma levels of TBARS, age-adjusted single-site ANCOVA analyses, involving one *RAD51C* SNP at a time were performed. Moreover, the subjects' lifetime tobacco consumption, which was found to differ between the groups (see Table 1), correlated significantly with blood plasma TBARS ($R_S = 0.248$; $p<0.005$), and was thus also involved in ANCOVA as confounder. Log-transformed levels of TBARS in blood plasma of controls and BrC cases with respect to carried genotype, under both additive and dominant genetic models, are presented in Table 4.

Age-adjusted ANCOVA involving lifetime smoking as confounder did not confirm the BrC status as the factor significantly affecting the blood plasma level of TBARS, despite the levels of TBARS in blood plasma of BrC females were slightly (but insignificantly) higher compared to the one among healthy controls (0.41±0.16 vs. 0.35±0.13 log-µM, *NS*; Table 4B).

Under additive genetic model, the main effects of rs12946522 (c.-1902T>G), rs16943176 (c.-118G>A) and rs12946397 (c.-26C>T), unlike the remaining four SNPs (i.e. rs302874 (c.-200A>G), rs302873 (c.-524C>G), rs17222691 (c.145+947C>T) and rs28363302 (c.146–706delC)), on blood plasma TBARS were all found to be statistically significant ($p<0.05$ for main effects of the three SNPs adjusted for age and lifetime tobacco consumption). No statistically significant interaction between the genetic variability of *RAD51C* and BrC was found, for any of investigated *RAD51C* SNPs. Post-hoc multiple comparisons showed that the significance of main effects of rs12946522, rs16943176 and rs12946397 on blood plasma level of TBARS was due to significantly higher levels of TBARS in heterozygotic females (in both BrC cases and controls taken together) compared to their respective wild-type homozygotic counterparts ($^{-1902}$TG vs. $^{-1902}$TT: 0.44±0.15 vs. 0.35±0.14 log-µM, $p<0.05$; $^{-118}$GA vs. $^{-118}$GG, $^{-26}$CT vs. $^{-26}$CC: 0.43±0.15 vs. 0.36±0.14 log-µM, $p<0.05$; Table 4B). Similar effects of the three SNPs with the same direction were observed in both BrC and control groups considered separately, but the resultant differences were not statistically significant (Table 4A).

Results of analyses assuming dominant genetic model confirm those described above as statistically significant main effects of rs12946522, rs16943176, rs12946397 and additionally also the rs17222691 on blood plasma levels of TBARS were found ($p<0.01$ and $p<0.05$ for age-and-tobacco-consumption-adjusted main effects of rs12946522, and rs16943176, rs12946397, rs17222691, respectively). It turned out that the blood plasma level of TBARS in females carrying rare-allele-containing genotypes was significantly higher compared to the one of respective wild-type homozygotes ($^{-1902}$TG&$^{-1902}$GG vs. $^{-1902}$TT: 0.43±0.15 vs. 0.35±0.14 log-µM, $p<0.01$; $^{-118}$GA&$^{-118}$AA vs. $^{-118}$GG and $^{-26}$CT&$^{-26}$TT vs. $^{-26}$CC: 0.43±0.15 vs. 0.36±0.14 log-µM, $p<0.01$; $^{145+947}$CT&$^{145+947}$TT vs. $^{145+947}$CC: 0.43±0.15 vs. 0.36±0.14 log-µM; $p<0.05$; Table 4B). Again, similar effects of the three SNPs with the same direction, although insignificant, were observed in the BrC and control subgroups (Table 4A).

Effect of *RAD51C* SNPs on DNA damage. Interaction with BrC

Overall levels of DNA strand breakage and total DNA damage in the groups of BrC cases and cancer-free controls are shown in Figure 2. The level of DNA strand breakage was significantly higher in BrC cases compared to controls ($p<0.001$) while the total DNA damage did not vary significantly between the groups. Again, to investigate how *RAD51C* SNPs interact with BrC in affecting the total DNA damage and the DNA strand breakage, age-adjusted single-site ANCOVA analyses were performed assuming only the dominant genetic model. Since the blood plasma levels of TBARS, which differed between compared groups (see Fig. 2), correlated significantly with the level of DNA strand breakage ($R_S = 0.184$; $p<0.05$), the subjects' blood plasma

Table 3. Observed frequencies of genotypes and haplotypes reconstructed based on SNPs located within the LD block identified in *RAD51C*, together with respective odds ratios (OR) and corresponding 95% confidence intervals in BrC cases and healthy controls.

SNP	BrC cases	Controls	OR [95% CI][a,b]	DNA damage control subset [c]
rs302874				
CC	55 (0.42)	69 (0.37)	A: 0.9 [0.7 – 1.3]	16 (0.40)
CT	56 (0.42)	92 (0.49)	D: 0.8 [0.5 – 1.2]	19 (0.48)
TT	21 (0.16)	27 (0.14)	R: 1.1 [0.6 – 2.1]	5 (0.13)
rs12946522				
TT	88 (0.67)	119 (0.64)	A: 0.8 [0.5 – 1.2]	29 (0.73)
TG	41 (0.31)	55 (0.29)	D: 0.9 [0.5 – 1.4]	8 (0.20)
GG	3 (0.02)	13 (0.07)	R: 0.5 [0.1 – 1.8]	3 (0.07)
rs302873				
CC	54 (0.41)	68 (0.36)	A: 0.9 [0.7 – 1.2]	15 (0.38)
CG	56 (0.42)	86 (0.46)	D: 0.8 [0.5 – 1.2]	17 (0.42)
GG	22 (0.17)	34 (0.18)	R: 0.9 [0.5 – 1.6]	8 (0.20)
rs16943176				
GG	86 (0.65)	118 (0.63)	A: 0.9 [0.6 – 1.3]	30 (0.74)
GA	43 (0.33)	63 (0.34)	D: 0.9 [0.6 – 1.5]	9 (0.23)
AA	3 (0.02)	7 (0.04)	R: 0.9 [0.2 – 3.7]	1 (0.03)
rs12946397				
CC	85 (0.64)	119 (0.63)	A: 0.9 [0.6 – 1.4]	30 (0.74)
CT	44 (0.33)	61 (0.32)	D: 1.0 [0.6 – 1.6]	9 (0.23)
TT	3 (0.02)	8 (0.04)	R: 0.7 [0.2 – 2.9]	1 (0.03)
rs17222691				
CC	88 (0.67)	119 (0.63)	A: 0.9 [0.6 – 1.3]	30 (0.74)
CT	41 (0.31)	62 (0.33)	D: 0.9 [0.5 – 1.4]	9 (0.23)
TT	3 (0.02)	7 (0.04)	R: 0.9 [0.2 – 3.7]	1 (0.03)
rs28363302				
CC	114 (0.86)	152 (0.80)	A: 0.7 [0.4 – 1.2]	32 (0.80)
C/del	17 (0.13)	36 (0.19)	D: 0.7 [0.4 – 1.4]	8 (0.20)
del/del	1 (0.01)	1 (0.01)	R: 1.3 [0.1 – 21.5]	0 (0.00)
Haplotype	**BrC cases**	**Controls**	**OR [95% CI] [d]**	
GCC	214 (0.811)	298 (0.793)	1.1 [0.8 – 1.7]	-
ATT	47 (0.178)	76 (0.202)	0.9 [0.6 – 1.3]	-
ATC	2 (0.008)	0 (0.000)	*NA*	-
GTC	1 (0.004)	1 (0.003)	1.4 [0.04 – 55.8]	-
ACC	0 (0.000)	1 (0.003)	*NA*	-

Data presented as absolute (relative) frequencies of individual genotypes observed in BrC cases, controls and in subjects randomized into DNA damage control subset. *NA* – not applicable.

[a] Genetic model employed in order to analyze the association between genotype distribution and cancer: A – direct comparison of the frequency of alleles; D – dominant genetic model; R – recessive genetic model;

[b] OR values adjusted for age and smoking status, together with 95% CI determined by logistic regression;

[c] Significant differences in genotype distributions between the whole control group and the DNA damage control subjects were sought for by the generalized Fisher exact (Fisher-Freeman-Halton) test. No significant differences were found;

[d] OR values and 95% CI determined by two-sided exact mid-P test.

levels of TBARS were accounted for in ANCOVA as confounder. Log-transformed levels of total DNA damage and DNA strand breakage with respect to carried genotype are provided in Figure 3.

The analysis did not reveal the main effects of BrC as well as any of the 7 *RAD51C* SNPs on the extent of total DNA damage as being statistically significant, so did it not find any significant interaction between these two factors (Table 5A). No significant differences in the subgroups of BrC cases and controls were observable either (Figure 3). On the other hand, DNA strand breakage was found to be significantly increased among BrC cases compared to controls ($p<0.005$ for main effect). Nevertheless, the

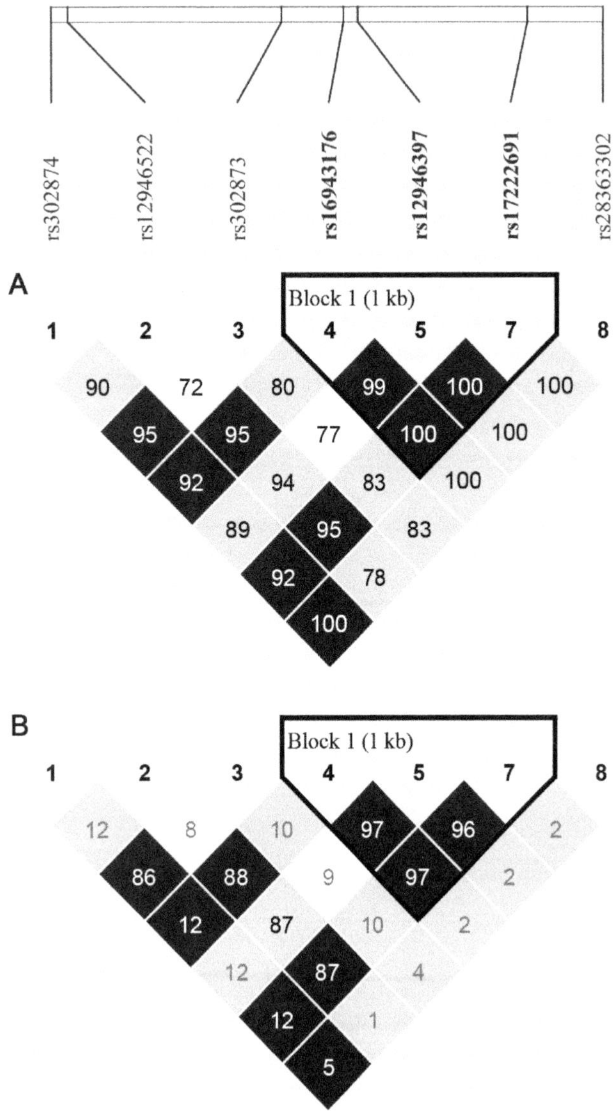

Figure 1. The map of LD between seven analyzed SNPs in non-coding regions of *RAD51C*. The values in the map are the normalized measures of allelic association |D'| (**A**) and correlation coefficients (r^2) (**B**) calculated for each pair of SNPs (both provided as percentages). The color scheme represent the corresponding confidence bounds for a given pair of SNPs: black – strong evidence of LD; grey – inconclusive; white – strong evidence of recombination [37]. Solid line indicates the identified 1 kb-long LD block, within which common and rare haplotypes were reconstructed, the frequency of which is provided in the Table 3. Algorithm employed for LD block identification is described in the *Material and Methods* section.

main effects of the 7 *RAD51C* SNPs on DNA strand breakage were not found to be statistically significant (Table 5B).

We subsequently analyzed the effect of *RAD51C* and BrC on the ratio of oxidatively generated DNA damage to DNA strand breakage (the *R*-value). The blood plasma level of TBARS was involved in age-adjusted ANCOVA as confounder due to significant correlation with *R*-value ($R_S = -0.323$; $p<0.001$). This analysis yielded the main effects of rs12946522, rs16943176, rs12946397 and rs17222691 on the ratio of oxidatively generated DNA damage to DNA strand breakage as statistically significant (age-and-TBARS-adjusted main effects: $p<0.005$ for rs16943176, $p<0.01$ in the case of rs12946522, rs12946397 and rs17222691; Table 6B). While in the carriers of respective wild-type genotypes the mean log-values of *R* ranged from −0.03 to −0.04, which corresponded to ratio of oxidatively generated DNA damage to DNA strand breakage between 0.93 and 0.91, the carriers of genotypes containing at least one respective rare allele presented significantly decreased log-values of *R* ranging from −0.28 to −0.31, corresponding to ratio of oxidatively generated DNA damage to DNA strand breakage of 0.49 to 0.52 ($p<0.0005$ for rs12946522 and rs16943176, $p<0.001$ for rs12946397 and $p<0.005$ for rs17222691; as compared to wild-types; Table 6B). Such effects of the four SNPs on *R*-value with the same direction were also found in the subgroups of BrC cases and healthy controls, but in the most of the cases, the resulting differences were not sufficient to prove their significance (Table 6A). No statistically significant main effects of the remaining three *RAD51C* SNPs on the ratio of oxidatively generated DNA damage to DNA strand breakage were observed. The main effect of BrC on *R*-value was found to be insignificant and so did the resultant between-group differences. No statistically significant interaction between BrC and *RAD51C* SNP influencing the *R*-value was either found.

Discussion

Since the first study by Meindl et al. in 2010 [13], *RAD51C* has been a subject of increasing interest and several subsequent studies employing different populations have generally delivered outcomes confirming that *RAD51C* harbors mutations associated to HBOC or unselected OC [14,18–22]. Despite the fact, that these mutations seem to occur with considerably lower frequency than it was originally suggested [14,19–21], *RAD51C* is nowadays considered a HBOC/OC susceptibility gene [20]. Notably, all of the studies available to date seem to be in unison reporting that these mutations are however absent or at least extremely rare in hereditary BrC.

Since the previous studies were predominantly focused on missense mutations, we conducted a study in which a case-control setup was employed to evaluate the role of seven common SNPs in non-coding regions of *RAD51C* in modulation of BrC risk. Single-site analyses did not provide any evidence in favor of the hypothesis that any of investigated SNPs may be of importance with respect to BrC risk. Analysis of reconstructed haplotypes also failed to confirm that higher structures resulting from non-random associations between SNPs within this region of *RAD51C* may alter the resultant BrC risk. Although such haplotypes were found to alter the HNC risk in our previous study [30], in the context of BrC our results seem to be in line with several recent studies, in which rs12946522, rs16943176, rs12946397 and rs17222691 were studied under the case-control setup or using the *in silico* methods in relation to BrC risk, all of which failed to confirm the significantly increased frequency of these SNPs among BrC patients [14,18,20,23,25,40,41]. The remaining three SNPs investigated in our study (rs302874, rs302873 and rs28363302) have not yet been studied earlier in relation to BrC, but our data seem to indicate that their involvement in BrC risk modulation is rather unlikely.

Nowadays, it is widely accepted that RAD51 paralogs are involved in HR-mediated step of DSB repair occurring during the S- and G_2-phase of the cell cycle [42,43], recovery of stalled or broken replication fork [44] and in repair of interstrand cross-links [12]. In addition to this, a recent study has proposed that RAD51, RAD51C and XRCC3 may all play their roles in protection of mitochondrial genome against oxidative damage as well [17]. Despite the fact that we did not find any evidence confirming a

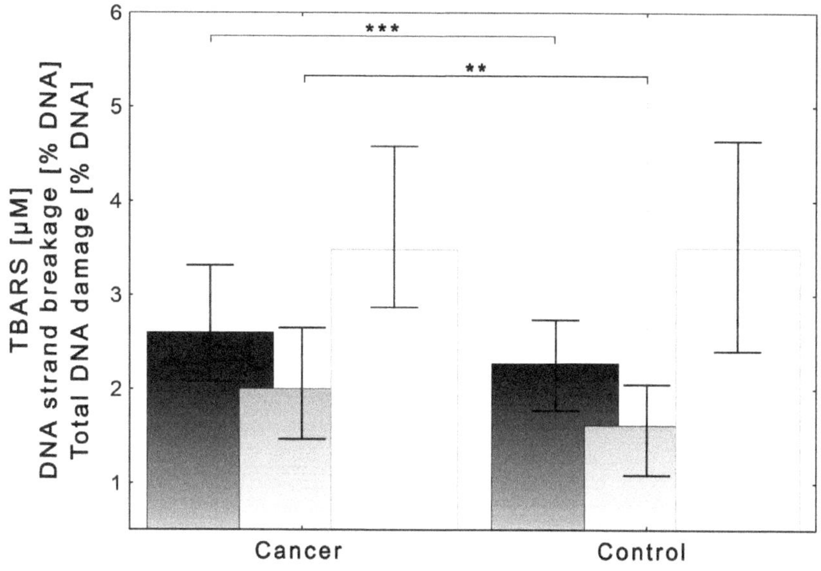

Figure 2. Levels of TBARS (dark columns), DNA strand breakage (grey columns) and total DNA damage (white columns) determined in whole blood samples from BrC cases and healthy control females. Data presented as medians (columns) and interquartile ranges (whiskers). Levels of TBARS among BrC cases (n = 132) vs. control females (n = 189): 2.6 [2.1–3.3] μM vs. 2.3 [1.8–2.7] μM, $p < 0.0001$, Mann-Whitney *U* test (***). Levels of DNA strand breakage and total DNA damage were assessed in the whole group of BrC cases and tested for differences against a subset of 40 control subjects randomly selected from the whole control group by means of the age-stratified randomization (*see Materials and Methods*). DNA strand breakage: BrC cases vs. controls: 2.0 [1.5–2.7] %DNA in comet tail vs. 1.6 [1.1–2.1] %DNA in comet tail, $p < 0.001$, Mann-Whitney *U* test (**). Total DNA damage: BrC cases vs. controls: 3.5 [2.9–4.6] %DNA in comet tail vs. 3.5 [2.4–4.6] %DNA in comet tail, *NS*. The age distribution in the control subset was verified to match with the one in the whole control group (*see Table 1*). The distribution of TBARS in the randomized subset of 40 controls did not differ significantly from the one observed in the whole control group (1.7 [1.5–2.1] μM vs. 2.3 [1.8–2.7] μM, *NS*) but differed significantly from the one in the BrC group (1.7 [1.5–2.1] μM vs. 2.6 [2.1–3.3] μM, $p < 0.001$, Kruskal-Wallis *H*-test post-hoc analysis).

direct link between genetic variability of RAD51C and BrC risk, such new and indeed intriguing notion made us to undertake further analyses aimed to find out, whether the role of RAD51C in protection against oxidative stress and oxidatively generated DNA damage can be extrapolated to nuclear DNA as well, and if so, whether it may be associated with BrC.

To our surprise, outcomes of our analyses seems to indicate that the variability in noncoding regions of *RAD51C* is linked to changes in blood plasma levels of TBARS, a widely-used marker of oxidative stress and thus that the role of this gene in certain modulation of oxidative stress in general cannot be ruled out. More precisely, we observed a blood plasma TBARS-increasing effect being linked to rare alleles of four out of seven investigated *RAD51C* SNPs (rs12946522, rs16943176, rs12946397 and rs17222691). Such effect was observed under dominant genetic model, in the case of which we obtained relatively straightforward outcomes with high power of statistical testing (reaching 90%) implying that heterozygotic and homozygotic carriers of rare alleles exhibit increased blood plasma levels of TBARS. Under additive genetic model, this effect was observed only among heterozygotic but not homozygotic carriers of rare alleles (compared to respective wild-type homozygotes), which may be due to relatively low number of rare homozygotes in some analyses: as shown in Table 3 there were only 3 homozygotic carriers of rare alleles for each of the four SNPs under discussion. Notably, such increased blood plasma level of TBARS was observed among both the controls and BrC cases, what seems to suggest that BrC and *RAD51C* genetic variability do not interact with each other in modulation of TBARS level, and thus the increased oxidative stress possibly caused by *RAD51C* genetic variability rather cannot be assumed to be linked to BrC. Nevertheless, one may speculate that the difference in blood plasma levels of TBARS between carriers of individual genotypes of rs12946522, rs16943176, rs12946397 and rs17222691 seems to be much more pronounced among control subjects than in BrC cases (see Table 4A), suggesting that the relationship between *RAD51C* SNPs and oxidative stress may differ between the groups of BrC and control subjects. This could possibly point to direct involvement of *RAD51C* in processes imposing conditions contributing to eventual BrC development, but unfortunately, our study did not provide sufficient evidence to prove significance of such interaction. Either way, further studies are required to elucidate whether such interaction is non-existent or the apparent lack of such is rather an effect of low number of rare homozygotes enrolled in our study.

Based on data obtained for biomarkers of DNA damage, our study seems to indicate that the situation concerning the effect of *RAD51C* genetic variability on DNA damage in peripheral blood leukocytes is much more complex. Generally speaking, none of the seven *RAD51C* SNPs investigated in our study were found to influence the level of total DNA damage. But intriguingly, under dominant genetic model, the contributions of oxidatively generated DNA damage and DNA strand breakage to the total pool of detected DNA damage seemed to be in function of *RAD51C* genetic variability. This hypothesis seems to be supported by the fact that the ratio of oxidatively generated DNA damage to DNA strand breakage was found to be significantly decreased among heterozygotic and homozygotic carriers of rs12946522, rs16943176, rs12946397 or rs17222691 rare alleles compared to carriers of their respective counterparts. This implies, that genetic variability at these four loci of *RAD51C* may somehow change the characteristics of observed DNA damage in whole blood leukocytes: according to observed changes in the *R*-value, the fraction of oxidatively generated DNA damage (out of the total

Table 4. Effect of *RAD51C* SNPs and BrC on blood plasma log-levels of TBARS.

A

	TBARS [log-μM]						
Controls	**rs302874**	**rs12946522**	**rs302873**	**rs16943176**	**rs12946397**	**rs17222691**	**rs28363302**
wt-homozygotes	0.37±0.12	0.31±0.11	0.37±0.12	0.32±0.11	0.32±0.11	0.32±0.11	0.35±0.14
heterozygotes	0.33±0.13	0.44±0.12	0.33±0.13	0.43±0.12	0.43±0.12	0.43±0.12	0.35±0.14
rare homozygotes	0.36±0.15	0.29±0.04	0.36±0.14	0.27±0.13	0.27±0.13	0.27±0.13	0.54
heterozygotes & *rare* homozygotes	0.34±0.13	0.42±0.13	0.34±0.13	0.42±0.13	0.42±0.13	0.42±0.13	0.35±0.11
BrC cases							
wt-homozygotes	0.40±0.15	0.39±0.14	0.40±0.15	0.39±0.15	0.39±0.15	0.40±0.15	0.42±0.15
heterozygotes	0.42±0.17	0.44±0.18	0.41±0.16	0.44±0.17	0.44±0.17	0.43±0.17	0.38±0.12
rare homozygotes	0.42±0.16	0.48±0.20	0.44±0.17	0.48±0.20	0.48±0.20	0.48±0.20	0.32
heterozygotes & *rare* homozygotes	0.42±0.16	0.45±0.18	0.42±0.16	0.45±0.17	0.45±0.17	0.44±0.17	0.36±0.11

B

	Summary of analysis						
Main effect: BrC status							
Controls	0.35±0.13						
BrC cases	0.41±0.16						
Main effect: *RAD51C* SNP	**rs302874**	**rs12946522** [a]	**rs302873**	**rs16943176** [b]	**rs12946397** [b]	**rs17222691** [c]	**rs28363302**
wt-homozygotes	0.39±0.14	0.35±0.14	0.39±0.14	0.36±0.14	0.36±0.14	0.36±0.14	0.38±0.15
heterozygotes	0.37±0.15	0.44±0.15 [d]	0.37±0.15	0.43±0.15[d]	0.43±0.15 [d]	0.43±0.15	0.36±0.13
rare homozygotes	0.39±0.15	0.38±0.16	0.40±0.16	0.43±0.19	0.43±0.19	0.43±0.19	0.43±0.15
heterozygotes & *rare* homozygotes	0.38±0.15	0.43±0.15 [e]	0.38±0.15	0.43±0.15 [e]	0.43±0.15 [e]	0.43±0.15 [f]	0.36±0.11

(**A**) Log-transformed levels of TBARS in blood plasma of healthy controls and BrC cases by carried genotype. (**B**) Summary of the analysis of main effects of *RAD51C* SNP and BrC on blood plasma levels of TBARS, adjusted to subjects' age and lifetime smoking. In each column data are presented as means ± SD. Identification of genotypes as wild-type (*wt*)-homozygotes, heterozygotes and *rare* homozygotes with reference to Table 3, in which individual genotypes for each SNP are ordered accordingly. The levels of significance of main effects and post-hoc multiple comparisons were inferred by ANCOVA and the *Scheffé* test, respectively. Main effects: [a] $p < 0.05$ and $p < 0.01$ under additive and dominant model, respectively; [b] $p < 0.05$ under additive and dominant models; [c] $p < 0.05$ under dominant model; Post-hoc comparisons: [d] $p < 0.05$ compared to *wt*-homozygotes; [e] $p < 0.01$ compared to *wt*-homozygotes; [f] $p < 0.05$ compared to *wt*-homozygotes.

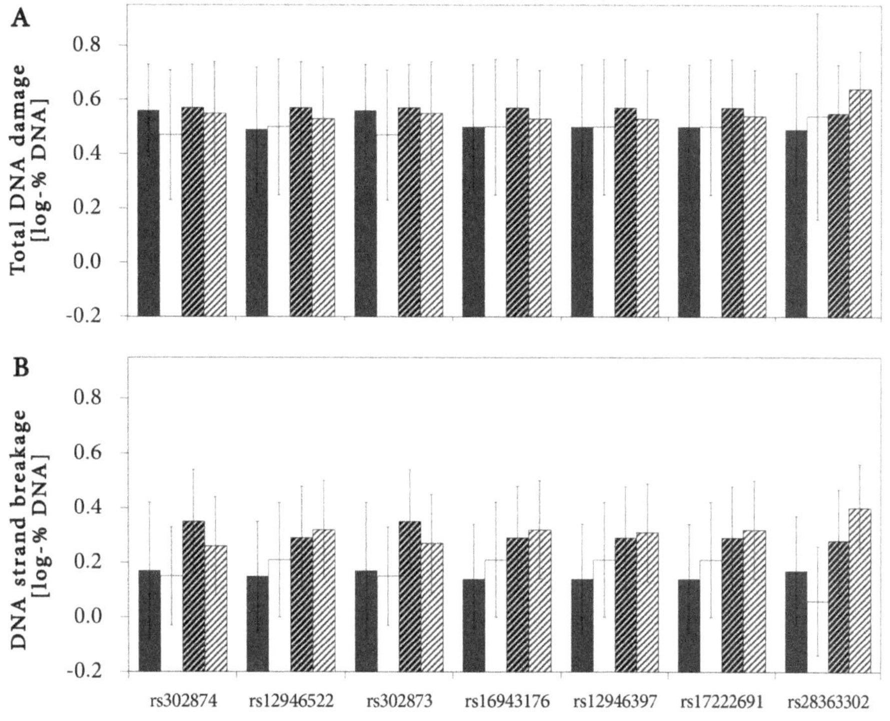

Figure 3. Log-transformed levels of total DNA damage (A) and DNA strand breakage (B) expressed as logarithmically-transformed relative amount of DNA in respective comet tails in whole blood leukocytes of healthy controls (solid) and BrC cases (stripes) carrying the respective wild-type (*wt-*; dark columns) or rare-allele containing (*var-*; light columns) genotypes. Only dominant genetic model was assumed. Identification of genotypes as *wild-type* or rare-allele containing (i.e. heterozygotic and *rare* homozygotes) with reference to Table 3, in which individual genotypes for each SNP are ordered accordingly. Data are presented as means (columns) ± SD (error bars). Logarithmical transformation was employed in order to normalize the distribution of raw comet assay data for the purpose of ANOVA/ANCOVA analysis. Total DNA damage data for *wt*-controls, *var*-controls, *wt*-cases and *var*-cases, respectively (log-%): **rs302874:** 0.56±0.17, 0.47±0.24, 0.57±0.16, 0.55±0.19; **rs12946522:** 0.49±0.23, 0.50±0.25, 0.57±0.17, 0.53±0.19; **rs302873:** 0.56±0.17, 0.47±0.24, 0.57±0.16, 0.55±0.19; **rs16943176:** 0.50±0.23, 0.50±0.25, 0.57±0.18, 0.53±0.18; **rs12946397:** 0.50±0.23, 0.50±0.25, 0.57±0.18, 0.53±0.18; **rs17222691:** 0.50±0.23, 0.50±0.25, 0.57±0.18, 0.54±0.17; **rs28363302:** 0.49±0.21, 0.54±0.38, 0.55±0.18, 0.64±0.14. DNA strand breakage data *wt*-controls, *var*-controls, *wt*-cases and *var*-cases: **rs302874:** 0.17±0.25, 0.15±0.18, 0.35±0.19, 0.26±0.18; **rs12946522:** 0.15±0.20, 0.21±0.21, 0.29±0.19, 0.32±0.18; **rs302873:** 0.17±0.25, 0.15±0.18, 0.35±0.19, 0.27±0.18; **rs16943176:** 0.14±0.20, 0.21±0.21, 0.29±0.19, 0.32±0.18; **rs12946397:** 0.14±0.20, 0.21±0.21, 0.29±0.19, 0.31±0.18; **rs17222691:** 0.14±0.20, 0.21±0.21, 0.29±0.19, 0.32±0.18; **rs28363302:** 0.17±0.20, 0.06±0.20, 0.28±0.19, 0.40±0.16. See Table 5 for the summary of statistical analysis.

DNA damage) dropped from some 48% among wild-types to some 34% among rare allele carriers, with this drop being statistically significant. Combined with increased blood plasma levels of TBARS observed among rare allele carriers, it all becomes even more intriguing: it seems that carriers of at least one rare allele of rs12946522, rs16943176, rs12946397 or rs17222691 present increased oxidative stress linked to increased proportion of DNA strand breakage (with relatively even distribution between oxidatively generated DNA damage and DNA strand breakage), while the respective wild-type carriers present decreased level of oxidative stress linked with DNA damage rather presenting the characteristics of oxidatively generated damage. On one hand, the link between *RAD51C* genetic variability and blood plasma levels of TBARS we observed in our study seems to indicate that this gene might indeed be involved in protection against oxidative damage, as it was suggested to be in the case of mitochondrial DNA [17]. On the other hand, simultaneous increase of the fraction of DNA strand breakage at the cost of oxidatively generated DNA damage due to genetic variability of *RAD51C* seems to support the crucial role of this gene in HR repair of DSBs, i.e. the protection of DNA against strand breakage instead. How could it be possible that increased level of oxidative stress marker is linked to decreased fraction of oxidatively generated DNA damage to the advance of DNA strand breakage? At first sight, this outcome might seem somewhat inconsistent, as one would anticipate the increased oxidative stress to come hand in hand with increased level of oxidatively damaged DNA. Nevertheless, it has earlier been suggested that direct oxidatively generated damage to DNA bases may not be the only possible mechanism by which reactive oxygen (ROS) and nitrogen (RNS) species impose their carcinogenic effect, as other alternative mechanisms have also been suggested (such as structural alterations in DNA/chromatin, decreased efficiency of DNA polymerase and DNA repair enzymes, and/or abnormal spatial configuration of DNA; see [45–47] for review). One can now easily envisage a situation, in which the increased amount of ROS/RNS does not directly damage DNA bases (or such damage is readily repaired), but causes structural/functional changes in DNA strand breaks-repairing enzymes (including RAD51C), which superposed to eventual suboptimal efficacy of the enzyme associated with rare allele may lead to increased levels of markers of DNA strand breakage. This would then point to superiority of the role of RAD51C in protection against DNA strand breakage over its role in protection against oxidatively generated damage. Nevertheless, a certain dose of inconsistency still remains due to contradictory associations of *RAD51C* rare alleles with the

Table 5. Summary of the analysis of effect of *RAD51C* SNPs and BrC on DNA damage.

A	**Total DNA damage [log-% DNA]**						
Main effect: BrC status							
Controls	0.50±0.23						
BrC cases	0.56±0.18						
Main effect: *RAD51C* SNP	**rs302874**	**rs12946522**	**rs302873**	**rs16943176**	**rs12946397**	**rs17222691**	**rs28363302**
wt-homozygotes	0.57±0.16	0.56±0.19	0.57±0.16	0.56±0.19	0.56±0.19	0.55±0.19	0.54±0.19
heterozygotes & *rare* homozygotes	0.54±0.20	0.53±0.20	0.54±0.20	0.53±0.19	0.53±0.19	0.53±0.18	0.63±0.18
B	**DNA strand breakage [log-% DNA]**						
Main effect: BrC status *							
Controls	0.15±0.20						
BrC cases	0.30±0.19 [a]						
Main effect: *RAD51C* SNP	**rs302874**	**rs12946522**	**rs302873**	**rs16943176**	**rs12946397**	**rs17222691**	**rs28363302**
wt-homozygotes	0.33±0.20	0.26±0.20	0.32±0.21	0.26±0.20	0.26±0.20	0.26±0.20	0.26±0.20
heterozygotes & *rare* homozygotes	0.24±0.19	0.30±0.19	0.24±0.19	0.30±0.19	0.29±0.19	0.31±0.19	0.33±0.21

The summary of analysis of main effects of *RAD51C* SNPs and BrC on total DNA damage **(A)** and DNA strand breakage **(B)** adjusted to subjects' age and blood plasma TBARS. In each column, logarithmically-transformed data are presented as means ± SD. Identification of subjects as wild-type (*wt*)-homozygotes, heterozygotes and *rare* homozygotes with reference to Table 3, in which individual genotypes for each SNP are ordered accordingly. Only dominant genetic model was assumed in the analysis. The levels of significance of main effects and post-hoc multiple comparisons were inferred by ANCOVA and the *Scheffé* test, respectively. Main effects (asterisks): * $p < 0.01$; Post-hoc comparisons (letters): [a] $p < 0.005$ compared to controls.

Table 6. The effect of *RAD51C* SNPs and BrC on ratio of oxidatively generated DNA damage to DNA strand breakage.

A	*log-R*						
	rs302874	**rs12946522**	**rs302873**	**rs16943176**	**rs12946397**	**rs17222691**	**rs28363302**
Controls							
wt-homozygotes	0.18±0.63	0.19±0.48	0.18±0.63	0.22±0.47	0.22±0.47	0.22±0.47	0.03±0.49
heterozygotes & *rare* homozygotes	0.06±0.51	−0.19±0.63	0.06±0.51	−0.19±0.63	−0.19±0.63	−0.19±0.63	0.45±0.75
BrC cases							
wt-homozygotes	−0.27±0.43	−0.08±0.34	−0.25±0.43	−0.08±0.34	−0.09±0.34	−0.10±0.37	−0.17±0.41
heterozygotes & *rare* homozygotes	−0.09±0.37	−0.33±0.47 [d]	−0.10±0.38	−0.31±0.47 [d]	−0.30±0.47	−0.29±0.44	−0.16±0.36
B	*Summary of analysis (log-R)*						
Main effect: BrC status							
Controls	0.10±0.54						
BrC cases	−0.17±0.40						
Main effect: *RAD51C* SNP	**rs302874**	**rs12946522** *	**rs302873**	**rs16943176** **	**rs12946397** *	**rs17222691** *	**rs28363302**
wt-homozygotes	−0.21±0.48	−0.03±0.38	−0.19±0.48	−0.03±0.39	−0.03±0.39	−0.04±0.41	−0.13±0.43
heterozygotes & *rare* homozygotes	−0.06±0.40	−0.31±0.49 [a]	−0.07±0.41	−0.30±0.49 [a]	−0.28±0.49 [b]	−0.28±0.47 [c]	−0.04±0.50

(A) Values of the ratio of oxidatively generated DNA damage to DNA strand breakage R in whole blood leukocytes of healthy controls and BrC cases, classified by carried genotype. **(B)** Summary of the analysis of main effects of *RAD51C* SNPs and BrC on R ratio adjusted to subjects' age and TBARS. Provided are the logarithmically-transformed values of R defined as FPG[%DNA]/SSB[%DNA]-1. Data are presented as means ± SD. Identification of subjects as wild-type (*wt*)-homozygotes, heterozygotes and *rare* homozygotes with reference to Table 3, in which individual genotypes for each SNP are ordered accordingly. Only dominant genetic model was assumed in the analysis. The levels of significance of main effects and post-hoc multiple comparisons were inferred by ANCOVA (with adjustment to subjects' age and blood plasma TBARS) and the *Scheffé* test, respectively. Main effects (asterisks): * $p < 0.01$; ** $p < 0.005$; Post-hoc comparisons (letters): [a] $p < 0.0005$ compared to *wt*-homozygotes; [b] $p < 0.001$ compared to *wt*-homozygotes; [c] $p < 0.005$ compared to *wt*-homozygotes; [d] $p < 0.05$ compared to *wt*-homozygotes.

biomarkers of oxidative stress and DNA damage. Moreover, *RAD51C* rare alleles were not found to increase the extent of DNA strand breakage directly, what also seems to be inconsistent with shifted ratio of the two types of DNA damage. Either way, it thus remains to be elucidated, whether such new function of *RAD51C* proposed in the context of mitochondrial genome may be extrapolated to nuclear DNA as well.

Of importance may be the outcome, that the effect of *RAD51C* SNPs on characteristics of DNA damage in leukocytes retained its level of significance even following the adjustment to differences in blood plasma TBARS. A question however arises as to what is the possible mechanism by which the genetic variability in non-coding regions of *RAD51C* could be involved in the protection of cells against DNA strand breaks. One possible explanation could be provided by the fact, that as predicted by is-rSNP algorithm [32], the majority of SNPs investigated in our study may be considered as regulatory, i.e. they are likely to alter the binding of transcription factors (TFs) to gene's promoter with high statistical significance (see Table 2). It is thus possible, that haplotypes reconstructed based on SNPs localized within the 1kb-long strong-LD region spanning from *RAD51C* promoter to its first intron also significantly alter the binding capacity of *RAD51C* promoter towards some of crucial TFs, leading to suboptimal transcription of *RAD51C* and eventually impaired capacity of the whole HR system. According to Transfac transcription factors position weight matrix database [48], there are more than 280 different TFs, the binding of which to *RAD51C* promoter may be significantly altered by SNPs localized within the 1-kb LD block (*data not shown*). However, no studies confirming these predictions experimentally are currently available.

One has to mention, that in or study, the BrC itself was not found to be the factor linked to increased level of oxidative stress or the total DNA damage, although it was found to be associated with increased extent of DNA strand breakage. This also seems to be in contrast to finding according to which the BrC itself does not significantly change the ratio of oxidatively generated DNA damage to DNA strand breakage. It is however interesting, that any differences in blood plasma levels of TBARS and total DNA damage in leukocytes between BrC cases and controls were readily explained by adjusting the analysis to differences in subjects' age and lifetime smoking, which is in line with a considerable wealth of knowledge supporting the view of both the age and lifetime smoking as oxidative stress-increasing factors [49,50].

Our study admittedly suffers from few limitations. One of them is undoubtedly the relatively low number of subjects enrolled, due to which the described effects of *RAD51C* SNPs on either the TBARS level or the characteristics of DNA damage were proven significant only on the level of main effects (i.e. analyzing all the subjects together irrespective of their BrC status), with respective differences in the groups of BrC cases and healthy controls analyzed separately not reaching the limit of statistical significance. Moreover, low abundance of rare alleles due to relatively small study size rendered the use of additive genetic model either impossible or leading to unreliable results. Therefore, it would definitely be of benefit to verify our outcomes in a larger study. Despite that, those SNPs for which significant associations with oxidative stress or DNA damage were found under dominant genetic model presented sufficiently high statistical power and, moreover, were proven to be not confounded by individual smoking history or the level of oxidative stress. The other limitation is comprised by significant differences in age between the BrC and control groups. According to the current theory of carcinogenesis, one would expect BrC itself to be linked with increased oxidative stress, what in fact was observed in our study. Although it is possible that certain confounding between the effects of BrC, subjects' age and their smoking statuses on blood plasma levels of TBARS and DNA damage markers might have taken place, such confounding probably did not affect the observed effect of *RAD51C* SNPs on TBARS and DNA damage, as it was identified to be independent of BrC status and robust enough to "sustain" the involvement of these confounders into the analysis.

Conclusion

The present study showed that SNPs localized in non-coding regions of *RAD51C* do not modulate the individual susceptibility to unselected BrC. Four of them (rs12946522, rs16943176, rs12946397 and rs17222691) may however affect the level of blood plasma TBARS and change the mutual proportions of oxidatively generated DNA damage and DNA strand breakage with no effect on total amount of DNA damage: while the wild-type homozygotes seem to be linked to significantly decreased levels of TBARS and relatively even proportion between oxidatively generated DNA damage and DNA strand breakage, the respective rare allele-containing genotypes are associated with significantly increased level of blood plasma TBARS and the DNA damage characteristics being significantly shifted towards the DNA strand breakage. As predicted by the *in silico* analysis, these SNPs may disrupt the binding of well-known transcription factors, what in turn may lead to altered capacity of DNA repair pathways in which the *RAD51C*-encoded protein takes its place. Significant shift of DNA damage characteristics towards DNA strand breakage among carriers of the rare alleles suggests that in the case of nuclear DNA, the role of this protein in HR strand break DNA damage response pathway could be superior to its possible role in protection against oxidative DNA damage recently suggested in the case of mitochondrial DNA. Taken together, although we did not find any evidence confirming that noncoding SNPs of *RAD51C* modulate the risk of unselected BrC, they may be responsible for altered oxidative stress status and characteristics of DNA damage. Either way, the mechanisms behind the involvement of protein encoded by this putative suppressor gene in protection against oxidative stress and DNA damage deserve further investigation.

Author Contributions

Conceived and designed the experiments: PG JG WW. Performed the experiments: PG EJ ET MS. Analyzed the data: PG. Contributed reagents/materials/analysis tools: OZQ. Wrote the paper: PG JG WW.

References

1. Ferlay J, Shin HR, Bray F, Forman D, Mathers C, et al. (2010) Estimates of worldwide burden of cancer in 2008: GLOBOCAN 2008. Int J Cancer 127: 2893–2917.
2. Fackenthal JD, Olopade OI (2007) Breast cancer risk associated with BRCA1 and BRCA2 in diverse populations. Nat Rev Cancer 7: 937–948.
3. Stratton MR, Rahman N (2008) The emerging landscape of breast cancer susceptibility. Nat Genet 40: 17–22.
4. Turnbull C, Rahman N (2008) Genetic predisposition to breast cancer: past, present, and future. Annu Rev Genomics Hum Genet 9: 321–345.
5. Levy-Lahad E (2010) Fanconi anemia and breast cancer susceptibility meet again. Nat Genet 42: 368–369.
6. Rahman N, Seal S, Thompson D, Kelly P, Renwick A, et al. (2007) PALB2, which encodes a BRCA2-interacting protein, is a breast cancer susceptibility gene. Nat Genet 39: 165–167.

7. Seal S, Thompson D, Renwick A, Elliott A, Kelly P, et al. (2006) Truncating mutations in the Fanconi anemia J gene BRIP1 are low-penetrance breast cancer susceptibility alleles. Nat Genet 38: 1239–1241.
8. Ripperger T, Gadzicki D, Meindl A, Schlegelberger B (2009) Breast cancer susceptibility: current knowledge and implications for genetic counselling. Eur J Hum Genet 17: 722–731.
9. Masson JY, Tarsounas MC, Stasiak AZ, Stasiak A, Shah R, et al. (2001) Identification and purification of two distinct complexes containing the five RAD51 paralogs. Genes Dev 15: 3296–3307.
10. Badie S, Liao C, Thanasoula M, Barber P, Hill MA, et al. (2009) RAD51C facilitates checkpoint signaling by promoting CHK2 phosphorylation. J Cell Biol 185: 587–600.
11. Liu Y, Masson JY, Shah R, O'Regan P, West SC (2004) RAD51C is required for Holliday junction processing in mammalian cells. Science 303: 243–246.
12. Somyajit K, Subramanya S, Nagaraju G (2012) Distinct roles of FANCO/RAD51C protein in DNA damage signaling and repair: implications for Fanconi anemia and breast cancer susceptibility. J Biol Chem 287: 3366–3380.
13. Meindl A, Hellebrand H, Wiek C, Erven V, Wappenschmidt B, et al. (2010) Germline mutations in breast and ovarian cancer pedigrees establish RAD51C as a human cancer susceptibility gene. Nat Genet 42: 410–414.
14. Vuorela M, Pylkas K, Hartikainen JM, Sundfeldt K, Lindblom A, et al. (2011) Further evidence for the contribution of the RAD51C gene in hereditary breast and ovarian cancer susceptibility. Breast Cancer Res Treat 130: 1003–1010.
15. De Leeneer K, Van Bockstal M, De Brouwer S, Swietek N, Schietecatte P, et al. (2012) Evaluation of RAD51C as cancer susceptibility gene in a large breast-ovarian cancer patient population referred for genetic testing. Breast Cancer Res Treat 133: 393–398.
16. Saleh-Gohari N, Bryant HE, Schultz N, Parker KM, Cassel TN, et al. (2005) Spontaneous homologous recombination is induced by collapsed replication forks that are caused by endogenous DNA single-strand breaks. Mol Cell Biol 25: 7158–7169.
17. Sage JM, Gildemeister OS, Knight KL (2010) Discovery of a novel function for human Rad51: maintenance of the mitochondrial genome. J Biol Chem 285: 18984–18990.
18. Osorio A, Endt D, Fernandez F, Eirich K, de la Hoya M, et al. (2012) Predominance of pathogenic missense variants in the RAD51C gene occurring in breast and ovarian cancer families. Hum Mol Genet 21: 2889–2898.
19. Romero A, Perez-Segura P, Tosar A, Garcia-Saenz JA, Diaz-Rubio E, et al. (2011) A HRM-based screening method detects RAD51C germ-line deleterious mutations in Spanish breast and ovarian cancer families. Breast Cancer Res Treat 129: 939–946.
20. Pelttari LM, Heikkinen T, Thompson D, Kallioniemi A, Schleutker J, et al. (2011) RAD51C is a susceptibility gene for ovarian cancer. Hum Mol Genet 20: 3278–3288.
21. Thompson ER, Boyle SE, Johnson J, Ryland GL, Sawyer S, et al. (2012) Analysis of RAD51C germline mutations in high-risk breast and ovarian cancer families and ovarian cancer patients. Hum Mutat 33: 95–99.
22. Loveday C, Turnbull C, Ruark E, Xicola RM, Ramsay E, et al. (2012) Germline RAD51C mutations confer susceptibility to ovarian cancer. Nat Genet 44: 475–476.
23. Zheng Y, Zhang J, Hope K, Niu Q, Huo D, et al. (2010) Screening RAD51C nucleotide alterations in patients with a family history of breast and ovarian cancer. Breast Cancer Res Treat 124: 857–861.
24. Akbari MR, Tonin P, Foulkes WD, Ghadirian P, Tischkowitz M, et al. (2010) RAD51C germline mutations in breast and ovarian cancer patients. Breast Cancer Res 12: 404.
25. Wong MW, Nordfors C, Mossman D, Pecenpetelovska G, Avery-Kiejda KA, et al. (2011) BRIP1, PALB2, and RAD51C mutation analysis reveals their relative importance as genetic susceptibility factors for breast cancer. Breast Cancer Res Treat 127: 853–859.
26. Pang Z, Yao L, Zhang J, Ouyang T, Li J, et al. (2011) RAD51C germline mutations in Chinese women with familial breast cancer. Breast Cancer Res Treat 129: 1019–1020.
27. Clague J, Wilhoite G, Adamson A, Bailis A, Weitzel JN, et al. (2011) RAD51C germline mutations in breast and ovarian cancer cases from high-risk families. PLoS One 6: e25632.
28. Pelttari LM, Nurminen R, Gylfe A, Aaltonen LA, Schleutker J, et al. (2012) Screening of Finnish RAD51C founder mutations in prostate and colorectal cancer patients. BMC Cancer 12:552.
29. Gresner P, Gromadzinska J, Polanska K, Twardowska E, Jurewicz J, et al. (2012) Genetic variability of Xrcc3 and Rad51 modulates the risk of head and neck cancer. Gene 504: 166–174.
30. Gresner P, Gromadzinska J, Twardowska E, Rydzynski K, Wasowicz W (2014) Rad51C: A novel suppressor gene modulates the risk of head and neck cancer. Mutat Res 762: 47–54.
31. Sherry ST, Ward MH, Kholodov M, Baker J, Phan L, et al. (2001) dbSNP: the NCBI database of genetic variation. Nucleic Acids Res 29: 308–311.
32. Macintyre G, Bailey J, Haviv I, Kowalczyk A (2010) is-rSNP: a novel technique for in silico regulatory SNP detection. Bioinformatics 26: i524–30.
33. Wasowicz W, Nève J, Peretz A (1993) Optimized steps in fluorometric determination of thiobarbituric acid-reactive substances in serum: importance of extraction pH and influence of sample preservation and storage. Clin Chem 39: 2522–2526.
34. Singh NP, McCoy MT, Tice RR, Schneider EL (1988) A simple technique for quantitation of low levels of DNA damage in individual cells. Exp Cell Res 175: 184–191.
35. McKelvey-Martin VJ, Green MH, Schmezer P, Pool-Zobel BL, De Meo MP, et al. (1993) The single cell gel electrophoresis assay (comet assay): a European review. Mutat Res 288: 47–63.
36. Collins AR, Duthie SJ, Dobson VL (1993) Direct enzymic detection of endogenous oxidative base damage in human lymphocyte DNA. Carcinogenesis 14: 1733–1735.
37. Barrett JC, Fry B, Maller J, Daly MJ (2005) Haploview: analysis and visualization of LD and haplotype maps. Bioinformatics 21: 263–265.
38. Lewontin RC (1995) The detection of linkage disequilibrium in molecular sequence data. Genetics 140: 377–388.
39. Gabriel SB, Schaffner SF, Nguyen H, Moore JM, Roy J, et al. (2002) The structure of haplotype blocks in the human genome. Science 296: 2225–2229.
40. Clague J, Wilhoite G, Adamson A, Bailis A, Weitzel JN, et al. (2011) RAD51C germline mutations in breast and ovarian cancer cases from high-risk families. PLoS One 6: e25632.
41. De LK, Van BM, De BS, Swietek N, Schietecatte P, et al. (2012) Evaluation of RAD51C as cancer susceptibility gene in a large breast-ovarian cancer patient population referred for genetic testing. Breast Cancer Res Treat 133: 393–398.
42. Johnson RD, Jasin M (2001) Double-strand-break-induced homologous recombination in mammalian cells. Biochem Soc Trans 29: 196–201.
43. Takata M, Sasaki MS, Sonoda E, Morrison C, Hashimoto M, et al. (1998) Homologous recombination and non-homologous end-joining pathways of DNA double-strand break repair have overlapping roles in the maintenance of chromosomal integrity in vertebrate cells. EMBO J 17: 5497–5508.
44. Ciccia A, Elledge SJ (2010) The DNA damage response: making it safe to play with knives. Mol Cell 40: 179–204.
45. Nakabeppu Y, Tsuchimoto D, Furuichi M, Sakumi K (2004) The defense mechanisms in mammalian cells against oxidative damage in nucleic acids and their involvement in the suppression of mutagenesis and cell death. Free Radic Res 38: 423–429.
46. Halliwell B (2007) Oxidative stress and cancer: have we moved forward? Biochem J 401: 1–11.
47. Halliwell B (2002) Effect of diet on cancer development: is oxidative DNA damage a biomarker? Free Radic Biol Med 32: 968–974.
48. Matys V, Kel-Margoulis O V, Fricke E, Liebich I, Land S, et al. (2006) TRANSFAC and its module TRANSCompel: transcriptional gene regulation in eukaryotes. Nucleic Acids Res 34: D108–10.
49. Liochev SI (2013) Reactive oxygen species and the free radical theory of aging. Free Radic Biol Med 60: 1–4.
50. Franco R, Panayiotidis MI, Kirkland SIEDJ, Mena S, Ortega A, et al. (2009) Oxidative stress in environmental-induced carcinogenesis. Mutat Res Toxicol Environ Mutagen 674: 36–44.

The Plasma B-Type Natriuretic Peptide Levels Are Low in Males with Stable Ischemic Heart Disease (IHD) Compared to Those Observed in Patients with Non-IHD

Kosuke Minai*, Takayuki Ogawa, Makoto Kawai, Kimiaki Komukai, Toshikazu Tanaka, Kazuo Ogawa, Tomohisa Nagoshi, Satoshi Arase, Satoshi Morimoto, Yasunori Inoue, Hiroshi Sekiyama, Akihiro Urabe, Seiichiro Matsuo, Kenichi Hongo, Michihiro Yoshimura

Division of Cardiology, Department of Internal Medicine, The Jikei University School of Medicine, Tokyo, Japan

Abstract

Objective: Although the plasma B-type natriuretic peptide (BNP) level is a marker of heart failure, it is unclear whether BNP *per se* plays a pivotal role for pathogenic mechanisms underlying the development of ischemic heart disease (IHD). In this study, we retrospectively examined the plasma BNP levels in stable patients with IHD and compared to stable patients with cardiovascular diseases other than IHD.

Methods: The study population was 2088 patients (1698 males and 390 females) who were admitted to our hospital due to IHD (n = 1,661) and non-IHD (n = 427) and underwent cardiac catheterization. Measurements of the hemodynamic parameters and blood sampling were performed.

Results: The plasma BNP levels were significantly lower in the IHD group than in the non-IHD group ($p<0.001$). The multiple regression analysis examining the logBNP values showed that age, a male gender, low left ventricular ejection fraction, low body mass index, serum creatinine, atrial fibrillation and IHD *per se* were significant explanatory variables. When the total study population was divided according to gender, the plasma BNP levels were found to be significantly lower in the IHD group than in the non-IHD group among males ($p<0.001$), but not females (p = NS). Furthermore, a multiple logistic regression analysis of IHD showed the logBNP value to be a significant explanatory variable in males (regression coefficient: −0.669, $p<0.001$), but not females (p = NS).

Conclusions: The plasma BNP levels were relatively low in stable patients with IHD compared with those observed in stable patients with non-IHD; this tendency was evident in males. Perhaps, the low reactivity of BNP is causally associated with IHD in males. We hope that this study will serve as a test of future prospective studies.

Editor: Yasuhiro Ikeda, Mayo Clinic, United States of America

Funding: The authors received no specific funding for this work.

Competing Interests: The authors have declared that no competing interests exist.

* Email: heart@jikei.ac.jp

Introduction

A-type natriuretic peptide and B-type natriuretic peptide (BNP), also known as atrial and brain natriuretic peptides, respectively, are cardiac hormones with a wide range of potent biological effects, including vasodilation, natriuresis and inhibition of the renin-angiotensin-aldosterone and sympathetic nervous systems [1–8]. BNP is selectively secreted from the ventricles, and the magnitude of secretion also varies as a function of the severity of heart failure. The BNP value is thus used as a biochemical marker of heart failure.

In addition, we previously reported that, in patients with acute myocardial infarction (AMI), the time course of the changes in the plasma BNP levels just after the onset of AMI exhibited a biphasic pattern, with the first peak occurring approximately 24 hours after the onset and the second peak 3–5 days after the onset. The second peak of plasma BNP was more marked in severe cases of AMI with heart failure [9].

The plasma immunoreactive BNP level is a sensitive biochemical marker of heart failure; although the precise molecular forms of BNP and its precursors have been discussed from different angles [10,11]. BNP increases the cyclic guanosine monophosphate (cGMP) levels [1]. cGMP activated by BNP is protective against cellular injury as it increase particulate guanylate cyclases [12]. BNP may also be beneficial for suppressing the progression of heart failure and atherosclerosis [13,14]. If the plasma BNP level is insufficiently increased for any reason, heart failure and atherosclerosis are likely

Table 1. Baseline characteristics and the past medical history and medication regimen of the study subjects.

	Total			Female			Male		
	Non-IHD (n = 427)	IHD (n = 1,661)	P Value	Non-IHD (n = 144)	IHD (n = 246)	P-Value	Non-IHD (n = 283)	IHD (n = 1,415)	P-Value
Age (yrs ± SD)	63.1±13.1	65.2±10.5	P<0.01	67.5±13.5	70.4±10.2	P<0.05	60.9±12.3	64.4±10.3	P<0.001
Male (%)	66.3	85.1	P<0.001						
Body mass index (kg/m2 ± SD)	23.2±3.6	24.3±3.4	P<0.001	21.9±3.2	23.0±3.5	P<0.01	23.7±3.6	24.5±3.4	P<0.001
Current smoker (%)	21.8	23.2	NS	8.3	12.6	NS	28.6	25.1	NS
Current+past smoker (%)	53.4	69.8	P<0.001	19.4	28.5	P<0.05	70.7	77.0	P<0.05
Hypertension (%)	64.6	76.5	P<0.001	66.0	77.6	P<0.05	64.0	76.3	P<0.001
Diabetes Mellitus (%)	28.8	45.1	P<0.001	27.1	42.7	P<0.01	29.7	45.5	P<0.001
Dyslipidemia (%)	45.7	75.9	P<0.001	43.1	74.0	P<0.001	47.0	76.3	P<0.001
s-Cr (mg/dl ± SD)	1.6±2.4	1.6±2.3	P = 0.001	1.6±2.5	1.5±2.3	NS	1.6±2.3	1.6±2.3	NS
HbA1c (% ± SD)	5.8±1.1	6.0±1.1	P<0.001	5.7±1.1	5.9±0.8	NS	5.8±1.1	6.1±1.1	P<0.001
BNP (pg/ml ± SD)	310.2±650.0	157.6±401.1	P<0.001	319.5±650.4	303.2±668.2	NS	305.5±650.9	132.3±327.4	P<0.001
HD & CAPD (%)	10.8	9.3	NS	13.2	13.0	NS	9.5	8.7	NS
LVEF (% ± SD)	56.0±14.4	57.7±10.8	P<0.05	59.3±12.3	59.5±11.6	NS	54.4±15.1	57.4±10.7	P = 0.001
Heart rate (beat/min ± SD) (At LVG)	74.0±16.4	70.6±13.5	P<0.001	73.3±14.0	72.5±14.3	NS	74.4±17.6	70.3±13.4	P<0.001
LVEDP (mmHg ± SD) (At PreLVG)	16.5±7.2	15.5±6.3	P<0.05	16.4±7.0	16.1±6.9	NS	16.6±7.3	15.5±6.1	P<0.05
LVESVI (ml/m² ± SD)	36.5±25.1	28.9±16.3	P<0.001	31.7±19.8	27.3±17.0	P<0.05	39.0±27.2	29.1±16.2	P<0.001
Prior MI (%)	0	38.5	P<0.001	0	35.8	P<0.001	0	38.9	P<0.001
Prior PCI (%)	0	44.6	P<0.001	0	35.8	P<0.001	0	46.1	P<0.001
Prior CABG (%)	0	12.5	P<0.001	0	15.9	P<0.001	0	12.0	P<0.001
Coronary spastic angina	0	8.5	P<0.001	0	12.6	P<0.001	0	7.8	P<0.001
Prior valve repair (%)	4.9	0.7	P<0.001	7.6	1.6	P<0.01	3.5	0.5	P<0.001
Valvular heart disease (%)	30.2	3.4	P<0.001	38.2	6.9	P<0.001	26.1	2.8	P<0.001
Congenital heart disease (%)	5.2	0.36	P<0.001	8.3	0.4	P<0.001	3.5	0.4	P<0.001
Cardiomyopathy (%)	22.7	2.0	P<0.001	20.8	3.3	P<0.001	23.7	1.8	P<0.001
AF (%)	20.6	5.5	P<0.001	19.4	4.9	P<0.001	21.2	5.7	P<0.001
Calcium-channel blockers (%)	39.1	60.6	P<0.001	43.1	59.8	P = 0.001	37.1	60.8	P<0.001
ACE-inhibitors (%)	15.0	21.3	P<0.01	14.6	18.3	NS	15.2	21.8	P<0.05
Angiotensin Receptor Blockers (%)	37.9	41.0	NS	44.4	42.7	NS	34.6	40.7	NS (P = 0.056)
Nitrates (%)	9.1	26.6	P<0.001	8.3	28.5	P<0.001	9.5	26.2	P<0.001
Nicorandil (%)	4.2	20.4	P<0.001	4.2	23.2	P<0.001	4.2	19.9	P<0.001

Table 1. Cont.

	Total			Female			Male		
	Non-IHD (n = 427)	IHD (n = 1,661)	P Value	Non-IHD (n = 144)	IHD (n = 246)	P-Value	Non-IHD (n = 283)	IHD (n = 1,415)	P-Value
Beta-blockers (%)	18.7	34.4	P<0.001	20.8	28.9	NS (P = 0.081)	17.7	35.3	P<0.001
Statins (%)	23.0	59.3	P<0.001	29.9	57.7	P<0.001	19.4	59.6	P<0.001
Fibrates (%)	3.3	3.4	NS	1.4	1.2	NS	4.2	3.8	NS
Diuretics (%)	32.1	19.1	P<0.001	38.2	28.5	P<0.05	29.0	17.5	P<0.001
Oral Hypoglycemic Agents (%)	11.5	23.5	P<0.001	9.7	18.3	P<0.05	12.4	24.5	P<0.001
insulin (%)	5.2	9.9	P<0.01	6.9	10.6	NS	4.2	9.8	P<0.01
Number of vessels disease (0–3)	0	0.95±0.97		0	0.96±0.96		0	0.95±097	

s-Cr, Serum creatinine; BNP, B-type natriuretic peptide; HD & CAPD, Hemodialysis & continuous ambulatory peritoneal dialysis; LVEF, Left ventricular ejection fraction; LVEDP, Left ventricular end-diastolic pressure; LVESVI, Left ventricular end-systolic volume Index; MI, Myocardial Infarction; PCI, Percutaneous coronary intervention; CABG, Coronary artery bypass graft; AF, Atrial Fibrillation.

to advance; therefore, low plasma BNP level, even in patients with high risk factors, may play a causative role in the pathogenetic mechanisms underlying the development of IHD and heart failure. However, the discussion regarding this issue has been insufficient to date, although genetic variations of BNP and related molecules have previously been reported [15–21]. It is also unclear whether the plasma BNP level actually varies according to the individual and whether individual changes in this parameter are associated with disease. Nevertheless, there were a few early reports showing dysregulation of ANP and BNP in patients prone to developing hypertension and other cardiovascular disease [22–24].

Here, we hypothesized that BNP contributes to a pathogenetic mechanism of IHD, and retrospectively examined a possible contribution by comparing the BNP levels between stable patients with IHD and stable patients with cardiovascular diseases other than IHD.

Methods

Study design

The study population was 2088 consecutive patients admitted to the Jikei University Hospital from January 2008 through January 2012 in whom cardiac catheterization, including left ventriculography, and blood sampling for the plasma BNP levels were performed and reviewed. The baseline patient characteristics, including the clinical parameters and the biochemical data, were collected retrospectively from the medical records. The study protocol was approved by the ethics committee of the Jikei University School of Medicine (24–355; 7121).

Recruitment of stable IHD patients and non-IHD patients in this study

The stable IHD patients consisted of 1,661 patients who had coronary stenosis newly diagnosed by angiography, or who had a medical history of coronary artery disease, such as previous myocardial infarction, post-percutaneous coronary intervention and coronary artery bypass graft. A total of 762 patients underwent only one cardiac catheterization, while 359 patients underwent catheterization twice, 50 patients three times, five patients four times, one patient five times and one patient underwent catheterization six times. In order to avoid a selection bias by choosing among the plural data in one patient, we used all consecutive data in this analysis (n = 1661). Patients with coronary spastic angina were included in the stable IHD group if the disease activity of coronary spasm was not clinically high. Coronary spasm was diagnosed by the acetylcholine provocation test. Patients with previously diagnosed coronary spastic angina were also included in the stable IHD group. In contrast, patients requiring urgent catheter intervention for AMI were excluded from this study because the plasma BNP levels are rapidly and extensively changes during the acute phase of AMI [9]. Similarly, patients with acute coronary syndrome were excluded from the stable IHD group in this study. In addition, Also, patients with chest pain syndrome of unknown origin and those with suspected microvascular angina were excluded from the stable IHD group because we were unable to appropriately define cardiac ischemia in such patients. Detailed information of the patients in the stable IHD group were summarized in Table 1.

The non-IHD group consisted of 427 patients; all of those had organic heart diseases such as valvular heart diseases, cardiomyopaty, congenital heart disease and others. All non-IHD patients were clinically stable and admitted to the hospital for evaluation of their underlying cardiac disease. A total of 406 patients underwent cardiac catheterization one time, while nine patients were

Table 2. Comparisons between female and male with and without IHD.

	Non-IHD			IHD		
	Female (n = 144)	**Male (n = 283)**	**P-Value**	**Female (n = 246)**	**Male (n = 1,415)**	**P-Value**
Age (yrs ± SD)	67.5±13.5	60.9±12.3	P<0.001	70.4±10.2	64.4±10.3	P<0.001
Body mass index (kg/m2 ± SD)	21.9±3.2	23.7±3.6	P<0.001	23.0±3.5	24.5±3.4	P<0.001
Current smoker (%)	8.3	28.6	P<0.001	12.6	25.1	P<0.001
Current+past smoker (%)	19.4	70.7	P<0.001	28.5	77.0	P<0.001
Hypertension (%)	66.0	64.0	NS	77.6	76.3	NS
Diabetes Mellitus (%)	27.1	29.7	NS	42.7	45.5	NS
Dyslipidemia (%)	43.1	47.0	NS	74.0	76.3	NS
s-Cr (mg/dl ± SD)	1.6±2.5	1.6±2.3	P<0.001	1.5±2.3	1.6±2.3	P<0.001
HbA1c (% ± SD)	5.7±1.1	5.8±1.1	NS	5.9±0.8	6.1±1.1	P<0.05
BNP (pg/ml ± SD)	319.5±650.4	305.5±650.9	P<0.05	303.2±668.2	132.3±327.4	P<0.001
HD & CAPD (%)	13.2	9.5	NS	13.0	8.7	P<0.05
LVEF (% ± SD)	59.3±12.3	54.4±15.1	P<0.001	59.5±11.6	57.4±10.7	P<0.01
Heart rate (beat/min ± SD) (At LVG)	73.3±14.0	74.4±17.6	NS	72.5±14.3	70.3±13.4	P<0.05
LVEDP (mmHg ± SD) (At Pre LVG)	16.4±7.0	16.6±7.3	NS	16.1±6.9	15.5±6.1	NS
LVESVI (ml/m^2 ± SD)	31.7±19.8	39.0±27.2	P<0.01	27.3±17.0	29.1±16.2	NS
Prior myocardial infarction (%)	0	0		35.8	38.9	NS
Prior PCI (%)	0	0		35.8	46.1	P<0.01
Prior CABG	0	0		15.9	12.0	NS
Coronary spastic angina	0	0		12.6	7.8	P<0.05
Prior valve repair (%)	7.6	3.5	NS	1.6	0.5	P<0.05
Valvular heart disease (%)	38.2	26.1	P = 0.01	6.9	2.8	P = 0.001
Congenital heart disease (%)	8.3	3.5	P<0.05	0.4	0.4	NS
Cardiomyopathy (%)	20.8	23.7	NS	3.3	1.8	NS
AF (%)	19.4	21.2	NS	4.9	5.7	NS
Calcium-channel blockers (%)	43.1	37.1	NS	59.8	60.8	NS
ACE-inhibitors (%)	14.6	15.2	NS	18.3	21.8	NS
Angiotensin Receptor Blockers (%)	44.4	34.6	P<0.05	42.7	40.7	NS
Nitrates (%)	8.3	9.5	NS	28.5	26.2	NS
Nicorandil (%)	4.2	4.2	NS	23.2	19.9	NS
Beta-blockers (%)	20.8	17.7	NS	28.9	35.3	P<0.05
Statins (%)	29.9	19.4	P<0.05	57.7	59.6	NS
Fibrates (%)	1.4	4.2	NS	1.2	3.8	P<0.05
Diuretics (%)	38.2	29.0	NS	28.5	17.5	P<0.001
Oral Hypoglycemic Agents (%)	9.7	12.4	NS	18.3	24.5	P<0.05
insulin (%)	6.9	4.2	NS	10.6	9.8	NS
Number of vessels disease (0–3)	0	0		0.96±0.96	0.95±097	NS

s-Cr, Serum creatinine; BNP, B-type natriuretic peptide; HD & CAPD, Hemodialysis & continuous ambulatory peritoneal dialysis; LVEF, Left ventricular ejection fraction; LVEDP, Left ventricular end-diastolic pressure; LVESVI, Left ventricular end-systolic volume Index; PCI, Percutaneous coronary intervention; CABG, Coronary artery bypass graft;AF, Atrial Fibrillation.

catheterized twice and one patient was catheterized three times. We used all consecutive data in this analysis just as we did in the IHD group (n = 427). We excluded patients suffering from acute heart failure at the time of cardiac cathetherization and blood sampling. Precise information including underlying cardiac disorders was also summarized in Table 1.

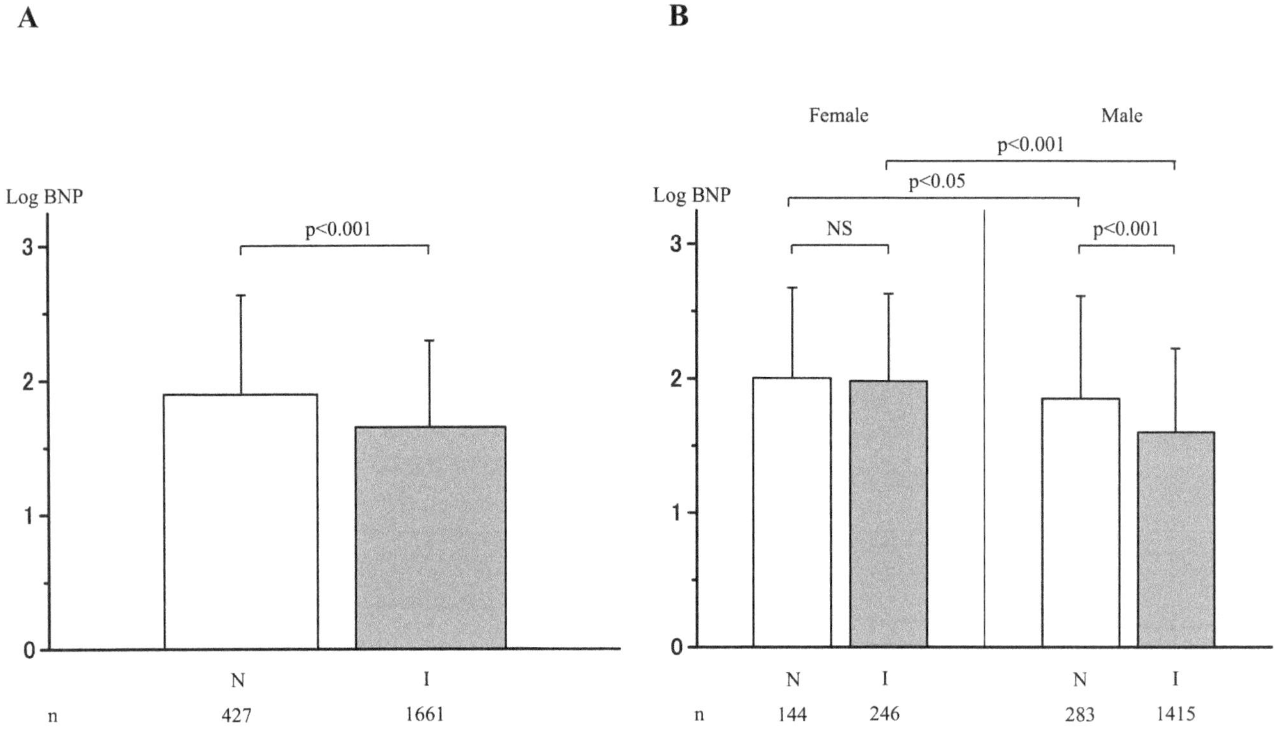

Figure 1. Comparison of the logBNP levels between the non-IHD and IHD groups. A: In the overall population. B: In males and females. N: non-ischemic heart disease group (non-IHD); I: ischemic heart disease group (IHD). BNP: B-type natriuretic peptide.

Measurement of the plasma BNP levels and other parameters

Whole blood (5 ml) was collected in tubes containing potassium EDTA (1 mg/ml blood). The plasma BNP level was determined by an enzyme-linked immunosorbent assay (non-extracted) using an antibody against human BNP (Shionogi Co. Ltd., Tokyo, Japan). Blood sampling was performed immediately before and after the cardiac catheterization whenever possible. The average interval between catheterization and blood sampling was 5.21±8.94 days; 1384 (66.3%) of patients had blood collected for BNP within 72 hours post catheterization. Of these patients, 830 underwent blood collection at the time of the procedure (during, immediately before or just after cardiac catheterization), 1185 underwent blood collection within 24 hours, and 1342 underwent blood collection within 48 hours.

The BMI was calculated as the body weight (kg) divided by the square of the height (m). Hypertension, diabetes mellitus and dyslipidemia were defined as described previously [25].

Statistical analysis

Continuous variables were expressed as the means ± SD. Categorical variables were expressed as percentages. Comparisons between groups were performed using Pearson's chi-square test for categorical variables and the Mann-Whitney U test or Student's t-test for continuous variables, where appropriate. To achieve a normal distribution, the BNP value was log-transformed before the analysis. To assess the dependent determinants of the log BNP, a multiple regression analysis was performed after the simple regression analysis. Age, gender (0 for females and 1 for males), IHD (0 for non-IHD and 1 for IHD), atrial fibrillation (0 for non-AF and 1 for AF), the LVEF, age, BMI, and s-Cr were included as

Table 3. The results of the simple regression analyses for the log BNP in all patients (n = 2088).

Explanatory variable	Regression coefficient	Standard regression coefficient	P	95%CI
Age	0.016	0.270	<0.001	0.014~0.019
Gender	−0.348	−0.203	<0.001	−0.420~−0.276
BMI	−0.047	−0.247	<0.001	−0.055~−0.039
s-Cr	0.119	0.415	<0.001	0.108~0.130
LVEF	−0.027	−0.478	<0.001	−0.030~−0.025
AF	0.597	0.251	<0.001	0.499~0.696
IHD	−0.243	−0.147	<0.001	−0.314~−0.173

BMI, Body mass index; s-Cr, Serum creatinine; LVEF, Left ventricular ejection fraction; AF, Atrial fibrillation; IHD, Ischemic heart disease.

Table 4. The results of the multiple regression analyses for the log BNP in all patients (n = 2088).

Explanatory variable	Regression coefficient	Standard regression coefficient	P	95%CI	VIF
Age	0.015	0.249	<0.001	0.013~0.017	1.125
Gender	−0.272	−0.159	<0.001	−0.327~−0.217	1.120
BMI	−0.015	−0.081	<0.001	−0.022~−0.009	1.128
s-Cr	0.095	0.333	<0.001	0.086~0.104	1.061
LVEF	−0.024	−0.414	<0.001	−0.026~−0.022	1.097
AF	0.325	0.137	<0.001	0.249~0.401	1.107
IHD	−0.115	−0.069	<0.001	−0.168~−0.061	1.131

BMI, Body mass index; s-Cr, Serum creatinine; LVEF, Left ventricular ejection fraction; AF, Atrial fibrillation; IHD, Ischemic heart disease.

variables in the multiple regression analysis. In addition, a gender-segregated multiple logistic regression analysis was performed to determine predictive factors for IHD using age, LVEF, BMI, s-Cr, atrial fibrillation (0 for non-AF and 1 for AF), and logBNP. A value of $p<0.05$ was considered to be statistically significant for all data that were statistically analyzed using the SPSS software package, version 21.0 (SPSS Inc., Chicago, IL).

Results

Clinical characteristics of the study subjects

Table 1 shows the clinical characteristic and the past medical history and medication regimen of the total 2088 patients.

High age, male gender, high BMI, smoking, hypertension, diabetes mellitus and dyslipidemia were more frequently seen in the IHD group than in the non-IHD group. The s-Cr was significantly higher in the non-IHD group than in the IHD group. The heart rate, LVESVI and LVEDP were lower in the IHD group than in the non-IHD group. The LVEF was slightly higher in the IHD group than in the non-IHD group. In this study, AF was more frequently detected in the non-IHD group than in the IHD group, which was due to the higher prevalence of valvular heart disease and cardiomyopathy in the non-IHD groups (precise data not shown in the Results).

The clinical characteristics are shown by gender in Table 2. It is important to compare the clinical characteristics between the females and males in the IHD group. For example, the LVEF was lower and the s-Cr was higher in males, whereas the age was lower and BMI values were higher in this group. With regard to the medical treatments, diuretics were used more frequently in females, and beta-blockers were used more frequently in males, while angiotensin-converting enzyme inhibitors/angiotensin II receptor blockers (ARBs) were used equally in females and males. Every patient had been prescribed the classes and doses of drugs based on his or her individual condition; therefore, it is difficult to compare the drugs more precisely. Nevertheless, the frequency in use and the amount used of major drugs such as enalapril, cavedilol or spironolactones was equivalent between females and males with or without IHD, while only the frequency of use and amount used of furosemide was significantly higher in males than in females (precise data not shown).

Comparison of the plasma BNP levels between the non-IHD and IHD groups and statistical analysis of the logBNP values in the total study population

The plasma BNP levels were significantly lower in the IHD group than in the non-IHD group as shown in Figure 1-A. In order to identify factors contributing to the difference in the plasma BNP levels between the IHD and non-IHD groups among the total study population, statistical analyses was performed, as shown in Table 3 and Table 4. Table 3 is the results of the simple regression analysis of the logBNP values using clinical factors as explanatory variables. Table 4 shows the results of the subsequent multiple regression analysis. Consequently, age, gender, BMI, s-Cr, LVEF, AF, and IHD were found to be significant determinants of the logBNP value. Among these factors, it is noteworthy that IHD *per se* was significantly and inversely correlated with the logBNP value.

Comparison of the plasma BNP levels between the non-IHD and IHD groups based on gender

Figure 1B shows that females with and without IHD had higher levels of plasma BNP compared to males with and without IHD.

Table 5. The results of the logistic regression analysis for IHD in females.

Explanatory variable	Regression coefficient	P	Odds ratio	Odds 95% CI
Log BNP	−0.085	NS (p = 0.719)	0.919	0.579~1.457
LVEF	−0.014	NS (p = 0.232)	0.986	0.963~1.009
Age	0.027	<0.01	1.028	1.007~1.048
BMI	0.101	<0.01	1.106	1.034~1.183
AF	−1.703	<0.001	0.182	0.086~0.388
s-Cr	−0.002	NS (p = 0.965)	0.998	0.901~1.105

BNP, B-type natriuretic peptide; LVEF, Left ventricular ejection fraction; BMI, Body mass index; AF, Atrial fibrillation; IHD, Ischemic heart disease; s-Cr, Serum creatinine.

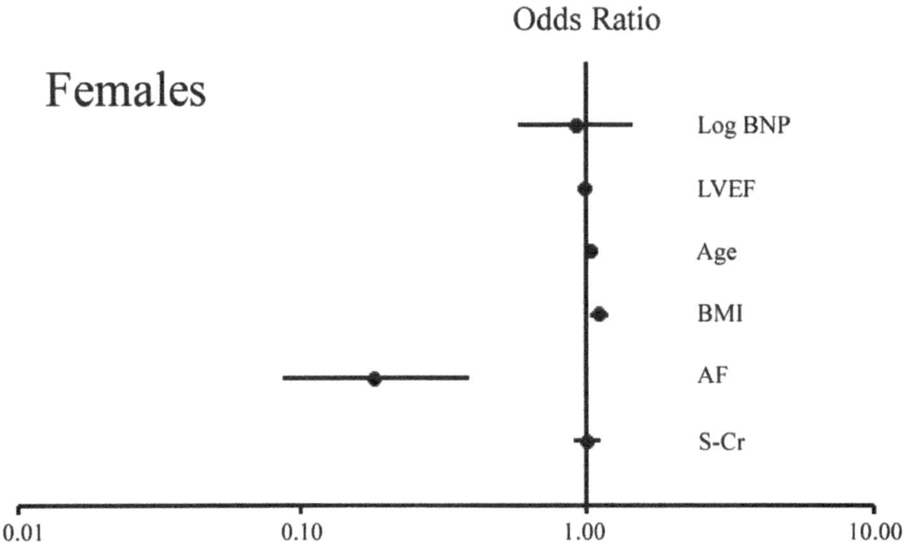

Figure 2. The Forest Plot displaying the odds ratio about risk of IHD in a females. BNP, B-type natriuretic peptide; LVEF, Left ventricular ejection fraction; BMI, Body mass index; AF, Atrial fibrillation; IHD, Ischemic heart disease; s-Cr, Serum creatinine.

The plasma BNP levels were similar in females with and without IHD ($p = NS$, actually $p = 0.725$). In contrast, the plasma BNP level was lower in males with IHD compared to males without IHD ($p<0.001$).

The results of the multiple logistic regression analysis for the determination of IHD

We finally examined the factors determining the presence of IHD; a multiple logistic regression analysis was performed for the determination of IHD by using the logBNP, LVEF, age, BMI, AF and s-Cr as explanatory variables in females and males. As shown in Tables 5 and Figure 2 (Females), and Table 6, and Figure 3 (Males), the trend between females and males was similar for age (significant in each gender), BMI (significant in each gender), AF (significant in each gender) and LVEF (not significant in each gender); however, the s-Cr was not significant in females ($p = NS$) but was significant in males ($p<0.05$). This result may suggest that chronic kidney disease is a more important risk factor for IHD in males than in females. It is noteworthy that the logBNP was not significantly associated with IHD in females ($p = NS$, actually $p = 0.719$), but was significantly and inversely associated with IHD in males (Regression coefficient: −0.669, $p < 0.001$). Thus, the logBNP may only correlate with IHD in males, and may have a possible causative role, although it is difficult to distinguish between cause and effect based on the present analysis.

Sub-analysis based on the presence or absence of AF

AF was found to be significantly associated with non-IHD in both females and males, as shown in Table 5 and Figure 2 (Females) and Table 6 and Figure 3 (Males). Therefore, an additional analysis would be necessary, and the study population was subsequently divided based on the presence or absence of AF: the AF (+) group and the AF (−) group. There were no significant differences in the plasma BNP levels between the non-IHD and IHD groups among the AF (+) or AF (−) females; however, the plasma BNP levels were significantly lower in the IHD group than in the non-IHD group among AF(+) or AF(−) males. The subgroup analysis of AF therefore suggested that the tendency toward a low plasma BNP level in IHD males was not affected by AF.

Discussion

In the beginning of the study, we found the plasma BNP levels to be specifically lower in the stable patients with IHD than in the stable patients with non-IHD among the total study population. In addition, the multiple regression analysis clearly showed for the

Table 6. The results of the logistic regression analysis for IHD in males.

Explanatory variable	Regression coefficient	P	Odds ratio	Odds 95% CI
Log BNP	−0.669	<0.001	0.512	0.388~0.677
LVEF	−0.007	NS (p = 0.318)	0.993	0.981~1.006
Age	0.049	<0.001	1.050	1.037~1.064
BMI	0.080	<0.001	1.083	1.039~1.128
AF	−1.351	<0.001	0.259	0.172~0.389
s-Cr	0.087	0.01	1.091	1.021~1.167

BNP, B-type natriuretic peptide; LVEF, Left ventricular ejection fraction; BMI, Body mass index; AF, Atrial fibrillation; IHD, Ischemic heart disease; s-Cr, Serum creatinine.

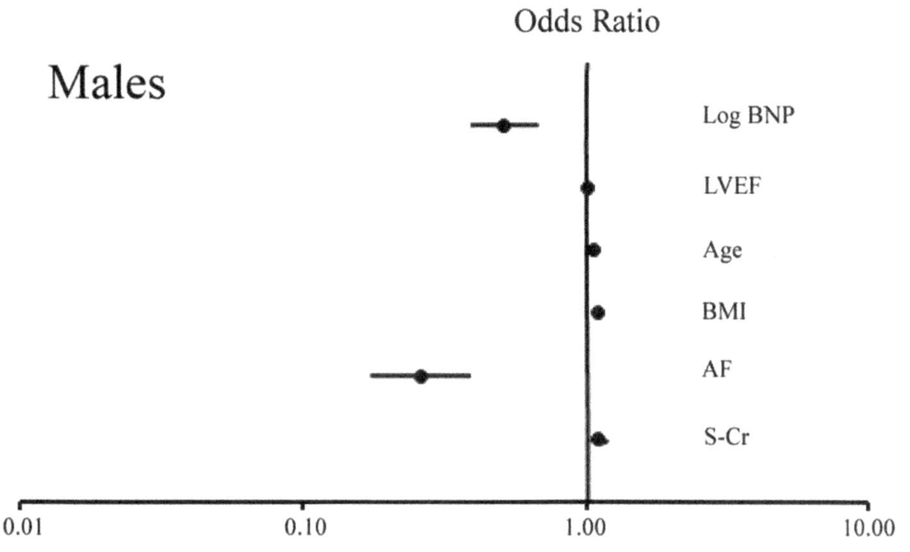

Figure 3. The Forest Plot displaying the odds ratio about risk of IHD in a males. BNP, B-type natriuretic peptide; LVEF, Left ventricular ejection fraction; BMI, Body mass index; AF, Atrial fibrillation; IHD, Ischemic heart disease; s-Cr, Serum creatinine.

first time that IHD *per se* is an independent determinant of the plasma BNP level, in addition to other known factors, such as age, male gender, low BMI, s-Cr, low LVEF and AF [26–31]. Furthermore, when the total study population was divided by gender, significant differences were identified between females and males. For example, it is noteworthy that the plasma BNP levels were significantly lower in the IHD group than in the non-IHD group among males only. In this analysis, the gender-difference observed in the plasma BNP levels in the IHD group was prominent even in consideration of the diverse clinical backgrounds. Therefore, unknown factors likely contributed to the observed gender difference. Next, by a multiple logistic regression analysis conversely performed using IHD as an objective variable and the logBNP as one of the explanatory variables, IHD was inversely determined by the logBNP only in males, but not in females. Hence the statistical analysis clarified that there is a substantial association between IHD *per se* and low plasma BNP level in males only. It is difficult to distinguish between cause and effect based on the present analyses; however, low plasma levels of BNP may be causally associated with IHD in males. In other words, the factor 'low reactivity of the plasma BNP level' may be a new risk factor for IHD in males. This way of thinking is supported by the previous reports showing that a deficiency of ANP and BNP was causatively associated with hypertension and other cardiovascular diseases [22–24].

BNP is biologically active and increases the cGMP levels. BNP is thus beneficial for suppressing the progression of heart failure, and probably atherosclerosis [13,14]. If the BNP level is insufficiently increased, low plasma BNP levels may have a causative role in IHD and heart failure. The reasons for the comparatively low plasma BNP levels or deteriorated response of BNP in IHD are unknown at present. Various factors such as neurohormones or genetic factors associated with gender differences may be linked to the current results. In addition, it is unknown whether a reduction of the synthesis or an augmented clearance of BNP affected the current results. As a next step, we need to examine the precise mechanisms responsible for the low plasma BNP levels seen only in male patients with IHD. The findings of the present and future studies may be able to provide a new strategy to prevent IHD and heart failure by increasing the endogenous natriuretic peptides using agents such as neutral endopeptidase inhibitors.

It is interesting to note a gender difference in the contribution of the plasma BNP level to the pathogenesis of IHD, as a gender difference have generally been reported to be negligible in patients with heart failure to date [27]. The results of this study may therefore help to answer the remaining questions regarding the impact of gender differences in the setting of IHD [32–37]. At present, it remains unknown whether IHD is the only or one of several cardiovascular diseases associated with the gender difference in the plasma BNP levels.

In general, the measurement of the plasma BNP levels is useful for early monitoring of asymptomatic ventricular dysfunction in patients with high risk factors. A value <18.4 pg/ml is considered to be ideal, and less than 40 pg/ml is considered to be within the normal range for patients without cardiac organic disorders visiting the hospital [27]. However, in this study, a considerable number of patients with a low EF (<55%) and low plasma BNP levels (<40 pg/ml) was seen in the IHD group compared with the non-IHD group among males; 153 patients (10.81%) vs. 16 patients (5.65%), $p<0.01$. On the other hand, there were few female patients with the same conditions; only two patients (0.81%) in the IHD group and nine patients (6.25%) in the non-IHD group, $p<0.01$ (precise data not shown in the Results). This indicates that clinicians should take care not to underestimate the degree of heart failure even if the plasma BNP levels are relatively low (less than 40 pg/ml) in male patients with IHD.

It is known that the BNP level increases with inflammation [38]. In this study, we examined the serum C-reactive protein (CRP) levels between 396 patients with IHD and 136 patients with non-IHD via blood samples obtained on the day of the catheterization. The average CRP level was 0.670±1.653 (95%CI: 0.390–0.950) in the non-IHD group and 0.521±1.109 (95%CI: 0.412–0.631) in the IHD group, which was not significantly different ($p=0.239$) (precise data not shown in the Results). Therefore, we thought that the inflammation status would not have influenced the present results.

To avoid a selection bias, the study population was consecutively and non-selectively recruited; therefore, all plural data from one patient were used in this analysis. We essentially performed the analysis by using 1,661 IHD patients and 427 non-IHD patients. However, by way of caution, we performed a similar statistical analysis by using only one dataset from each patient (1178 IHD patients and 416 non-IHD patients) who underwent cardiac catheterization for the first time during this protocol. As a result, the plasma BNP levels were found to be significantly lower in the IHD group than in the non-IHD group ($p<0.001$), the same as in the full dataset. In addition, when the total study population was divided by gender, the plasma BNP levels were significantly lower in the IHD group than in the non-IHD group only in males ($p<0.001$), but not in females (p = NS). Thus, the findings of the full dataset and the data from just individual cases were the same.

Finally, this is only a pilot retrospective study of the possible contribution of a low plasma BNP level to the pathogenesis of IHD. Therefore, a prospective study is needed to examine whether male patients with very low levels of plasma BNP, even under conditions of high risk factors, are more likely to develop IHD, for example, by comparing the rates of acute ischemic attack, the progression of IHD and the severity of stenosis in IHD patients grouped by the plasma BNP level.

Study Limitation

First, the number of females was small compared with that of males (1698 males and 390 females); thus, it is difficult to draw any definitive conclusions regarding the gender difference in the contribution of the plasma BNP level to IHD. A larger study including more females is required to arrive at an absolute conclusion. Second, while the plasma BNP level was the primary outcome measurement of the study, the samples were collected on a wide range intervals, and up to 33.7% of the subjects underwent blood collection more than 72 hours after cardiac catheterization. It is ideal to perform simultaneous sampling with hemodynamic measurements during cardiac catheterization; however, this was a retrospective study, and blood sampling for the purpose of measuring the plasma BNP levels was performed in the clinical setting based on the discretion of the attending physician. For this reason, there was a time delay in blood sampling in some patients. However, no statistical differences were noted in the timing of sampling between females and males; the patients who underwent blood sampling after more than 72 hours included 125 females (32.1% of the total 390 females) and 579 males (34.1% of the total 1,698 males) (P = NS). Therefore, we do not believe that the time lag in sampling in some cases largely affected the present findings.

Conclusions

The plasma BNP levels were relatively low in stable patients with IHD compared with that observed in the stable patients with non-IHD; this tendency was more evident in males. Perhaps, the low reactivity of BNP is causally associated with IHD in males. We hope this study serves as a test of a prospective study in the future.

Acknowledgments

We thank Mr. Brian Quinn (Japan Medical Communication) for his kind advice regarding the use of the English language.

Author Contributions

Conceived and designed the experiments: KM MY. Performed the experiments: KM TO TT KO TN SA S. Morimoto YI HS AU. Analyzed the data: KM TO MK KK TT S. Matsuo KH MY. Contributed reagents/materials/analysis tools: KM MK MY. Wrote the paper: KM TO KK TT MY.

References

1. Sudoh T, Kangawa K, Minamino N, Matsuo H (1988) A new natriuretic peptide in porcine brain. Nature 332: 78–81.
2. Mukoyama M, Nakao K, Hosoda K, Suga S, Saito Y, et al. (1991) Brain natriuretic peptide as a novel cardiac hormone in humans. Evidence for an exquisite dual natriuretic peptide system, atrial natriuretic peptide and brain natriuretic peptide. J Clin Invest 87: 1402–1412.
3. Yasue H, Yoshimura M, Sumida H, Kikuta K, Kugiyama K, et al. (1994) Localization and mechanism of secretion of B-type natriuretic peptide in comparison with those of A-type natriuretic peptide in normal subjects and patients with heart failure. Circulation 90: 195–203.
4. Omland T, Aakvaag A, Bonarjee VV, Caidahl K, Lie RT, et al. (1996) Plasma brain natriuretic peptide as an indicator of left ventricular systolic function and long-term survival after acute myocardial infarction. Comparison with plasma atrial natriuretic peptide and N-terminal proatrial natriuretic peptide. Circulation 93: 1963–1969.
5. Tsutamoto T, Wada A, Maeda K, Hisanaga T, Maeda Y, et al. (1997) Attenuation of compensation of endogenous cardiac natriuretic peptide system in chronic heart failure: prognostic role of plasma brain natriuretic peptide concentration in patients with chronic symptomatic left ventricular dysfunction. Circulation 96: 509–516.
6. Richards AM, Nicholls MG, Espiner EA, Lainchbury JG, Troughton RW, et al. (2003) B-type natriuretic peptides and ejection fraction for prognosis after myocardial infarction. Circulation 107: 2786–2792.
7. Suzuki S, Yoshimura M, Nakayama M, Mizuno Y, Harada E, et al. (2004) Plasma level of B-type natriuretic peptide as a prognostic marker after acute myocardial infarction: a long-term follow-up analysis. Circulation 110: 1387–1391.
8. Wang TJ, Larson MG, Levy D, Benjamin EJ, Leip EP, et al. (2004) Plasma natriuretic peptide levels and the risk of cardiovascular events and death. N Engl J Med 350: 655–663.
9. Morita E, Yasue H, Yoshimura M, Ogawa H, Jougasaki M, et al. (1993) Increased plasma levels of brain natriuretic peptide in patients with acute myocardial infarction. Circulation 88: 82–91.
10. Hawkridge AM, Heublein DM, Bergen HR III, Cataliotti A, Burnett JC Jr, et al. (2005) Quantitative mass spectral evidence for the absence of circulating brain natriuretic peptide (BNP-32) in severe human heart failure. Proc Natl Acad Sci U S A 102: 17442–17447.
11. Nishikimi T, Okamoto H, Nakamura M, Ogawa N, Horii K, et al. (2013) Direct immunochemiluminescent assay for proBNP and total BNP in human plasma proBNP and total BNP levels in normal and heart failure. PLoS One 8: e53233.
12. Gorbe A, Giricz Z, Szunyog A, Csont T, Burley DS, et al. (2010) Role of cGMP-PKG signaling in the protection of neonatal rat cardiac myocytes subjected to simulated ischemia/reoxygenation. Basic Res Cardiol 105: 643–650.
13. Ogawa Y, Itoh H, Tamura N, Suga S, Yoshimasa T, et al. (1994) Molecular cloning of the complementary DNA and gene that encode mouse brain natriuretic peptide and generation of transgenic mice that overexpress the brain natriuretic peptide gene. J Clin Invest 93: 1911–1921.
14. Nishikimi T, Maeda N, Matsuoka H (2006) The role of natriuretic peptides in cardioprotection. Cardiovasc Res 69: 318–328.
15. Costello-Boerrigter LC, Boerrigter G, Ameenuddin S, Mahoney DW, Slusser JP, et al. (2011) The effect of the brain-type natriuretic peptide single-nucleotide polymorphism rs198389 on test characteristics of common assays. Mayo Clin Proc 86: 210–218.
16. Szabo G, Molvarec A, Stenczer B, Rigo J Jr, Nagy B (2011) Natriuretic peptide precursor B gene (TTTC)(n) microsatellite polymorphism in pre-eclampsia. Clin Chim Acta 412: 1371–1375.
17. Ellis KL, Newton-Cheh C, Wang TJ, Frampton CM, Doughty RN, et al. (2011) Association of genetic variation in the natriuretic peptide system with cardiovascular outcomes. J Mol Cell Cardiol 50: 695–701.
18. Choquet H, Cavalcanti-Proenca C, Lecoeur C, Dina C, Cauchi S, et al. (2009) The T-381C SNP in BNP gene may be modestly associated with type 2 diabetes: an updated meta-analysis in 49 279 subjects. Hum Mol Genet 18: 2495–2501.
19. Poreba R, Poczatek K, Gac P, Poreba M, Gonerska M, et al. (2009) SNP rs198389 (T-381 C) polymorphism in the B-type natriuretic peptide gene promoter in patients with atherosclerotic renovascular hypertension. Pol Arch Med Wewn 119: 219–224.
20. Weber M, Burian M, Dragutinovic I, Moellmann H, Nef H, et al. (2008) Genetic polymorphism of the type A human natriuretic peptide receptor (NPR-A) gene contributes to the interindividual variability in the BNP system. Eur J Heart Fail 10: 482–489.

21. Vassalle C, Andreassi MG, Prontera C, Fontana M, Zyw L, et al. (2007) Influence of ScaI and natriuretic peptide (NP) clearance receptor polymorphisms of the NP System on NP concentration in chronic heart failure. Clin Chem 53: 1886–1890.
22. Ferrari P, Weidmann P, Ferrier C, Dietler R, Hollmann R, et al. (1990) Dysregulation of atrial natriuretic factor in hypertension-prone man. J Clin Endocrinol Metab 71: 944–951.
23. Belluardo P, Cataliotti A, Bonaiuto L, Giuffre E, Maugeri E, et al. (2006) Lack of activation of molecular forms of the BNP system in human grade 1 hypertension and relationship to cardiac hypertrophy. Am J Physiol Heart Circ Physiol 291: H1529–1535.
24. Macheret F, Boerrigter G, McKie P, Costello-Boerrigter L, Lahr B, et al. (2011) Pro-B-type natriuretic peptide(1-108) circulates in the general community: plasma determinants and detection of left ventricular dysfunction. J Am Coll Cardiol 57: 1386–1395.
25. Komukai K, Ogawa T, Yagi H, Date T, Sakamoto H, et al. (2008) Decreased renal function as an independent predictor of re-hospitalization for congestive heart failure. Circ J 72: 1152–1157.
26. Nakane T, Kawai M, Komukai K, Kayama Y, Matsuo S, et al. (2012) Contribution of extracardiac factors to the inconsistency between plasma B-type natriuretic peptide levels and the severity of pulmonary congestion on chest X-rays in the diagnosis of heart failure. Intern Med 51: 239–248.
27. Kawai M, Yoshimura M, Harada M, Mizuno Y, Hiramitsu S, et al. (2013) Determination of the B-type natriuretic peptide level as a criterion for abnormalities in japanese individuals in routine clinical practice: the J-ABS Multi-Center Study (Japan Abnormal BNP Standard). Intern Med 52: 171–177.
28. Cataliotti A, Malatino LS, Jougasaki M, Zoccali C, Castellino P, et al. (2001) Circulating natriuretic peptide concentrations in patients with end-stage renal disease: role of brain natriuretic peptide as a biomarker for ventricular remodeling. Mayo Clin Proc 76: 1111–1119.
29. Redfield MM, Rodeheffer RJ, Jacobsen SJ, Mahoney DW, Bailey KR, et al. (2002) Plasma brain natriuretic peptide concentration: impact of age and gender. J Am Coll Cardiol 40: 976–982.
30. Wang TJ, Larson MG, Levy D, Leip EP, Benjamin EJ, et al. (2002) Impact of age and sex on plasma natriuretic peptide levels in healthy adults. Am J Cardiol 90: 254–258.
31. Knudsen CW, Riis JS, Finsen AV, Eikvar L, Muller C, et al. (2004) Diagnostic value of a rapid test for B-type natriuretic peptide in patients presenting with acute dyspnoe: effect of age and gender. Eur J Heart Fail 6: 55–62.
32. Njolstad I, Arnesen E, Lund-Larsen PG (1996) Smoking, serum lipids, blood pressure, and sex differences in myocardial infarction. A 12-year follow-up of the Finnmark Study. Circulation 93: 450–456.
33. Jousilahti P, Vartiainen E, Tuomilehto J, Puska P (1999) Sex, age, cardiovascular risk factors, and coronary heart disease: a prospective follow-up study of 14 786 middle-aged men and women in Finland. Circulation 99: 1165–1172.
34. Yarnell JW, Beswick AD, Sweetnam PM, Riad-Fahmy D (1993) Endogenous sex hormones and ischemic heart disease in men. The Caerphilly prospective study. Arterioscler Thromb 13: 517–520.
35. Malkin CJ, Pugh PJ, Jones TH, Channer KS (2003) Testosterone for secondary prevention in men with ischaemic heart disease? Qjm 96: 521–529.
36. Schuit SC, Oei HH, Witteman JC, Geurts van Kessel CH, van Meurs JB, et al. (2004) Estrogen receptor alpha gene polymorphisms and risk of myocardial infarction. Jama 291: 2969–2977.
37. Rod NH, Kristensen TS, Diderichsen F, Prescott E, Jensen GB, et al. (2010) Cortisol, estrogens and risk of ischaemic heart disease, cancer and all-cause mortality in postmenopausal women: a prospective cohort study. Int J Epidemiol 39: 530–538.
38. Inoue T, Kawai M, Nakane T, Nojiri A, Minai K, et al. (2010) Influence of low-grade inflammation on plasma B-type natriuretic peptide levels. Intern Med 49: 2659–2668.

12

Factors Influencing the Measurement of Plasma/Serum Surfactant Protein D Levels by ELISA

Preston E. Bratcher[1,5*], Amit Gaggar[1,2,3,4,5]

1 Department of Medicine and Division of Pulmonary, Allergy, and Critical Care Medicine, University of Alabama at Birmingham, Birmingham, Alabama, United States of America, 2 Gregory Fleming James Cystic Fibrosis Research Center, University of Alabama at Birmingham, Birmingham, Alabama, United States of America, 3 University of Alabama at Birmingham, UAB Lung Health Center, Birmingham, Alabama, United States of America, 4 Medicine Service, United States Department of Veterans Affairs Medical Center, Birmingham, Alabama, United States of America, 5 Program in Protease and Matrix Biology, University of Alabama at Birmingham, Birmingham, Alabama, United States of America

Abstract

Background: Extensive variations in human surfactant protein D (SP-D) levels in circulation as measured by ELISA exist in the published literature. In order to determine the source of these variations, factors influencing the measurement by ELISA were explored.

Materials and Methods: Peripheral blood from healthy individuals was collected into various vacutainers during the same blood draw. Recombinant SP-D was diluted into different matrices and used for a standard curve. Samples were analyzed by capture ELISA using one of two distinct detection antibodies.

Results: The type of matrix had some effects on detection of recombinant SP-D. The type of anticoagulant used and dilution factor had very little effect, except for in plasma collected in EDTA vacutainers. The extent of variation in published values seemed to be due to the ELISA configuration employed, and, in agreement with this, we found that by switching the detection antibody, there was a 50% decrease in the extrapolated SP-D value of serum and plasma samples. Storage of samples resulted in slight changes in measured SP-D levels.

Conclusions: The ELISA configuration employed to measure circulating levels of SP-D has a significant effect on the extrapolated values. In both configurations tested, the use of EDTA as a coagulant resulted in inconsistent values, and we, therefore, suggest the avoidance of this anticoagulant when assaying for SP-D by ELISA. While the demonstrated effects of several factors on measurement of SP-D may not account for all the disparities amongst the previous studies, they stress that variations in methodologies for measuring the same protein can result in very inconsistent results.

Editor: Nades Palaniyar, The Hospital for Sick Children and The University of Toronto, Canada

Funding: This work is supported by the National Institutes of Health (HL102371 to AG and 5T32HL105346-02 to PEB). The funders had no role in study design, data collection and analysis, decision to publish, or preparation of the manuscript.

Competing Interests: The authors have declared that no competing interests exist.

* Email: bratcher@uab.edu

Introduction

Surfactant protein D (SP-D) is a pulmonary collectin involved in regulation of inflammation, innate immune defense, and surfactant homeostasis. It is expressed by Clara cells and alveolar type II cells in the lung. SP-D has a multimeric structure which gives it the ability to agglutinate pathogens, as well as aid in the clearance of apoptotic cells, cellular debris, and foreign particles in the lung [reviewed in [1]].

Circulating levels of SP-D have been examined for their potential use as a biomarker in various diseases including dermatitis [2,3], acute lung injury (ALI)/acute respiratory distress syndrome (ARDS) [4–13], periodontitis [14], interstitial pulmonary fibrosis (IPF) [10,12,15–23], chronic obstructive pulmonary disease (COPD) [15,24–36], emphysema [37], cystic fibrosis (CF) [15,38,39], coronary disease [40,41], sclerosis [42–46], cancer [47,48], sarcoidosis [21,49], allergies [28,50–52], rheumatoid arthritis [53,54], and respiratory infections [18,55–60]. SP-D levels have also been proposed to correlate with genetic elements [61–63], body mass index (BMI) [64–68], age [65], circadian rhythm [69], and with particle exposure [70,71] and cigarette smoking habits [25,27,28,31,37,72–77]. In addition, there have been studies examining the levels of SP-D in subjects with Turner syndrome [78], paraquat intoxication [79], swimming in variably treated waters [80], lung transplant patients [81], patients undergoing neurosurgical operations [82], drowning victims [83], polymyositis/dermatomyositis [84], dementia [85], lupus [86], and sleep apnea [87].

Similarly to CC-16 and KL-6, SP-D is thought to be a marker of pulmonary leak into the vasculature [88], and therefore alveolar destruction would result in an increase in levels of these pulmonary proteins in the blood. However, protein levels in lung do not always correlate with protein levels in blood [35], suggesting the possibility of alternative mechanisms affecting SP-D levels in circulation.

Various commercially available kits and non-commercially available ELISA configurations have been used to compare SP-D levels in plasma and serum from normal, healthy controls and the various disease states described above. Interestingly, there is a very substantial discrepancy between the reported values of the healthy control populations between studies, as well as in the magnitude of the range of values in this population. While the ELISA configuration used to measure SP-D seemed to have a large impact on the values reported, there are significant variations in the healthy control SP-D levels and range amongst reports using the same configuration. The purpose of this study is to determine factors affecting the measurement of SP-D by ELISA that may, therefore, explain the variations of serum and plasma SP-D levels reported in the published literature.

Materials and Methods

Study subjects, peripheral blood collection, and processing

All human studies were approved by the University of Alabama at Birmingham Institutional Review Board for Human Use with all subjects providing written consent. Peripheral blood was collected from healthy volunteers by venipuncture into serum, heparin sulfate, K_2EDTA, and sodium citrate vacutainers (BD Biosciences) during a single draw. Samples were kept at room temperature until blood in the serum tube was coagulated. Afterwards, samples were centrifuged at 400xg for 10 minutes to separate blood cells from serum or plasma. Samples were either directly aliquoted and stored at -80°C or given an additional round of centrifugation at 3000xg for 10 minutes to separate platelets from serum or plasma. All serum and plasma sample values depicted in figures were free of platelets. All experiments had 6 samples per group except for the experiments depicted in Figures 2 and 4.

Measurement of SP-D concentration by ELISA and data analysis

Mouse antihuman SP-D capture antibody, biotinylated mouse antihuman SP-D detection antibody, streptavidin conjugated to horse radish peroxidase, and recombinant human SP-D standard were purchased as a kit from R&D Systems (Catalog # DY1920) and used according to the manufacturer's protocol. For experiments testing the effects of different matrices on the detection of recombinant human SP-D, a concentrated stock was made in PBS with 1% BSA from separately purchased recombinant human SP-D expressed in NSO cells (R&D Systems, Catalog # 1920-SP-050). For studies comparing detection antibodies, polyclonal goat antihuman SP-D antibody (R&D systems, Catalog # AF1920) was used instead with a monoclonal mouse antigoat conjugated to horse radish peroxidase (Sigma) used as a secondary. All sample values were extrapolated from a second order polynomial curve fit of 9 concentrations of the standard (two-fold dilutions with a high concentration of 40 ng/mL) diluted in 1% BSA PBS. Statistical analyses were performed as described in the figure legends using Prism 5 (GraphPad Software), and all reported p values are two-tailed. All error bars represent standard deviation.

Results

Variations in previously reported SP-D levels

In order to determine the mean and range of SP-D levels in the serum/plasma of normal, healthy individuals, we performed a non-exhaustive search of the literature which revealed more than 60 publications in which these values were described. Interestingly, an unexpected amount of variation on these reported values was observed. When grouping according to the ELISA configuration used, one configuration consistently resulted in significantly higher values than the two other configurations for which multiple references were obtained (Figure 1a). For each configuration, a substantial range of means/medians was observed in the healthy control population. In addition to the variations seen in the averages, the spectrum of values in all populations ranged from 55.9 pg/mL [22] to 3.9653 μg/mL [89], representing a more than 70,000 fold difference. When examining the range of values seen in healthy subjects from each individual study and grouping according to the ELISA configuration used, a large variation in range was observed (Figure 1b). Overall, the study with the smallest range for any population (as a percentage of the average) reported a 95% confidence interval of 95.7–109.0 [54], while the study containing the population with the largest range reported a standard deviation of 327% of the mean value [42].

Based on the above observations, we can infer that the largest difference in the measured levels of SP-D is due to the ELISA configuration employed, but that there are still significant differences between the averages of healthy individuals from studies using the same configurations. In order to compare the results of various studies in another manner, we examined the fold change from healthy populations for the four diseases/conditions for which a substantial number of publications were available (IPF, CF, cigarette smoking, and systemic sclerosis). This would allow us to control for ELISA configurations employed, technical protocol followed for the ELISA as well as for sample collection and processing, and any differences in the populations (as controls have been appropriately matched). The expectation was that the fold change from healthy would be very similar for each disease/condition. However, large differences in the extent of this change were observed (Figure 1c).

Influence of matrix on detection of recombinant SP-D

In order to determine if the matrix used to generate the serial dilutions of recombinant human standard (rhSP-D) had any effects upon measurement, we compared values produced by dilutions in PBS, solutions of BSA (in PBS), and solutions of FBS (diluted in PBS) (Figure 2). At higher concentrations of protein (i.e. 5% BSA, 50% FBS, and 100% FBS), a decrease in the amount of rhSP-D detected was observed, with the amount measured in samples containing 10 ng/mL rhSP-D being the most variable of any samples measured in this assay. Using the manufacturer's recommended matrix (1% BSA) produced results very similar to a 10% FBS matrix, with both giving very consistent measurements and the greatest values. The values for PBS matrix gave similarly consistent measurements, but at a slightly lower value. This effect may be due to adsorption of rhSP-D without a carrier protein to the tubes used for serial dilutions [90]. Serum Matrix (Millipore), which had background levels of SP-D, also inhibited detection of recombinant SP-D at higher concentrations. All further standard curves were established by serial dilutions of recombinant SP-D in 1% BSA in PBS.

Influence of anticoagulant on extrapolated SP-D level

One factor that was found to differ between studies and could, therefore, be a source of variation of reported healthy population values, was the type of anticoagulant (or lack thereof) in the collection container. When blood was simultaneously collected in various vacutainers, serum and heparin plasma gave similar measurements of SP-D, while citrate plasma gave values

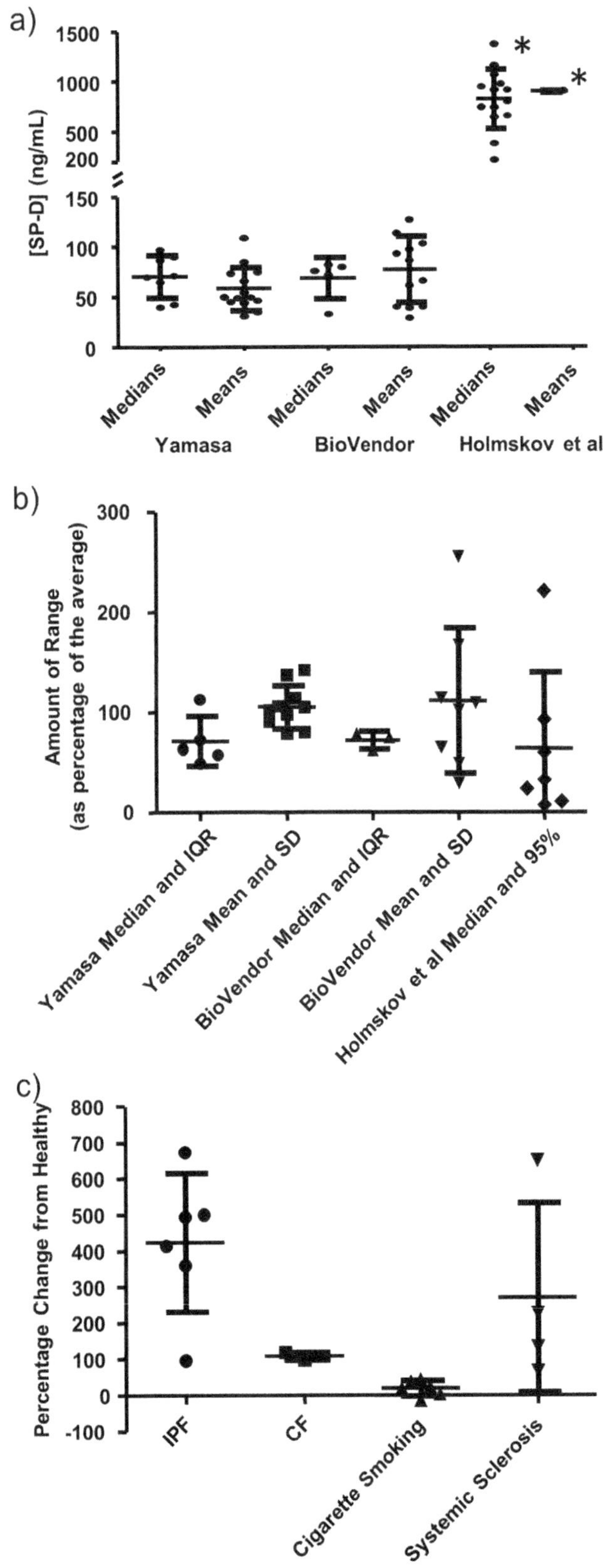

Figure 1. Published values for [SP-D] in the blood. a) A substantial amount of variation in the average [SP-D] in the serum/plasma of healthy control population exists between studies using the same or different ELISA configurations. Three configurations (Yamasa [12,13,17–19,21,25,28,38,43–45,49,50,59,61,77,84,89], BioVendor [14,31–36,46,52,56,64,65,72,75,76,79,80], and Holmskov et al. [3,39,53–55,58,62,66,69,70,78,85,86]) were compared. b) The range of healthy control [SP-D] greatly varied from study to study. Values shown are either median and interquartile range (IQR), median and 95% confidence interval (95%), or mean and standard deviation (SD). c) The calculated fold increase from the average healthy [SP-D] and average [SP-D] during IPF [12,16–19,21], CF [15,38,39], cigarette smoking [28,31,72–75], or sclerosis [42–44,46] was different between publications. An asterisk (*) denotes $p \leq 0.001$ by one-way ANOVA with Tukey's multiple comparison test.

significantly lower than serum values (Figure 3). EDTA plasma gave the most inconsistent results, and values were also significantly lower than serum values.

Influence of calcium on detection of SP-D by ELISA

In order to determine if calcium concentration in the sample had a significant effect upon the measurement of SP-D, rhSP-D was assayed in serially diluted $CaCl_2$ or EDTA. The detection of rhSP-D was only slightly effected by the changes in calcium concentration in the sample (Figure 4a). Additionally, we examined the effects of calcium concentration in the human samples by adding calcium to EDTA plasma samples and by adding EDTA to serum samples. While reconstituting the free calcium in the EDTA samples had little effect, the addition of EDTA to the serum samples had a dramatic effect that was inconsistent amongst the patient samples.

While many ELISAs employ the use of PBS lacking divalent cations as a buffer during the detection of antibody-captured antigens, the ELISA configuration employed by Holmskov et al. uses a Tris-buffered saline solution containing 5 mM calcium chloride, as the monoclonal detection antibody binds to SP-D in the presence of calcium [58]. In addition, it was previously demonstrated that SP-D has the ability to bind to various immunoglobulins in a calcium-dependent manner [91]. In order to determine the effects of calcium in the context of SP-D detection by ELISA, ELISAs were performed with antibodies diluted in buffer with or without calcium. We examined these effects on both recombinant SP-D and SP-D in plasma with either the ELISA kit's detection antibody or a polyclonal goat anti-SP-D antibody produced by the same manufacturer. In all cases but one, the addition of 5 mM calcium to the dilution and wash buffer resulted in a small (~17%) but significant increase in SP-D concentration relative to detection in the absence of calcium (Figure 4b). It is important to note that with the kit reagents, since the relative increase in detection of recombinant SP-D and SP-D in plasma in the presence of calcium is very similar, the extrapolated SP-D concentration in plasma when using a standard curve of recombinant SP-D should not significantly change. Interestingly, while the inclusion of calcium increased the recognition of native SP-D by the polyclonal antibody, it had no effect on the detection of recombinant SP-D by this antibody. Although it is beyond the scope of this study, future work will explore whether this effect is due to an increase in antibody recognition of antigen, increase in non-specific binding of antibodies by captured SP-D, or an increase through another mechanism.

Influence of detection antibody on extrapolated SP-D level

Given that some of the variation seen in the published literature might be explained by the use of different antibodies, we detected SP-D in serum and plasma samples using either the ELISA kit's detection antibody or the polyclonal goat anti-SP-D antibody. While there is no significant difference between detection by the

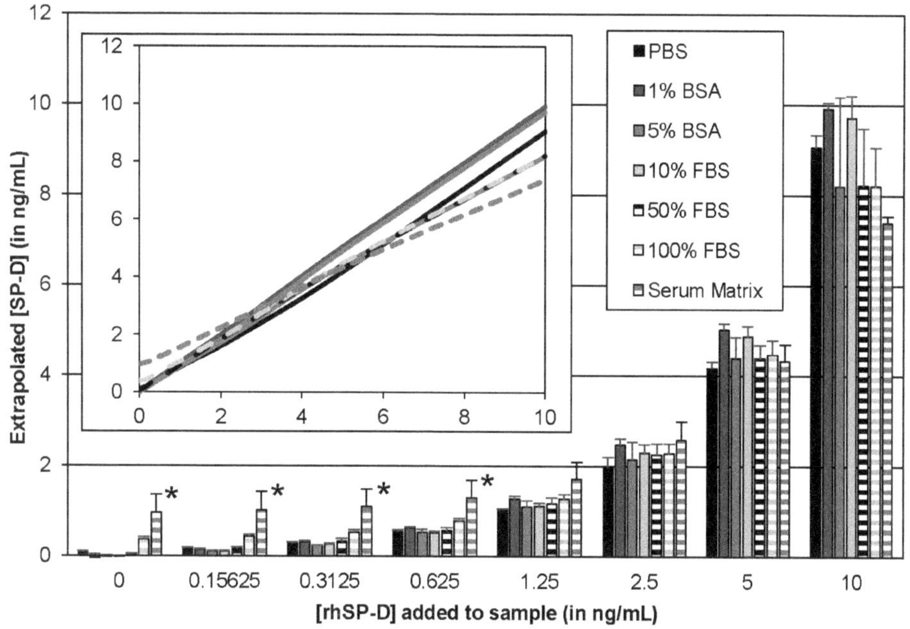

Figure 2. Use of various diluents for the recombinant SP-D standard. A 1 µg/mL recombinant SP-D stock was diluted 1:99 in various matrices and then serially diluted 2 fold in the same matrix. Mean and standard deviation for three independent experiments are shown. An asterisk (*) denotes values are significantly different ($p \leq 0.01$) from both the 1% BSA and 10% FBS values by one-way ANOVA using Tukey's multiple comparison test.

kit antibody versus the polyclonal goat antibody with regard to the type of collection tube used, overall, there is a ~50% reduction in the extrapolated value produced by detection with the polyclonal goat antibody compared to the kit antibody (Figure 5). In both cases, the same capture antibody was employed, and it is therefore possible that using a different capture antibody could have a similar effect on varying the extrapolated SP-D concentration in the sample.

Influence of sample dilution on extrapolated SP-D level

Another factor that fluctuated from study to study was whether the sample was assayed neat or the sample was prediluted (and the amount the sample was diluted). Given this fact and that diluting recombinant SP-D into 100% FBS had some influence in the detection of said SP-D, we compared SP-D values detected in undiluted and diluted samples. There was a very minimal difference between values produced by undiluted and 10 fold diluted serum, citrate plasma, and heparin plasma (Figure 6). Ten fold diluted EDTA plasma, however, produced a significantly higher extrapolated SP-D value when compared to the same sample undiluted. This same effect was seen when the polyclonal goat antibody tested above was used for detection (data not shown).

Influence of storage condition on extrapolated SP-D level

While the most common processing technique involved separating the blood cells (but not platelets) from serum and plasma and storing this sample at −80°C until assayed, some variations in processing and storage were present. To address this, we assayed serum and heparin plasma without platelets immediately after processing or after storage at 4°C, −20°C, or −80°C (Figure 7); there were no significant differences between conditions. Additionally, there were

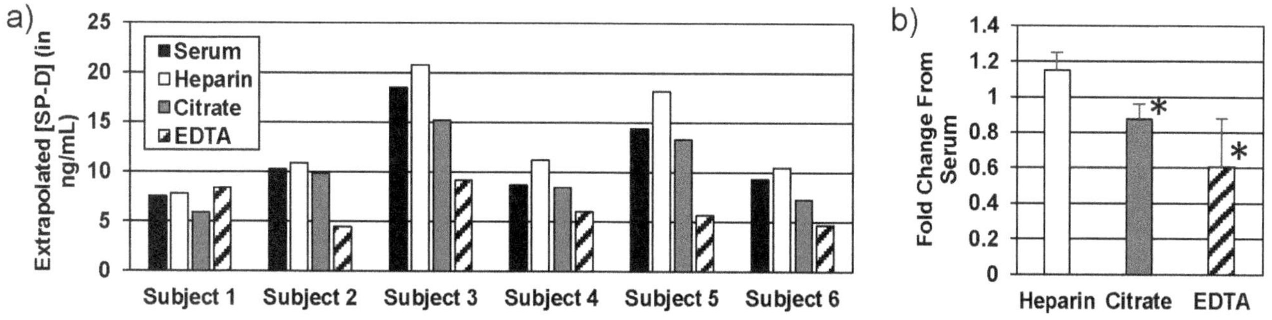

Figure 3. Detection of SP-D in serum and plasma collected using various anticoagulants. a) SP-D concentrations were measured in samples collected into four different vacutainers during a single blood draw. b) Measured values of samples were normalized to the SP-D concentration in serum for each patient in order to compare the effect of the anticoagulant on the measured SP-D concentration. An asterisk (*) denotes values are significantly different by Wilcoxon signed rank test (for EDTA, $p = 0.0156$, and for Citrate, $p = 0.0078$).

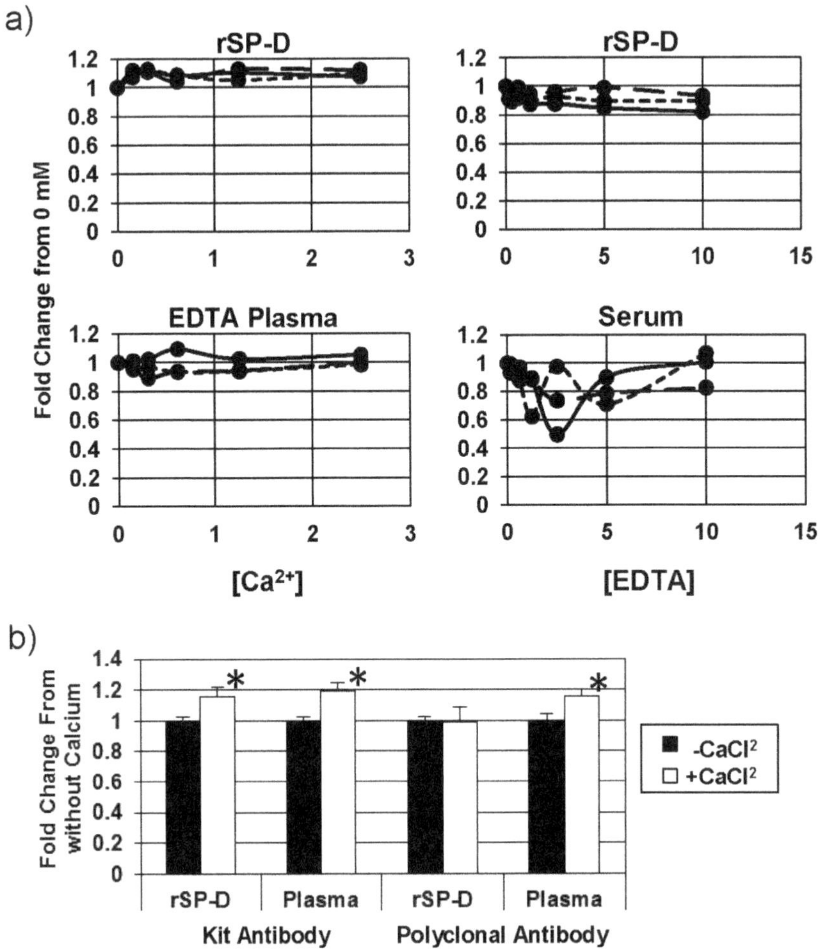

Figure 4. Influence of calcium concentration on detection of recombinant SP-D and native SP-D in serum and plasma. a) Recombinant SP-D (rSP-D), serum, and EDTA plasma were assayed in twofold dilutions of $[Ca^{2+}]$ or [EDTA] (concentrations are displayed in mM). For the inclusion of calcium with recombinant SP-D, Hank's Balanced Salt Solution (HBSS) was used as a buffer instead of PBS. Recombinant SP-D was assayed at 5 ng/mL while serum and plasma were diluted twofold. Each line represents an independent experiment. b) ELISAs were performed with detection reagents diluted in HBSS without calcium chloride ($-CaCl^2$) or with 5 mM calcium chloride ($+CaCl^2$). Wash buffer also either lacked or included calcium chloride. Recombinant SP-D was assayed at 10 ng/mL and Heparin plasma from four subjects was pooled, and sample values were extrapolated from a single standard curve under the conditions lacking calcium. n = 3 samples per group.

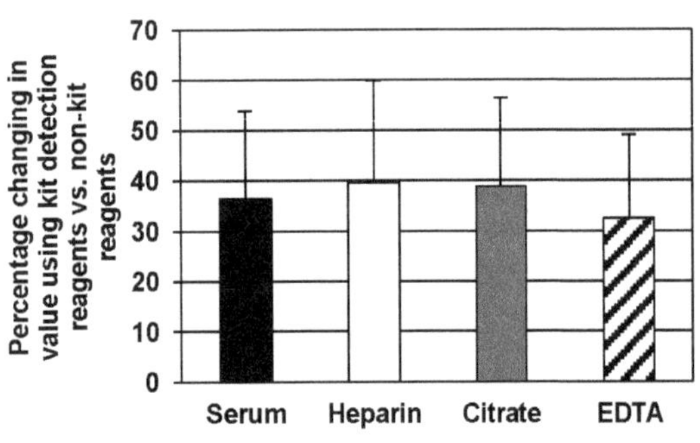

Figure 5. Comparison of SP-D values using two different detection antibodies. Serum, plasmas, and recombinant SP-D standard were detected using either kit reagents or non-kit reagents as described in the methods. SP-D concentrations in human samples were extrapolated from the standard curve as detected with the corresponding reagents. All values were significantly different ($p<0.05$) by Wilcoxon signed rank test.

only subtle differences between a sample stored at −20°C and −80°C, and depending on whether the sample went through a freeze/thaw (FT) cycle, contained platelets or not, or was spun after thawing to separate any precipitates/debris (data not shown). SP-D concentrations of samples stored at −20°C and −80°C for two weeks were not different from the same samples at one week (data not shown).

Discussion

This study provides experimental evidence that variations in the anticoagulant used and ELISA configuration can have dramatic effects upon the measured SP-D level. Storage and processing of samples as well as diluent used for the standard have minor effects on the level of SP-D extrapolated by ELISA. Although these results may partially explain the variations seen in reported SP-D values in the blood, it is important to note the caveats associated with this review of the literature. For the comparison of healthy control groups amongst various studies, it is possible that differences in ethnic background and/or geographical location from which subjects were recruited may contribute to the

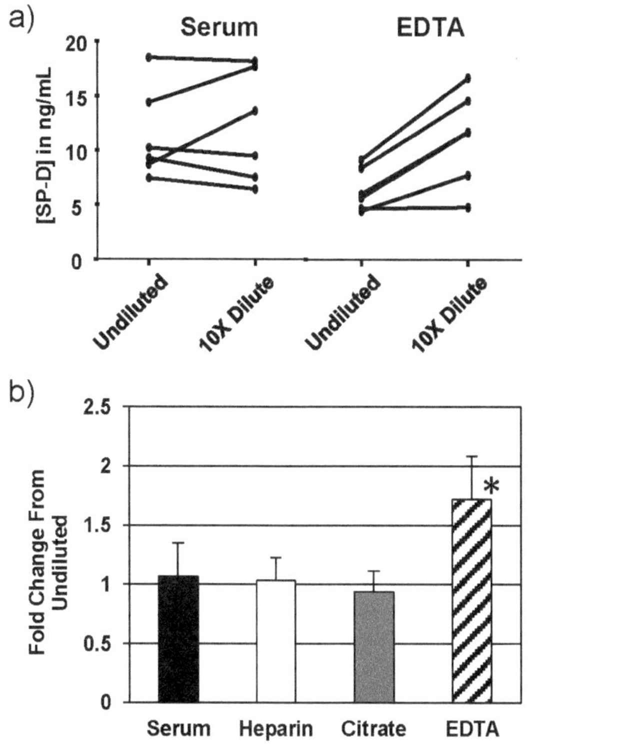

Figure 6. Comparison of SP-D values using neat and diluted samples. a) Serum and plasma samples were assayed as both undiluted and diluted tenfold in PBS. The extrapolated value in the tenfold diluted sample was multiplied by 10 in order to compare to the original, undiluted sample. b) Measured values of diluted samples were normalized to the SP-D concentration in the corresponding undiluted sample in order to compare the effect of the anticoagulant on the measured SP-D concentrations in these conditions. An asterisk (*) denotes p = 0.0313 by Wilcoxon signed rank test.

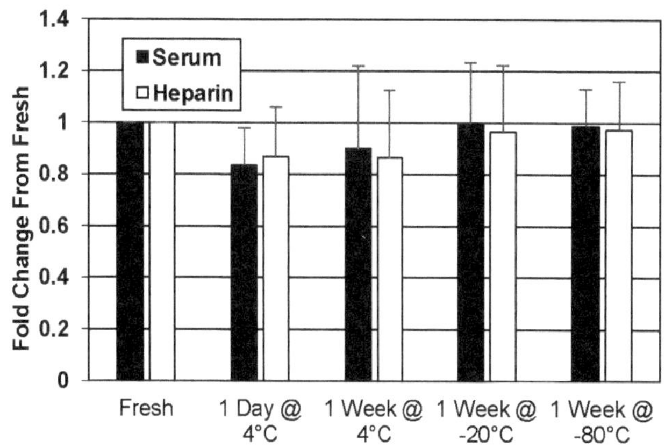

Figure 7. Comparison of SP-D values in samples stored in various conditions. Serum and heparin plasma samples collected during a single draw were either analyzed fresh or aliquoted and stored at 4°C, −20°C, or −80°C.

variations seen when the same ELISA configuration was employed, as could the type of anticoagulant. However, we would expect the range of samples between healthy populations of different studies to be similar. In addition, assuming that an appropriately matched control population was used for comparison to the disease population, the fold change between healthy and disease should be more similar than what was observed in the literature.

Measuring SP-D by ELISA presents a problem due to its multimeric structure. For each molecule (a complete dodecamer) of multimerized protein, there are at least 12 of the same epitopes present. Due to this property, it is not necessary to use discrete antibodies in a sandwich ELISA format to capture and then detect SP-D; even the same monoclonal antibody could be used for both. However, this may cause a difference in read out compared to using antibodies that detect different epitopes, due to the fact that the degree of multimerization has been shown to vary in the lungs during different disease states [92] and using the same monoclonal antibody would fail to detect a monomer. Even using two monoclonals that recognize distinct epitopes to measure SP-D in its native state would be confounded by differences in the degree of multimerization. For example, if an antibody against the carbohydrate recognition domain of SP-D was used to capture and an antibody against the neck region of SP-D was used to detect, a single, captured monomer of SP-D would be able to bind a single anti-neck antibody. However, a single, captured dodecamer would be able to bind 12 anti-neck antibodies. In order to accurately establish absolute concentrations by ELISA, it would be important that the multimeric structure of the standard was equivalent to that of the samples, as there could be differences in antigen binding in higher order multimers due to steric hinderance. Unfortunately, we did not have the necessary resources to examine the influence of the degree of multimerization on ELISA measurements.

In addition to the possible effects caused by its multimeric nature, there is evidence in the literature to variable post-translational modifications of SP-D in native samples. These modifications may, in fact, mask the epitope recognized by an ELISA antibody. This may account for one of the largest differences seen in the reported ELISA measurements of SP-D in serum/plasma, as the highest concentrations of SP-D came from the non-commercially available ELISA which used purified, native SP-D as a standard; this is opposed to almost all others, which used recombinantly expressed SP-D as a standard. Regardless of whether the antibodies used were raised against recombinant SP-D or purified native, because the post-translational modifications can vary from one patient to the next, this presents a significant obstacle to accurate measurements of natural SP-D using antibodies.

The results of this study demonstrate the influence that the antibody may have on the SP-D concentration as measured by ELISA. In our experiments, it is important to note that the same recombinant standard and human serum/plasma samples were analyzed. Given the confounders mentioned above, it is possible that the antibody from the kit recognizes an epitope that is not post-translationally modified or altered in human serum/plasma SP-D, while several of the epitopes recognized by the polyclonal antibody are modified in human serum/plasma SP-D, but were unmodified in the recombinantly expressed SP-D (which was used as the immunogen). This would result in the observed relative decrease in binding of the native SP-D from the blood compared to the recombinant SP-D.

Accuracy of SP-D measurements is critically important to the validation of this protein as a biomarker in pulmonary disease. Standardization of sample processing and storage, including the avoidance of EDTA as an anticoagulant, is necessary to ensure consistent results. Although absolute values may vary greatly due to the ELISA configuration employed, relative differences in SP-D concentrations amongst various disease groups should be consistent throughout the published literature. We are currently exploring alternative methods to quantify SP-D levels in the blood, as we believe this is necessary in order to establish the absolute concentration.

Acknowledgments

The authors would like to thank Tarek Abdalla for his assistance with sample collection and processing.

Author Contributions

Conceived and designed the experiments: PEB. Performed the experiments: PEB. Analyzed the data: PEB. Contributed reagents/materials/analysis tools: PEB AG. Wrote the paper: PEB AG.

References

1. Kishore U, Greenhough TJ, Waters P, Shrive AK, Ghai R, et al. (2006) Surfactant proteins SP-A and SP-D: structure, function and receptors. Mol Immunol 43: 1293–1315.
2. Maeda M, Ichiki Y, Aoyama Y, Kitajima Y (2001) Surfactant protein D (SP-D) and systemic scleroderma (SSc). J Dermatol 28: 467–474.
3. Hohwy T, Otkjaer K, Madsen J, Soerensen G, Nielsen O, et al. (2006) Surfactant protein D in atopic dermatitis and psoriasis. Exp Dermatol 15: 168–174.
4. Eisner MD, Parsons P, Matthay MA, Ware L, Greene K, et al. (2003) Plasma surfactant protein levels and clinical outcomes in patients with acute lung injury. Thorax 58: 983–988.
5. Watkins TR, Rubenfeld GD, Martin TR, Nester TA, Caldwell E, et al. (2008) Effects of leukoreduced blood on acute lung injury after trauma: a randomized controlled trial. Crit Care Med 36: 1493–1499.
6. Todd DA, Marsh MJ, George A, Henderson NG, Barr H, et al. (2010) Surfactant phospholipids, surfactant proteins, and inflammatory markers during acute lung injury in children. Pediatr Crit Care Med 11: 82–91.
7. Ware LB, Koyama T, Billheimer DD, Wu W, Bernard GR, et al. (2010) Prognostic and pathogenetic value of combining clinical and biochemical indices in patients with acute lung injury. Chest 137: 288–296.
8. Determann RM, Millo JL, Waddy S, Lutter R, Garrard CS, et al. (2009) Plasma CC16 levels are associated with development of ALI/ARDS in patients with ventilator-associated pneumonia: a retrospective observational study. BMC Pulm Med 9: 49.
9. Determann RM, Royakkers AA, Haitsma JJ, Zhang H, Slutsky AS, et al. (2010) Plasma levels of surfactant protein D and KL-6 for evaluation of lung injury in critically ill mechanically ventilated patients. BMC Pulm Med 10: 6.
10. Collard HR, Calfee CS, Wolters PJ, Song JW, Hong SB, et al. (2010) Plasma biomarker profiles in acute exacerbation of idiopathic pulmonary fibrosis. Am J Physiol Lung Cell Mol Physiol 299: L3–7.
11. Ware LB, Koyama T, Zhao Z, Janz DR, Wickersham N, et al. (2013) Biomarkers of lung epithelial injury and inflammation distinguish severe sepsis patients with acute respiratory distress syndrome. Crit Care 17: R253.
12. Greene KE, King TE Jr, Kuroki Y, Bucher-Bartelson B, Hunninghake GW, et al. (2002) Serum surfactant proteins-A and -D as biomarkers in idiopathic pulmonary fibrosis. Eur Respir J 19: 439–446.
13. Greene KE, Wright JR, Steinberg KP, Ruzinski JT, Caldwell E, et al. (1999) Serial changes in surfactant-associated proteins in lung and serum before and after onset of ARDS. Am J Respir Crit Care Med 160: 1843–1850.
14. Glas J, Beynon V, Bachstein B, Steckenbiller J, Manolis V, et al. (2008) Increased plasma concentration of surfactant protein D in chronic periodontitis independent of SFTPD genotype: potential role as a biomarker. Tissue Antigens 72: 21–28.
15. Sims MW, Beers MF, Ahya VN, Kawut SM, Sims KD, et al. (2011) Effect of single vs bilateral lung transplantation on plasma surfactant protein D levels in idiopathic pulmonary fibrosis. Chest 140: 489–496.
16. Honda Y, Kuroki Y, Matsuura E, Nagae H, Takahashi H, et al. (1995) Pulmonary surfactant protein D in sera and bronchoalveolar lavage fluids. Am J Respir Crit Care Med 152: 1860–1866.
17. Nagae H, Takahashi H, Kuroki Y, Honda Y, Nagata A, et al. (1997) Enzyme-linked immunosorbent assay using F(ab')2 fragment for the detection of human pulmonary surfactant protein D in sera. Clin Chim Acta 266: 157–171.
18. Ohnishi H, Yokoyama A, Kondo K, Hamada H, Abe M, et al. (2002) Comparative study of KL-6, surfactant protein-A, surfactant protein-D, and monocyte chemoattractant protein-1 as serum markers for interstitial lung diseases. Am J Respir Crit Care Med 165: 378–381.
19. Kuwano K, Maeyama T, Inoshima I, Ninomiya K, Hagimoto N, et al. (2002) Increased circulating levels of soluble Fas ligand are correlated with disease activity in patients with fibrosing lung diseases. Respirology 7: 15–21.
20. Takahashi H, Shiratori M, Kanai A, Chiba H, Kuroki Y, et al. (2006) Monitoring markers of disease activity for interstitial lung diseases with serum surfactant proteins A and D. Respirology 11 Suppl: S51–54.
21. Lin FC, Chen YC, Chang SC (2008) Clinical importance of bronchoalveolar lavage fluid and blood cytokines, surfactant protein D, and Kerbs von Lungren 6 antigen in idiopathic pulmonary alveolar proteinosis. Mayo Clin Proc 83: 1344–1349.
22. Ando M, Miyazaki E, Ito T, Hiroshige S, Nureki SI, et al. (2010) Significance of serum vascular endothelial growth factor level in patients with idiopathic pulmonary fibrosis. Lung 188: 247–252.
23. Ichiyasu H, Ichikado K, Yamashita A, Iyonaga K, Sakamoto O, et al. (2012) Pneumocyte biomarkers KL-6 and surfactant protein D reflect the distinct findings of high-resolution computed tomography in nonspecific interstitial pneumonia. Respiration 83: 190–197.
24. Tkacova R, McWilliams A, Lam S, Sin DD (2010) Integrating lung and plasma expression of pneumo-proteins in developing biomarkers in COPD: a case study of surfactant protein D. Med Sci Monit 16: CR540–544.
25. Ilumets H, Mazur W, Toljamo T, Louhelainen N, Nieminen P, et al. (2011) Ageing and smoking contribute to plasma surfactant proteins and protease imbalance with correlations to airway obstruction. BMC Pulm Med 11: 19.
26. Celli BR, Locantore N, Yates J, Tal-Singer R, Miller BE, et al. (2012) Inflammatory biomarkers improve clinical prediction of mortality in chronic obstructive pulmonary disease. Am J Respir Crit Care Med 185: 1065–1072.
27. Um SJ, Lam S, Coxson H, Man SF, Sin DD (2013) Budesonide/formoterol enhances the expression of pro Surfactant Protein-B in lungs of COPD patients. PLoS One 8: e83881.
28. Mutti A, Corradi M, Goldoni M, Vettori MV, Bernard A, et al. (2006) Exhaled metallic elements and serum pneumoproteins in asymptomatic smokers and patients with COPD or asthma. Chest 129: 1288–1297.
29. Sin DD, Leung R, Gan WQ, Man SP (2007) Circulating surfactant protein D as a potential lung-specific biomarker of health outcomes in COPD: a pilot study. BMC Pulm Med 7: 13.
30. Sin DD, Man SF, Marciniuk DD, Ford G, FitzGerald M, et al. (2008) The effects of fluticasone with or without salmeterol on systemic biomarkers of inflammation in chronic obstructive pulmonary disease. Am J Respir Crit Care Med 177: 1207–1214.
31. Lomas DA, Silverman EK, Edwards LD, Locantore NW, Miller BE, et al. (2009) Serum surfactant protein D is steroid sensitive and associated with exacerbations of COPD. Eur Respir J 34: 95–102.
32. Shakoori TA, Sin DD, Ghafoor F, Bashir S, Bokhari SN (2009) Serum surfactant protein D during acute exacerbations of chronic obstructive pulmonary disease. Dis Markers 27: 287–294.
33. Winkler C, Atochina-Vasserman EN, Holz O, Beers MF, Erpenbeck VJ, et al. (2011) Comprehensive characterisation of pulmonary and serum surfactant protein D in COPD. Respir Res 12: 29.
34. Ju CR, Liu W, Chen RC (2012) Serum surfactant protein D: biomarker of chronic obstructive pulmonary disease. Dis Markers 32: 281–287.
35. Ozyurek BA, Ulasli SS, Bozbas SS, Bayraktar N, Akcay S (2013) Value of serum and induced sputum surfactant protein-D in chronic obstructive pulmonary disease. Multidiscip Respir Med 8: 36.
36. El-Deek SE, Makhlouf HA, Saleem TH, Mandour MA, Mohamed NA (2013) Surfactant protein d, soluble intercellular adhesion molecule-1 and high-sensitivity C-reactive protein as biomarkers of chronic obstructive pulmonary disease. Med Princ Pract 22: 469–474.
37. Atkinson JJ, Lutey BA, Suzuki Y, Toennies HM, Kelley DG, et al. (2011) The role of matrix metalloproteinase-9 in cigarette smoke-induced emphysema. Am J Respir Crit Care Med 183: 876–884.
38. Krane M, Griese M (2003) Surfactant protein D in serum from patients with allergic bronchopulmonary aspergillosis. Eur Respir J 22: 592–595.
39. Olesen HV, Holmskov U, Schiotz PO, Sorensen GL (2010) Serum-surfactant SP-D correlates inversely to lung function in cystic fibrosis. J Cyst Fibros 9: 257–262.
40. Hill J, Heslop C, Man SF, Frohlich J, Connett JE, et al. (2011) Circulating surfactant protein-D and the risk of cardiovascular morbidity and mortality. Eur Heart J 32: 1918–1925.
41. Engels GE, Gu YJ, van Oeveren W, Rakhorst G, Mariani MA, et al. (2013) The utility of lung epithelium specific biomarkers in cardiac surgery: a comparison of biomarker profiles in on- and off-pump coronary bypass surgery. J Cardiothorac Surg 8: 4.
42. Elhaj M, Charles J, Pedroza C, Liu X, Zhou X, et al. (2013) Can serum surfactant protein D or CC-chemokine ligand 18 predict outcome of interstitial lung disease in patients with early systemic sclerosis? J Rheumatol 40: 1114–1120.
43. Takahashi H, Kuroki Y, Tanaka H, Saito T, Kurokawa K, et al. (2000) Serum levels of surfactant proteins A and D are useful biomarkers for interstitial lung disease in patients with progressive systemic sclerosis. Am J Respir Crit Care Med 162: 258–263.

44. Asano Y, Ihn H, Yamane K, Yazawa N, Kubo M, et al. (2001) Clinical significance of surfactant protein D as a serum marker for evaluating pulmonary fibrosis in patients with systemic sclerosis. Arthritis Rheum 44: 1363–1369.
45. Yanaba K, Hasegawa M, Takehara K, Sato S (2004) Comparative study of serum surfactant protein-D and KL-6 concentrations in patients with systemic sclerosis as markers for monitoring the activity of pulmonary fibrosis. J Rheumatol 31: 1112–1120.
46. Hant FN, Ludwicka-Bradley A, Wang HJ, Li N, Elashoff R, et al. (2009) Surfactant protein D and KL-6 as serum biomarkers of interstitial lung disease in patients with scleroderma. J Rheumatol 36: 773–780.
47. Sasaki R, Soejima T, Matsumoto A, Maruta T, Yamada K, et al. (2001) Clinical significance of serum pulmonary surfactant proteins a and d for the early detection of radiation pneumonitis. Int J Radiat Oncol Biol Phys 50: 301–307.
48. Takahashi H, Imai Y, Fujishima T, Shiratori M, Murakami S, et al. (2001) Diagnostic significance of surfactant proteins A and D in sera from patients with radiation pneumonitis. Eur Respir J 17: 481–487.
49. Janssen R, Sato H, Grutters JC, Bernard A, van Velzen-Blad H, et al. (2003) Study of Clara cell 16, KL-6, and surfactant protein-D in serum as disease markers in pulmonary sarcoidosis. Chest 124: 2119–2125.
50. Koopmans JG, van der Zee JS, Krop EJ, Lopuhaa CE, Jansen HM, et al. (2004) Serum surfactant protein D is elevated in allergic patients. Clin Exp Allergy 34: 1827–1833.
51. Higashi A, Higashi N, Tsuburai T, Takeuchi Y, Taniguchi M, et al. (2005) Involvement of eicosanoids and surfactant protein D in extrinsic allergic alveolitis. Eur Respir J 26: 1069–1073.
52. Vizcaya D, Mirabelli MC, Orriols R, Anto JM, Barreiro E, et al. (2013) Functional and biological characteristics of asthma in cleaning workers. Respir Med 107: 673–683.
53. Hoegh SV, Lindegaard HM, Sorensen GL, Hoj A, Bendixen C, et al. (2008) Circulating surfactant protein D is decreased in early rheumatoid arthritis: a 1-year prospective study. Scand J Immunol 67: 71–76.
54. Christensen AF, Sorensen GL, Horslev-Petersen K, Holmskov U, Lindegaard HM, et al. (2010) Circulating surfactant protein -D is low and correlates negatively with systemic inflammation in early, untreated rheumatoid arthritis. Arthritis Res Ther 12: R39.
55. Wu YP, Liu ZH, Wei R, Pan SD, Mao NY, et al. (2009) Elevated plasma surfactant protein D (SP-D) levels and a direct correlation with anti-severe acute respiratory syndrome coronavirus-specific IgG antibody in SARS patients. Scand J Immunol 69: 508–515.
56. Bejvl I, Weseslindtner L, Strassl R, Jaksch P, Kundi M, et al. (2013) Analysis of plasma surfactant protein D levels in lung transplant recipients. Transpl Infect Dis 15: 645–651.
57. Arai Y, Obinata K, Sato Y, Hisata K, Tadokoro R, et al. (2001) Clinical significance of the serum surfactant protein D and KL-6 levels in patients with measles complicated by interstitial pneumonia. Eur J Pediatr 160: 425–429.
58. Leth-Larsen R, Nordenbaek C, Tornoe I, Moeller V, Schlosser A, et al. (2003) Surfactant protein D (SP-D) serum levels in patients with community-acquired pneumonia small star, filled. Clin Immunol 108: 29–37.
59. Kawasaki Y, Endo K, Suyama K, Sato M, Ito M, et al. (2011) Serum SP-D levels as a biomarker of lung injury in respiratory syncytial virus bronchiolitis. Pediatr Pulmonol 46: 18–22.
60. Nishida S, Fukazawa R, Imai T, Takeda S, Hayakawa J, et al. (2011) Serum KL-6 and surfactant protein D in children with 2009 pandemic H1N1 influenza infection. Pediatr Int 53: 910–914.
61. Al-Salmi QA, Walter JN, Colasurdo GN, Sockrider MM, Smith EO, et al. (2005) Serum KL-6 and surfactant proteins A and D in pediatric interstitial lung disease. Chest 127: 403–407.
62. Heidinger K, Konig IR, Bohnert A, Kleinsteiber A, Hilgendorff A, et al. (2005) Polymorphisms in the human surfactant protein-D (SFTPD) gene: strong evidence that serum levels of surfactant protein-D (SP-D) are genetically influenced. Immunogenetics 57: 1–7.
63. Fernandez-Real JM, Valdes S, Manco M, Chico B, Botas P, et al. (2010) Surfactant protein d, a marker of lung innate immunity, is positively associated with insulin sensitivity. Diabetes Care 33: 847–853.
64. Wutzler S, Lehnert T, Laurer H, Lehnert M, Becker M, et al. (2011) Circulating levels of Clara cell protein 16 but not surfactant protein D identify and quantify lung damage in patients with multiple injuries. J Trauma 71: E31–36.
65. Engstrom G, Lindberg C, Gerhardsson de Verdier M, Nihlen U, Anderson M, et al. (2012) Blood biomarkers and measures of pulmonary function–a study from the Swedish twin registry. Respir Med 106: 1250–1257.
66. Sorensen GL, Hjelmborg JV, Leth-Larsen R, Schmidt V, Fenger M, et al. (2006) Surfactant protein D of the innate immune defence is inversely associated with human obesity and SP-D deficiency infers increased body weight in mice. Scand J Immunol 64: 633–638.
67. Hoegh SV, Sorensen GL, Tornoe I, Lottenburger T, Ytting H, et al. (2010) Long-term stability and circadian variation in circulating levels of surfactant protein D. Immunobiology 215: 314–320.
68. Leth-Larsen R, Garred P, Jensenius H, Meschi J, Hartshorn K, et al. (2005) A common polymorphism in the SFTPD gene influences assembly, function, and concentration of surfactant protein D. J Immunol 174: 1532–1538.
69. Zhao XM, Wu YP, Wei R, Cai HX, Tornoe I, et al. (2007) Plasma surfactant protein D levels and the relation to body mass index in a chinese population. Scand J Immunol 66: 71–76.
70. Hoffmann HJ, Iversen M, Brandslund I, Sigsgaard T, Omland O, et al. (2003) Plasma C3d levels of young farmers correlate with respirable dust exposure levels during normal work in swine confinement buildings. Ann Agric Environ Med 10: 53–60.
71. Van Miert E, Sardella A, Nickmilder M, Bernard A (2012) Respiratory effects associated with wood fuel use: a cross-sectional biomarker study among adolescents. Pediatr Pulmonol 47: 358–366.
72. Wang SX, Liu P, Wei MT, Chen L, Guo Y, et al. (2007) Roles of serum clara cell protein 16 and surfactant protein-D in the early diagnosis and progression of silicosis. J Occup Environ Med 49: 834–839.
73. Kobayashi H, Kanoh S, Motoyoshi K (2008) Serum surfactant protein-A, but not surfactant protein-D or KL-6, can predict preclinical lung damage induced by smoking. Biomarkers 13: 385–392.
74. Van Miert E, Sardella A, Bernard A (2011) Biomarkers of early respiratory effects in smoking adolescents. Eur Respir J 38: 1287–1293.
75. Shiels MS, Chaturvedi AK, Katki HA, Gochuico BR, Caporaso NE, et al. (2011) Circulating markers of interstitial lung disease and subsequent risk of lung cancer. Cancer Epidemiol Biomarkers Prev 20: 2262–2272.
76. Aul R, Armstrong J, Duvoix A, Lomas D, Hayes B, et al. (2012) Inhaled LPS challenges in smokers: a study of pulmonary and systemic effects. Br J Clin Pharmacol 74: 1023–1032.
77. Haddam N, Samira S, Dumont X, Taleb A, Haufroid V, et al. (2009) Lung epithelium injury biomarkers in workers exposed to sulphur dioxide in a non-ferrous smelter. Biomarkers 14: 292–298.
78. Gravholt CH, Leth-Larsen R, Lauridsen AL, Thiel S, Hansen TK, et al. (2004) The effects of GH and hormone replacement therapy on serum concentrations of mannan-binding lectin, surfactant protein D and vitamin D binding protein in Turner syndrome. Eur J Endocrinol 150: 355–362.
79. Gil HW, Hong JR, Park JH, Seo YS, Yang JO, et al. (2007) Plasma surfactant D in patients following acute paraquat intoxication. Clin Toxicol (Phila) 45: 463–467.
80. Fernandez-Luna A, Gallardo L, Plaza-Carmona M, Garcia-Unanue J, Sanchez-Sanchez J, et al. (2013) Respiratory function and changes in lung epithelium biomarkers after a short-training intervention in chlorinated vs. ozone indoor pools. PLoS One 8: e68447.
81. Shah RJ, Bellamy SL, Localio AR, Wickersham N, Diamond JM, et al. (2012) A panel of lung injury biomarkers enhances the definition of primary graft dysfunction (PGD) after lung transplantation. J Heart Lung Transplant 31: 942–949.
82. Duda I, Grzybowska K, Jedrzejowska-Szypulka H, Lewin-Kowalik J (2012) The sitting position during neurosurgical procedures does not influence serum biomarkers of pulmonary parenchymal injury. BMC Surg 12: 24.
83. Kamada S, Seo Y, Takahama K (2000) A sandwich enzyme immunoassay for pulmonary surfactant protein D and measurement of its blood levels in drowning victims. Forensic Sci Int 109: 51–63.
84. Ihn H, Asano Y, Kubo M, Yamane K, Jinnin M, et al. (2002) Clinical significance of serum surfactant protein D (SP-D) in patients with polymyositis/dermatomyositis: correlation with interstitial lung disease. Rheumatology (Oxford) 41: 1268–1272.
85. Nybo M, Andersen K, Sorensen GL, Lolk A, Kragh-Sorensen P, et al. (2007) Serum surfactant protein D is correlated to development of dementia and augmented mortality. Clin Immunol 123: 333–337.
86. Hoegh SV, Voss A, Sorensen GL, Hoj A, Bendixen C, et al. (2009) Circulating surfactant protein D is decreased in systemic lupus erythematosus. J Rheumatol 36: 2449–2453.
87. Aihara K, Oga T, Harada Y, Chihara Y, Handa T, et al. (2011) Comparison of biomarkers of subclinical lung injury in obstructive sleep apnea. Respir Med 105: 939–945.
88. Hermans C, Bernard A (1999) Lung epithelium-specific proteins: characteristics and potential applications as markers. Am J Respir Crit Care Med 159: 646–678.
89. Stapleton RD, Dixon AE, Parsons PE, Ware LB, Suratt BT, et al. (2010) The association between BMI and plasma cytokine levels in patients with acute lung injury. Chest 138: 568–577.
90. Bratcher PE, Gaggar A (2013) Characterization and prevention of the adsorption of surfactant protein D to polypropylene. PLoS One 8: e73467.
91. Nadesalingam J, Reid KB, Palaniyar N (2005) Collectin surfactant protein D binds antibodies and interlinks innate and adaptive immune systems. FEBS Lett 579: 4449–4453.
92. Kotecha S, Davies PL, Clark HW, McGreal EP (2013) Increased prevalence of low oligomeric state surfactant protein D with restricted lectin activity in bronchoalveolar lavage fluid from preterm infants. Thorax 68: 460–467.

Whole Exome Sequencing Identifies Novel Genes for Fetal Hemoglobin Response to Hydroxyurea in Children with Sickle Cell Anemia

Vivien A. Sheehan[1]*, Jacy R. Crosby[2,3], Aniko Sabo[4], Nicole A. Mortier[5], Thad A. Howard[5], Donna M. Muzny[4], Shannon Dugan-Perez[4], Banu Aygun[6], Kerri A. Nottage[7], Eric Boerwinkle[3,4], Richard A. Gibbs[4], Russell E. Ware[5], Jonathan M. Flanagan[1]

1 Hematology Center, Department of Pediatrics, Baylor College of Medicine, Houston, Texas, United States of America, **2** The University of Texas Graduate School of Biomedical Sciences at Houston, Department of Biostatistics, Bioinformatics, and Systems Biology, University of Texas, Houston, Texas, United States of America, **3** Human Genetics Center, University of Texas, Houston, Texas, United States of America, **4** Human Genome Sequencing Center, Baylor College of Medicine, Houston, Texas, United States of America, **5** Division of Hematology, Cincinnati Children's Hospital Medical Center, Cincinnati, Ohio, United States of America, **6** Steven and Alexandra Cohen Children's Medical Center of New York, New Hyde Park, New York, United States of America, **7** Department of Hematology, St. Jude Children's Research Hospital, Memphis, Tennessee, United States of America

Abstract

Hydroxyurea has proven efficacy in children and adults with sickle cell anemia (SCA), but with considerable inter-individual variability in the amount of fetal hemoglobin (HbF) produced. Sibling and twin studies indicate that some of that drug response variation is heritable. To test the hypothesis that genetic modifiers influence pharmacological induction of HbF, we investigated phenotype-genotype associations using whole exome sequencing of children with SCA treated prospectively with hydroxyurea to maximum tolerated dose (MTD). We analyzed 171 unrelated patients enrolled in two prospective clinical trials, all treated with dose escalation to MTD. We examined two MTD drug response phenotypes: HbF (final %HbF minus baseline %HbF), and final %HbF. Analyzing individual genetic variants, we identified multiple low frequency and common variants associated with HbF induction by hydroxyurea. A validation cohort of 130 pediatric sickle cell patients treated to MTD with hydroxyurea was genotyped for 13 non-synonymous variants with the strongest association with HbF response to hydroxyurea in the discovery cohort. A coding variant in *Spalt-like transcription factor*, or *SALL2*, was associated with higher final HbF in this second independent replication sample and *SALL2* represents an outstanding novel candidate gene for further investigation. These findings may help focus future functional studies and provide new insights into the pharmacological HbF upregulation by hydroxyurea in patients with SCA.

Editor: Wilbur Lam, Emory University/Georgia Insititute of Technology, United States of America

Funding: This work was supported by the National Human Genome Research Institute (U54-HGOO3273)(EB, RAG), National Heart, Lung and Blood Institute (U01-HL078787, R01-HL090941)(REW), Doris Duke Charitable Foundation (2010036)(REW), and the Russell and Diana Hawkins Family Foundation Discovery Fellowship (JRC). The funders had no role in study design, data collection and analysis, decision to publish, or preparation of the manuscript.

Competing Interests: The authors have declared that no competing interests exist.

* Email: vsheehan@bcm.edu

Introduction

Sickle cell anemia (SCA) is an inherited blood disorder, affecting 1 in 400 African Americans, causing significant morbidity and mortality. Although a monogenic disease, individuals with SCA (usually homozygous HbSS) exhibit wide variability in their laboratory and clinical phenotypes. One of the most powerful and reproducible modifiers of disease severity is an individual's endogenous level of fetal hemoglobin (HbF) [1]. If produced in sufficient amounts, HbF is able to prevent the intracellular polymerization of deoxygenated sickle hemoglobin (HbS), which is the nidus of the clinical disease process [2,3]. Pharmacologic induction of HbF is clinically beneficial, and the most widely used and safest method for increasing HbF levels in patients with SCA is treatment with hydroxyurea. Currently, it is the only FDA-approved pharmacologic treatment for induction of HbF in adult patients with SCA, and is approved by the European Medicines Agency for both children and adults with SCA. Hydroxyurea significantly reduces pain and acute chest episodes, the need for blood transfusions and hospitalizations, and most importantly, reduces mortality [4–6]. While hydroxyurea has suspected disease modulating effects outside of HbF induction, the majority of its benefit is directly related to the amount of HbF produced in response to the drug [7,8]. There is an inverse relationship between levels of drug-induced HbF and number of pain episodes, hospitalizations, and overall mortality [9,10].

Several clinical studies have shown that individual hematological responses to hydroxyurea treatment are highly variable, with induced HbF levels ranging from 10% to greater than 30% HbF even for compliant patients on similar dosing regimens [11–14].

Previous efforts to identify predictors associated with final HbF produced in response to hydroxyurea have identified higher baseline HbF values, higher white blood cell count (WBC), and absolute reticulocyte count (ARC) as important factors [13,15,16]. However, none of these parameters can accurately predict the degree of HbF induction by hydroxyurea in an individual patient. From analysis of sibling pairs, it is known that the degree of HbF induction by hydroxyurea has a strong heritable component [17], indicating that genetic modifiers may have a large effect on drug response. Identification of specific genetic variants associated with HbF induction may elucidate reasons for this phenotypic variability and provide new insights into the drug's mechanisms of action related to HbF induction.

The aim of this study was to use a whole exome sequencing (WES) pharmacogenomics approach to identify genetic predictors of HbF response to hydroxyurea. Using two prospective pediatric cohorts with robust HbF phenotype data and standardized dose escalation regimen to MTD as a discovery cohort, we undertook a novel unbiased screen to test the entire exome for variants that are associated with hydroxyurea-induced HbF response levels (as measured by maximum %HbF at MTD [final HbF] or the change in %HbF from baseline to final [ΔHbF]). We focused on genetic variants with predicted functional effects on protein coding regions and identified several non-synonymous mutations that may influence the HbF response to hydroxyurea in children with SCA. We then validated a coding variant in *SALL2* in an unrelated, "real-world" cohort of children treated with hydroxyurea.

Results

Patient characteristics

Overall, both cohorts showed robust response to hydroxyurea with evidence of substantial individual variability in drug response (Table 1). All discovery cohort samples were genotyped for variants in *BCL11A* (rs1427407, rs4671393, rs11886868, rs7599488) and *HBSIL-MYB* (rs9399137, rs9402686); we found an association with baseline HbF for all *BCL11A* variants tested other than rs7599488. There was no significant association between the *BCL11A* variants tested and final HbF. No association with baseline, final or HbF was seen for either *HBSIL-MYB* variants tested. Linear association was performed with *BCL11A* variants as a covariate, without a significant change in associations.

At the time of hydroxyurea initiation, the average age of the 171 patients in the discovery cohort was 10.4±4.5 years of age. The average age of the 130 patients in the validation cohort was 8.1±4.0 years. All patients were treated under a similar dose escalation to MTD regimen according to protocol, or similar institutional guidelines 18, 19. After a minimum of 6 months on hydroxyurea therapy, all patients reached a stable MTD (average 25.1±4.5 mg/kg/day in the discovery cohort, 27.1±4.3 mg/kg/day in the validation cohort) with predictable laboratory benefits (Table 1). The mean increase in HbF was 19.5±6.6% in the discovery cohort and 13.9±7.0% in the validation cohort, reflecting slight differences between the two groups of patients. There was evidence of consistent myelosuppression across both cohorts, however. The baseline HbF, distribution of ΔHbF at MTD and final HbF at MTD were all similar to prior reports (Figure 1, A–C). [15,20].

Whole exome sequencing

All 171 samples in the discovery cohort passed stringent WES quality control parameters with an average of 92% of the targeted

Table 1. Comparison of discovery and validation cohorts.

	Discovery Cohort		Validation Cohort		Discovery Cohort		Validation Cohort	
Age (years)	10.4	±4.5	8.1	±4.0	-		-	
WBC (x10^9/L)	13.5	±4.2	13.1	±5.7	6.5	±2.0	6.9	±2.0
ANC (x10^9/L)	7.2	±3.2	6.2	±4.3	3.0	±1.2	2.7	±0.9
Hb (g/dL)	9.1	±0.9	8.0	±1.7	9.4	±1.0	9.5	±1.3
ARC (x10^9/L)	0.28	±0.13	0.29	±0.12	0.17	±0.09	0.12	±0.05
MCV (fL)	86.1	±4.8	82.1	±8.3	116.4	±13.0	97.7	±11.1
HbF (%)	8.0	±4.9	11.9	±5.9	27.6	±7.3	25.8	±8.2
ΔHbF (%)		-		-	19.5	±6.6	13.9	±7.0
HU dose (mg/kg/day)		-		-	25.1	±4.5	27.1	±4.3

WBC: white blood cell count; ANC: absolute neutrophil count; ARC: absolute reticulocyte count; MCV: mean corpuscular volume; HU: hydroxyurea.
The discovery cohort was composed of 120 patients from HUSTLE and 51 from SWiTCH. The validation cohort was collected from patients treated at TCCH.

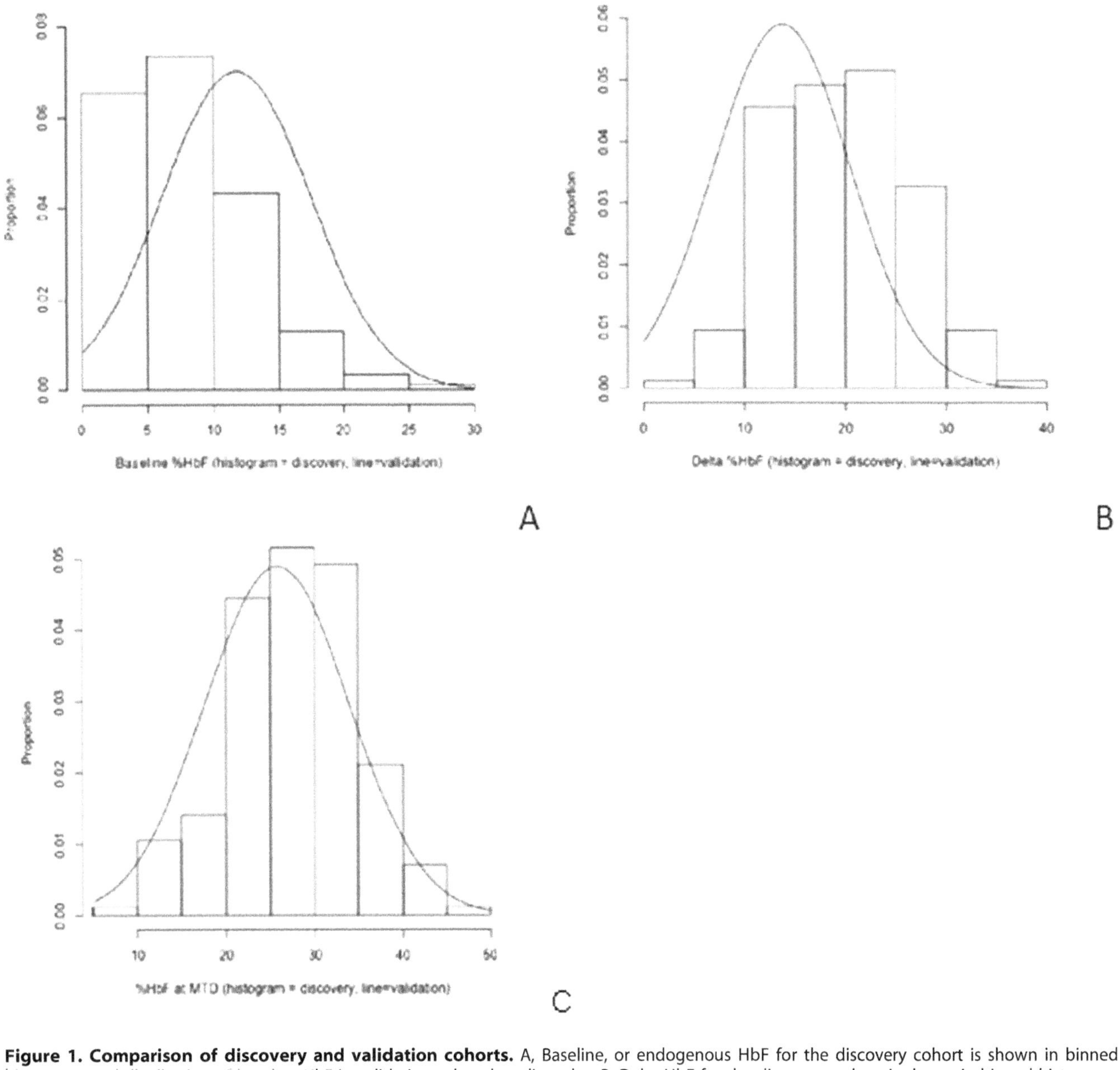

Figure 1. Comparison of discovery and validation cohorts. A, Baseline, or endogenous HbF for the discovery cohort is shown in binned histogram, and distribution of baseline HbF in validation cohort by a line plot. B, Delta HbF for the discovery cohort is shown in binned histogram, and distribution of delta HbF in validation cohort by a line plot. C, Final, or MID HbF for the discovery cohort is shown in binned histogram, and distribution of final, or MID in validation cohort by a line plot.

exonic regions sequenced at greater than 20× coverage per individual. We identified a total of 278,639 autosomal variants, and 127,238 of these variants were non-synonymous or splice site variants expected to introduce an amino acid change in their encoded proteins (Table S1). For single variant association testing, we further filtered the non-synonymous variants (n = 127,238) for those with a minor allele frequency (MAF) greater than or equal to 2% (n = 38,012). We corrected for any population stratification using principal component analysis (PCA) performed by the EIGENSTRAT method.

As our phenotypes of interest are continuous variables, we used linear regression analysis to test the association of the 38,012 common (MAF≥2%) non-synonymous variants using final HbF, and ΔHbF as independent, continuous variables. In addition, we attempted to find rare variants with MAF<2% associated with drug response by performing burden analysis with SKAT and T2 tests using the ΔHbF and final HbF phenotypes, but none of the gene level p-values were significant.

We identified 12 variants associated with ΔHbF with a p-value less than 5×10^{-4} (Table 2). In addition, we identified 13 variants associated with final HbF, also with a p-value less than 5×10^{-4} (Table 3). Although none of the p-values achieved genome wide significance level ($p<1.3X10^{-6}$), these results offered suggestive signals of potential associations. We used the existing methods of SIFT and PolyPhen2 [21] for predicting the functional impact of each non-synonymous variant to estimate which of the 25 variants had a predicted damaging or benign effect on encoded protein function (Tables 2 and 3).

From these 25 variants, we identified 13 variants with strongest association with response to hydroxyurea and predicted to

Table 2. Variants associated with ΔHbF on hydroxyurea.

Gene	SNP ID	Amino Acid Change	Protein Function Prediction	MAF (%)	Function	Beta Value	SE	P-value
EML1	rs141631682	Gly109Asp	Damaging	2	Microtubule assembly	10.9	2.7	7.41×10^{-5}
SESN1	rs2273668	Leu103Ile	Damaging	2	Peroxiredoxin reduction	9.3	2.3	8.88×10^{-5}
PAPLN	rs17126352	Val416Ile	Benign	3	Metalloprotease	7.1	1.8	1.35×10^{-4}
DCHS2	rs61746132	Pro1676Lys	Damaging	12	Calcium dependent cell adhesion	3.9	1.0	1.73×10^{-4}
KRT80	rs61749462	Arg364Ser	Damaging	3	Keratin 80	8.0	2.1	1.80×10^{-4}
SALL2	rs61743453	Pro840Arg	Damaging	4	Transcription factor	6.7	1.8	2.37×10^{-4}
NOM1	rs61742645	Arg779Cys	Benign	2	PP1 interacting protein	8.7	2.3	2.43×10^{-4}
N4BP2L2	rs35108810	Asp246Val	Damaging	15	*ELA2* transcription inhibitor	−3.3	0.9	3.47×10^{-4}
RNF113B	rs16955011	Val92Met	Damaging	18	Ring finger protein	3.1	0.8	3.76×10^{-4}
FTSJ2	rs55904231	Ser11Phe	Benign	7	RNA methyltransferase	5.2	1.4	3.76×10^{-4}
RHPN2	rs28626308	Arg70Gln	Damaging	7	Rho GTPase binding protein	5.2	1.4	3.91×10^{-4}
ADAR	rs17843865	Tyr587Cys	Benign	4	Adenosine deaminase	−6.4	1.8	4.65×10^{-4}

Variants selected were predicted damaging, with a p-value <0.001 in the discovery cohort, n = 171, composed of patients from HUSTLE and SWiTCH trials.

introduce an amino acid change that has a damaging effect on protein structure or function. We genotyped these 13 variants by TaqMan PCR in our independent validation cohort of 130 patients with SCA. We found that one of the 13 variants, located in the *SALL2* gene, maintained association with hydroxyurea response. In the discovery cohort, the P840R variant in the *SALL2* gene (rs61743453) was associated with a higher change in HbF in response to hydroxyurea ($p = 2.37\times10^{-4}$, beta value 6.7). In the validation cohort, this same P840R variant was associated with a higher final HbF, with a p-value of 0.05, and a beta value of 4.2. Using Fisher's combined probability test method, a meta analysis of the association of the *SALL2* variant with ΔHbF in the discovery and validation sample groups (n = 301) leads to a combined p-value of 8.30×10^{-4}. The meta analysis of the association of *SALL2* with final HbF in the discovery and validation sample groups resulted in a combined p-value of 1.48×10^{-4}.

Discussion

Many individuals with SCA are prescribed hydroxyurea, and there is evidence that genetic modifiers affect individual response [17,22]. In order to identify novel candidate genes and variants associated with hydroxyurea response, we sequenced the exomes of 171 individuals enrolled in two prospective clinical trials and related their sequence variant data to HbF response. This discovery cohort was obtained from patients treated on protocol, with the highest level of drug compliance supervision, including monthly pill counts. Our validation cohort (n = 130) was treated under guidelines similar to that of the discovery cohort. As expected, individual MTD was achieved at different hydroxyurea doses, within a range of 10–35 mg/kg/d, reflecting the typical range in bioavailability among patients. There was no correlation between hydroxyurea dose and HbF response ($p = 0.56$), supporting the conclusion that differences in pharmacokinetics and pharmacodynamics affect HbF levels achieved on hydroxyurea [22].

Whole exome sequencing permitted analysis of genes beyond a usual set of *a priori* biologic candidate genes for this phenotype and variants across a broad allele frequency spectrum. We identified multiple non-synonymous variants associated with ΔHbF or final HbF (Tables 2 and 3) in the discovery cohort. We then performed genotyping on a validation cohort for 13 candidate variants with the lowest p-values and were also predicted to be damaging. Of the 13 variants genotyped, the variant in SALL2 was associated with a higher HbF in the discovery cohort, and a higher final HbF at MTD in the discovery cohort. The validated variant in *SALL2* represents a novel variant not previously implicated in -globin expression or HbF response to hydroxyurea. Further studies of other sickle cell cohorts treated with hydroxyurea are needed to confirm this promising association.

SALL2 is a multi-zinc finger transcription factor implicated in hematopoietic cell maturation and cell cycle arrest [23]. It contains the same conserved 12 amino acid N-terminal motif as BCL11A [24,25]. This motif has been shown to be essential for binding of the nucleosome remodeling and deacetylase co-repressor complex, or NuRD, which includes the histone deacelylases HDAC1 and HDAC2. Both HDAC1 and HDAC2 have been shown to act as co-repressors of gamma globin [26]. The variant identified here (rs61743453), causes a proline to arginine change at residue 840 and is predicted to bedamaging to protein function. This P840R SALL2 variant was associated with a higher HbF response to hydroxyurea (Figure 2). Further function-

Table 3. Variants associated with final HbF on hydroxyurea.

Gene	SNP ID	Amino Acid Change	Protein Function Prediction	MAF (%)	Function	Beta Value	SE	P-value
RSPH3	rs61750777	Ala154Val	Damaging	6	Radial spoke protein	−6.5	1.6	6.55×10^{-5}
OLR1	rs11053646	Lys167Asn	Benign	2	Opioid receptor	3.4	0.9	1.22×10^{-4}
SEC31B	rs11819496	Arg478Thr	Damaging	2	ER transport	−12.0	3.1	1.55×10^{-4}
COPE	rs34510432	Arg85 His	Damaging	2	ER transport	9.9	2.6	1.88×10^{-4}
RNF113B	rs16955011	Val92Met	Damaging	18	Ring finger protein	3.4	0.9	1.93×10^{-4}
CDHR3	rs6967330	Cys529Tyr	Benign	29	Calcium dependent cell adhesion	3.1	0.8	2.58×10^{-4}
ETAA1	rs3770655	Pro771Ser	Benign	89	Ewing's tumor associated antigen	4.3	1.2	2.84×10^{-4}
TTLL10	rs113596156	Arg35Gln	Benign	2	Polyglycylase	9.8	2.7	2.91×10^{-4}
DOCK1	rs869801	Ala1793Thr	Benign	21	Cytokinesis	−3.5	1.0	3.60×10^{-4}
MYBBP1A	rs899441	Lys637Glu	Benign	6	MYB associated	−5.4	1.5	4.26×10^{-4}
MARCH10	rs116835087	Gly587Ser	Damaging	6	Membrane-associated ring finger	−6.0	1.7	4.33×10^{-4}
PKD1L1	rs11972142	Thr879Ala	Benign	15	Polycystic kidney disease like	3.6	1.0	4.78×10^{-4}
ADCY10	rs16859886	Thr234Met	Benign	12	Adenyl cyclase	3.9	1.1	4.96×10^{-4}

Variants selected were predicted damaging, with a p-value <0.001 in the discovery cohort, $n=171$, composed of patients from HUSTLE and SWiTCH trials.

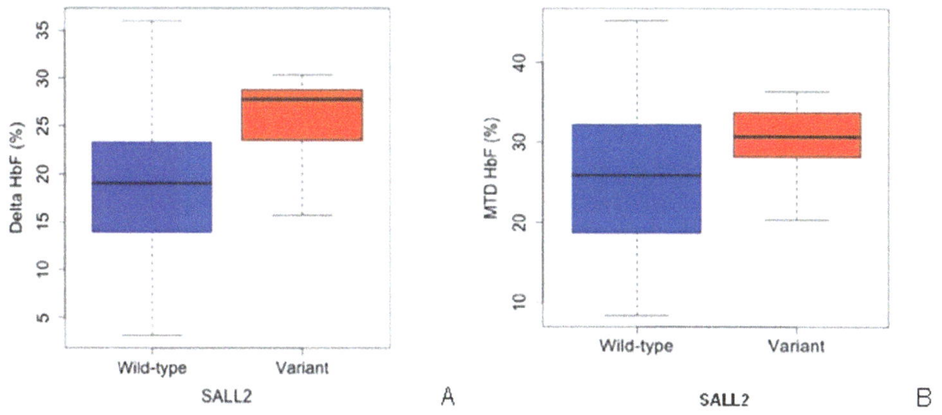

Figure 2. Effect of *SALL2* variant rs61743453 on HbF response to hydroxyurea. A, Effect of rs61743453 on delta HbF in discovery cohort. B, Effect of rs61743453 on MTD HbF in validation cohort. Variant refers to the Pro840Arg variant; no individuals were homozygous for this change.

al studies will help establish the role of SALL2 in HbF induction in the context of hydroxyurea.

Despite the relatively small sample size, we used the best genotype-phenotype pairs available from prospectively treated pediatric patients from two clinical trials for the discovery cohort. We assembled a validation cohort from patients treated with hydroxyurea according to standard of care and expert guidelines in a pediatric hematology center with an established sickle cell program.

This study may have failed to detect loci with modest effects because of low statistical power and some associations identified in the discovery cohort may have failed validation given the small size of the validation cohort. Accordingly, all of the mutations identified in the discovery cohort may represent coding variants worth pursuing in future studies. The data presented here bodes well for the success of larger collaborative efforts aimed at identifying genetic modifiers of hydroxyurea response, and serves as a call for coordinated collaboration among pediatric sickle cell centers to increase sample size and increase the odds for novel discovery and translational potential.

Methods

Subjects

The discovery cohort was composed of 171 unrelated children with SCA; 120 were enrolled in the Hydroxyurea Study of Long-Term Effects (HUSTLE, NCT00305175); and 51 were enrolled in the NHLBI-sponsored Stroke with Transfusions Changing to Hydroxyurea (SWiTCH, NCT00122980). HUSTLE was a single center trial investigating long term effects of hydroxyurea in SCA, while SWiTCH was a multi-center trial investigating the use of hydroxyurea on stroke prevention. HUSTLE and SWiTCH study patient samples were used with approval from the Baylor College of Medicine Internal Review Board, protocol H-29047. Patients and their families in both clinical trials provided written consent for DNA sample collection, storage and sequencing. Texas Children's Hospital Hematology Center patients and their families provided written consent to whole exome sequencing, posting of sequences to dbGAP, and data collection under BCM Internal Review Board protocol H31356. All DNA samples and data in this study were denominalized for analysis. All 171 individuals had a known baseline HbF level measured at greater than 3 years of age, were initially treated with hydroxyurea at 20 mg/kg, and then dose-escalated to mild myelosuppression using a standardized regimen [18,19].

The validation cohort contained 130 unrelated children with SCA followed at the Texas Children's Hospital Hematology Center (TCHHC). All patients receiving hydroxyurea at TCHHC were approached for enrollment in an Internal Review Board-approved protocol for genetic analysis. They were treated with hydroxyurea using institutional guidelines rather than a specific protocol, but all were escalated to MTD following a standardized regimen as previously described [19]. All patients were treated with hydroxyurea for at least 6 months prior to the designated MTD timepoint. Total HbF levels for both discovery and validation cohorts were measured by HPLC.

Ethics Statement

All patients and their families gave informed consent for genomic DNA sample collection, storage, and sequencing. The WES genomic analyses were approved by the Baylor College of Medicine Institutional Review Board. All DNA samples and data in this study were denominalized for analysis.

Whole exome sequencing

DNA concentrations were quantified using picogreen fluorescent detection method (Quant-iT, Invitrogen). For each DNA sample, the entire exome was captured using the NimbleGen VCRome 2.1 capture reagent followed by sequencing on an Illumina platform using standard chemistries. The sequencing reads were mapped to Hg19 reference genome using the BWA [27]. Sample level genome variants were identified and annotated using the Human Genome Sequencing Center's integrated Mercury pipeline which includes quality score recalibration and insertion/deletion (Indel) realignment, genome variant identification by AtlasSNP [28], and annotation using Cassandra software. A project level variant call format (VCF) was generated for all the samples, and included variants that were present in at least one sample. Variants with more than 5% missed genotyping calls were excluded from analysis. Error threshold for alignment was two base errors per read with penalties for indels (maximum of 1) are much more costly than the penalties for SNVs (maximum of 2). We allowed for read-trimming to 35 bp.

WES genotyping of variants of interest with heterozygosity scores less than 0.45 were verified by TaqMan genotyping. TaqMan genotyping assays were performed on an Applied Biosystem's StepOne instrument (AB, Foster City, CA). After 40 amplification cycles, threshold cycle values were automatically calculated, and the individual SNP genotypes were called by the StepOne v2.0 software (AB, Foster City, CA).

Statistical Analysis

Linear regression analysis was used to test the association of the filtered variants using final HbF and ΔHbF as independent, continuous variables. The ΔHbF and final HbF phenotypes both had normal distributions, indicating they were suitable for linear regression analysis (Figure 1); values were adjusted for age and gender. Principal component analysis (PCA) was performed using the EIGENSTRAT method, and applied to all models. Quality control filtering steps, including SNP missingness check, removal of sex chromosomes, monomorphic site, synonymous and intronic variant removal, excess heterozygosity filter and minor allele frequency (MAF) cut-off of 2% and the impact of these filtering steps on the total number of SNPs, are described in Table S1.

To analyze the effect of rare variants (MAF<2%) on the phenotypes ΔHbF and final HbF, we used two gene based tests, a simple burden test (T2) and SKAT [29,30]. In SKAT and T2 testing, a collection of rare variants within a single gene are tested for association with the phenotype. The T2 considers those rare variants with MAF less than 2% and assumes that the effects of all variants are in the same direction. SKAT is a kernel-based test that considers rare variants having effects in either direction [29,31]. Both tests considered only non-synonymous variants.

Validation

Genomic DNA from 130 patients from TCHHC collected as a validation cohort were genotyped by TaqMan or Sanger sequencing for 13 SNPs with the lowest p-values that were identified as associated with HbF response to hydroxyurea, non-synonymous, and damaging. The relationship between genotype and HbF response to hydroxyurea was analyzed with a one directional t-test.

Supporting Information

Table S1 Quality control filters used in WES analysis. Sex chromosomes were removed, as gender did not impact HbF response to hydroxyurea. Sites with heterzygousto homozygous ration>0.4 were removed.Variants with MAF<2% were analyzed by burden testing.

Acknowledgments

We thank all the patients and families, as well as the clinical investigators and research staff, for their participation in the SWiTCH and HUSTLE trials. We would like to thank the patients, their families, and the research staff at Texas Children's Hematology Center for their participation in FWES, which provided the validation cohort.

Author Contributions

Conceived and designed the experiments: VAS JMF EB RAG REW. Performed the experiments: TAH AS DMM SDP. Analyzed the data: JRC EB. Contributed reagents/materials/analysis tools: RAG EB. Wrote the paper: VAS JMF REW EB. Clinical trial data analysis and sample collection: BA KAN NAM REW.

References

1. Platt OS, Brambilla DJ, Rosse WF, Milner PF, Castro O, et al. (1994) Mortality in sickle cell disease. Life expectancy and risk factors for early death. N Engl J Med 330: 1639–1644.
2. Cheetham RC, Huehns ER, Rosemeyer MA (1979) Participation of haemoglobins A, F, A2 and C in polymerisation of haemoglobin S. J Mol Biol 129: 45–61.
3. Powars DR, Weiss JN, Chan LS, Schroeder WA (1984) Is there a threshold level of fetal hemoglobin that ameliorates morbidity in sickle cell anemia? Blood 63: 921–926.
4. Steinberg MH, McCarthy WF, Castro O, Ballas SK, Armstrong FD, et al. (2010) The risks and benefits of long-term use of hydroxyurea in sickle cell anemia: A 17.5 year follow-up. Am J Hematol 85: 403–408.
5. Voskaridou E, Christoulas D, Bilalis A, Plata E, Varvagiannis K, et al. (2010) The effect of prolonged administration of hydroxyurea on morbidity and mortality in adult patients with sickle cell syndromes: results of a 17-year, single-center trial (LaSHS). Blood 115: 2354–2363.
6. Lobo CL, Pinto JF, Nascimento EM, Moura PG, Cardoso GP, et al. (2013) The effect of hydroxcarbamide therapy on survival of children with sickle cell disease. Br J Haematol 161: 852–860.
7. Lebensburger J, Johnson SM, Askenazi DJ, Rozario NL, Howard TH, et al. (2011) Protective role of hemoglobin and fetal hemoglobin in early kidney disease for children with sickle cell anemia. Am J Hematol 86: 430–432.
8. Lebensburger JD, Pestina TI, Ware RE, Boyd KL, Persons DA (2010) Hydroxyurea therapy requires HbF induction for clinical benefit in a sickle cell mouse model. Haematologica 95: 1599–1603.
9. Steinberg MH, Barton F, Castro O, Pegelow CH, Ballas SK, et al. (2003) Effect of hydroxyurea on mortality and morbidity in adult sickle cell anemia: risks and benefits up to 9 years of treatment. JAMA 289: 1645–1651.
10. Smith WR, Ballas SK, McCarthy WF, Bauserman RL, Swerdlow PS, et al. (2011) The association between hydroxyurea treatment and pain intensity, analgesic use, and utilization in ambulatory sickle cell anemia patients. Pain Med 12: 697–705.
11. Maier-Redelsperger M, de Montalembert M, Flahault A, Neonato MG, Ducrocq R, et al. (1998) Fetal hemoglobin and F-cell responses to long-term hydroxyurea treatment in young sickle cell patients. The French Study Group on Sickle Cell Disease. Blood 91: 4472–4479.
12. Kinney TR, Helms RW, O'Branski EE, Ohene-Frempong K, Wang W, et al. (1999) Safety of hydroxyurea in children with sickle cell anemia: results of the HUG-KIDS study, a phase I/II trial. Pediatric Hydroxyurea Group. Blood 94: 1550–1554.
13. Zimmerman SA, Schultz WH, Davis JS, Pickens CV, Mortier NA, et al. (2004) Sustained long-term hematologic efficacy of hydroxyurea at maximum tolerated dose in children with sickle cell disease. Blood 103: 2039–2045.
14. Ware RE, Aygun B (2009) Advances in the use of hydroxyurea. Hematology Am Soc Hematol Educ Program: 62–69.
15. Ware RE, Eggleston B, Redding-Lallinger R, Wang WC, Smith-Whitley K, et al. (2002) Predictors of fetal hemoglobin response in children with sickle cell anemia receiving hydroxyurea therapy. Blood 99: 10–14.
16. Green NS, Ender KL, Pashankar F, Driscoll C, Giardina PJ, et al. (2013) Candidate sequence variants and fetal hemoglobin in children with sickle cell disease treated with hydroxyurea. PLoS One 8: e55709.
17. Steinberg MH, Voskaridou E, Kutlar A, Loukopoulos D, Koshy M, et al. (2003) Concordant fetal hemoglobin response to hydroxyurea in siblings with sickle cell disease. Am J Hematol 72: 121–126.
18. Ware RE, Helms RW (2011) Stroke With Transfusions Changing to Hydroxyurea (SWiTCH). Blood 119: 3925–3932.
19. Ware RE (2009) How I use hydroxyurea to treat young patients with sickle cell anemia. Blood 115: 5300–5311.
20. Steinberg MH (2001) Modulation of fetal hemoglobin in sickle cell anemia. Hemoglobin 25: 195–211.
21. Flanagan SE, Patch AM, Ellard S (2010) Using SIFT and PolyPhen to predict loss-of-function and gain-of-function mutations. Genet Test Mol Biomarkers 14: 533–537.
22. Ware RE, Despotovic JM, Mortier NA, Flanagan JM, He J, et al. (2011) Pharmacokinetics, pharmacodynamics, and pharmacogenetics of hydroxyurea treatment for children with sickle cell anemia. Blood 118: 4985–4991.
23. Chai L (2011) The role of HSAL (SALL) genes in proliferation and differentiation in normal hematopoiesis and leukemogenesis. Transfusion 51 Suppl 4: 87S–93S.
24. Sankaran VG, Menne TF, Xu J, Akie TE, Lettre G, et al. (2008) Human fetal hemoglobin expression is regulated by the developmental stage-specific repressor BCL11A. Science 322: 1839–1842.
25. Lauberth SM, Rauchman M (2006) A conserved 12-amino acid motif in Sall1 recruits the nucleosome remodeling and deacetylase corepressor complex. J Biol Chem 281: 23922–23931.
26. Bradner JE, Mak R, Tanguturi SK, Mazitschek R, Haggarty SJ, et al. (2010) Chemical genetic strategy identifies histone deacetylase 1 (HDAC1) and HDAC2 as therapeutic targets in sickle cell disease. Proc Natl Acad Sci U S A 107: 12617–12622.
27. Li H, Durbin R (2009) Fast and accurate short read alignment with Burrows-Wheeler transform. Bioinformatics 25: 1754–1760.

28. Challis D, Yu J, Evani US, Jackson AR, Paithankar S, et al. (2012) An integrative variant analysis suite for whole exome next-generation sequencing data. BMC Bioinformatics 13: 8.
29. Lee S, Wu MC, Lin X (2012) Optimal tests for rare variant effects in sequencing association studies. Biostatistics 13: 762–775.
30. Li B, Leal SM (2008) Methods for detecting associations with rare variants for common diseases: application to analysis of sequence data. Am J Hum Genet 83: 311–321.
31. Morgenthaler S, Thilly WG (2007) A strategy to discover genes that carry multi-allelic or mono-allelic risk for common diseases: a cohort allelic sums test (CAST). Mutat Res 615: 28–56.

14

Impact of Early Reoperation following Living-Donor Liver Transplantation on Graft Survival

Yoshikuni Kawaguchi[1], Yasuhiko Sugawara[1]*, Nobuhisa Akamatsu[1], Junichi Kaneko[1], Tsuyoshi Hamada[3], Tomohiro Tanaka[2], Takeaki Ishizawa[1], Sumihito Tamura[1], Taku Aoki[1], Yoshihiro Sakamoto[1], Kiyoshi Hasegawa[1], Norihiro Kokudo[1]

1 Artificial Organ and Transplantation Surgery Division, Department of Surgery, Graduate School of Medicine, University of Tokyo, Tokyo, Japan, **2** Organ Transplantation Service, University of Tokyo, Tokyo, Japan, **3** Department of Gastroenterology, Graduate School of Medicine, University of Tokyo, Tokyo, Japan

Abstract

Background: The reoperation rate remains high after liver transplantation and the impact of reoperation on graft and recipient outcome is unclear. The aim of our study is to *evaluate the impact of early reoperation following living-donor liver transplantation* (LDLT) on graft and recipient survival.

Methods: Recipients that underwent LDLT (n = 111) at the University of Tokyo Hospital between January 2007 and December 2012 were divided into two groups, a reoperation group (n = 27) and a non-reoperation group (n = 84), and case-control study was conducted.

Results: Early reoperation was performed in 27 recipients (24.3%). Mean time [standard deviation] from LDLT to reoperation was 10 [9.4] days. Female sex, Child-Pugh class C, Non-HCV etiology, fulminant hepatitis, and the amount of intraoperative fresh frozen plasma administered were identified as possibly predictive variables, among which females and the amount of FFP were identified as independent risk factors for early reoperation by multivariable analysis. The 3-, and 6- month graft survival rates were 88.9% (95%confidential intervals [CI], 70.7–96.4), and 85.2% (95%CI, 66.5–94.3), respectively, in the reoperation group (n = 27), and 95.2% (95%CI, 88.0–98.2), and 92.9% (95%CI, 85.0–96.8), respectively, in the non-reoperation group (n = 84) (the log-rank test, p = 0.31). The 12- and 36- month overall survival rates were 96.3% (95%CI, 77.9–99.5), and 88.3% (95%CI, 69.3–96.2), respectively, in the reoperation group, and 89.3% (95%CI, 80.7–94.3) and 88.0% (95%CI, 79.2–93.4), respectively, in the non-reoperation group (the log-rank test, p = 0.59).

Conclusions: Observed graft survival for the recipients who underwent reoperation was lower compared to those who did not undergo reoperation, though the result was not significantly different. Recipient overall survival with reoperation was comparable to that without reoperation. The present findings enhance the importance of vigilant surveillance for postoperative complication and surgical rescue at an early postoperative stage in the LDLT setting.

Editor: Guy Brock, University of Louisville, United States of America

Funding: This work was supported by a Grant-in-aid for Scientific Research from the Ministry of Education, Culture, Sports, Science and Technology of Japan and from the Ministry of Health, Labor and Welfare of Japan (AIDS Research). The funders had no role in study design, data collection and analysis, decision to publish, or preparation of the manuscript.

Competing Interests: The authors have declared that no competing interests exist.

* Email: yasusugatky@yahoo.co.jp

Introduction

Continuous advances in surgical techniques, postoperative management, and immunosuppression have improved the safety of liver transplantation (LT) and patient survival [1–5]. In fact, overall survival rates in the later period of experience are reportedly better than those in the earlier period [6]. The Japanese Liver Transplantation Society reported overall survival rates for deceased-donor LT (DDLT) (n = 98) of 80.5% at 1 year, 77.8% at 3 years, and 76.0% at 5 years, and overall survival rates for living-donor LT (LDLT) (n = 6097) of 83.4% at 1 year, 79.3% at 3 years, and 76.9% at 5 years based on the data from 1998 to 2010 [7]. Similar survival rates are reported in Europe (83% at 1 year, and 71% at 5 years [1995–2000]) [8] and the United States (83.3% at 1 year [2002–2004], and 67.4% at 5 years [1997–2000]) [9].

Despite improved graft and recipient survival, the reoperation rate among LT recipients remains high, ranging from 9.2% to 34% [10–13], compared to that for liver resection, which ranges from 2.5% to 10.9% [14–16]. While several studies about the post-LT complication rates, including early reoperation, have been reported, there are few reports of the factors associated with early reoperation and the influence of early reoperation on LT recipient outcome. Recent reports indicate that early reoperation is a risk factor for impaired recipient outcome in both LDLT [12] and DDLT [10] recipients.

In the present study, we conducted a retrospective analysis investigating the incidence and cause of early reoperation, the factors associated with early reoperation, and the impact of early reoperation on graft and recipient survival among 111 consecutive adult LDLT recipients.

Patients and Methods

Patients

Between January 1996 and December 2012, 500 patients, including 77 pediatric patients, underwent LDLT at the University of Tokyo Hospital. Considering the technical standardization and establishment of criteria for reoperation, 111 consecutive adult LDLT cases between January 2007 and December 2012 were the subjects of the present study. The clinical records of these patients were retrospectively reviewed. The data of blood tests were based on the results in recipients' admission for the transplantation. All operations and reoperations were performed after obtaining informed consent from the patients and approval by the local ethics committee of the University of Tokyo.

Graft selection criteria and surgical treatment

The indication for LDLT and the type of liver graft were determined according to the ratio of the remnant liver volume to the total liver volume in living donors, and that of the graft volume to the standard liver volume (SLV) [17] in recipients [4]. Briefly, 40% of the recipient SLV was the minimum requirement for the graft and the donor remnant liver volume needed to be over 30% of total liver volume of the donor. Our detailed donor selection criteria and surgical procedures for both the donor and recipient are described elsewhere [18].

Postoperative management

All recipients were transferred to the intensive care unit with respirator support after the initial LDLT procedure. Recipients with an uneventful course were transferred to the surgical ward around postoperative day (POD) 5.

Routine postoperative investigations were as follows; blood tests (complete blood count, biochemical measurements, and coagulation profiles) were performed three or four times daily until POD 3, and twice daily between POD 4 and POD 14, chest and abdominal radiographs were examined twice daily until POD 3 and once daily between POD 4 and POD 14, Doppler ultrasonography to examine flow in the graft vessels was performed at least twice daily until POD 14 to detect abnormal flow in the hepatic artery/portal vein/hepatic vein, thrombi in the graft vessels, and intraabdominal fluid collection.

Indications for blood transfusions were as follows: red blood cell concentrate if the hemoglobin level or hematocrit was less than 6 g/dL and 15%, respectively, FFP if the prothrombin time-international normalized ratio (PT-INR) was greater than 2.00, and platelet concentrate if the platelet count was less than $3.0\times10^4/\mu L$.

The basic immunosuppression regimen consisted of tacrolimus and steroids for all recipients, and the doses of each drug were gradually tapered for 6 months after LDLT. Our detailed protocol of immunosuppression is described elsewhere [2].

Anticoagulation regimen after LDLT

To prevent early vascular thrombosis, anticoagulation therapy was started just after transplantation and continued until POD 14 in all recipients. The regimen was started with dalteparin (25 IU/kg/d), which was administered until POD 2. On POD 3, the anticoagulant drug was changed to heparin (unfractionated heparin sodium, 5000 U/d), the dose of which was adjusted to achieve a targeted activated clotting time of between 130 and 160 seconds.

Definitions for early reoperation and early graft loss

Early reoperation in our study was defined as surgical intervention after LDLT between just after transplant and the day of initial discharge. Early graft loss was defined as graft loss occurring within 6 months after LDLT.

Indications for early reoperation after LDLT

Indications for early reoperation were generally divided into three categories, postoperative bleeding, vessel flow problems, and biliary complications. Reoperation for postoperative bleeding was indicated for recipients with postoperative bleeding with hemodynamic instability, hemorrhage above Grade B defined by International Study Group of Liver Surgery [19], or suspected intraabdominal hematoma infection. Vessel flow problems included hepatic arterial thrombosis, portal venous thrombosis, and decreased or hepatofugal portal flow developing during the early postoperative period, all which were detected by Doppler US. Biliary complications, which we initially attempted to treat with interventional strategies, were indicated for early reoperation in cases with massive biliary leakage resulting in biliary peritonitis or biliary obstruction with intrahepatic biliary dilatation just after LDLT.

Ethics Statement

All LDLTs were performed after individually obtaining informed consent from recipients and donors. LDLT program at the University of Tokyo Hospital has been approved by its Institutional Review Board, and all aspects of the procedures have been conducted according to the principles expressed in the Declaration of Helsinki. The current human subject research was approved as project number G3515 by Graduate School of Medicine and Faculty of Medicine, the University of Tokyo Research Ethics Committee and Human Genome, Gene Analysis Research Ethics Committee. All subjects have been properly instructed and participated by signing the appropriate informed consent paperwork. In the preparation of this manuscript, all efforts have been made to protect patient privacy and anonymity.

Statistical analysis

Continuous variables are expressed as mean values (with standard deviations). Categorical variables are expressed as number (%), and were compared between groups using Fisher's exact test or the chi-square test, as appropriate. Graft and overall survival were measured from the time of LT. Survival curves were constructed using the Kaplan-Meier method, and compared using the log-rank test. Factors with $p<0.10$ in a Cox proportional hazard model as a univariable analysis were considered potential risk factors and were further analyzed in a multivariable Cox model. Hazard ratios (HR) and 95% confidential intervals (CI) were calculated for each factor. A p value of less than 0.05 was considered to indicate statistical significance. Statistical analysis was performed with JMP software (version 9.0.2; SAS Institute Inc., Cary, NC).

Results

Patient characteristics

The characteristics of the 111 consecutive patients are summarized in Table 1. The cohort included 50 males and 61 females (male:female, reoperation group; 7: 20, non-reoperation group; 43: 41). Mean [standard deviation (SD)] age was 51 [12] years (reoperation group; 49.9 [13.2] years, non-reoperation group; 50.7 [11.6] years). Mean [SD] Child-Pugh score was 9.3 [1.9] (reoperation group; 9.6 [1.9], non-reoperation group 9.1 [1.9]) and the mean [SD] model for end-stage liver disease score was 16.8 [7.3] (reoperation group; 17.6 [7.0], non-reoperation group; 16.6 [7.4]). There was no significant difference in the indications between the reoperation group and the non-reoperation group (Table 2). The indications for LT were liver cirrhosis caused by hepatitis C virus infection (reoperation group vs. non-reoperation group, 5 [18.5%] vs. 32 [38.1%], p = 0.052), liver cirrhosis caused by hepatitis B virus infection (2 [7.4%] vs. 13 [15.5%], p = 0.35), primary biliary cirrhosis (5 [18.5%] vs. 15 [17.8%], p>0.99), primary sclerosing cholangitis (5 [18.5%] vs. 15 [17.8%], p>0.99), alcoholic cirrhosis (2 [7.4%] vs. 5 [6.0%], p = 0.68), biliary atresia (1 [3.7%] vs. 2 [2.4%], p = 0.57), autoimmune hepatitis (1 [3.7%] vs. 2 [2.4%], p = 0.57), fulminant hepatitis (6 [22.3%] vs. 7 [8.3%], p = 0.07), and others (5 [18.5%] vs. 2 [2.4%]).

Profiles of early reoperation

Early reoperations after LDLT (reoperation group) were performed in 27 recipients (24.3%) on POD 10 [9.4]. Among them, 19 cases (70.4%) were performed within 10 days after LDLT and 5 cases (18.5%) required multiple reoperations. Table 3 lists the reasons for reoperation, which comprised mainly postoperative bleeding (n = 13, 48%), vessel problems (n = 8, 30%), and biliary complications (n = 5, 19%). One recipient underwent reoperation for strangulated bowel obstruction. Early graft loss subsequent to early reoperation occurred in 4 cases. Two recipients had graft loss subsequent to reoperation for portal venous thrombosis and simultaneous hepatic artery and portal venous thrombosis, and both underwent successful retransplantation. The remaining two recipients underwent reoperation for biliary problems, one for severe biliary leakage and the other for biliary stricture with severe cholangitis, both of which finally resulted in graft loss; only one recipient was saved by retransplantation.

Table 1. Characteristics of reoperation and non-reoperation cases after LDLT.

Variables			Total (n = 111)	Reoperation Group (n = 27, 24.3%)	Non-reoperation Group (n = 84, 75.7%)
Recipient factors					
	Age, y*		50.5 [12.0]	49.9 [13.2]	50.7 [11.6]
	Sex (female), n (%)		61 (55.0)	20 (74.1)	41 (48.8)
	Child-Pugh score, pts*		9.3 [1.9]	9.6 [1.9]	9.1 [1.9]
	MELD score, pts*		16.8 [7.3]	17.6 [7.0]	16.6 [7.4]
	Preoperative status (hospitalized), n (%)		5 (4.5)	1 (3.7)	4 (4.8)
	Preoperative blood data*				
		Albumin level, g/dL	2.9 [0.4]	2.8 [0.3]	2.9 [0.5]
		Serum creatinine, mg/dL	0.8 [0.5]	0.8 [0.3]	0.8 [0.6]
		Total bilirubin, mg/dL	8.9 [9.1]	8.9 [8.5]	9.0 [9.4]
		PT-INR	1.51 [0.68]	1.60 [0.46]	1.49 [0.74]
		Platelet count, $\times 10^4/\mu L$	8.8 [6.5]	8.9 [7.3]	8.7 [6.2]
Donors factors					
	Age, years*		39.6 [12.7]	38.6 [13.5]	39.6 [12.5]
	Sex (female), n (%)		60 (54.1)	15 (55.6)	45 (53.6)
	Graft type (LL: RL:PS)		40: 67: 4	12: 14: 1	28: 53: 3
	GV/SLV, %		45.4 [9.7]	45.5 [11.1]	45.4 [9.3]
	GV, g		528 [126]	504 [129]	536 [125]
Operative factors*					
	Operative time, min		788 [132]	801 [206]	783[99]
	Operative blood loss, L		5.5 [7.9]	7.7 [15.2]	4.8 [2.7]
	Transfusion				
		Red blood cell concentrate, U	9.5 [12.3]	13.6 [22.2]	8.2 [6.2]
		Fresh frozen plasma, U	21.2 [19.2]	29.8 [33.8]	18.4 [9.8]
		Platelet concentrate, U	24.6 [19.7]	25.9 [24.5]	24.2 [18.1]
	Biliary reconstruction, duct-to-duct, n (%)		99 (89.2)	25 (92.6)	74 (88.1)

Abbreviations: LDLT, living-donor liver transplantation; LL, left lobe; MELD, model for end-stage liver disease; PT-INR, international normalized ratio of prothrombin time; PS, posterior sector; RL, right lobe; GV, graft volume; SLV, standard liver volume.* mean [standard deviation].

Table 2. Comparison of primary disease between reoperation and non-reoperation cases after LDLT.

Variables	Total (n = 111)	Reoperation Group (n = 27, 24.3%)	Non-reoperation Group (n = 84, 75.7%)	p value
Liver cirrhosis-HCV	37 (33.4)	5 (18.5)	32 (38.1)	0.052
Liver cirrhosis-HBV	15 (13.5)	2 (7.4)	13 (15.5)	0.35
PBC	20 (18.1)	5 (18.5)	15 (17.8)	>0.99
PSC	6 (5.4)	0 (0)	6 (7.1)	0.33
Alcoholic cirrhosis	7 (6.3)	2 (7.4)	5 (6.0)	0.68
Biliary atresia	3 (2.7)	1 (3.7)	2 (2.4)	0.57
Autoimmune hepatitis	3 (2.7)	1 (3.7)	2 (2.4)	0.57
Fulminant hepatitis	13 (11.6)	6 (22.3)	7 (8.3)	0.07
Others	7 (6.3)	5 (18.5)	2 (2.4)	N.A.

Abbreviations: HCV, hepatitis C virus; HBV, hepatitis B virus; PBC, primary biliary cirrhosis, PBC; PSC, Primary sclerosing cholangitis; LDLT, living-donor liver transplantation; N.A., not applicable. n (%).

Risk factors for early reoperation

The results of analyses to identify risk factors for early reoperation in a Cox proportional hazard model were shown in Table 4. Recipient female sex (hazards ratio [HR] 2.63, 95% confidential intervals [CI] 1.17–6.72, p = 0.02), Child-Pugh class C (HR 2.27, 95% CI 1.04–5.29, p = 0.04), Non-HCV etiology (HR 2.44, 95%CI 1.00–7.28, p = 0.05), fulminant hepatitis (HR 2.78, 95%CI 1.02–6.49, p = 0.05), and the amount of fresh frozen plasma (FFP) administered (HR 1.01, 95% CI 1.00–1.02, p = 0.04) were demonstrated to be potential risk factors for early reoperation with p<0.10 in the univariable Cox model. Subsequent multivariable Cox model revealed that female sex (HR 2.90, 95% CI 1.18–8.27, p = 0.02) and the amount of FFP (HR 1.02, 95%CI 1.00–1.03, p = 0.03) were independent risk factors for early reoperation.

Graft and recipient survival in each group

Among the present cohort, early graft loss occurred in 10 cases, 4 in the reoperation group and 6 in the non-reoperation group. Mean follow-up time was 48.2 [25.9] months in the reoperation group and 50.6 [24.1] months in the non-reoperation group (p = 0.679). The3-, 6-, 12-, and 36- month graft survival rates were 88.9% (95%CI, 70.7–96.4), 85.2%, (95%CI, 66.5–94.3), 85.2% (95%CI, 66.5–94.3), and 77.1% (95%CI, 57.4–89.4), respectively, in the reoperation group (n = 27), and 95.2% (95%CI, 88.0–98.2), 92.9% (95%CI, 85.0–96.8), 89.3% (95%CI, 80.7–94.3), and 88.1% (95%CI, 79.2–93.4), respectively, in the non-reoperation group (n = 84). The 1- and 3-year overall survival rates were 96.3% (95%CI, 77.9–99.5), and 88.3% (95%CI, 69.3–96.2), respectively, in the reoperation group, and 89.3% (95%CI,

Table 3. Reasons of reoperation after LDLT.

Variables		Number of cases (n = 27)	Early graft loss, n (%)
Postoperative bleeding		13	
	Graft surface	4	0
	Diaphragm	3	0
	Hepatic artery	3	0
	Hilar plate	1	0
	Drain insertion site	1	0
	Undetected	1	0
Vessels		8	
	HAT	2	0
	PVT	3	1(33)
	Simultaneous HAT and PVT	1	1(100)
	Regurgitant portal flow	1	0
	The portal steal phenomenon in APOLT	1	0
Biliary tract		5	
	Biliary peritonitis	4	1 (25)
	Biliary stenosis	1	1 (100)
Others		1	
	Incarcerated obstruction of the jejunum	1	0

Abbreviations: LDLT, living-donor liver transplantation; HAT, hepatic artery thrombosis; PVT, portal vein thrombosis; APOLT, auxiliary partial orthotopic liver transplantation.

Table 4. Univariable and multivariable Cox proportional hazards model analysis to identify risk factors for early reoperation.

Variables			Univariable analysis			Multivariable analysis		
			HR	95% CI	p value	HR	95% CI	p value
Recipient factors								
	Age, years		0.99	0.97–1.03	0.72			
	Sex, female		2.63	1.17–6.72	0.02	2.90	1.18–8.27	0.02
	Child-Pugh, C vs A, B		2.27	1.04–5.29	0.04	1.47	0.61–3.67	0.39
	MELD score		1.01	0.96–1.06	0.57			
	Preoperative blood data							
		Albumin level, g/dL	0.87	0.37–1.99	0.75			
		Serum creatinine, mg/dL	0.71	0.22–1.47	0.43			
		Total bilirubin, mg/dL	1.00	0.95–1.04	0.97			
		PT-INR	1.17	0.67–1.62	0.50			
		Platelet count, $\times 10^4/\mu L$	1.00	0.94–1.06	0.87			
	Primary disease							
		Non-HCV vs others	2.44	1.00–7.28	0.05	1.59	0.60–4.98	0.37
		Fulminant hepatitis vs others	2.78	1.02–6.49	0.05	2.44	0.84–6.45	0.10
Donors factors								
	Age, years		0.99	0.96–1.02	0.69			
	Sex, female		1.15	0.40–1.86	0.72			
	GV/SLV, %		1.00	0.96–1.04	0.87			
	GV, g		1.00	0.99–1.00	0.18			
Operative factors								
	Operative time, min		1.00	1.00–1.003	0.58			
	Operative blood loss, L		1.00	1.00–1.00004	0.16			
	Transfusion							
		RCC, U	1.02	1.00–1.03	0.10			
		FFP, U	1.01	1.00–1.02	0.04			
		PC, U	1.00	0.98–1.02	0.74			
	Biliary duct-to-duct		1.61	0.48–9.98	0.49	1.02	1.00–1.03	0.03

Abbreviations: LDLT, living-donor liver transplantation; MELD, model for end-stage liver disease; PT-INR, international normalized ratio of prothrombin time; GV, graft volume; SLV, standard liver volume; RCC, red blood cell concentrate; FFP, fresh frozen plasma; PC, platelet concentration.

80.7–94.3) and 88.0% (95%CI, 79.2–93.4), respectively, in the non-reoperation group. Graft and recipient survival did not differ significantly between groups (the log-rank test, p = 0.31, and 0.59, respectively) (Figure 1). A multivariable Cox proportional hazards model was applied to evaluate the risk of early reoperation for graft survival adjusting for other potential risk factors (female sex; HR 2.67, 95%CI 1.02–8.27, p = 0.05, GV/SLV; HR 1.05, 95%CI 1.00–1.09, p = 0.06) (Table 5). Reoperation was not a significant risk factor for graft survival (HR 1.28, 95% CI 0.45–3.29, p = 0.63). No significant risk factors for overall survival were identified in a Cox proportional hazards model. The duration of postoperative hospital stay was significantly longer in the reoperation group than in non-reoperation group (99 [117] vs. 52 [29]; p<0.01).

Discussion

In the present study, 24% (27/111) of LDLT recipients required early reoperation, comparable to previous reports [10–12]. The causes of reoperation, most of which were categorized as postoperative bleeding, vascular complications, and biliary complications, were also consistent with those in previous reports [10–12]. Early reoperation places additional surgical stress on each recipient, which may theoretically have a negative impact on both the graft and recipient. Previous reports have indicated an impaired graft/overall survival rate of recipients with early reoperation [10,12]. In the current study, early reoperation also tended to lead decreased graft survival rate. However, overall survival rates for recipients who underwent reoperation were comparable to those who did not, and therefore, our results

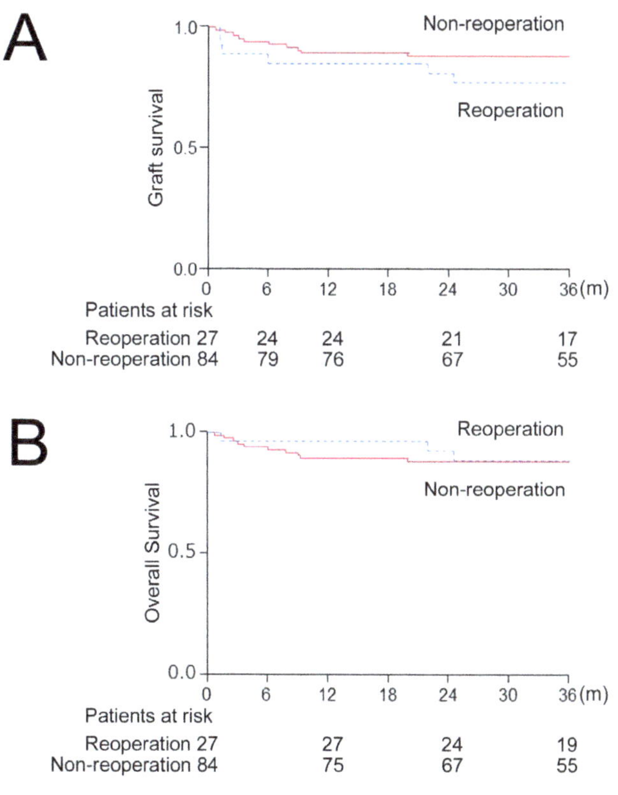

Figure 1. Graft and overall survival. (**A**) Graft survival rates for the reoperation group and the non-reoperation group. p = 0.31(the log-rank test). (**B**) Overall survival rates for the reoperation group and the non-reoperation group. p = 0.59 (the log-rank test).

enhance the importance of vigilant surveillance for early postoperative complication and early surgical rescue.

The reoperation rate after LT is reported to be high, ranging from 9.2% to 34% [10–13], while the reoperation rate after liver resection is reported to be as low as 2.5% to 10.9% [14–16]. In fact, at our institute, reoperations were performed for only 3 cases (2.7%) among 111 corresponding donors for biliary leakage (2 cases, 1.8%) and postoperative bleeding (1 case, 0.9%). The reasons for the increased rate of reoperation after LT could be attributed to poor recipient preoperative condition with hepatic failure, the administration of particular drugs such as immunosuppressants and anticoagulants, and the need for meticulous vessel reconstructions, including the hepatic vein, hepatic artery, portal vein, and bile duct [20–22]. The reoperation rate is reported to be even higher for LDLT than for DDLT [11,20,23].

Regarding risk factors for early reoperation, female sex, Child-Pugh class C, Non-HCV etiology, fulminant hepatitis, and the amount of intraoperative FFP administered were identified as possibly predictive variables, among which female sex and the amount of intraoperative FFP were identified as independent risk factors by multivariable analysis. Hendriks et al. [10] and Kappa et al. [13] reported that intraoperative blood loss predicted early reoperation. Child-Pugh class C and the amount of intraoperative FFP, which represent poor recipient liver function and have been associated with poor recipient outcome [24,25], can reasonably be associated with early reoperation after liver transplantation, although, to the best of our knowledge, this is the first report demonstrating a higher early reoperation rate in more seriously ill recipients. Although there is no previous reports supporting the reason for female sex as a predictive risk factors of reoperation in liver transplantation, in the setting of coronary stenting, there is the preponderance of evidence supporting that female had increased risk of in-hospital death and complications [26,27]. One possible reason in our study is that female recipient has significant smaller body and graft size in comparison with male (body height; female vs male, 156.6 [7.1] cm vs 170.5 [5.9] cm, p<0.01, body weight; 52.8 [8.4] kg vs 69.1 [9.9] kg, p<0.01, and graft size; 486.6 [127.7] g vs 579.4 [105.0] g, p<0.01), which might indicate the possible technical complications in smaller vessel reconstructions as reported in liver transplantation in children [28].

One concern for patients with liver failure and LT recipients is hemostatic balance [29]. While routine laboratory tests of these patients show bleeding diathesis, they are actually in hemostatic balance, because both pro- and antihemostatic factors are affected, the latter of which are not well reflected in routine coagulation testing [30]. This balance, however, can easily be tipped toward a hypo- or hypercoagulable state [31]. Our results demonstrating the high incidence of postoperative hemorrhage and vessel thrombosis as the cause for reoperation despite close monitoring with heparin administration, are representative of this situation. Further studies to investigate the ideal balance of coagulability are needed to reduce the incidence of early reoperation after LDLT.

Recently, Yoshiya et al. [12] of the Kyushu group and Hendriks et al. [10] reported that early reoperation was significantly associated with poor graft and/or recipient survival after LDLT and DDLT, respectively. In the present study, observed graft survival for the recipients who underwent reoperation was also lower compared to those who did not, though the result was not significantly different. Overall survival in the reoperation group was comparable to that in the non-reoperation group (Figure 1). These results in our study imply the importance of vigilant surveillance for early complications and early surgical interventions to improve graft/overall survival of recipients. However, the

Table 5. Univariable and multivariable Cox proportional hazards model analysis for graft survival.

Variables			Univariable analysis			Multivariable analysis		
			HR	95% CI	p value	HR	95% CI	p value
Reoperation			1.54	0.54–3.89	0.40	1.28	0.45–3.29	0.63
Recipient factors								
	Age, years		0.99	0.96–1.03	0.51			
	Sex, female		2.67	1.02–8.27	0.05	2.54	0.95–7.94	0.06
	Child-Pugh, C vs A, B		1.00	0.40–2.50	0.99			
	MELD score		1.05	0.99–1.11	0.14			
	Preoperative blood data							
		Albumin level, g/dL	0.92	0.33–2.44	0.87			
		Serum creatinine, mg/dL	1.36	0.66–2.12	0.34			
		Total bilirubin, mg/dL	1.03	0.98–1.07	0.28			
		PT-INR	1.23	0.69–1.70	0.40			
		Platelet count, $\times 10^4/\mu L$	1.01	0.93–1.07	0.86			
	Primary disease							
		Non-HCV vs others	1.11	0.32–2.28	0.83			
		Fulminant hepatitis vs others	2.37	0.67–6.53	0.16			
Donors factors								
	Age, years		0.95	0.38–2.38	0.90			
	Sex, female		1.15	0.40–1.86	0.72			
	GV/SLV, %		1.05	1.00–1.09	0.06	1.04	1.00–1.09	0.06
	GV, g		1.00	1.00–1.004	0.70			
Operative factors								
	Operative time, min		1.00	1.00–1.002	0.61			
	Operative blood loss, L		1.00	1.00–1.00003	0.40			
	Transfusion							
		RCC, U	0.99	0.92–1.02	0.60			
		FFP, U	1.00	0.96–1.01	0.85			
		PC, U	0.99	0.97–1.02	0.64			
	Biliary duct-to-duct		0.65	0.21–2.77	0.51			

Abbreviations: LDLT, living-donor liver transplantation; MELD, model for end-stage liver disease; PT-INR, international normalized ratio of prothrombin time; GV, graft volume; SLV, standard liver volume; RCC, red blood cell concentrate; FFP, fresh frozen plasma; PC, platelet concentration.

different results between our study (4 early graft losses [14.8%] in 27 recipients with reoperation) and the Kyushu group study (10 graft losses [34.5%] in 26 recipients with reoperation) need further investigation. The learning curve, as suggested by Kyushu group, as well as the radiologic and hematologic assays used to detect early complications, and differences in the criteria for reoperation might partially explain the discrepancy.

The main limitations of our study are its retrospective nature, the small number of cases, and biases caused by learning curves of surgical techniques and postoperative management. The early reoperation group was a small inhomogenous cohort with various causes for reoperation, which may make the data inadequate to support the findings with a multivariable analysis. Further analyses with a large number of patients in a well-designed multicenter study are needed to clarify the impact of early reoperation on outcome.

In conclusion, observed graft survival for the recipients who underwent reoperation was lower compared to those who did not undergo reoperation, though the result was not significantly different. Recipient overall survival with reoperation was comparable to that without reoperation. Independent risk factors for reoperation were recipient female sex and the amount of intraoperative FFP in our study. The present findings enhance the importance of vigilant surveillance for early postoperative complication and early surgical rescue at a postoperative period in the LDLT setting.

Supporting Information

Checklist S1 This study was conducted based on the STROBE statement.

Author Contributions

Conceived and designed the experiments: YK Y. Sugawara. Performed the experiments: NA JK TH TT. Analyzed the data: TI ST TA Y. Sakamoto. Contributed reagents/materials/analysis tools: KH. Wrote the paper: YK Y. Sugawara NK.

References

1. Starzl TE, Klintmalm GB, Porter KA, Iwatsuki S, Schroter GP (1981) Liver transplantation with use of cyclosporin a and prednisone. N Engl J Med 305: 266–269.
2. Sugawara Y, Makuuchi M, Kaneko J, Ohkubo T, Imamura H, et al. (2002) Correlation between optimal tacrolimus doses and the graft weight in living donor liver transplantation. Clin Transplant 16: 102–106.
3. Sugawara Y, Makuuchi M, Akamatsu N, Kishi Y, Niiya T, et al. (2004) Refinement of venous reconstruction using cryopreserved veins in right liver grafts. Liver Transpl 10: 541–547.
4. Kokudo N, Sugawara Y, Imamura H, Sano K, Makuuchi M (2005) Tailoring the type of donor hepatectomy for adult living donor liver transplantation. Am J Transplant 5: 1694–1703.
5. Pomposelli JJ, Verbesey J, Simpson MA, Lewis WD, Gordon FD, et al. (2006) Improved survival after live donor adult liver transplantation (LDALT) using right lobe grafts: program experience and lessons learned. Am J Transplant 6: 589–598.
6. Jain A, Reyes J, Kashyap R, Dodson SF, Demetris AJ, et al. (2000) Long-term survival after liver transplantation in 4,000 consecutive patients at a single center. Ann Surg 232: 490–500.
7. (2010) Liver transplantation in Japan: registry by the Japanese Liver Transplantation Society. Jap J Transpl 46: 524–536.
8. Adam R, McMaster P, O'Grady JG, Castaing D, Klempnauer JL, et al. (2003) Evolution of liver transplantation in Europe: report of the European Liver Transplant Registry. Liver Transpl 9: 1231–1243.
9. The Organ Procurement and Transplantation Network. http://optn.transplant.hrsa.gov/accessed on 2014 July 14.
10. Hendriks HG, van der Meer J, de Wolf JT, Peeters PM, Porte RJ, et al. (2005) Intraoperative blood transfusion requirement is the main determinant of early surgical re-intervention after orthotopic liver transplantation. Transpl Int 17: 673–679.
11. Freise CE, Gillespie BW, Koffron AJ, Lok AS, Pruett TL, et al. (2008) Recipient morbidity after living and deceased donor liver transplantation: findings from the A2ALL Retrospective Cohort Study. Am J Transplant 8: 2569–2579.
12. Yoshiya S, Shirabe K, Kimura K, Yoshizumi T, Ikegami T, et al. (2012) The Causes, Risk Factors, and Outcomes of Early Relaparotomy After Living-Donor Liver Transplantation. Transplantation Journal 94: 947–952.
13. Kappa SF, Gorden DL, Davidson MA, Wright JK, Guillamondegui OD (2010) Intraoperative blood loss predicts hemorrhage-related reoperation after orthotopic liver transplantation. Am Surg 76: 969–973.
14. Schroeder RA, Marroquin CE, Bute BP, Khuri S, Henderson WG, et al. (2006) Predictive indices of morbidity and mortality after liver resection. Ann Surg 243: 373–379.
15. Barbas AS, Turley RS, Mallipeddi MK, Lidsky ME, Reddy SK, et al. (2013) Examining reoperation and readmission after hepatic surgery. J Am Coll Surg 216: 915–923.
16. Imamura H, Seyama Y, Kokudo N, Maema A, Sugawara Y, et al. (2003) One thousand fifty-six hepatectomies without mortality in 8 years. Arch Surg 138: 1198–1206; discussion 1206.
17. Urata K, Kawasaki S, Matsunami H, Hashikura Y, Ikegami T, et al. (1995) Calculation of child and adult standard liver volume for liver transplantation. Hepatology 21: 1317–1321.
18. Sugawara Y, Makuuchi M, Kaneko J, Ohkubo T, Matsui Y, et al. (2003) Living-donor liver transplantation in adults: Tokyo University experience. J Hepatobiliary Pancreat Surg 10: 1–4.
19. Rahbari NN, Garden OJ, Padbury R, Maddern G, Koch M, et al. (2011) Post-hepatectomy haemorrhage: a definition and grading by the International Study Group of Liver Surgery (ISGLS). HPB (Oxford) 13: 528–535.
20. Duailibi DF, Ribeiro MA Jr (2010) Biliary complications following deceased and living donor liver transplantation: a review. Transplant Proc 42: 517–520.
21. Soong RS, Chan KM, Chou HS, Wu TJ, Lee CF, et al. (2012) The risk factors for early infection in adult living donor liver transplantation recipients. Transplant Proc 44: 784–786.
22. Arshad F, Lisman T, Porte RJ (2013) Hypercoagulability as a contributor to thrombotic complications in the liver transplant recipient. Liver Int 33: 820–827.
23. Khalaf H (2010) Vascular complications after deceased and living donor liver transplantation: a single-center experience. Transplant Proc 42: 865–870.
24. Onaca NN, Levy MF, Sanchez EQ, Chinnakotla S, Fasola CG, et al. (2003) A correlation between the pretransplantation MELD score and mortality in the first two years after liver transplantation. Liver Transpl 9: 117–123.
25. Kamath PS, Wiesner RH, Malinchoc M, Kremers W, Therneau TM, et al. (2001) A model to predict survival in patients with end-stage liver disease. Hepatology 33: 464–470.
26. Anderson ML, Peterson ED, Brennan JM, Rao SV, Dai D, et al. (2012) Short- and long-term outcomes of coronary stenting in women versus men: results from the National Cardiovascular Data Registry Centers for Medicare & Medicaid services cohort. Circulation 126: 2190–2199.
27. Peterson ED, Lansky AJ, Kramer J, Anstrom K, Lanzilotta MJ (2001) Effect of gender on the outcomes of contemporary percutaneous coronary intervention. Am J Cardiol 88: 359–364.
28. Sanada Y, Wakiya T, Hishikawa S, Hirata Y, Yamada N, et al. (2013) Risk factors and treatments for hepatic arterial complications in pediatric living donor liver transplantation. J Hepatobiliary Pancreat Sci.
29. Lisman T, Caldwell SH, Burroughs AK, Northup PG, Senzolo M, et al. (2010) Hemostasis and thrombosis in patients with liver disease: the ups and downs. J Hepatol 53: 362–371.
30. Tripodi A, Primignani M, Chantarangkul V, Dell'Era A, Clerici M, et al. (2009) An imbalance of pro- vs anti-coagulation factors in plasma from patients with cirrhosis. Gastroenterology 137: 2105–2111.
31. Lisman T, Porte RJ (2009) Hepatic artery thrombosis after liver transplantation: more than just a surgical complication? Transpl Int 22: 162–164.

15

Effects of Intraosseous Erythropoietin during Hemorrhagic Shock in Swine

Vesna Borovnik-Lesjak[1], Kasen Whitehouse[1], Alvin Baetiong[1], Yang Miao[1], Brian M. Currie[1], Sathya Velmurugan[1], Jeejabai Radhakrishnan[2], Raúl J. Gazmuri[3]*

1 Resuscitation Institute at Rosalind Franklin University of Medicine and Science, North Chicago, Illinois, United States of America, **2** Department of Medicine and Resuscitation Institute at Rosalind Franklin University of Medicine and Science, North Chicago, Illinois, United States of America, **3** Department of Medicine, Department of Physiology and Biophysics, and Resuscitation Institute at Rosalind Franklin University of Medicine and Science, and Critical Care Medicine at the Captain James A. Lovell Federal Health Care Center, North Chicago, Illinois, United States of America

Abstract

Objective: To determine whether erythropoietin given during hemorrhagic shock (*HS*) ameliorates organ injury while improving resuscitation and survival.

Methods: Three series of 24 pigs each were studied. In an initial series, 50% of the blood volume (BV) was removed in 30 minutes and normal saline (threefold the blood removed) started at minute 90 infusing each third in 30, 60, and 150 minutes with shed blood reinfused at minute 330 ($HS\text{-}50_{BV}$). In a second series, the same $HS\text{-}50_{BV}$ protocol was used but removing an additional 15% of BV from minute 30 to 60 ($HS\text{-}65_{BV}$). In a final series, blood was removed as in $HS\text{-}65_{BV}$ and intraosseous vasopressin given from minute 30 (0.04 U/kg min^{-1}) until start of shed blood reinfusion at minute 150 ($HS\text{-}65_{BV}+VP$). Normal saline was reduced to half the blood removed and given from minute 90 to 120 in half of the animals. In each series, animals were randomized 1:1 to receive erythropoietin (1,200 U/kg) or control solution intraosseously after removing 10% of the BV.

Results: In $HS\text{-}50_{BV}$, O_2 consumption remained near baseline yielding minimal lactate increases, 88% resuscitability, and 60% survival at 72 hours. In $HS\text{-}65_{BV}$, O_2 consumption was reduced and lactate increased yielding 25% resuscitability. In $HS\text{-}65_{BV}+VP$, vasopressin promoted hemodynamic stability yielding 92% resuscitability and 83% survival at 72 hours. Erythropoietin did not affect resuscitability or subsequent survival in any of the series but increased interleukin-10, attenuated lactate increases, and ameliorated organ injury based on lesser troponin I, AST, and ALT increases and lesser neurological deficits in the $HS\text{-}65_{BV}+VP$ series.

Conclusions: Erythropoietin given during HS in swine failed to alter resuscitability and 72 hour survival regardless of HS severity and concomitant treatment with fluids and vasopressin but attenuated acute organ injury. The studies also showed the efficacy of vasopressin and restrictive fluid resuscitation for hemodynamic stabilization and survival.

Editor: Raghavan Raju, Georgia Regents University, United States of America

Funding: This research was supported by the Telemedicine and Advanced Technology Research Center (TATRC) at the U.S. Army Medical Research and Materiel Command (USAMRMC) Fort Detrick, MD under contract number: W81XWH-11-2-0019. Funding was received by RJG. The funders had no role in study design, data collection and analysis, decision to publish, or preparation of the manuscript.

Competing Interests: The authors have declared that no competing interests exist.

* Email: raul.gazmuri@rosalindfranklin.edu

Introduction

Acute hemorrhage resulting from traumatic injury is responsible for a high percentage of death in military personnel engaged in combat operations [1]. A recent report including 4,596 battlefield fatalities from Operation Iraqi Freedom and Operation Enduring Freedom between October 2001 and June 2011 showed that 87.3% of all injury related deaths occurred before arriving to a medical treatment facility [2]. Of these deaths, 24.3% were deemed potentially survivable with acute mortality associated with hemorrhage in 90.9%. The current acute management of hemorrhage focuses on hemostasis, hemodynamic stabilization, and rapid transfer to a medical treatment facility.

Erythropoietin (EPO) – a hormone best known for its effect on red blood cell production – has been shown to protect organs and tissues from ischemia and reperfusion injury including the heart [3–7], brain [8,9], spinal cord [10,11], kidney [12–14], liver [13–15], and skin [16,17]. We have reported beneficial effects of EPO for resuscitation from cardiac arrest in animal models [18–20] and in human victims of sudden cardiac arrest [21]. These effects were in part associated with non-genomic activation of mitochondrial protective pathways (e.g., Akt and PKC_{ε}) leading to lesser myocardial injury and dysfunction during and after resuscitation

[20]. We hypothesized that similar benefits could be elicited in other low-flow states such as hemorrhagic shock (HS) and ameliorate organ injury improving resuscitability and survival. This hypothesis was supported by rat models of HS in which pretreatment with EPO improved survival associated with lesser reductions in mean aortic pressure and lesser increases in lactic acid, tumor necrosis factor (TNF)-α, and interleukin (IL)-6 [14] along with lesser injury to the liver and kidneys [13,14], and by studies – also in rats – showing that EPO given during HS attenuated intestinal mucosal injury and bacterial translocation [22] along with maintaining intestinal microcirculatory blood flow [23]. Although – to the best of our knowledge – the effects of EPO during HS have not been investigated in large animal models (i.e., swine, sheep, and dog), EPO has been shown to exert tissue protection in swine models of liver [15] and spinal cord [11] ischemia.

We developed a model of HS in swine – an animal higher in the phylogenic scale and thus of greater translational relevance – and investigated the effects of EPO incorporating logistic constraints expected to limit care in far forward combat operations. We used a protocol of controlled bleeding as the initial approach in a multi-year project to first characterize the effects of the proposed interventions without the confounding elements of uncontrolled bleeding and tissue injury (to be incorporated in future series). We conducted three successive series of 24 animals each in which animals were randomized 1:1 to receive EPO (1,200 U/kg) or control solution. The series had in common (a) removal of blood to a target percentage of the estimated blood volume (simulating bleeding and hemostasis in the field); (b) delivery of EPO through the intraosseous route upon removal of 10% of the animal's blood volume (simulating early drug delivery using a low-skill technique); (c) fluid resuscitation with 0.9% NaCl (normal saline) initiated after a period of untreated HS (simulating delayed access to rescuers); (d) shed blood reinfusion at the end of HS (simulating arrival to a medical post), and (e) contingent on the series, recovery from anesthesia and 72 hour observation. The first series modeled low severity HS; the second series modeled high severity HS; and the third series modeled high severity HS with use of vasopressin to augment resuscitability while examining the role of limited fluid resuscitation.

Materials and Methods

The studies were approved by the Institutional Animal Care and Use Committee (IACUC) at Rosalind Franklin University of Medicine and Science (approval number 12–23) and by the United States Army Medical Research and Materiel Command Animal Care and Use Review Office (ACURO) and were conducted according to institutional guidelines.

Animal Housing and Husbandry

Animals were group housed in pens at the Biological Resource Facility (AAALAC accredited facility) at the Rosalind Franklin University of Medicine and Science in which lights are set at the recommended illumination levels of a 12/12-hour cycle controlled via automatic timers. Temperature was maintained at 61–81°F. Resting mats were provided and Aspen Sani-Chip bedding from a certified vendor (Harlan Laboratories, Indiana) was used. Health assessment for general health and well-being, possible injuries, or death was performed daily by animal care technicians and the day before/during/after the experiment by the investigator.

Animal Preparation

Basic Preparation. Male domestic pigs (32–48 kg, age ~11 weeks) were sedated with ketamine hydrochloride (30 mg·kg^{-1} intramuscularly). Anesthesia was induced with propofol (2 mg·kg^{-1} through an ear vein) and the animal intubated with a size 8 tracheal tube initiating positive pressure ventilation with a volume controlled ventilator (840 Ventilator System, Nellcor Puritan Bennett, Boulder, CO) set to deliver a tidal volume of 10 mL·kg^{-1}, peak flow of 60 l·min^{-1}, and FiO_2 of 0.5. Respiratory rate was adjusted at baseline to maintain the end-expired PCO_2 ($P_{ET}CO$) between 35 and 45 mmHg (Capnogard, Novometrix Medical Systems, Wallingford, CT). Anesthesia was continued using isoflurane (1.75% to 2.75%) and a 1:1 mixture of nitrous oxide and oxygen. The electrocardiogram was recorded through defibrillator adhesive skin pads. All procedures were performed using sterile technique. A 7 F high-fidelity micro-tip catheter transducer (Millar Instruments, Houston, TX) was advanced through the right femoral artery into the descending thoracic aorta for pressure measurement (Figure 1). A 7 F thermodilution balloon-tipped pulmonary artery catheter was advanced through the left cephalic vein or through the left internal jugular vein (when the cephalic vein was used to access the great cardiac vein as described under *Experimental Series*) into the pulmonary artery for measuring core temperature and thermodilution cardiac output along with pressures in the right atrium and pulmonary artery. A 6 F high-fidelity micro-tip pressure transducer pigtail catheter (Millar Instruments, Houston, TX) was advanced through the surgically exposed left carotid artery for measuring left ventricular pressure. A 23 F cannula (Bio-Medicus, Medtronic, Minneapolis, MN) was advanced through the left external jugular vein into the right atrium and used for blood withdrawal into a blood transfer bag. Core temperature was maintained between 37.5°C and 38.5°C with water-circulated blanket (Blanketrol II, Cincinnati SubZero, Cincinnati, OH).

Hemorrhagic Shock Protocol

The animal's blood volume was estimated at 60 ml/kg-body weight and a predetermined percentage was withdrawn into a heparinized transfer bag (heparin 10 U·ml^{-1} of blood) using a roller pump (model 313S, Watson Marlow, Inc., Wilmington, MA) controlled by a custom-developed software in LabVIEW 6.0. The heparinized transfer bag was placed on an electronic scale (model 2200, Doran Scales, Inc., Batavia, IL) connected to the LabVIEW

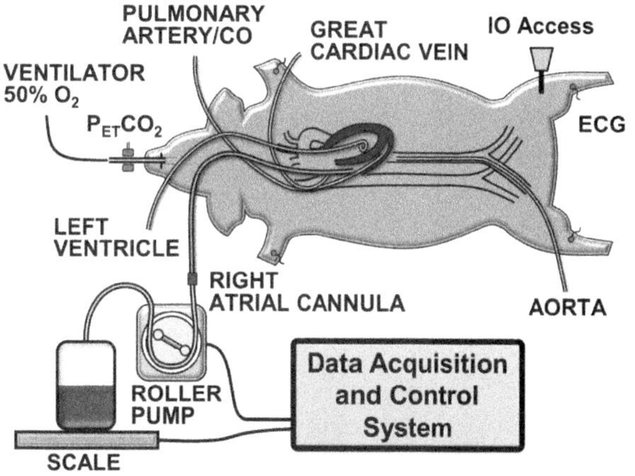

Figure 1. Swine model of hemorrhagic shock. CO, cardiac output; IO, intraosseous; $P_{ET}CO_2$, end-tidal PCO_2; ECG, electrocardiogram.

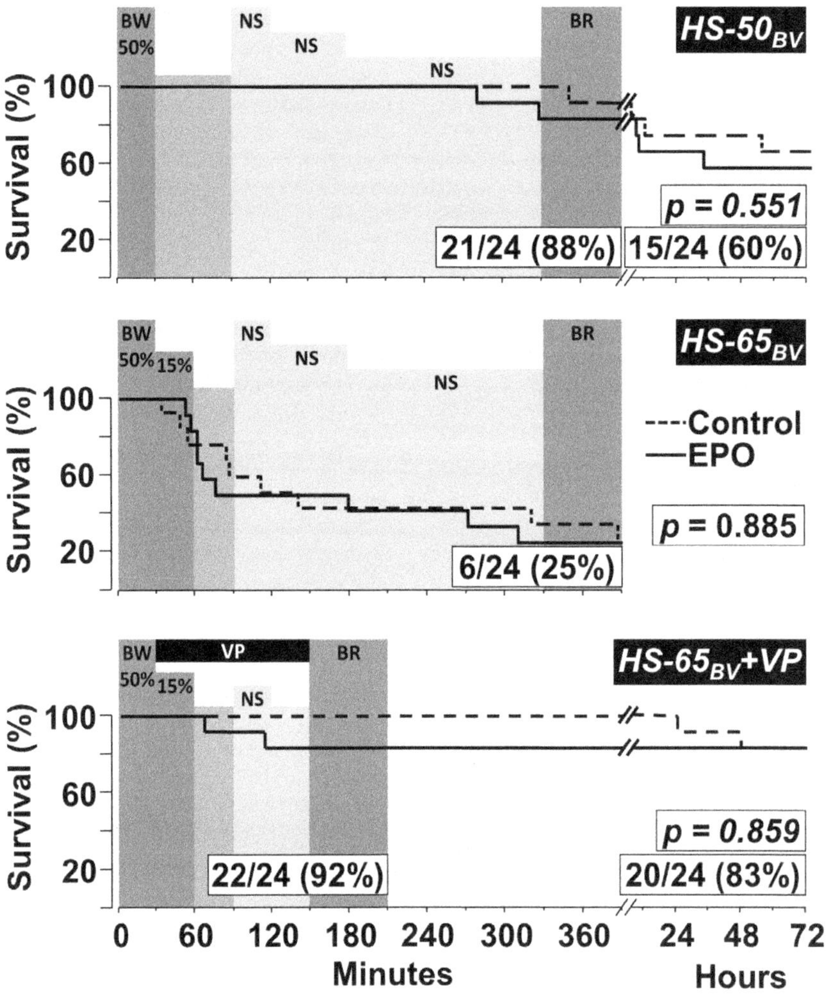

Figure 2. Survival curves comparing pigs treated with EPO and controls. Series *HS-50*$_{BV}$ and *HS-65*$_{BV}$*+VP* include 72 hour survival. The *p*-values for survival differences between groups were calculated using the Gehan-Breslow test and are shown within each graph along with the resuscitation and survival rates for the combined EPO and control groups. The shaded horizontal bars successively represent; the percentage of blood withdrawn (BW), the interval of hemorrhagic shock after blood withdrawal without fluid administration, the administration of normal saline (NS) as described in the Method, and blood reinfusion (BR). Shown in *65*$_{BV}$*+VP* is the vasopressin infusion (VP).

software to gravimetrically monitor the rate of blood withdrawal (blood density = 1.06 g/ml) and automatically adjust the pump rate as needed (Figure 1). The withdrawn blood was kept in a water bath at 37.5°C until reinfusion. Resuscitation was subsequently attempted by administration of normal saline followed by reinfusion of the shed blood using a blood transfusion filter (PALL Biomedical, Port Washington, NY). The volume, timing, and use of additional drugs varied as described under *Experimental Series*. In each series, pigs were randomized 1:1 to receive a 1,200 U/kg bolus of erythropoietin (Epogen [epoetin alpha]; 20,000 U/ml, Amgen) or normal saline vehicle (control) into the left tibia upon 10% removal of the blood volume (6 minutes from the start of blood removal). The investigators were blind to the treatment assignment and the group identification was revealed only after completion of the data analysis in each series.

At the completion of resuscitation in the first and third series, all catheters were removed, vessels ligated, and the skin wounds stapled, all under sterile conditions. The animal was allowed to recover from anesthesia and the endotracheal tube removed after resumption of spontaneous breathing and returned to its pen. The animal was then monitored every 60 minutes until it was able to right itself to sternal recumbency and thereafter every 4 hours for the initial 24 hours and at a minimum interval of 8 hours until completion of the 72 hours. A fentanyl dermal patch was used for analgesia throughout the 72 hour post-resuscitation period. If additional analgesia was needed, 2.2 mg/kg of flunixin meglumine was administered intramuscularly. The neurological status was evaluated at 24, 48, and 72 hours post-resuscitation using a neurological deficit score (0 = best; 420 = worst) [24]. The pig was euthanized at 72 hours by intravenous injection of euthanasia solution (pentobarbital sodium and phenytoin sodium; 5 ml, Vedco Inc., St Joseph, MO), or earlier – for humanitarian reason – in the event of moderate to severe of pain and distress unalleviated by analgesic agents, inability to eat or drink unassisted after 24 hours post-surgery, non-weight bearing or paralysis after 24 hours, depression or lethargy after 48 hours, profuse diarrhea, infection not resolved with antimicrobial therapy, lack of righting reflex, or cyanosis with difficulty breathing. The choice of drugs, route of administration, surgical preparation, and method of euthanasia were based on the recommendations by ACLAM board certified DVMs.

Table 1. Baseline Characteristics.

Variable	*HS-50_{BV}* CTR	*HS-50_{BV}* EPO	*HS-65_{BV}* CTR	*HS-65_{BV}* EPO	*HS-65_{BV}+VP* CTR	*HS-65_{BV}+VP* EPO
n	12	12	12	12	12	12
Weight (kg)	39.6±3.7	37.5±4.2	34.6±1.5	35.4±1.2	39.4±2.4	38.1±2.5
Preparation Time (min)	170±36	174±41	123±59	114±21	119±22	113±21
Temperature (°C)	38.1±0.4	38.0±0.4	38.0±0.3	38.0±0.2	38.2±0.3	38.2±0.2
Respiration Rate (bpm)	31±5	31±4	35±2	36±1	36±2	35±2
End-tidal CO_2 (mmHg)	38±2	38±2	40±2	42±2	38±3	37±3
Mean Arterial Pressure (mmHg)	62±8	62±8	59±6	63±9	61±7	68±9
Cardiac Index (ml/min·m^{-2})	4.6±0.6	4.4±1.1	3.9±0.6	4.2±1.1	4.8±0.8	4.9±0.8
Heart Rate (bpm)	98±20	92±9	98±10	106±16	105±20	100±12
Blood Withdrawal Index (ml/m^2)	1398±70	1370±43	1909±162	1972±316	1814±39	1796±39

Values are mean ± SD. $HS\text{-}50_{BV}$, blood volume withdrawal 50%; $HS\text{-}65_{BV}$, blood volume withdrawal 65%; $HS\text{-}65_{BV}+VP$, blood volume withdrawal 65% and vasopressin infusion. CTR, control; EPO, erythropoietin. There were no statistically significant differences between groups within each series.

After euthanasia, the whole left lung was weighed before and after drying in the oven at 70°C for at least 72 hours for calculations of the wet/dry ratio in the last series.

Sample Size

The sample size of 12 pigs per group was based on extrapolation from work in similar animal models intended to identify biologically robust differences in survival effects and continuous variables with a power>0.60 at an α level of 0.05.

Experimental Series

Experiments were performed between 9 AM to 5 PM in a large animal surgical suite located inside the university Biological Resource Facility. Three consecutive series of 24 experiments each were conducted. The sequence of interventions are described below and depicted in Figure 2. In the first series, 50% of the estimated blood volume was withdrawn in 30 minutes ($HS\text{-}50_{BV}$). Animals remained untreated for 60 minutes after which normal saline – threefold the blood volume removed – was infused delivering sequentially a third of each in 30, 60, and 150 minutes followed by infusion of the shed blood in 60 minutes. The $HS\text{-}50_{BV}$ protocol triggered a vigorous adaptive response that enabled maintaining oxygen consumption close to baseline resulting in minimal lactate increases and high resuscitability and survival without differences between EPO and control. To test EPO under greater HS severity, a second series was conducted withdrawing an additional 15% of the blood volume in 30 minutes after completing the initial 50% of blood volume removal for a total of 65% of blood volume removed ($HS\text{-}65_{BV}$). Animals remained untreated for 30 minutes after which the same $HS\text{-}50_{BV}$ protocol for fluid resuscitation and blood reinfusion was applied. In this series, an additional 7 F angiographic catheter was advanced with the aid of fluoroscopy from the left cephalic vein into the great cardiac vein to assess effect on myocardial metabolism [25]. The $HS\text{-}65_{BV}$ protocol was indeed severe, reducing resuscitability to only 25%, but again showing no difference between EPO and control. A third series was then conducted using the same $HS\text{-}65_{BV}$ protocol for blood withdrawal but infusing arginine vasopressin to prevent death by maintaining a higher coronary perfusion ($HS\text{-}65_{BV}+VP$). Vasopressin (Pitressin, JHP Pharmaceuticals, Rochester, MI) was given intraosseously as a bolus (0.04 U·kg^{-1}) upon completion of the initial 50% of blood volume removal followed by a continuous infusion (0.04 U·kg^{-1}·min^{-1}) using a syringe pump (PHD 2000 Syringe Pump Series, Harvard Apparatus, Holliston, MA) until start of blood reinfusion.

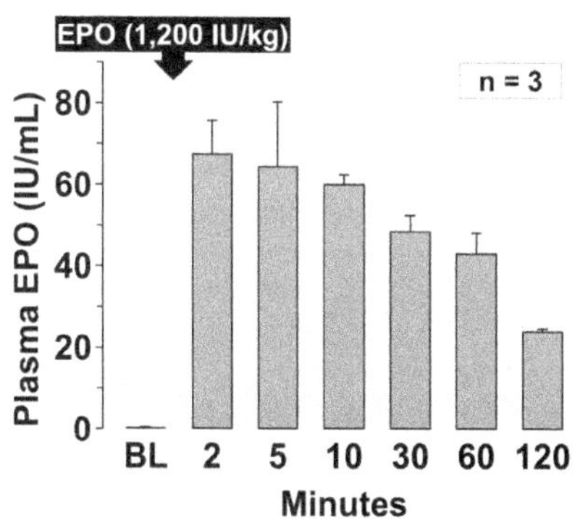

Figure 3. Plasma levels of EPO measured in 3 representative experiments from the $HS\text{-}50_{BV}$ series. Values are mean ± SEM.

In $HS\text{-}65_{BV}+VP$, we also assessed the effect of less or no fluid resuscitation [26] under conditions of shorter HS duration. Thus, animals were also randomized 1:1 to receive either normal saline infusion – half of the blood volume withdrawn in 30 minutes – or no fluid at all. Blood was reinfused starting at 150 minutes (Figure 2). The addition of vasopressin dramatically improved resuscitability, allowing examination of survival and impact on organ function by blood sampling every 24 hours from the superior vena cava after sedation with ketamine hydrochloride (30 mg·kg^{-1} intramuscularly). Pigs were euthanized at 72 hours.

Experimental Outcomes

The primary outcome was survival at 390 minutes in series $HS\text{-}65_{BV}$ (without recovery from anesthesia) and survival at 72 hours in series $HS\text{-}50_{BV}$ and in series $HS\text{-}65_{BV}+VP$ (with recovery from anesthesia). Secondary outcomes included: (1) hemodynamic and metabolic function, (2) myocardial function, (3) organ injury including the heart, brain, lung, liver, and kidney, (4) plasma cytokines, and (5) blood cell count.

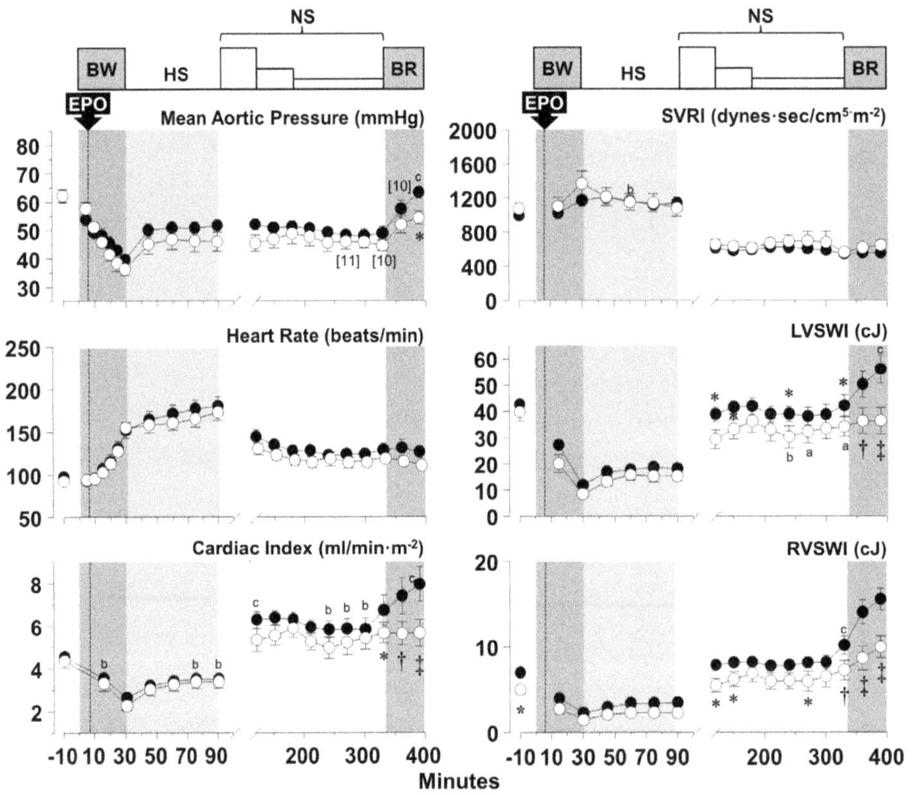

Figure 4. Hemodynamic and myocardial effects of EPO (open circles, n = 12) and vehicle control (closed circles, n = 12) in series *HS-50*$_{BV}$. Numbers in brackets indicate when the number of animals decreased from the preceding time point consequent to death of the animal. BL, baseline; BW, blood withdrawal; HS, hemorrhagic shock; NS, normal saline; BR, blood reinfusion; Ao, aortic pressure; SVRI, systemic vascular resistance index; LVSWI, left ventricular stroke work index; RVWI, right ventricular stroke work index. Values are shown as mean ± SEM. Differences between groups were analyzed by two-way repeated measures ANOVA. There were no overall significant treatment effects. However, there were overall statistically significant interactions between treatment and time for Ao mean ($p = 0.033$), cardiac index ($p < 0.001$), LVSWI ($p = 0.001$), and RVSWI ($p < 0.001$). $^{*}p \leq 0.05$, $^{\dagger}p \leq 0.01$, and $^{\ddagger}p \leq 0.001$ denote statistically significant differences between groups at the specified time points. $^{a}p \leq 0.05$, $^{b}p \leq 0.01$, and $^{c}p \leq 0.001$ denote significant differences *vs* baseline using the Holm-Sidak test for multiple comparisons showing the differences only when they occurred in one of the two groups.

Measurements

Blood analysis. Blood samples were collected from the aorta and pulmonary artery in all three series with the addition of great cardiac vein in *HS-65*$_{BV}$. Blood samples were processed on site for pH, PO_2, PCO_2, hemoglobin, and lactate using a cartridge based device (OPTI CCA-TS Blood Gas and Electrolyte Analyzer, OPTI Medical Systems, Roswell, GA) and for common hemoglobin types (oxy-, met-, carboxy-, and reduced-) using a co-oximeter (AVOXimeter 4000, AVOX systems Inc., San Antonio, TX). O_2 content in the aorta (CaO_2), pulmonary artery (CvO_2), and great cardiac vein ($CgcvO_2$) was calculated according to the following equation:

$$O_2Content\left(\frac{ml}{dl}\right) = Hemoglobin\left(\frac{g}{dl}\right) \times 1.39\left(\frac{ml}{g}\right) \times S_FO_2 + 0.003\left(\frac{ml}{dl}\cdot mmHg^{-1}\right) \times PO_2(mmHg)$$

where 1.39 denotes ml of O_2 bound to 1 g of hemoglobin (Hufner's number), S_FO_2 the fraction of oxyhemoglobin relative to the four hemoglobin types, and 0.003 the O_2 solubility coefficient. Aortic blood samples were also taken and processed for complete blood count and chemistry (blood urea nitrogen [BUN], creatinine, alanine aminotransferase [ALT], aspartate aminotransferase [AST], and troponin I) at the Captain James A. Lovell Federal Health Care Center, North Chicago, IL.

Plasma EPO. In series *HS-50*$_{BV}$, the serum level of EPO was measured in three animals that received EPO and in one control using a double-antibody "sandwich" enzyme-linked immunosorbent assay kit (MD Bioproducts, St Paul, MN) targeted to human EPO according to the manufacturer instructions. The EPO level in serum samples (diluted 100 times) was calculated using a standard curve generated with EPO calibrators included in the kit (0, 10.3, 24.8, 48, 156, and 523 mU/ml). The final plasma concentration was determined by applying the dilution factors and a conversion factor whereby one U/ml of EPO [Epogen (epoetin alpha), Amgen] equaled 0.798 U/ml of the calibrator.

Hemodynamic Measurements. Thermodilution cardiac output was measured in duplicate after bolus injection of normal saline (5 ml) into the right atrium (HP-Philips M012AT cardiac output module, Amsterdam, The Netherlands). Cardiac output was normalized to body surface area using the Kelley equation (body surface area [m^2] $= 0.073 \cdot$body-weight$^{2/3}$ [kg]) [27]. Aortic and left ventricular pressure signals were calibrated with a built-in calibration system (PCU-2000, Millar). Other pressure signals were zeroed to mid-cavity level. All signals were sampled and digitized at 250 Hz using a 16-bit data acquisition board

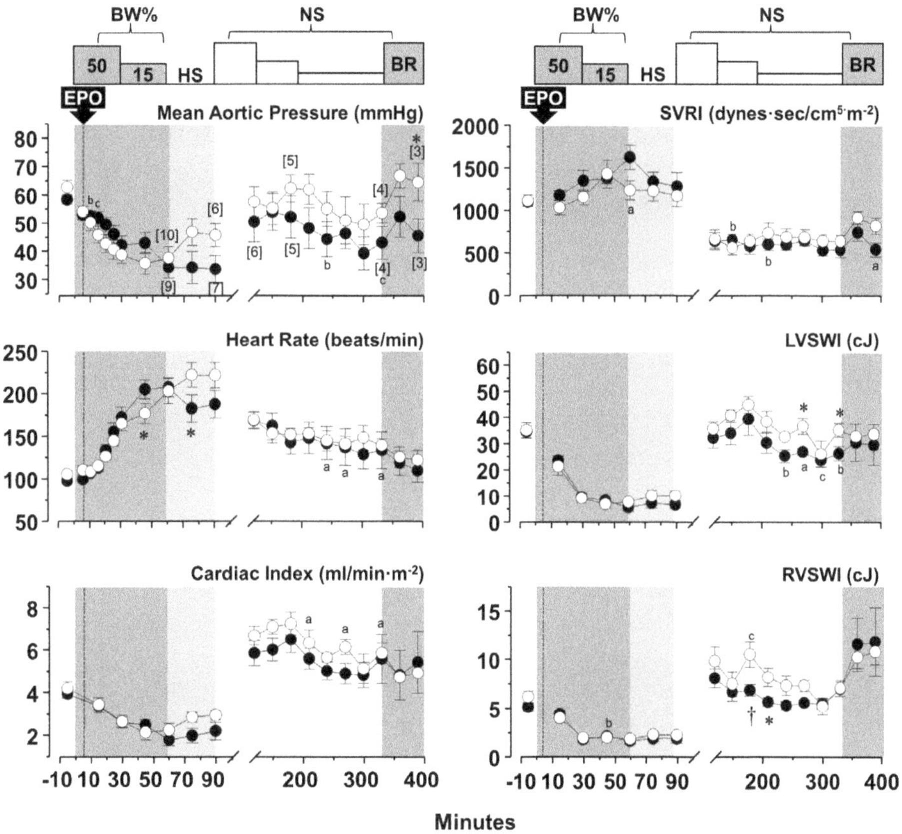

Figure 5. Hemodynamic and myocardial effects of EPO (open circles, n = 12) compared with vehicle control (closed circles, n = 12) in series *HS-65*$_{BV}$. Numbers in brackets indicate when the number of animals decreased from the preceding time point consequent to death of the animal. BL, baseline; BW, blood withdrawal; HS, hemorrhagic shock; NS, normal saline; BR, blood reinfusion; Ao, aortic pressure; SVRI, systemic vascular resistance index; LVSWI, left ventricular stroke work index; RVWI, right ventricular stroke work index. Values are shown as mean ± SEM. Differences between groups were analyzed by two-way repeated measures ANOVA. There were no overall significant treatment effects. However, there was an overall statistically significant interaction between treatment and time for Ao mean ($p = 0.002$). *$p \leq 0.05$, †$p \leq 0.01$, and ‡$p \leq 0.001$ denote statistically significant differences between groups at the specified time points. $^{a}p \leq 0.05$, $^{b}p \leq 0.01$, and $^{c}p \leq 0.001$ denote significant differences *vs* baseline using the Holm-Sidak test for multiple comparisons showing the differences only when they occurred in one of the two groups.

(AT-MIO-16XE-50; National Instruments, Austin, TX) and analyzed using custom developed software (Labview 6.0, National Instruments).

Cytokine Measurements. In the *HS-65*$_{BV}$*+VP* series, plasma levels of IL-6, IL-8, IL-10, and TNF-α were measured by a prototype 4-plex porcine cytokine electrochemiluminescence assay kit (Lot# Z00X2801, Meso Scale Discovery) using a QuickPlex SQ 120 multiplex imager (Meso Scale Discovery). The assay was performed as recommended by the manufacturer. Standards were prepared using IL-6, IL-8, IL-10, and TNF-α calibrators provided in the assay kit after a series of dilutions representing concentrations of 10,000 pg/ml, 2500 pg/ml, 625 pg/ml, 156.3 pg/ml, 39.1 pg/ml, 9.8 pg/ml, 2.4 pg/ml, and 0 pg/ml. Plasma collected at baseline, end of blood withdrawal, 24 hours after resuscitation, and 72 hours after resuscitation previously stored at −80°C was thawed in ice and centrifuged at 2,320 *g* for 10 minutes. Twenty five microliters of the plasma was used for the assay. All standards and samples were run in duplicates. Concentrations were calculated from a 4-parameter logistic equation standard curve using Discovery Workbench software (Meso Scale Discovery). Lower limit of detection (LLOD) of the assay was 2 pg/ml for IL-6, 5 pg/ml for IL-8, 1 pg/ml for IL-10, and 4 pg/ml for TNF-α. The coefficient of variation between the duplicate samples was <5%.

Cardiac Function. Indices of cardiac function were derived from left ventricular pressures, reporting the maximal rate of left ventricular pressure increase (dP/dt_{max}) and pressure decrease (dP/dt_{min}), the stroke volume index (SVI), and the left and right ventricular stroke work (LVSWI and RVSWI), corresponding to SVI times the difference between the systolic and end-diastolic left ventricular pressures (LVSWI) and SVI times the difference between the mean pulmonary and right atrial pressures (RVSWI) expressed in centijoules (cJ) by multiplying by 0.013332 [28].

Statistical Analysis

SigmaPlot 11.0 (Systat Software, Point Richmond, CA) was used for statistical analysis. For all repetitive variables, two-way repeated measures ANOVA was used to test for the treatment effect between groups and their interaction over time identifying differences at specified time points when present. For clarity, statistical results are presented only at time points shown in tables and figures, but reflect analysis of all available time points. Kaplan-Meier survival curves were plotted and statistical differences assessed using the Gehan-Breslow test. The hematological data from survivors in the *HS-50*$_{BV}$ and *HS-65*$_{BV}$*+VP series* were pooled; analyzing changes from baseline to 72 hours post-resuscitation within each treatment group by paired *t*-test and differences between groups by unpaired *t*-test. The data were

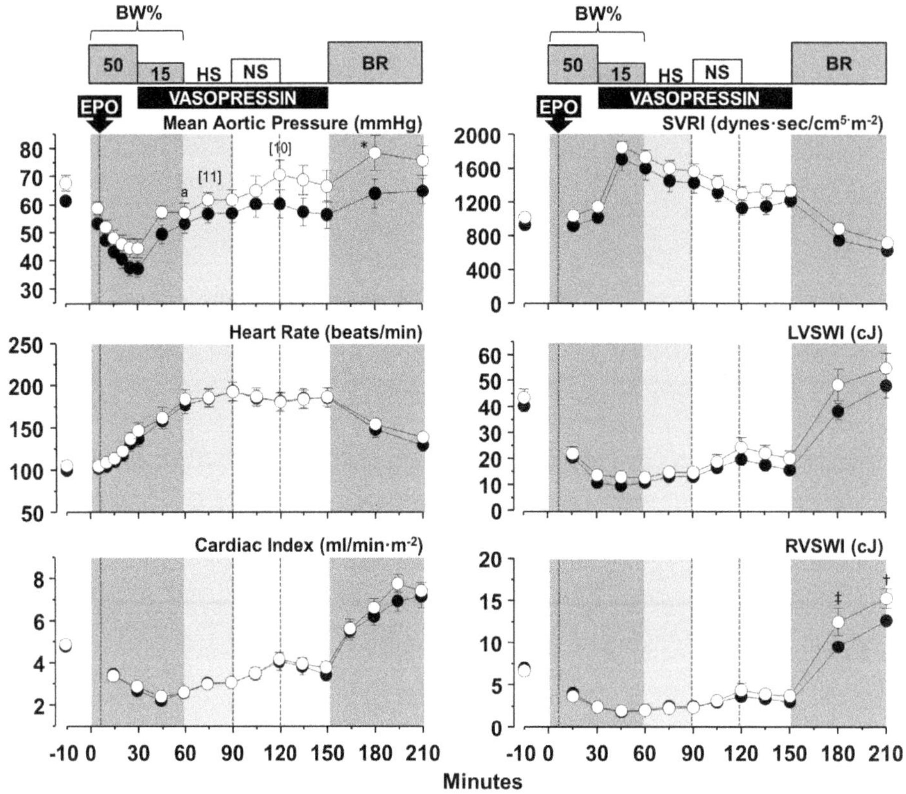

Figure 6. Hemodynamic and myocardial effects of EPO (open circles, n = 12) compared with vehicle control (closed circles, n = 12) in *HS-65$_{BV}$+VP*. Numbers in brackets indicate when the number of animals decreased from the preceding time point consequent to death of the animal. BL, baseline; BW, blood withdrawal; HS, hemorrhagic shock; NS, normal saline; BR, blood reinfusion; Ao, aortic pressure; SVRI, systemic vascular resistance index; LVSWI, left ventricular stroke work index; RVWI, right ventricular stroke work index. Values are shown as mean ± SEM. Differences between groups were analyzed by two-way repeated measures ANOVA. There was an overall statistically significant treatment effect for LVSWI ($p = 0.035$) and an overall statistically significant interaction between treatment and time for Ao mean ($p = 0.002$). *$p \leq 0.05$, †$p \leq 0.01$, and ‡$p \leq 0.001$ denote statistically significant differences between groups at the specified time points. $^{a}p \leq 0.05$, $^{b}p \leq 0.01$, and $^{c}p \leq 0.001$ denote significant differences *vs* baseline using the Holm-Sidak test for multiple comparisons showing the differences only when they occurred in one of the two groups.

presented as means ± SD unless otherwise stated. A two-tailed probability value of $p<0.05$ was considered significant.

Results

No unexpected adverse events occurred. Demise occurred attributed to hemorrhagic shock consequent to hemodynamic compromise during the acute phase and to organ dysfunction during the 72 hour observation interval.

Baseline

No significant differences between EPO and control groups were observed at baseline within each series as shown on Table 1 and on each successive tables and figures, except for RVSWI in *HS-50$_{BV}$*.

EPO plasma levels

Plasma levels of EPO averaging 3 representative experiments from series *HS-50$_{BV}$* are shown in Figure 3 confirming the adequacy of the intraosseous route yielding levels in excess of 20 U/ml for at least 120 minutes after administering 1,200 U/kg.

Resuscitation and survival

The initial resuscitation rate for all three series and subsequent 72 hour survival for *HS-50$_{BV}$* and *HS-65$_{BV}$ +VP* are shown in Figure 2. For the EPO and the control group combined; *HS-50$_{BV}$* resulted in 88% initial resuscitation and 60% survival; *HS-65$_{BV}$* resulted in only 25% initial resuscitation (noticing that demise started after removing more than 50% of the blood volume); and *HS-65$_{BV}$ +VP* resulted in 92% initial resuscitation (preventing demise after exceeding 50% of blood volume withdrawal) and 83% survival. EPO had no effect on initial resuscitation or subsequent survival in any of the three series.

Hemodynamic and myocardial function

Blood removal triggered a chronotropic response that attenuated reductions in cardiac index and aortic blood pressure yielding a relatively stable hemodynamic state after completion of blood removal despite marked reduction in left and right ventricular work indexes, attributed mainly to reduced preload (Figures 4–6). Administration of normal saline, three-fold the volume of blood removed in series *HS-50$_{BV}$* and *HS-65$_{BV}$*, markedly increased cardiac index (to levels higher than baseline), normalized left and right ventricular work indexes, and reduced the chronotropic response without substantial change in aortic pressure (Figures 4

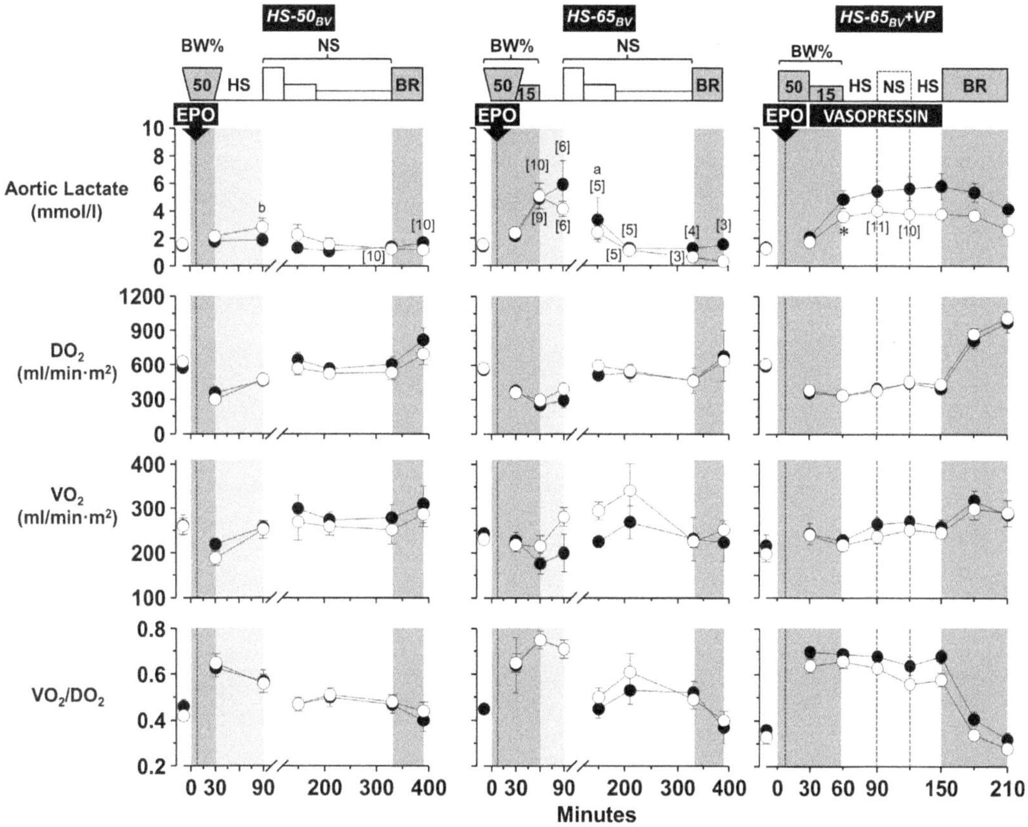

Figure 7. Metabolic effects of EPO (open circles) compared with vehicle control (closed circles) in series *HS-50$_{BV}$*, *HS-65$_{BV}$*, and *HS-65$_{BV}$+VP*. Numbers in brackets indicate when the number of animals decreased from the preceding time point. BW, blood withdrawal; HS, hemorrhagic shock; NS, normal saline; BR, blood reinfusion. Values are shown as mean ± SEM. Differences between groups were analyzed by two-way repeated measures ANOVA for each series separately. There were no overall significant treatment effects. However, there was an overall statistically significant interaction between treatment and time for lactate in series *HS-65$_{BV}$+VP* ($p = 0.007$). *$p \leq 0.05$ denotes statistically significant differences between groups at the specified time points. $^{a}p \leq 0.05$ and $^{b}p \leq 0.01$ denote significant differences *vs* baseline using the Holm-Sidak test for multiple comparisons showing the differences only when they occurred in one of the two groups.

and 5). Administration of vasopressin in *HS-65$_{BV}$+VP* with or without normal saline (equal to half the volume of blood removed) increased systemic vascular resistance and aortic pressure with a modest increase in cardiac index and left and right stroke work indexes (Figure 6). Blood reinfusion maintained or increased cardiac index, aortic pressure, and work indexes in *HS-50$_{BV}$* and *HS-65$_{BV}$*; whereas in *HS-65$_{BV}$+VP* the predominant effect was increase in cardiac index and work indices (Figure 4–6). Relatively minor effects that varied contingent on the series were observed in relation to EPO. In *HS-50$_{BV}$*, EPO appeared to blunt the hemodynamic and myocardial response to HS and the subsequent fluid resuscitation and blood reinfusion interval (Figure 4). The opposite effect was observed in *HS-65$_{BV}$* and *HS-65$_{BV}$+VP* in which favorable hemodynamic and myocardial response were more prominent in the EPO group during HS and the subsequent fluid resuscitation and blood reinfusion intervals (Figure 5 and 6).

Oxygen metabolism and lactatemia

The chronotropic response along with the expected increase in systemic oxygen extraction in *HS-50$_{BV}$* allowed adequate adaptation to HS evidenced by minimal lactatemia and high resuscitation and survival rates (Figure 7 and Figure 2, *HS-50$_{BV}$*). Greater blood volume removal in *HS-65$_{BV}$* exhausted the adaptive response evidenced by higher systemic oxygen extraction, higher levels of lactic acid, and substantial demise after removing more than 50% of the blood volume (Figure 7 and Figure 2, *HS-65$_{BV}$*). Use of vasopressin in *HS-65$_{BV}$+VP* enabled survival despite similar exhaustion of the adaptive response and was attributed to maintaining a higher aortic pressure required for coronary perfusion (Figure 7 and Figure 2, *HS-65$_{BV}$+VP*). Relatively minor metabolic effects related to EPO were observed, highlighting an attenuation of lactate increase in *HS-65$_{BV}$+VP* (Figure 7).

Myocardial metabolism

In *HS-65$_{BV}$*, potential myocardial metabolic effects produced by severe HS were assessed measuring myocardial oxygen, lactate, and pCO_2 differences across the coronary circuit. As shown in Table 2, HS was not associated with myocardial ischemia (despite ischemia in other organs evidenced by lactatemia), with EPO and control groups behaving similarly.

Effects of fluid resuscitation

The effect of low-volume fluid administration was assessed in the *HS-65$_{BV}$+VP series* and shown in Figure 8 and Table 3. Fluid administration promoted an increase in cardiac index, mean aortic pressure, and left ventricular dP/dt_{max} (Figure 8) accompanied by attenuation of systemic oxygen extraction and faster normalization of lactic acidosis (Table 3). Of the 12 animals that received fluids, 11 were resuscitated and remained alive at 72 hours. Of the 12

Table 2. Myocardial Metabolic Effects of EPO in *HS-65*$_{BV}$.

	Baseline	End BW 50%	End BW 15%	End HS	NS	End NS	End BR
	−10 min	**30 min**	**60 min**	**90 min**	**210 min**	**330 min**	**390 min**
Ao O_2 Content (ml/dl)							
CTR	14.1±1.2	13.9±1.9	13.7±1.3[9]	12.6±2.7[6]	9.3±1.4[5]	8.1±1.3[4]	12.2±1.8[3]
EPO	13.6±1.3	13.6±1.4	13.3±1.4[10]	13.3±1.4[6]	8.8±1.0[5]	7.9±0.9[3]	13.0±1.0
GCV O_2 Content (ml/dl)							
CTR	3.6±1.6	3.5±1.5	2.5±0.6^c	2.7±0.6^c	3.0±0.4^c	1.3±1.5	4.01±1.4
EPO	2.8±0.8	2.8±0.8	2.6±1.3	2.6±0.3	2.9±0.9	2.9±0.3	4.04±1.3
O_2 Extraction Ratio ([Ao-GCV]/Ao)							
CTR	0.75±0.10	0.76±0.09	0.81±0.05	0.78±0.04	0.67±0.03	0.66±0.07	0.67±0.08
EPO	0.80±0.05	0.79±0.05	0.80±0.09	0.80±0.02	0.66±0.11	0.63±0.04	0.69±0.11
GCV-Ao Lactate Gradient (mmol/l)							
CTR	−0.8±0.5	−1.2±0.7	−0.9±0.7	−1.1±0.6	0.1±0.3	−0.0±0.7	−0.5±0.5
EPO	−0.9±0.5	−1.5±0.5	−1.6±0.4	−1.3±0.8	0.0±0.4	−0.2±0.1	0.0±0.0
GCV-Ao pCO_2 Gradient (mmHg)							
CTR	13±4	15±4	19±4^a	16±4	12±6	11±9	10±3
EPO	15±3	14±2	16±10	18±3	13±4	9±2	12±3

Numbers in brackets indicate when the sample size decreased from the initial twelve animals. BW, blood withdrawal; HS, hemorrhagic shock; NS, normal saline; BR, blood reinfusion; EPO, erythropoietin; CTR, control; Ao, aorta; GCV, great cardiac vein. Values are mean ± SD. The data was analyzed using two-way repeated measures ANOVA. There were no overall significant treatment effects and no overall statistically significant interactions between treatment and time. $^a p \leq 0.05$; $^c p \leq 0.001$ denote significant differences *vs* baseline using the Holm-Sidak test for multiple comparisons showing the differences only when they occurred in one of the two groups.

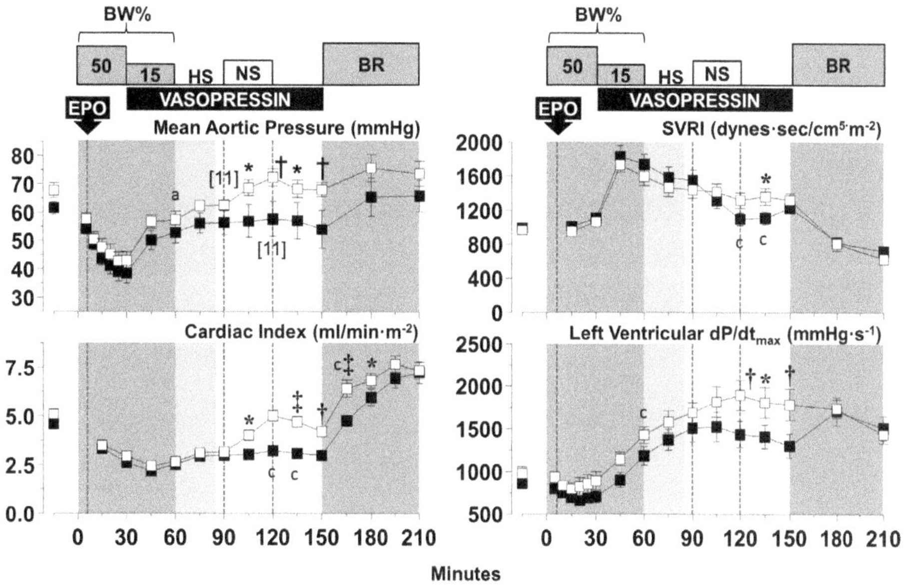

Figure 8. Hemodynamic effects of fluid resuscitation (open symbols, n = 12) and no fluid resuscitation (closed symbols, n = 12) in series *HS-65*$_{BV}$*+VP*. Numbers in brackets indicate when the number of animals decreased from the preceding time point consequent to death of the animal. BL, baseline; BW, blood withdrawal; HS, hemorrhagic shock; NS, normal saline; BR, blood reinfusion; Ao, aortic pressure; SVRI, systemic vascular resistance index. Values are shown as mean ± SEM. Differences between groups were analyzed by two-way repeated measures ANOVA. There was an overall statistically significant treatment effect for cardiac index ($p = 0.021$). There were also overall statistically significant interactions between treatment and time for cardiac index ($p < 0.001$) and SVRI ($p < 0.001$). *$p \leq 0.05$, †$p \leq 0.01$, and ‡$p \leq 0.001$ denote statistically significant differences between groups at the specified time points. [a]$p \leq 0.05$, and [c]$p \leq 0.001$ denote significant differences *vs* baseline using the Holm-Sidak test for multiple comparisons showing the differences only when they occurred in one of the two groups.

Table 3. Metabolic Effect of Fluid Resuscitation in *HS-65*$_{BV}$*+VP*.

	Baseline	End BW 65%	HS/NS	End HS	End BR
	−10 min	60 min	120 min	150 min	210 min
Aortic Lactate (mmol/l)					
NS	1.3±0.7	3.9±1.0	4.0±1.0[11] *	3.9±0.9*	2.7±1.0*
No NS	1.3±0.5	4.0±2.4	5.6±3.1[11]	5.8±3.3	4.1±1.9
Aortic pH					
NS	7.48±0.05	7.41±0.06	7.33±0.03	7.37±0.04	7.40±0.03
No NS	7.47±0.04	7.38±0.06	7.33±0.06	7.34±0.02	7.37±0.02
Aortic O_2 Content (ml/dl)					
NS	12.7±1.3	13.3±1.3	10.1±1.1‡	10.9±1.0*[c]	13.0±0.6
No NS	12.1±2.1	12.8±1.8[a]	12.4±1.7	12.4±1.5	14.1±1.9[c]
Venous O_2 Content (ml/dl)					
NS	8.1±1.2	4.6±1.1	4.7±0.7	4.7±0.9	9.2±0.7
No NS	8.0±1.4	4.0±1.3	4.2±1.6	3.8±1.6	9.8±2.3
VO_2/DO_2 (ratio)					
NS	0.36±0.10	0.66±0.08	0.54±0.04*	0.57±0.07*	0.29±0.04*[a]
No NS	0.33±0.09	0.69±0.08	0.67±0.11	0.70±0.11	0.31±0.12

Numbers in brackets indicate when the sample size decreased from the initial twelve animals. Values are mean ± SD. BW, blood withdrawal; HS, hemorrhagic shock; NS, normal saline; BR, blood reinfusion; VO_2/DO_2, oxygen consumption divided by oxygen delivery. The data was analyzed using two-way repeated measures ANOVA. There were overall statistically significant interactions between treatment and time for aortic pH ($p = 0.043$), aortic O_2 content ($p \leq 0.001$), and VO_2/DO_2 ratio ($p \leq 0.001$). There was no overall statistically significant treatment effect. *$p \leq 0.05$ and ‡$p \leq 0.001$ denote statistically significant differences between groups at the specified time point. [a]$p \leq 0.05$ and [c]$p \leq 0.001$ denote statistically significant differences *vs* baseline using the Holm-Sidak test for multiple comparisons showing the differences only when they occurred in one of the two groups.

Table 4. Effect of EPO on Organ Function in $HS\text{-}65_{BV}$+*VP*.

	Baseline	Post-Resuscitation		
	−10 min	**24 h**	**48 h**	**72 h**
Creatinine (mg/dl)				
CTR	1.3±0.2	1.5±1.4	1.4±1.7 [11]	0.9±0.1^{b} [10]
EPO	1.0±0.2	0.9±0.2 [10]	0.9±0.2	0.9±0.1
Blood Urea Nitrogen (mg/dl)				
CTR	10±5	22±22	15±24	7±2
EPO	9±3	9±3	7±3	7±2
AST (U/l)				
CTR	35±7	400±501^{c}	188±204	113±118
EPO	32±6	168±101†	85±43	67±26
ALT (U/l)				
CTR	51±10	126±109^{c}	107±51^{c}	100±36
EPO	53±8	82±24*	86±26	58±23^{c}
Troponin I (ng/ml)				
CTR	0.22±0.18	1.47±2.40^{c}	0.48±1.06	0.22±0.24
EPO	0.15±0.09	0.41±0.29	0.20±0.47	0.12±0.09*
Neurologic Deficit Score				
CTR	0±0	26±45^{a}	15±45	2±6
EPO	0±0	13±35	0±0	0±0

Numbers in brackets indicate when the sample size decreased from the initial twelve animals. Values are mean ± SD. CTR, control; EPO, erythropoietin. The data was analyzed using two-way repeated measures ANOVA. There was no overall significant treatment effect and no overall statistically significant interactions between treatment and time. $^{*}p \le 0.05$ and $^{\dagger}p \le 0.01$ denote statistically significant differences between groups at the specified time points. $^{a}p \le 0.05$, $^{b}p \le 0.01$, and $^{c}p \le 0.001$ denote statistically significant differences *vs* baseline using the Holm-Sidak test for multiple comparisons showing the differences only when they occurred in one of the two groups.

Table 5. Effect of EPO on Plasma Cytokines in $HS\text{-}65_{BV}$+*VP*.

	Baseline	End BR	Post-Resuscitation	
	−10 min	**210 min**	**24 h**	**72 h**
IL-6 (pg/ml)				
CTR	42±28 [34;25]	79±55 [63; 34]	794±2515 [59, 53]	115±152 [66; 43]
EPO	30±28 [16;43]	106±73 [94; 57]	58±72 [25;30]	34±24 [26;28]
IL-8 (pg/ml)				
CTR	18±13 [14;22]	34±4 [24;27]	17±22 [6;15]	10±5 [12;8]
EPO	18±14 [15;15]	18±12 [15;17]	7±4 [5;3]	8±5 [7;2]
IL-10 (pg/ml)				
CTR	23±50; [8;8]	70±81 [33;28]	16±14 [11;9]	11±9 [8;4]
EPO	12±7 [12;9]	207±281 [70; 174]^{b†}	15±16 [7;8]	10±6 [8;3]
TNF-α (pg/ml)				
CTR	31±12 [30;9]	31±9 [33;10]	24±13 [24;11]	29±11 [28;12]
EPO	24±7 [21;6]	37±26 [27;15]^{a}	20±8 [18;4]	24±5 [22;5]

Samples were available for each of the 12 control (CTR) pigs including the 10 that survived at 72 hours; but, for only 10 of the erythropoietin (EPO) treated pigs, which included all the survivors. Values are mean ± SD showing also the median with interquartile range in brackets as values for several time events were not normally distributed. BR, blood reinfusion; IL, interleukin; TNF-α, tumor necrosis factor-α. The data was analyzed using two-way repeated measures ANOVA. There was no overall statistically significant treatment effect. There was a statistically significant time effect for IL-8 ($p = 0.011$), IL-10 ($p \le 0.001$) and TNF-α ($p = 0.006$) and there was a borderline statistically significant interactions between treatment and time for IL-10 ($p = 0.062$). $^{\dagger}p \le 0.003$ denotes a statistically significant difference between groups at the specified time point. $^{a}p \le 0.05$, $^{b}p \le 0.001$ denote statistically significant differences from baseline within each group using the Holm-Sidak test for multiple comparisons.

Table 6. Effect of Fluid Resuscitation on Plasma Cytokines in *HS-65*$_{BV}$*+VP*.

	Baseline	End BR	Post-Resuscitation	
	−10 min	210 min	24 h	72 h
IL-6 (pg/ml)				
NS	30±22 [23;23]	62±27 [57; 24]	40±23 [38;20]	42±25 [38;33]
No NS	43±33 [33;45]	120±77 [101; 68]	880±2620 [83; 132]	115±164 [69; 61]
IL-8 (pg/ml)				
NS	16±14 [10;17]	16±11 [17;17]	9±9 [5;4]	8±4 [6;5]
No NS	20±11 [19;13]	37±42 [32;27] *	16±23 [5;9]	11±5 [11;9]
IL-10 (pg/ml)				
NS	25±53 [9;11]	84±120 [38;35]	8±4 [7;4]	10±6 [9;3]
No NS	11±5 [9;6]	181±262 [67; 206][a]*	23±17 [14;28]	12±9 [8;3]
TNF-α (pg/ml)				
NS	28±15 [21;16]	30±10 [29;10]	26±13 [25;17]	30±11 [27;13]
No NS	27±5 [27;5]	38±24 [31;16]	18±7 [19;5]	23±4 [22;3]

Samples were available for all 11 pigs in each group that survived the initial 24 hours and for all the 9 that survived at 72 hours from the group without fluid resuscitation. Values are mean ± SD showing also the median with interquartile range in brackets as values for several time events were not normally distributed. BR, blood reinfusion; NS, normal saline; IL, interleukin; TNF-α, tumor necrosis factor-α. The data was analyzed using two-way repeated measures ANOVA. There was no overall statistically significant treatment effect. There was a statistically significant time effect for IL-8 ($p = 0.008$), IL-10 ($p \leq 0.001$), and TNF-α ($p = 0.008$). *$p \leq 0.05$ denotes a statistically significant difference between groups at the specified time points. [a]$p \leq 0.001$ denotes a statistically significant difference from baseline using the Holm-Sidak test for multiple comparisons.

animals that did not receive fluids, 11 were also resuscitated but only 9 were alive at 72 hours; a difference however that was not statically significant.

Organ injury and function

The post-resuscitation effect on various organs was assessed daily in *HS-65*$_{BV}$*+VP*. As shown in Table 4, EPO treated animals had an attenuated increase in AST, ALT, troponin I, and less neurological deficit at some point during the post-resuscitation phase. There were statistically insignificant differences suggesting less kidney injury in the EPO group. There was no difference in the percentage of lung water at 72 hours between EPO and control pigs (81.0±0.6% *vs* 81.8±1.0%).

Plasma cytokines

Plasma IL-6, IL-8, IL-10, and TNF-α were measured in the *HS-65*$_{BV}$*+VP* series, analyzing the effects of EPO (Table 5) and the effects of fluid resuscitation (Table 6). Overall there was a time effect with increases in IL-8 and IL-10 by the end of blood reinfusion reversing to baseline by 72 hours. Most prominently, EPO was associated with an increase in IL-10 by the end of blood reinfusion (Table 5). Administration of normal saline blunted increases in IL-8 and in IL-10 (Table 6).

Hematological effects

Pooled data from animals that survived in the *HS-50*$_{BV}$ and *HS-65*$_{BV}$*+VP* series (18 animals in control group and 17 in EPO group) showed no differences between treatment groups at baseline with cell counts within normal for swine [29]. Red blood cell count and hematocrit increased relative to baseline in both

Table 7. Hematological Effects of EPO in *HS-50*$_{BV}$ and *HS-65*$_{BV}$*+VP*.

		Baseline	72 h Post-Resuscitation
Red Blood Cells (10^6/µl)	CTR	5.5±0.4[[18]]	6.0±0.8[a]
	EPO	5.6±0.6[[17]]	6.8±0.7*[c]
Hematocrit (%)	CTR	31.5±1.7	34.4±4.8[a]
	EPO	31.6±2.1	39.3±4.5*[c]
White Blood Cells (10^3/µl)	CTR	18.0±4.0	20.9±4.9
	EPO	20.0±3.5	21.0±5.5
Platelets (10^3/µl)	CTR	312±68	332±106
	EPO	304±85	397±164[a]

Values are mean ± SD. CTR, control; EPO, erythropoietin. Data was pooled from *HS-50*$_{BV}$ and *HS-65*$_{BV}$*+VP series*. Numbers in bracket indicate pooled sample size. Unpaired *t*-test was used to compare differences in the pooled hematological data between treatment groups at given time points. *$p \leq 0.05$. Paired *t*-test was used to compare pooled hematological data from *HS-50*$_{BV}$ and *HS-65*$_{BV}$*+VP series* at baseline and post-resuscitation within each treatment group. [a]$p \leq 0.05$ and [c]$p \leq 0.001$. There were no statistically significant differences between groups at baseline.

groups at 72 hours post-resuscitation but to a greater extent in the EPO group (Table 7). Over the same time interval, platelet count increased but only in the EPO group whereas the white blood cell count remained unchanged.

Discussion

The present study failed to demonstrate a beneficial (or detrimental) effect of EPO on initial resuscitability or subsequent survival in a swine model of HS regardless of its severity. The work was conducted in three consecutive HS series modeling mild severity, high severity with high fatality despite aggressive fluid resuscitation, and high severity with low fatality associated with vasopressin infusion and low-fluid or no-fluid resuscitation. EPO in the last series featuring high severity with low fatality increased plasma levels of the anti-inflammatory cytokine IL-10, attenuated lactatemia, and lessened transient injury to the liver, heart, and brain based on enzyme release and clinical neurological deficit. In addition, the study addressed several current aspects of HS management showing the efficacy of vasopressin infusion and restrictive fluid resuscitation.

EPO Effect

The dose of EPO chosen for the present experiments (1,200 U/kg) was extrapolated from a dose previously used in a study targeting sudden cardiac arrest victims (90,000 U) [21]. A lower dose (12,000 U) was deemed effective in a pilot human assessing potential protection after acute myocardial infarction [30]. In the present study, we confirmed that the chosen EPO dose – delivered through the intraosseous route – reached the bloodstream (Figure 3) attaining plasma levels that exceeded 30 U/ml for the initial 60 minutes decreasing to approximately 20 U/ml after 120 minutes. Only a brief exposure to EPO is required to trigger a sustained protective effect during HS [31] and levels above 5 U/ml are sufficient to elicit cytoprotection [32]. Accordingly, the lack of effects of EPO on resuscitability and survival occurred despite a sustained presence of EPO in the bloodstream and evidence of biological activity given the significant increase in hematocrit and platelets after 72 hours (Table 5).

The lack of impact on initial resuscitability from HS likely reflected the mechanism of death. Animals died preceded by progressive reductions in blood pressure that at some point precipitously compromised coronary perfusion and cardiac function. However, there was no evidence of protracted myocardial ischemia before demise upon which EPO could have exerted an acute "protective" effect, as previously reported during resuscitation from cardiac arrest [20]. The lack of myocardial ischemia was shown in series $HS\text{-}65_{BV}$ (the series with the highest HS severity and mortality), in which the lactate gradient across the coronary circuit was negative (i.e., lactate utilization) and the PCO_2 gradient was not increased [25], both indicating absence of myocardial ischemia (Table 2). At the same time, substantial systemic lactic acidosis developed in series $HS\text{-}65_{BV}$ and series $HS\text{-}65_{BV}+VP$, indicating critical reductions in oxygen delivery prompting anaerobic metabolism in other tissues. In $HS\text{-}65_{BV}+VP$, EPO attenuated increases in lactic acid, consistent with a beneficial effect at the mitochondrial level as we have reported in a rat model of cardiac arrest [20]. Likewise, there was attenuation of markers of organ injury in EPO treated pigs in the $HS\text{-}65_{BV}+VP$ series. The protective effects at the cell level reported by us [20] and others [32] in rats involve at the very least Akt activation (phosphorylation); a kinase that plays a key role in cell survival and other adaptive responses including mitochondrial bioenergetic function and enhanced myocardial contractility [33,34]. In addition, plasma IL-10 was higher in pigs that received EPO at the end of blood reinfusion. IL-10 mediates anti-inflammatory effects and EPO can increase production of IL-10 [35–37]; pointing to the pleiotropic effect of EPO and mediation of additional effects that could be potentially beneficial for HS. The levels of IL-6 and IL-8 (pro-inflammatory cytokines) were lower at 24 and 72 hours in pigs treated with EPO but the differences were not statistically significant.

Studying the potential clinical relevance of these effects at the organ level was beyond the scope of the present study. In clinical settings, patients are exposed to repetitive injuries after stabilization (i.e., biological, infectious, sterile, etc.) and information on whether organ susceptibility to subsequent injuries could be ameliorated by EPO would be of substantial clinical interest.

Hemodynamic Response to Hemorrhagic Shock

A prominent (adaptive) chronotropic response maintained the cardiac index in $HS\text{-}50_{BV}$ at ~80% of baseline, enabling increases in oxygen extraction to preserve aerobic metabolism and thereby yielding only minor increases in lactic acid. In series $HS\text{-}65_{BV}$ and $HS\text{-}65_{BV}+VP$, however, the cardiac index was maintained at ~62% of baseline and the oxygen extraction reached its maximum level prompting systemic lactic acidosis; most likely from tissues excluded from the circulation following redistribution of blood flow towards vital organs. Accordingly, in this swine model, the critical transition from "compensated" to "uncompensated" HS occurred after removing 50% of the blood volume.

Vasopressin

Hemodynamic crises, including HS, trigger the release of vasopressin as part of a prominent neuroendocrine stress response. However, the endogenous vasopressin response is time-limited and exogenous administration has been suggested for hemodynamic stabilization in sepsis [38,39] and HS [40,41]. In models of HS, vasopressin was comparably superior to fluid administration or epinephrine [42,43] and has been proposed as the "preferred" vasopressor agent for hemodynamic stabilization during HS [41]. In a small clinical study in civilians suffering traumatic injury with hypotension, vasopressin infusion reduced the need of resuscitation fluids [44]. Clinicaltrials.gov lists two studies examining the effects of vasopressin in civilians with HS; the AVERT Shock study by Sims, C and the VITRIS study by Wenzel, V. [45].

These reasons prompted us to select vasopressin in our last series ($HS\text{-}65_{BV}+VP$), with the dose chosen according to a previous study by Voelckel *et al.*, also in swine [42]. The timing for initiation of vasopressin infusion was based on series $HS\text{-}65_{BV}$, noticing that demise began to occur after removing greater than 50% of the blood volume (Figure 2). The effect of vasopressin infusion on resuscitability was impressive, increasing from 25% (in $HS\text{-}65_{BV}$) to 92% (in $HS\text{-}65_{BV}+VP$) for the same degree of blood volume removal (Figure 2). Moreover, 83% of the animals in $HS\text{-}65_{BV}+VP$ were alive at 72 hours and with essentially no organ dysfunction (Table 4).

Fluid Resuscitation

There is growing consensus that aggressive fluid resuscitation during HS can be detrimental [46]. Coagulation is compromised consequent to dilution of clotting factors and reduced activity by hypothermia and acidosis. Concomitantly, the endogenous fibrinolytic system is activated, tilting the hemostatic balance toward bleeding [47]. Excessive fluid also drives edema formation, which may affect the lungs and other tissues [48]. Large amounts of normal saline can precipitate hyperchloremic acidosis which has been associated with increased risk of renal injury [49] and activation of inflammatory cascades [50]. For this and other (logistic) reasons, resuscitation with minimal or no fluid is gaining acceptance. The Tactical Combat Casualty Care Guidelines recommend fluid administration during HS only when there is altered mental status (in the absence of head injury) and weak or absent peripheral pulses.

In our initial two series (i.e., $HS\text{-}50_{BV}$ and $HS\text{-}65_{BV}$), we administered normal saline 3 times the amount of blood removed according to the old paradigm resulting in a substantial increase in cardiac index (*via* preload increase) exceeding baseline levels. However, despite high initial resuscitability, the 72 hour survival was less than in the more severe $HS\text{-}65_{BV}\text{+}VP$ series suggesting that excess fluid could have been detrimental. In the $HS\text{-}65_{BV}\text{+}VP$ series, we examined the current paradigm and administered normal saline half the amount of blood removed in half of the animals and no fluids in the other half observing no differences in resuscitability or survival. Normal saline, however, had as positive effect on cardiac index, aortic pressure, and left ventricular dP/dt_{max} while reducing systemic oxygen extraction and the generation of lactic acid (Figure 8, Table 3). Thus, there was hemodynamic and metabolic benefit elicited by fluid administration which could be critical under conditions of more severe HS and when vasopressin alone is not sufficient.

Limitations

Extrapolation of the current findings to real-life battlefield resuscitation from hemorrhagic shock is limited by several factors. Upmost is modeling HS without additional tissue injury. Although HS can occur in military and (more so) in civilian settings with low-grade or unassociated tissue injury, HS in the battlefield occurs typically accompanied by substantial tissue injury. Tissue injury compounds the severity of HS partly by the specific organ dysfunction, wound contamination, and amplification of the inflammatory response. In addition, the rate of blood withdrawal was controlled by a predetermined algorithm and did not follow the natural profile of bleeding after injury. The present studies, however, allowed assessing the effects of the studied interventions on severe HS without the confounding effects of tissue injury and uncontrolled bleeding. In subsequent series we incorporated the elements of tissue injury and uncontrolled bleeding by using a liver laceration model. Other limitations include the use of anesthesia, masking some of the physiologic responses to hypovolemic shock. The naturally occurring neuropeptide in swine is lysine vasopressin whereas in humans it is arginine vasopressin (the one used in the present studies). Thus, potency may vary contingent on specific receptors and vascular beds and translation of these findings to humans will need to consider human dose-responses. Despite these limitations, our model reproduced key characteristics of resuscitation from hemorrhagic shock and provided mechanistic information under highly controlled conditions that would be difficult to obtain in a more realistic model.

Conclusions

EPO given during HS in a swine model of HS failed to alter resuscitability and 72 hour survival regardless of HS severity and concomitant treatment with fluids and vasopressin. EPO, however, attenuated lactate increases and acute injury to the liver, heart, and brain based on enzyme release and neurological deficit scores. The studies also showed that vasopressin infusion with restrictive fluid administration is highly effective for hemodynamic stabilization and subsequent survival.

Supporting Information

Datafile S1 Hemodynamic and metabolic data from the three hemorrhagic shock series.

Checklist S1 ARRIVE guidelines checklist.

Acknowledgments

This research was supported by the Telemedicine and Advanced Technology Research Center (TATRC) at the U.S. Army Medical Research and Materiel Command (USAMRMC) Fort Detrick, MD under contract number: W81XWH-11-2-0019.

We also thank the Pathology Laboratory and the Pharmacy Services at Captain James A. Lovell Federal Health Care Center for their support processing blood samples and facilitating the purchase of the various drugs used in the project.

Non-Endorsement Disclaimer: The views, opinions and/or findings contained in this report are those of the author(s) and should not be construed as an official Department of the Army position, policy or decision unless so designated by other documentation.

Author Contributions

Conceived and designed the experiments: RJG. Performed the experiments: VBL KW BMC. Analyzed the data: VBL KW BMC RJG. Contributed reagents/materials/analysis tools: AB YM SV JR. Wrote the paper: VBL RJG.

References

1. Kauvar DS, Lefering R, Wade CE (2006) Impact of hemorrhage on trauma outcome: an overview of epidemiology, clinical presentations, and therapeutic considerations. J Trauma 60: S3–11.
2. Eastridge BJ, Mabry RL, Seguin P, Cantrell J, Tops T, et al. (2012) Death on the battlefield (2001-2011): implications for the future of combat casualty care. J Trauma Acute Care Surg 73: S431–S437.
3. Cai Z, Manalo DJ, Wei G, Rodriguez ER, Fox-Talbot K, et al. (2003) Hearts from rodents exposed to intermittent hypoxia or erythropoietin are protected against ischemia-reperfusion injury. Circulation 108: 79–85.
4. Moon C, Krawczyk M, Ahn D, Ahmet I, Paik D, et al. (2003) Erythropoietin reduces myocardial infarction and left ventricular functional decline after coronary artery ligation in rats. Proc Natl Acad Sci U S A 100: 11612–11617.
5. Parsa CJ, Matsumoto A, Kim J, Riel RU, Pascal LS, et al. (2003) A novel protective effect of erythropoietin in the infarcted heart. J Clin Invest 112: 999–1007.
6. Tramontano AF, Muniyappa R, Black AD, Blendea MC, Cohen I, et al. (2003) Erythropoietin protects cardiac myocytes from hypoxia-induced apoptosis through an Akt-dependent pathway. Biochem Biophys Res Commun 308: 990–994.
7. Vilarinho KA, de Oliveira PP, Saad MJ, Eghtesady P, Filho LM, et al. (2013) Erythropoietin protects the systolic function of neonatal hearts against ischaemia/reperfusion injury. Eur J Cardiothorac Surg 43: 156–162.
8. Brines ML, Ghezzi P, Keenan S, Agnello D, de Lanerolle NC, et al. (2000) Erythropoietin crosses the blood-brain barrier to protect against experimental brain injury. Proc Natl Acad Sci U S A 97: 10526–10531.
9. Siren AL, Fratelli M, Brines M, Goemans C, Casagrande S, et al. (2001) Erythropoietin prevents neuronal apoptosis after cerebral ischemia and metabolic stress. Proc Natl Acad Sci U S A 98: 4044–4049.
10. Celik M, Gokmen N, Erbayraktar S, Akhisaroglu M, Konakc S, et al. (2002) Erythropoietin prevents motor neuron apoptosis and neurologic disability in experimental spinal cord ischemic injury. Proc Natl Acad Sci U S A 99: 2258–2263.
11. Simon F, Scheuerle A, Groger M, Vcelar B, McCook O, et al. (2011) Comparison of carbamylated erythropoietin-FC fusion protein and recombinant human erythropoietin during porcine aortic balloon occlusion-induced spinal cord ischemia/reperfusion injury. Intensive Care Med 37: 1525–1533.
12. Vesey DA, Cheung C, Pat B, Endre Z, Gobe G, et al. (2004) Erythropoietin protects against ischaemic acute renal injury. Nephrol Dial Transplant 19: 348–355.

13. Abdelrahman M, Sharples EJ, McDonald MC, Collin M, Patel NS, et al. (2004) Erythropoietin attenuates the tissue injury associated with hemorrhagic shock and myocardial ischemia. Shock 22: 63–69.
14. Wu WT, Lin NT, Subeq YM, Lee RP, Chen IH, et al. (2010) Erythropoietin protects severe haemorrhagic shock-induced organ damage in conscious rats. Injury 41: 724–730.
15. Shimoda M, Sawada T, Iwasaki Y, Mori S, Kijima H, et al. (2009) Erythropoietin strongly protects the liver from ischemia-reperfusion injury in a pig model. Hepatogastroenterology 56: 470–475.
16. Buemi M, Vaccaro M, Sturiale A, Galeano MR, Sansotta C, et al. (2002) Recombinant human erythropoietin influences revascularization and healing in a rat model of random ischaemic flaps. Acta Derm Venereol 82: 411–417.
17. Bohr S, Patel SJ, Shen K, Vitalo AG, Brines M, et al. (2013) Alternative erythropoietin-mediated signaling prevents secondary microvascular thrombosis and inflammation within cutaneous burns. Proc Natl Acad Sci U S A 110: 3513–3518.
18. Singh D, Kolarova JD, Wang S, Ayoub IM, Gazmuri RJ (2007) Myocardial protection by erythropoietin during resuscitation from ventricular fibrillation. Am J Ther 14: 361–368.
19. Borovnik-Lesjak V, Whitehouse K, Baetiong A, Artin B, Radhakrishnan J, et al. (2013) High-dose erythropoietin during cardiac resuscitation lessens postresuscitation myocardial stunning in swine. Transl Res 162: 110–121.
20. Radhakrishnan J, Upadhyaya MP, Ng M, Edelheit A, Moy HM, et al. (2013) Erythropoietin facilitates resuscitation from ventricular fibrillation by signaling protection of mitochondrial bioenergetic function in rats. Am J Transl Res 5: 316–326.
21. Grmec S, Strnad M, Kupnik D, Sinkovic A, Gazmuri RJ (2009) Erythropoietin facilitates the return of spontaneous circulation and survival in victims of out-of-hospital cardiac arrest. Resuscitation 80: 631–637.
22. Kao NR, Xenocostas A, Driman DK, Rui T, Huang W, et al. (2011) Recombinant human erythropoietin improves gut barrier function in a hemorrhagic shock and resuscitation rat model. J Trauma 71: S456–S461.
23. Kao RL, Xenocostas A, Rui T, Huang W, Martin CM (2010) The effect of erythropoietin on microcirculation perfusion and tissue bioenergetics of the small intestine in a hemorrhagic shock and resuscitation rat model. J Trauma 68: 1342–1348.
24. Berg RA, Otto CW, Kern KB, Sanders AB, Hilwig RW, et al. (1994) High-dose epinephrine results in greater early mortality after resuscitation from prolonged cardiac arrest in pigs: a prospective, randomized study. Crit Care Med 22: 282–290.
25. Gudipati CV, Weil MH, Gazmuri RJ, Deshmukh HG, Bisera J, et al. (1990) Increases in coronary vein CO2 during cardiac resuscitation. J Appl Physiol 68: 1405–1408.
26. Morrison CA, Carrick MM, Norman MA, Scott BG, Welsh FJ, et al. (2011) Hypotensive resuscitation strategy reduces transfusion requirements and severe postoperative coagulopathy in trauma patients with hemorrhagic shock: preliminary results of a randomized controlled trial. J Trauma 70: 652–663.
27. Kelley KW, Curtis SE, Marzan GT, Karara HM, Anderson CR (1973) Body surface area of female swine. J Anim Sci 36: 927–930.
28. Faybik P, Lahner D, Schramm W (2010) A longstanding error by Ernest Henry Starling (author reply 1584–5). Resuscitation 81: 1584–1585.
29. Jonasson R, Johannisson A, Jacobson M, Fellstrom C, Jensen-Waern M (2004) Differences in lymphocyte subpopulations and cell counts before and after experimentally induced swine dysentery. J Med Microbiol 53: 267–272.
30. Ozawa T, Toba K, Suzuki H, Kato K, Iso Y, et al. (2010) Single-dose intravenous administration of recombinant human erythropoietin is a promising treatment for patients with acute myocardial infarction - randomized controlled pilot trial of EPO/AMI-1 study -. Circ J 74: 1415–1423.
31. Brines M, Cerami A (2008) Erythropoietin-mediated tissue protection: reducing collateral damage from the primary injury response. J Intern Med 264: 405–432.
32. Nandra KK, Collino M, Rogazzo M, Fantozzi R, Patel NS, et al. (2013) Pharmacological preconditioning with erythropoietin attenuates the organ injury and dysfunction induced in a rat model of hemorrhagic shock. Dis Model Mech 6: 701–709.
33. Beiser DG, Wojcik KR, Zhao D, Orbelyan GA, Hamann KJ, et al. (2010) Akt1 genetic deficiency limits hypothermia cardioprotection following murine cardiac arrest. Am J Physiol Heart Circ Physiol 298: H1761–H1768.
34. Huang HH, Shao ZH, Li CQ, Vanden Hoek TL, Li J (2014) Baicalein protects cardiomyocytes against mitochondrial oxidant injury associated with JNK inhibition and mitochondrial Akt activation. Am J Chin Med 42: 79–94.
35. Bryl E, Mysliwska J, Debska-Slizien A, Rachon D, Bullo B, et al. (1998) The influence of recombinant human erythropoietin on tumor necrosis factor alpha and interleukin-10 production by whole blood cell cultures in hemodialysis patients. Artif Organs 22: 177–181.
36. Liu X, Xie W, Liu P, Duan M, Jia Z, et al. (2006) Mechanism of the cardioprotection of rhEPO pretreatment on suppressing the inflammatory response in ischemia-reperfusion. Life Sci 78: 2255–2264.
37. Jia HB, Jin Y, Ji Q, Hu YF, Zhou ZQ, et al. (2009) Effects of recombinant human erythropoietin on neuropathic pain and cerebral expressions of cytokines and nuclear factor-kappa B. Can J Anaesth 56: 597–603.
38. Guzman JA, Rosado AE, Kruse JA (2003) Vasopressin vs norepinephrine in endotoxic shock: systemic, renal, and splanchnic hemodynamic and oxygen transport effects. J Appl Physiol 95: 803–809.
39. Russell JA, Fjell C, Hsu JL, Lee T, Boyd J, et al. (2013) Vasopressin compared with norepinephrine augments the decline of plasma cytokine levels in septic shock. Am J Respir Crit Care Med 188: 356–364.
40. Voelckel WG, Convertino VA, Lurie KG, Karlbauer A, Schochl H, et al. (2010) Vasopressin for hemorrhagic shock management: revisiting the potential value in civilian and combat casualty care. J Trauma 69 Suppl 1: S69–S74.
41. Anand T, Skinner R (2012) Arginine vasopressin: The future of pressure-support resuscitation in hemorrhagic shock. J Surg Res 178: 321–329.
42. Voelckel WG, Raedler C, Wenzel V, Lindner KH, Krismer AC, et al. (2003) Arginine vasopressin, but not epinephrine, improves survival in uncontrolled hemorrhagic shock after liver trauma in pigs. Crit Care Med 31: 1160–1165.
43. Raedler C, Voelckel WG, Wenzel V, Krismer AC, Schmittinger CA, et al. (2004) Treatment of uncontrolled hemorrhagic shock after liver trauma: fatal effects of fluid resuscitation versus improved outcome after vasopressin. Anesth Analg 98: 1759–1766.
44. Cohn SM, McCarthy J, Stewart RM, Jonas RB, Dent DL, et al. (2011) Impact of low-dose vasopressin on trauma outcome: prospective randomized study. World J Surg 35: 430–439.
45. Lienhart HG, Wenzel V, Braun J, Dorges V, Dunser M, et al. (2007) [Vasopressin for therapy of persistent traumatic hemorrhagic shock: The VITRIS.at study]. Anaesthesist 56: 145–8, 150.
46. Bougle A, Harrois A, Duranteau J (2013) Resuscitative strategies in traumatic hemorrhagic shock. Ann Intensive Care 3: 1.
47. Nunez TC, Young PP, Holcomb JB, Cotton BA (2010) Creation, implementation, and maturation of a massive transfusion protocol for the exsanguinating trauma patient. J Trauma 68: 1498–1505.
48. Madigan MC, Kemp CD, Johnson JC, Cotton BA (2008) Secondary abdominal compartment syndrome after severe extremity injury: are early, aggressive fluid resuscitation strategies to blame? J Trauma 64: 280–285.
49. Shaw AD, Bagshaw SM, Goldstein SL, Scherer LA, Duan M, et al. (2012) Major complications, mortality, and resource utilization after open abdominal surgery: 0.9% saline compared to Plasma-Lyte. Ann Surg 255: 821–829.
50. Volta CA, Trentini A, Farabegoli L, Manfrinato MC, Alvisi V, et al. (2013) Effects of two different strategies of fluid administration on inflammatory mediators, plasma electrolytes and acid/base disorders in patients undergoing major abdominal surgery: a randomized double blind study. J Inflamm (Lond) 10: 29.

Reduced Heme Levels Underlie the Exponential Growth Defect of the *Shewanella oneidensis hfq* Mutant

Christopher M. Brennan[1☯¤a], Nicholas Q. Mazzucca[1☯], Taylor Mezoian[1], Taylor M. Hunt[1], Meaghan L. Keane[1¤b], Jessica N. Leonard[1¤c], Shelby E. Scola[2], Emma N. Beer[1], Sarah Perdue[1¤d], Brett J. Pellock[1*]

1 Department of Biology, Providence College, Providence, Rhode Island, United States of America, **2** Department of Chemistry and Biochemistry, Providence College, Providence, Rhode Island, United States of America

Abstract

The RNA chaperone Hfq fulfills important roles in small regulatory RNA (sRNA) function in many bacteria. Loss of Hfq in the dissimilatory metal reducing bacterium *Shewanella oneidensis* strain MR-1 results in slow exponential phase growth and a reduced terminal cell density at stationary phase. We have found that the exponential phase growth defect of the *hfq* mutant in LB is the result of reduced heme levels. Both heme levels and exponential phase growth of the *hfq* mutant can be completely restored by supplementing LB medium with 5-aminolevulinic acid (5-ALA), the first committed intermediate synthesized during heme synthesis. Increasing expression of *gtrA*, which encodes the enzyme that catalyzes the first step in heme biosynthesis, also restores heme levels and exponential phase growth of the *hfq* mutant. Taken together, our data indicate that reduced heme levels are responsible for the exponential growth defect of the *S. oneidensis hfq* mutant in LB medium and suggest that the *S. oneidensis hfq* mutant is deficient in heme production at the 5-ALA synthesis step.

Editor: Roy Martin Roop II, East Carolina University School of Medicine, United States of America

Funding: Research reported in this publication was supported by an Institutional Development Award (IDeA) from the National Institute of General Medical Sciences of the National Institutes of Health under grant number 2 P20 GM103430. IDeA website address: http://www.nigms.nih.gov/Training/IDeA/Pages/default.aspx. BJP's funding was awarded as a sub-project of the above grant through Rhode Island IDeA Network for Excellence in Biomedical Research (RI-INBRE, http://web.uri.edu/inbre/). The funders had no role in study design, data collection and analysis, decision to publish, or preparation of the manuscript.

Competing Interests: The authors have declared that no competing interests exist.

* Email: bpellock@providence.edu

☯ These authors contributed equally to this work.

¤a Current address: Department of Biology, Massachusetts Institute of Technology, Cambridge, Massachusetts, United States of America
¤b Current address: Liver Diseases Branch, National Institute of Diabetes and Digestive and Kidney Diseases (NIDDK), National Institutes of Health, Bethesda, Maryland, United States of America
¤c Current address: Department of Psychiatry and Human Behavior, Brown Medical School, Providence, Rhode Island, United States of America
¤d Current address: Department of Biochemistry, Molecular Biology and Biophysics, University of Minnesota, Saint Paul, Minnesota, United States of America

Introduction

The RNA chaperone Hfq is a highly conserved protein that mediates interactions between many regulatory sRNA molecules and their mRNA targets in bacteria (for reviews see [1–4]). Hfq protein monomers form a homohexameric ring capable of binding both regulatory small, noncoding RNAs (sRNAs) and their target mRNAs [5,6]. These Hfq-RNA interactions stabilize sRNAs and help the sRNAs locate and interact with their mRNA targets. Because sRNA expression and subsequent changes in target gene expression help bacteria adapt to changing environmental conditions, Hfq plays key roles in regulating a wide variety of cellular functions.

Genetic loss-of-function studies have been widely employed to elucidate how Hfq functions to help regulate bacterial gene expression networks (for example see [7–10]). Consistent with a role in a multitude of cellular processes, loss of Hfq is typically pleiotropic, and *hfq* mutants exhibit a diverse array of bacterium-specific phenotypes. This suggests that, despite its high level of conservation, Hfq has evolved distinct roles in closely related bacteria. However, a common theme in the study of Hfq is that *hfq* mutants are typically less efficient at responding to the challenges of growth and stress conditions, which is consistent with the role of Hfq as a functional mediator for adaptive sRNAs. Though reduced sRNA function likely contributes to many *hfq* mutant phenotypes, the mechanisms by which loss of Hfq results in particular mutant phenotypes often remain obscure.

A null mutant of *hfq* in the dissimilatory metal-reducing bacterium *Shewanella oneidensis* was recently characterized [10]. Loss of *hfq* in *S. oneidensis* results in slow exponential phase growth, reduced stationary phase culture density, slow anaerobic growth, a reduced capacity for chromium reduction, and a greatly increased sensitivity to oxidative stress. *S. oneidensis* is of particular interest because anaerobically growing cells are capable of transferring electrons to a wide variety of extracellular terminal electron acceptors, including many soluble and insoluble metals [11,12]. This capability has sparked interest in *S. oneidensis* as a potential bioremediating organism as well as an organism capable of producing electrical current in microbial fuel cells [13,14]. Because bacteria in nature likely experience frequent metabolic changes, understanding how Hfq and sRNAs mediate adaptive cellular processes will provide useful insights into the genetic and physiological control mechanisms of *S. oneidensis*.

Heme molecules participate in a variety of important cellular processes. For example, heme is a key prosthetic group in cytochrome proteins used in electron transport chains. Heme also has other important physiological roles in iron storage and oxidative stress resistance. The importance of heme in bacterial growth is underscored by the fact that bacteria that are unable to synthesize heme, including many pathogens, must acquire it from their external environments [15]. Heme availability is particularly important for electron transport in *S. oneidensis*, which can potentially encode 42 different c-type cytochromes that are thought to confer the ability to use a diverse array of terminal electron acceptors [16,17]. The predominant form of heme in *S. oneidensis* is heme C [18], which is covalently attached to two cysteine residues in cytochrome proteins by the activity of the heme lyase protein CcmF [19].

Heme biosynthesis is a well-conserved process (for reviews see [15,20]). The first committed step in heme synthesis is the production of 5-aminolevulinic acid (5-ALA). In mammalian cells, yeast, and the α-proteobacteria, the HemA protein (5-ALA synthase) catalyzes the synthesis of 5-ALA in a single step from glycine and succinyl-CoA (the C_4 pathway). In other organisms (the remaining eubacteria, plants, Archaea, and algae), 5-ALA is produced in a two step process (the C_5 pathway). First, glutamyl tRNA reductase (GtrA/HemA) uses NADPH as a cofactor to reduce glutamate supplied by a charged glutamyl tRNA to a glutamate-1-semialdehyde (GSA) intermediate. GSA is then converted to 5-ALA by the enzyme GSA aminotransferase (HemL). Following 5-ALA synthesis, heme is produced using seven additional conserved enzyme-catalyzed reactions.

Regulation of heme biosynthesis in bacteria is largely focused on the activity of the first enzyme in the heme biosynthetic pathway (reviewed in [20]). Though bacteria modulate production of GtrA/HemA on the transcriptional level, this regulation is generally modest. In contrast, bacteria appear to exert a much larger influence on glutamyl tRNA reductase activity by post-tranlationally regulating GtrA/HemA protein stability. For example, in *Salmonella typhimurium*, heme binds to the GtrA/HemA protein and promotes its proteolytic degradation via the Lon and ClpAP proteases [21]. Thus, high heme levels negatively regulate the first committed step in heme biosynthesis via anabolite repression.

In this study, we report the serendipitous discovery that reduced heme levels underlie the exponential growth phase defect of the *S. oneidensis hfq* mutant. Restoring heme levels in the *hfq* mutant by nutritional supplementation with 5-aminolevulinic acid or by exogenous production of the *S. oneidensis* glutamyl tRNA reductase (hereafter referred to as *gtrA* or GtrA to reflect the naming convention proposed by Panek and O'Brian [15]), the first enzyme in the heme biosynthesis pathway, restores exponential growth to wild type levels. Thus, the slow growth of the *S. oneidensis hfq* mutant in LB is due to reduced heme levels and not a combination of pleiotropic factors. In addition, the defect in heme synthesis in the *S. oneidensis hfq* mutant occurs at or before the 5-ALA synthesis step. Our findings represent an important advance in understanding the link between the *S. oneidensis hfq* mutant slow growth phenotype and a defect in a specific metabolic pathway.

Results

Growth on blood agar substantially rescues the small colony defect of the *S. oneidensis hfq* mutant

Colonies formed by an *S. oneidensis hfq* mutant on LB plates are substantially smaller than colonies formed by cells containing a wild type copy of *hfq* (Figure 1A, [10]). Because the *hfq* mutant is highly sensitive to peroxide stress, we tested trypticase soy agar (TSA) medium containing 5% sheep blood as a potential qualitative measure to assay whether the *hfq* mutant produces higher levels of reactive oxygen species. Though the *hfq* mutant did not produce more heme oxidation (α hemolysis) than wild type cells, we were surprised to observe that growth on sheep blood agar substantially rescued the colony size defect of the *hfq* mutant (Figure 1B). The *hfq* mutant small colony defect on TSA without blood (Figure S1A) was comparable to the phenotype observed on LB (Figure 1A).

Heme or 5-aminolevulinic acid substantially rescues the small colony phenotype of the *S. oneidensis hfq* mutant

Because most bacteria have the capacity to scavenge iron from hemoglobin to support vital cellular functions [27], we determined whether the addition of iron to the medium at concentrations approximating those found in trypticase soy agar plates containing 5% sheep blood could rescue the growth defect of the *hfq* mutant. Addition of 50 μM $FeCl_3$ to LB plates, which already contain ~17 μM iron [28], did not substantially alter the size of the *hfq* mutant colonies or the wild type colonies (Figure 1C), suggesting that iron is not the factor present in blood that rescues growth of the *hfq* mutant. An alternative possibility is that the *hfq* mutant might be defective in iron uptake, but not heme uptake, allowing the cells to scavenge iron by importing heme. However, exponentially growing *hfq* mutant and wild type cells contained similar levels of free iron per cell (Figure 1D). In addition, for both the MR-1 wild type and *hfq* mutant cultures we observed the same pattern of free iron levels. At lower cell densities, iron levels per cell are highest, but after culture density reaches an ABS_{600} of ~4.0, the free iron content of the cells decreases (Figure S2C). Taken together, these data suggest that rescue of the *hfq* mutant small colony phenotype is due to a factor other than iron.

Since *hfq* mutant colonies are noticeably less pigmented than colonies of strains with a wild type copy of *hfq* (Figure 1A), and because the pink hue of *Shewanella* is largely the result of reduced heme in cytochrome proteins [29,30], we hypothesized that growth rescue of the *hfq* mutant was due to the heme present in mammalian blood. Addition of 50 μM heme in the form of purified porcine hemin substantially rescued the small colony phenotype and partially restored the pink color of the *hfq* mutant (Figure 1E). This suggests that heme, but not iron alone, rescues the growth of the *hfq* mutant.

Synthesis of 5-aminolevulinic acid (5-ALA) is the first committed step in heme biosynthesis. 5-ALA synthesis is a critical focal point for regulation of heme biosynthesis, since 5-ALA is used exclusively for heme production [20]. Because exogenously-supplied heme partially rescues the *hfq* mutant small colony phenotype, we hypothesized that a defect in 5-ALA synthesis, and thus heme biosynthesis, results in slow growth of the *hfq* mutant. Addition of 50 μM 5-ALA to LB plates rescued the colony size defect of the *hfq* mutant to a similar extent as addition of 50 μM heme (Figure 1F). Because eight 5-ALA molecules are used to synthesize one heme molecule, we also determined whether higher levels of 5-ALA would increase the degree of colony size rescue. However addition of 400 μM 5-ALA rescued *hfq* mutant growth to a similar extent as 50 μM 5-ALA (Figure S1B).

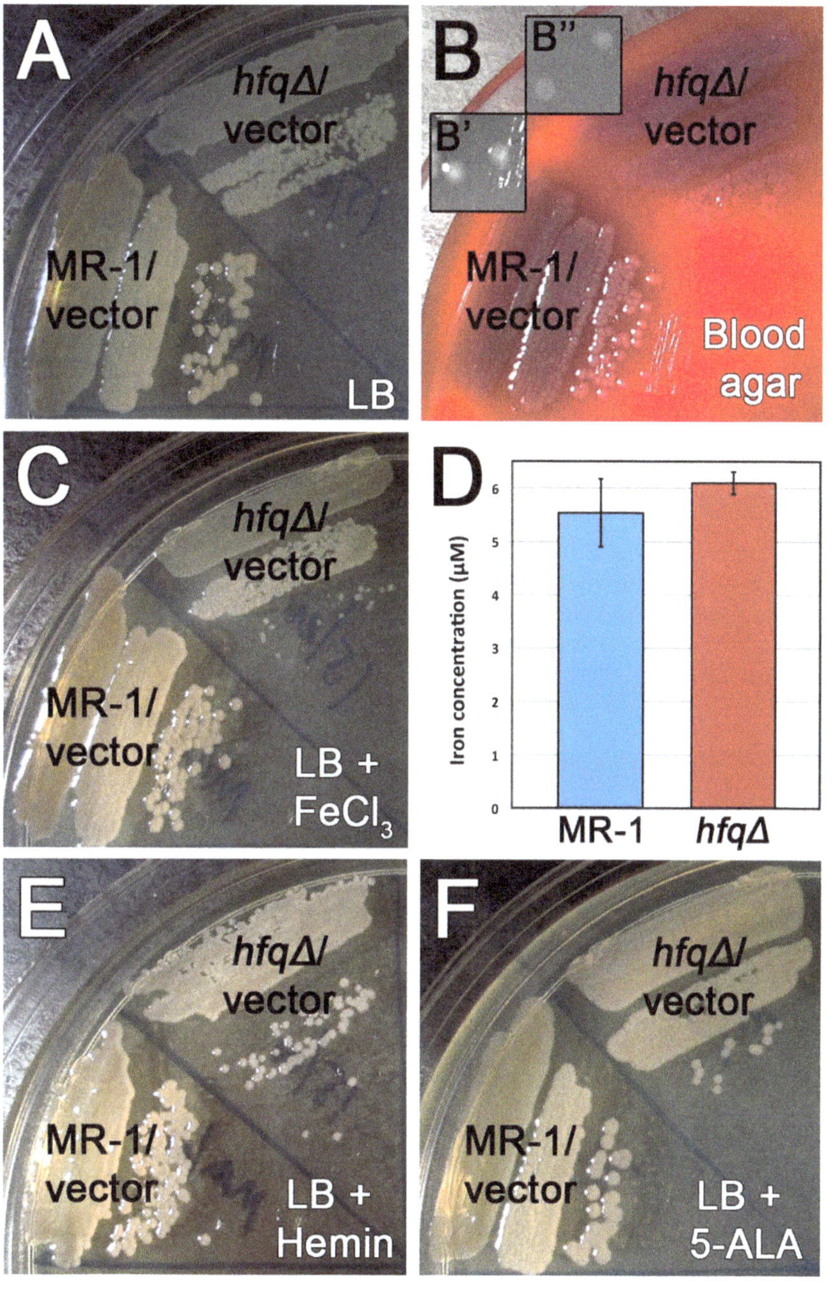

Figure 1. Heme or 5-ALA supplementation substantially rescues the colony size phenotype of the *hfq* mutant. Colony size comparisons of MR-1/pBBR1-MCS2 (vector), and *hfqΔ*/pBBR1-MCS2 (vector) streaked to single colonies on (A) LB Km, (B) TSA containing 5% sheep blood [including higher magnification insets for colony size comparison: (B') MR-1/pBBR1-MCS2 (vector) colonies and (B'') *hfqΔ*/pBBR1-MCS2 (vector) colonies], (C) LB Km supplemented with 50 μM $FeCl_3$, (E) LB Km supplemented with 50 μM hemin, or (F) LB Km supplemented with 50 μM 5-aminolevulinic acid (5-ALA). Plates were photographed following 23–25 hours of growth at 30°C. (D) Quantification of total free iron in wild type MR-1 and *hfqΔ* mutant cells using the ferrozine reagent. Concentration of detectable free iron was computed as described in Materials and Methods. Data presented is the mean of three independent cultures. Error bars indicate standard deviations. The difference between iron levels in MR-1 and the *hfqΔ* mutant is not statistically significant ($P = 0.22$ in an unpaired two-tailed Student's t-test).

Nutritional rescue by 5-ALA of the growth defect of the *hfq* mutant suggests that loss of *hfq* creates a heme-specific growth phenotype. This model is supported by our observation that increasing the nutritional content of LB by doubling the concentrations of the tryptone and yeast extract components failed to rescue the *hfq* mutant growth defect (Figure S1C). Because glutamyl $tRNA^{Glu}$ supplies the glutamate that is converted into 5-ALA, we also determined whether supplementing LB with a mixture of glutamate, arginine, and serine could rescue the *hfq* mutant growth defect. However, addition of these amino acids at the concentrations they are found in modified M1 medium (see Materials and Methods) did not rescue *hfq* mutant colony size beyond that seen on LB alone (Figure S1D). Taken together, our data suggest that the *hfq* mutant is defective in heme biosynthesis at the 5-ALA synthesis step.

The *hfq* mutant contains reduced levels of heme

The pigmentation difference between wild type *S. oneidensis* colonies and *hfq* mutant colonies on LB plates (Figure 1A) is more striking when cell pellets of the two strains are compared (Figure 2A). To determine whether the reduced pigmentation of *hfq* mutant cells is in fact due to reduced levels of heme, we performed the pyridine hemochrome assay [23] on exponentially growing wild type MR-1 and *hfq* mutant cells. In this assay, the reduced form of heme C, the dominant heme species in *S. oneidensis* [18], produces an absorbance peak at 550 nm. The height of the 550 nm absorbance peak as measured from the absorbance trough at 535 nm is directly proportional to the amount of heme in the sample [23]. Analyses of the heme spectra from wild type and *hfq* mutant cultures (Figure 2B) and subsequent statistical analyses of the quantities of heme present in the samples (Figure 2C) indicated that exponentially growing wild type cells contain significantly more heme than *hfq* mutant cells.

Increasing expression of *gtrA* rescues the small colony phenotype of the *S. oneidensis hfq* mutant

That addition of 5-ALA to the growth medium substantially rescued the small colony phenotype of the heme deficient *hfq* mutant suggests that a deficiency in heme production might be the result of a defect in 5-ALA synthesis. In *S. oneidensis*, 5-ALA is synthesized in a putative two-step process involving the genes *gtrA* and *hemL* (Figure 3A). GtrA protein converts glutamate donated by glutamyl $tRNA^{Glu}$ into glutamate-1-semialdehyde, which is then converted into 5-ALA by the HemL protein. Since 5-ALA is used exclusively for heme production, we hypothesized that the heme biosynthesis defect of the *hfq* mutant is due to reduced function of the *gtrA* gene, the *hemL* gene, or both.

If lowered *gtrA* and/or *hemL* function underlies the heme biosynthesis defect of the *hfq* mutant, then increasing expression of *gtrA*, *hemL*, or both should rescue the mutant growth defect. To test this, we constructed arabinose-inducible plasmid expression vectors containing the *gtrA* gene, the *hemL* gene, or both the *gtrA* and *hemL* genes. We then constructed wild type and *hfq* mutant strains containing these plasmids and determined whether expression of *gtrA*, *hemL*, or both altered growth of these strains relative to wild type and *hfq* mutant strains containing the empty vector.

Exogenous expression of *gtrA* alone completely rescued the small colony phenotype of the *hfq* mutant (Figure 3B and 3C). In contrast, *hfq* mutant colonies expressing *hemL* alone were indistinguishable in size from *hfq* mutant colonies with vector alone (Figure 3D and 3E). Expressing both *gtrA* and *hemL* rescued *hfq* colony size to a similar extent as expressing *gtrA* alone (Figure S3). Taken together, our data suggest that reduced *gtrA* function underlies the colony size defect of the *hfq* mutant.

Increasing heme availability via nutritional supplementation or genetic manipulation rescues the exponential growth defect of the *hfq* mutant

The small colony phenotype of the *hfq* mutant could be due to one or more *S. oneidensis hfq* mutant phenotypes, including the defect in exponential phase growth and/or saturation at a lower terminal density [10]. To determine how nutritional supplementation and genetic manipulation of the heme biosynthetic pathway influence culture growth kinetics and increase the size of *hfq* mutant colonies, we performed detailed analyses of both the growth kinetics and heme content of wild type and *hfq* mutant

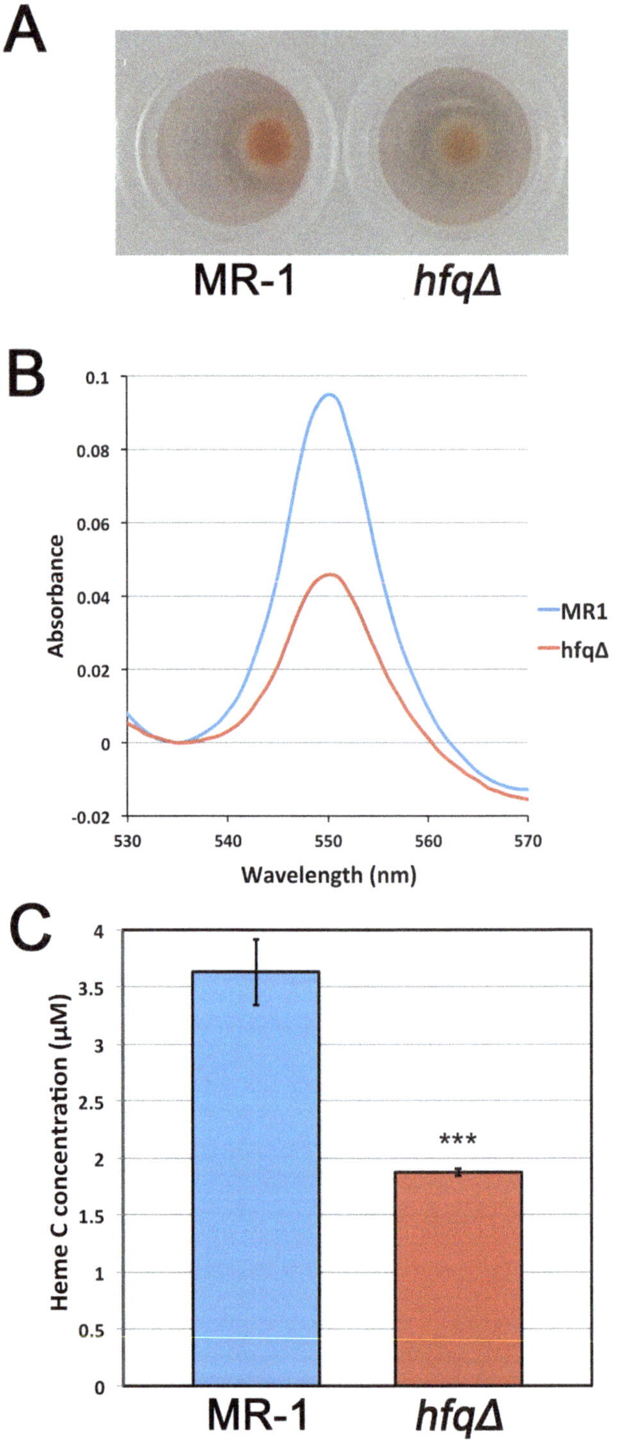

Figure 2. The *hfq* mutant is deficient in heme production. (A) Comparison of exponentially-growing MR-1 wild type and *hfqΔ* mutant cell pellet pigmentation. Both cell pellets are comprised of similar numbers of cells. (B) Superimposed heme assay subtraction spectra (reduced – oxidized) from single samples of exponentially-growing MR-1 wild type and *hfqΔ* mutant cultures. Data presented is typical of the difference observed for the two strains. (C) Quantification of heme concentrations from MR-1 wild type and *hfqΔ* mutant cultures. Concentration of detectable heme was computed as described in Materials and Methods. Data presented is the mean of three independent cultures. Error bars indicate standard deviations. *** indicate that the difference in heme levels between MR-1 and the *hfqΔ* mutant is statistically significant ($P<0.001$ in an unpaired two-tailed Student's t-test).

cultures in which we manipulated heme availability via nutritional or genetic means.

Addition of 50 μM 5-ALA to LB liquid medium completely rescued the exponential phase growth defect of the *hfq* mutant (Figure 4A) and restored heme levels in the *hfq* mutant to wild type levels (Figure 4B). However, by 7–8 hours of culture growth, when heme levels in the unsupplemented *hfq* mutant were indistinguishable from those in wild type cells (Figure 4B and 4D), absorbance values for the *hfq* mutant plus 5-ALA stopped increasing and were no longer coincident with the MR-1 cultures (Figure 4A). The terminal density of stationary phase *hfq* mutant cultures was significantly increased by addition of 5-ALA, but these cultures never achieved the terminal density of wild type cultures (Figure 4A). This suggests that factors independent of heme levels are at least partially responsible for the reduced terminal density of the *hfq* mutant.

Increasing *gtrA* expression using an inducible plasmid vector also completely rescued the *hfq* mutant exponential phase growth defect in LB liquid medium, as growth of the *hfq* mutant expressing *gtrA* was indistinguishable from growth of wild type cells expressing *gtrA* (Figure 4C). We consistently observed that expression of *gtrA* slightly slows the growth of both the *hfq* mutant and wild type cells, indicating that exogenous *gtrA* expression mildly compromises growth of *S. oneidensis* cultures. Expression of *gtrA* restored heme levels in exponentially growing *hfq* mutant cells to wild type levels (Figure 4D). Similar to nutritional rescue of *hfq* mutant growth, genetic rescue of growth waned between 7–8 hours (Figure 4C).

These data indicate that the exponential phase growth defect of the *hfq* mutant is strongly linked to heme levels 2–3 fold lower (see Figures 2C, 4B, and 4D) than those found in wild type cells. This heme deficiency persists only until cultures begin to enter stationary phase, at which point the heme levels in the mutant cells are equivalent to those found in wild type cells (Figure 4B and 4D). Increasing heme availability rescues exponential growth of the *S. oneidensis hfq* mutant in LB, indicating that slow growth is due to reduced heme levels. In addition, our genetic and nutritional data strongly suggest that the *S. oneidensis hfq* mutant's heme defect occurs at the 5-ALA synthesis step.

The *hfq* mutant contains modestly reduced levels of *gtrA* mRNA

To begin to elucidate the mechanism by which Hfq regulates *gtrA* function, we analyzed relative *gtrA* mRNA levels in exponentially growing wild type and *hfq* mutant cells. In 4 hour old cultures, we observed a modest, but significant reduction in *gtrA* mRNA levels in the *hfq* mutant relative to the wild type strain. When *gtrA* expression levels were normalized to 16S rRNA levels, the *hfq* mutant contained 0.63 fold the quantity ($P < 0.00002$) of *gtrA* mRNA detected in wild type cultures (Data S1). When we independently normalized *gtrA* expression levels to *recA* mRNA levels, we observed that the *hfq* mutant contained 0.69 fold the quantity ($P < 0.0014$) of *gtrA* mRNA detected in wild type cultures (Data S1). Thus, our data suggest that loss of *hfq* results in reduced *gtrA* transcription, an increased *gtrA* mRNA turnover rate, or both.

Discussion

Here we report that the exponential growth defect of the *S. oneidensis hfq* mutant in LB medium is due to reduced levels of heme during exponential phase growth. The lowered heme levels are likely due to a defect in the 5-ALA synthesis step, as addition of 5-ALA to the medium or increased *gtrA* expression completely restores growth, while increasing the nutrient pool available to the cells does not restore growth. The fact that growth in nutritionally supplemented solid medium was not as robust as rescue in nutritionally supplemented liquid medium could be the result of local depletion of resources surrounding colonies on solid medium. However, increasing supplement concentrations did not further increase growth rescue on solid medium, suggesting that the difference in degree of growth rescue between solid and liquid

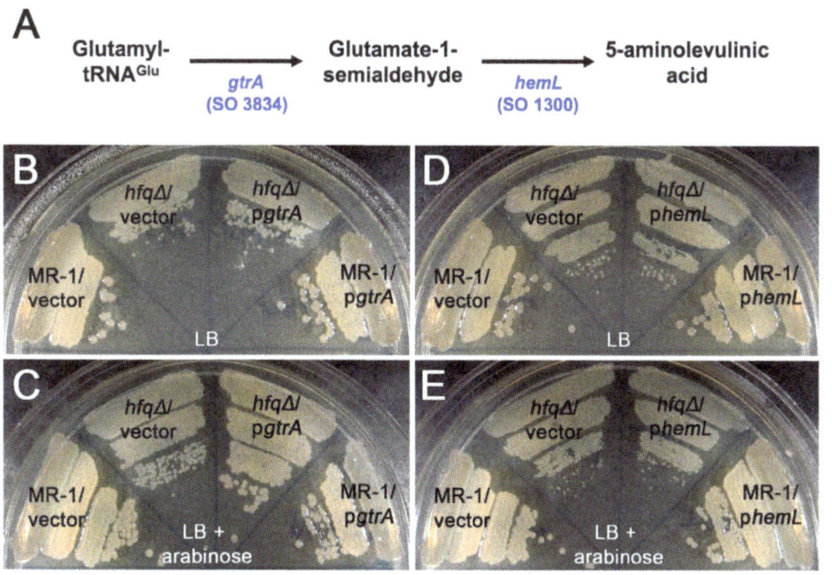

Figure 3. Exogenous *gtrA* expression rescues the colony size defect of the *hfq* mutant. (A) Putative two step pathway for the biosynthesis of 5-aminolevulinic acid in *Shewanella oneidensis* MR-1. (B and C) Colony size comparisons of MR-1/pBBAD-SP (vector), MR-1/pBBAD-*gtrA* (p*gtrA*), *hfqΔ*/pBBAD-SP (vector), and *hfqΔ*/pBBAD-*gtrA* (p*gtrA*), streaked to single colonies on (B) LB Km and (C) LB Km containing 0.005% arabinose. (D and E) Colony size comparisons of MR-1/pBBAD-SP (vector), MR-1/pBBAD-p*hemL* (p*hemL*), *hfqΔ*/pBBAD-SP (vector), and *hfqΔ*/pBBAD-p*hemL* (p*hemL*), on (D) LB Km and (E) LB Km containing 0.005% arabinose. Plates were photographed following 24 hours of growth at 30°C.

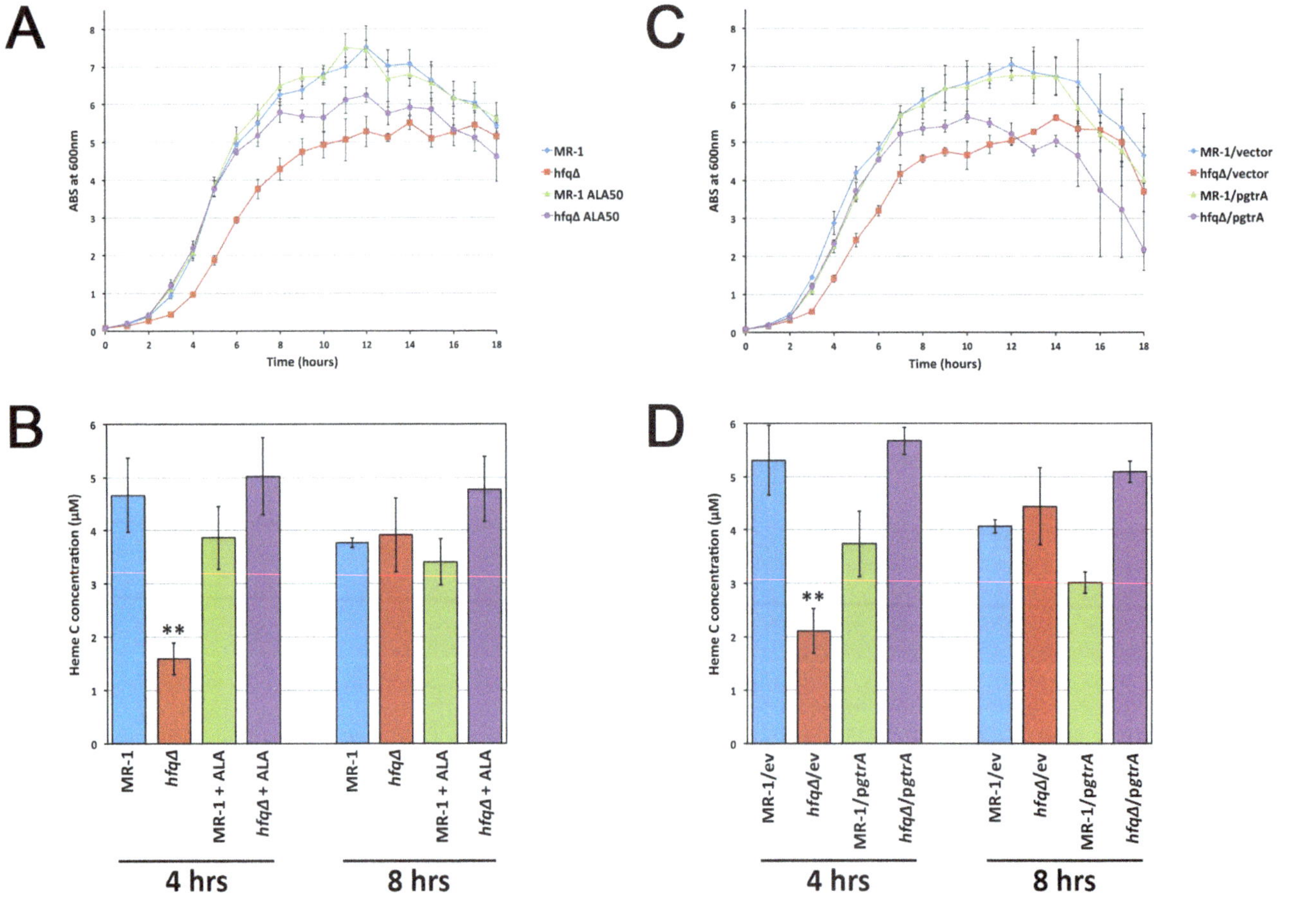

Figure 4. Restoring heme biosynthesis rescues the exponential phase growth defect of the *hfq* mutant. (A) Growth curves for MR-1/pBBAD-SP (MR-1) and *hfqΔ*/pBBAD-SP (*hfqΔ*) grown in either LB Km liquid medium or in LB Km liquid medium supplemented with 50 µM 5-ALA. (B) Heme content analysis of cells from MR-1/pBBAD-SP (MR-1) and *hfqΔ*/pBBAD-SP (*hfqΔ*) cultures grown for either 4 hours or 8 hours in either LB Km liquid medium or in LB Km liquid medium supplemented with 50 µM 5-ALA. (C) Growth curves for the wild type MR-1 strain and *hfqΔ* mutant strains containing either pBBAD-SP (vector/ev) or p*gtrA* grown in either LB Km or in LB Km containing 0.005% arabinose. (D) Heme content analysis of MR-1 and *hfqΔ* mutant cells containing either pBBAD-SP (vector/ev) or p*gtrA* grown in either LB Km or in LB Km containing 0.005% arabinose. Results presented for both growth curve and heme assays are the means from three independent cultures. Error bars in panels (A) and (C) indicate a 99% confidence interval ($P = 0.01$). Error bars in panels (B) and (D) indicate standard deviations. ** indicates that the difference between heme levels at 4 hours between MR1 and the *hfqΔ* mutant are statistically significant ($P < 0.0025$ in an unpaired two-tailed Student's t-test).

medium is likely a reflection of differences in growth in the two media types.

That the *hfq* mutant exponential growth phenotype in LB is due to a deficiency in a single metabolic pathway is striking because loss of Hfq compromises many cellular processes. *S. oneidensis hfq* mutant cells growing in LB are partially auxotrophic for heme during exponential growth. Any other deficiencies that might influence exponential growth of the *hfq* mutant are not apparent when grown in LB liquid. A heme deficiency also contributes to the slow growth of the *hfq* mutant in medium other than LB, since heme supplementation of modified M1, a less rich defined medium, also substantially rescues the *hfq* colony size defect (Figure S4A and S4B). However in M1 medium, we observe a more modest rescue of *hfq* mutant growth with 5-ALA supplementation than we observe in LB (Figure S4C). This suggests that the *hfq* mutant has a reduced ability to convert 5-ALA into heme when it is grown on modified M1 medium. Indeed, supplementation of M1 medium with 400 µM ALA inhibits growth of the *hfq* mutant, possibly as the result of buildup of heme biosynthetic intermediates, some of which are toxic [31]. Thus, growth in less nutritionally rich medium appears to expose additional metabolic deficiencies of the *hfq* mutant.

Once *hfq* mutant cells reach the end of exponential phase, their heme levels are similar to those observed in similarly aged wild type cells. Thus, a heme deficiency cannot fully explain other *hfq* mutant phenotypes, such as the reduced stationary phase density or the late stationary phase survival defect of *hfq* mutant cultures. However, the terminal densities of *hfq* mutant cultures in which the heme defect has been rescued are significantly higher than the terminal densities of *hfq* mutant cultures alone. This indicates that the terminal density of a culture is in part, but not wholly, determined by the extent of its exponential phase growth. Further investigations into the mechanisms by which Hfq regulates heme levels should provide insight into why the *hfq* mutant has lower heme levels during exponential phase growth but not at the beginning of stationary phase.

An attractive model to explain slow exponential phase growth in the *hfq* mutant is that lower heme levels reduce the electron transport capacity of the cells, since heme is the redox center of cytochrome proteins. Reduced cytochrome function and diminished electron transport could also account for the slower chromium reduction kinetics and reduced anaerobic growth of the *hfq* mutant. Low heme levels could explain other *S. oneidensis hfq* mutant phenotypes. For example, because heme is a key part of the active site of the hydrogen peroxide degrading enzyme catalase, reduced heme availability could compromise catalase activity, making the *hfq* mutant more sensitive to oxidative stress. Heme is also a key part of the iron storage protein bacterioferritin, raising the possibility that changes in heme availability during exponential phase could impact iron homeostasis in the *hfq* mutant. However, regardless of bacterioferritin function, the levels of free iron in both wild type and *hfq* mutant cells are similar, suggesting that iron homeostasis may be minimally affected by loss of Hfq under the conditions tested.

Though Hfq appears to regulate heme production at the 5-ALA synthesis step, the mechanism by which loss of *hfq* results in lowered GtrA activity and thus reduced heme levels is not yet clear. Considering the modest reduction in *gtrA* mRNA levels in the *hfq* mutant during exponential growth, Hfq could function to stimulate transcription of *gtrA* and/or promote *gtrA* mRNA stability. However, though there is a statistically significant difference in *gtrA* mRNA levels between wild type and *hfq* mutant cells, it is not clear whether a ~1.5 fold difference in *gtrA* expression is biologically significant in regard to heme levels. This raises the possibility that *S. oneidensis* regulates *gtrA* activity posttranscriptionally. For example, Hfq could promote the function of an unidentified sRNA that positively regulates the translation of *gtrA* mRNA by releasing attenuation due to a secondary structure that blocks the putative ribosome binding site. It is also possible that loss of Hfq could result in an increased heme or GtrA turnover rate, leading to lower steady state heme levels in exponentially growing *hfq* mutant cells. It is clear from our analyses that the regulatory mechanisms controlling heme levels in the *hfq* mutant differ substantially from those in wild type cells. We are currently investigating the mechanism(s) by which Hfq regulates heme levels in *S. oneidensis*.

Materials and Methods

Growth media, strains, and culture conditions

Unless otherwise specified, cultures were grown in LB medium (10g/L tryptone, 5g/L yeast extract, 10g/L NaCl) supplemented with kanamycin (Km). Other media used included modified M1 medium [10,11], LB with double the normal quantities of tryptone and yeast extract (20g/L tryptone, 10g/L yeast extract, 10g/L NaCl), LB supplemented with 135.9 µM L-glutamic acid, 114.8 µM L-arginine, and 190.3 µM DL-serine, the concentrations of amino acids found in modified M1 medium [10,11], trypticase soy agar (TSA), TSA supplemented with 5% sheep blood (Becton Dickinson), LB supplemented with 50 µM iron (in the form of $FeSO_4$ or $FeCl_3$), LB or M1 supplemented with 50 µM or 400 µM 5-aminolevulinic acid, and LB or M1 supplemented with 50 µM porcine hemin.

S. oneidensis strains used in this study are wild type strain MR-1 [11] and the MR-1 *hfqΔ* mutant [10] and their derivatives. *S. oneidensis* cultures and cultures containing both *E. coli* and *S. oneidensis* were grown at 30°C, while *E. coli* cultures were grown at 37°C. Antibiotics were used at the following concentrations: kanamycin (Km), 25 µg/mL; gentamicin (Gm), 5 µg/mL.

Bacteria grown on plates were streaked to single colonies in four phases from frozen permanent stocks or from colonies on streak plates that had been inoculated from frozen permanent stocks and grown overnight. For growth curves, overnight aerobic 5 mL LB Km cultures of *S. oneidensis* strains inoculated from frozen permanent stocks were diluted in LB Km to an ABS_{600} ≅0.1 and outgrown aerobically to mid exponential phase (ABS_{600} ≅0.4–1.0). These log phase cultures were then diluted to an ABS_{600} ≅0.1 in LB Km and grown aerobically in 125 mL Erlenmeyer flasks shaken at 250RPM. Culture turbidity (ABS_{600}) was measured at regular intervals.

Detection of free intracellular iron

Free, intracellular iron was detected via a modified version of a previously described protocol [22]. Overnight LB Km cultures of *S. oneidensis* strains were diluted to an ABS_{600} ≅0.1 and outgrown in LB Km. The equivalent of 5 mL of culture at an ABS_{600} of 1.0 was harvested for each strain after 4 hours of growth. Cells were pelleted in Eppendorf tubes and washed once by resuspending in sterile 0.85% (w/v) saline. The washed pellets were then resuspended in 1 mL of Bacterial Protein Extraction Reagent (B-PER, Thermo Scientific) containing 100 µg/mL lysozyme and incubated at room temperature for 15 minutes with regular mixing. 100 µL of 10 mM ferrozine reagent [3-(2-pyridyl)-5,6-diphenyl-1,2,4-triazine-4′, 4″-disulfonic acid sodium salt] (Sigma Aldrich) in 0.1 M ammonium acetate was added to each sample and mixed. 800 µL of this solution was then mixed with 150 µL of 1.4 M hydroxylamine hydrochloride in a fresh Eppendorf tube and incubated for 15 minutes at room temperature to reduce Fe(III) to Fe(II). The solution was then neutralized by adding 50 µL of 10 M ammonium acetate, pH 9.5. Samples were incubated for at least 4 hours at room temperature to allow full color development. Each sample was then pelleted for 2 minutes at maximum speed in a microcentrifuge. 600 µL of the supernatant was then transferred to a cuvette for ABS_{562} measurement in a spectrophotometer zeroed using a sample with assay reagents only. This assay is quantitative, as there is a linear relationship between iron concentration and ABS_{562} values (Figure S2A). Hemin alone did not produce a signal using this protocol (Figure S2B).

Detection of total intracellular heme

Bacterial heme was detected via a modified version of a previously described protocol [23]. Overnight LB Km cultures of *S. oneidensis* strains were diluted to an ABS_{600} ≅0.1 and outgrown in LB Km. The equivalent of 10 mL of culture at an ABS_{600} of 1.0 was harvested in duplicate for each strain at the indicated time points. Cells were pelleted in Eppendorf tubes and washed once by resuspending in sterile 0.85% (w/v) saline. The washed pellets were then resuspended in 840 µL of Bacterial Protein Extraction Reagent (B-PER, Thermo Scientific) containing 100 µg/mL lysozyme and incubated at room temperature for 15 minutes with regular mixing. 200 µL of pyridine and 100 µL of 1.0 M NaOH was then mixed with each sample. One paired sample was oxidized by addition of 10 µL of 1 M potassium ferricyanide. The second paired sample was reduced by addition of 2–5 mg of sodium hydrosulfite powder. After zeroing the spectrophotometer with a sample with assay reagents only, an absorbance spectrum for each sample at 400–700 nm was obtained. A subtraction spectrum for each sample pair was generated by subtracting the oxidized spectrum from the reduced spectrum. Heme concentration was calculated using the absorbance difference between the peak at 550 nm and the trough at 535 nm from the subtraction spectrum and the millimolar extinction coefficient for heme C of 23.97 [23].

Construction of plasmid vectors and arabinose induction

pBBAD-SP is an arabinose-inducible expression vector derived from the Km^r broad host range vector pBBR1-MCS2 [24]. A ~1.7 kb fragment containing the *araC* gene, the P_{BAD} promoter, the multiple cloning site, and the transcriptional terminators from pBAD18 [25] was PCR amplified using the primers TCCGAGA-TCTTTATGACAACTTGACGGCTACATC and AGCGCTC-GAGAACAAAAGAGTTTGTAGAAACGCAAAAAGG. This PCR fragment was restricted with both *Bgl*II and *Xho*I and then ligated to *Bam*HI and *Xho*I-restricted pBBR1-MCS2.

To construct plasmid vectors expressing *gtrA* (So_3834) alone, *hemL* (So_1300) alone, or both *gtrA* and *hemL* from *S. oneidensis* under control of an arabinose-inducible promoter, the appropriate open reading frame(s) was/were PCR amplified and cloned into pBBAD-SP. To construct pBBAD-*gtrA*, a *gtrA* PCR product generated using the 5′ primer GGCGAATTCCATAGGGCCC-TAAGGAGGAAAAAAAATGAGCCTTGTAGCAATC and the 3′ primer GGCAAGCTTCCTTCATTTAACTCGCTAACC was digested with *Eco*RI and *Hin*dIII and ligated to *Eco*RI and *Hin*dIII-restricted pBBAD-SP. To construct pBBAD-*hemL*, a *hemL* PCR product generated using the 5′ primer GGCGAATTCCATAGGG-CCCTAAGGAGGAAAAAAAATGACCCGTTCCGAAGC and the 3′ primer GGCAAGCTTGTAAATACTTAGTTTGCCGC was digested with *Eco*RI and *Hin*dIII and ligated to *Eco*RI and *Hin*dIII-restricted pBBAD-SP. To construct pBBAD-*gtrA+hemL*, a *gtrA* PCR product was generated using the 5′ primer GGCGA-ATTCCATAGGGCCCTAAGGAGGAAAAAAAATGAGCCT-TGTAGCAATC and the 3′ primer GGCGAATTCCCTTCATT-TAACTCGCTAACC, while a *hemL* PCR product was generated using the 5′ primer GGCGAATTCCATAGGGCCCTAAGGAG-GAAAAAAAATGACCCGTTCCGAAGC and the 3′ primer GG-CAAGCTTGTAAATACTTAGTTTGCCGC. The *gtrA* PCR product was digested with *Eco*RI, while the *hemL* PCR product was digested with both *Eco*RI and *Hin*dIII. These two fragments were ligated to pBBAD-SP restricted with *Eco*RI and *Hin*dIII to generate an arabinose-inducible *gtrA-hemL* synthetic operon.

S. oneidensis strains (wild type MR-1 and *hfq* mutant) containing the plasmids described above were constructed by first transforming the plasmids into the tra^+ *E. coli* strain S17-1 λ*pir* [26]. The plasmids were then mobilized into *S. oneidensis* via conjugal transfer. MR-1 transconjugants were isolated from modified M1 plates [10] containing Km, while *hfq* mutant transconjugants were isolated from LB Km Gm plates.

Induction of heme biosynthesis genes cloned downstream of the P_{BAD} promoter was accomplished by addition of 0.005% (w/v) arabinose to the medium. This arabinose concentration was selected to optimize growth rescue and minimize negative effects of exogenous *gtrA* expression (see Figure 4C). The slight rescue of the *hfq* mutant growth phenotype by the pBBAD-*gtrA* plasmid (Figure 3B) and the significant rescue by the pBBAD-*gtrA+hemL* plasmid (Figure S3A) without arabinose present suggests that there is a low level of expression from the P_{BAD} promoter in *S. oneidensis* on LB medium in the absence of induction.

Preparation of total RNA and QRT-PCR analysis

Aerobic, 5 mL LB Km cultures of *S. oneidensis* strains inoculated from frozen permanent stocks and grown overnight were diluted in LB Km to an ABS_{600} ≅0.1 and outgrown aerobically until harvest 4 hours later. Total RNA was prepared using the RNeasy Protect Bacterial RNA Kit (Qiagen) following manufacturer instructions.

cDNA reaction mixtures were prepared with the AffinityScript QPCR cDNA synthesis kit (Agilent Technologies) according to manufacturer's instructions. cDNA synthesis was primed using random oligonucleotide nonamers provided in the cDNA synthesis kit, and 100 ng of total RNA was used as the template for each 20 µL reverse transcription (RT) reaction. RT reactions were incubated at 25°C for 5′, 42°C for 15′, 55°C for 15′, 95°C for 5′, and then held at 4°C. Reactions were used immediately or stored at −20°C for later use.

Target-specific primers for QPCR reactions (Table S1) were selected using the PrimerQuest tool available on the Integrated DNA Technologies (IDT) web site. QPCR reactions were performed using the Brilliant II SYBR Green QPCR Master Mix reagent and the Mx3000P QPCR System (both from Agilent Technologies) as per manufacturer instructions. For each target, up to three different sets of QPCR primers were evaluated for quantitative amplification and amplification efficiency using four serial dilutions of cDNA samples spanning a 64 fold concentration range. For *gtrA* and *recA* primers, cDNA dilutions used were undiluted, 1/4, 1/16, and 1/64, while for 16S primers dilutions were 1/16, 1/64, 1/256, and 1/1024. Technical data for primer sets selected for QPCR analyses are contained in Data S1. All primers were used at a concentration of 600 nM.

Quantitative RT-PCR analyses were performed on three independent biological replicates. Three technical replicates were analyzed for each biological replicate. QPCR reactions for *recA* and *gtrA* were performed using 1/4 dilutions of cDNA, while 16S rRNA reactions were performed using 1/256 dilutions of the cDNA. Threshold cycle (Ct) values were determined as per the software defaults. *gtrA* data was individually normalized to either 16S rRNA levels or *recA* mRNA levels. All amplification data were efficiency corrected using the primer pair standard curve data found in Data S1 and Table S1, and relative target quantities were calculated as per the software specifications. Statistical analyses of QPCR data were performed using unpaired two-tailed Student's t-tests to compare the means of the technical replicate data for the three biological replicates. Technical data for the QPCR reactions is contained in Data S1. Despite the multiple physiological differences associated with loss of Hfq, both 16S rRNA and recA mRNA levels were similar between exponentially-growing wild type and hfq mutant cells for each of the biological replicates (Data S1).

Supporting Information

Data S1 Data from QPCR experiments and primer set efficiency analyses.

Data S2 Data for Figure 1D. Raw and processed data for total free iron assays.

Data S3 Data for Figure 2B and 2C. Raw and processed data for heme assays.

Data S4 Data for Figure 4. Raw and processed data for growth curves and heme assays.

Data S5 Data for Figure S2. Raw and processed data from iron assay standard curve and from total free iron assays.

Figure S1 Growth of wild type and *hfq* mutant strains on different media. Colony size comparisons of MR-1/pBBR1-MCS2 (vector) and *hfqΔ*/pBBR1-MCS2 (vector) streaked to single colonies on (A) trypticase soy agar (TSA), (B) LB Km supplemented with 400 µM 5-ALA, (C) LB Km containing double the normal concentrations of tryptone and yeast extract (2X LB), and (D) LB Km supplemented with DL-serine, L-glutamic acid, and L-arginine (LB + AAs - see Materials and Methods).

Figure S2 Total iron detection: standard curve and cell culture trends. (A) Standard curve generated from ferrozine assays performed using known concentrations of $FeCl_3$. The blue trend line from a linear regression analysis with the y-intercept set at zero indicates that the assay is quantitative within the indicated concentration range ($ABS_{562} = 0.0182$ * [Fe] in the sample). For this data set the coefficient of determination (R^2) = 0.99705. (B) Results of iron assays using samples containing either 5 μM $FeSO_4$ or 5 μM hemin. Data is the mean of three independent samples. Error bars indicate standard deviation. **** indicates that the difference between iron detected is statistically significant ($P<0.0001$ in an unpaired two-tailed Student's t-test). (C) Plot of ferrozine assay results (ABS_{562} values) from iron assays versus culture densities (ABS_{600} values) at time of harvest. Data is pooled from multiple independent experiments using both MR-1 wild type cells (blue data points) and *hfq* mutant cells (red data points).

Figure S3 Exogenous expression of both *gtrA* and *hemL* rescues the colony size defect of the *hfq* mutant. Colony size comparisons of MR-1/pBBAD-SP (vector), MR-1/pBBAD-p*gtrA+hemL* (p*gtrA+hemL*), *hfqΔ*/pBBAD-SP (vector), and *hfqΔ*/pBBAD-p*gtrA+hemL* (p*gtrA+hemL*) streaked to single colonies on (A) LB Km and (B) LB Km containing 0.005% arabinose. Plates were photographed following 24 hours of growth at 30°C.

Figure S4 Growth of wild type and *hfq* mutant strains on solid M1 medium supplemented with heme or 5-ALA. Colony size comparisons of MR-1/pBBR1-MCS2 (vector) and *hfqΔ*/pBBR1-MCS2 (vector) streaked to single colonies on (A) M1 Km medium, (B) M1 Km medium supplemented with 50 μM hemin, (C) M1 Km medium supplemented with 50 μM 5-aminolevulinic acid (5-ALA), and (D) M1 Km medium supplemented with 400 μM 5-ALA. Plates were photographed following 72 hours of growth at 30°C.

Table S1 Oligonucleotide primers used for QPCR analyses.

Acknowledgments

We thank Fr. Nicanor Austriaco, O.P. and Jennifer Gervais for thoughtful discussions and critical reading of the manuscript. We also thank Marla Tipping for technical assistance with the QRT-PCR analyses.

Author Contributions

Conceived and designed the experiments: CMB NQM TMH BJP. Performed the experiments: CMB NQM TM TMH MLK JNL SES ENB BJP. Analyzed the data: CMB NQM TMH BJP. Contributed reagents/materials/analysis tools: SP. Wrote the paper: CMB NQM TM TMH BJP.

References

1. De Lay N, Schu DJ, Gottesman S (2013) Bacterial small RNA-based negative regulation: Hfq and its accomplices. The Journal of Biological Chemistry 288: 7996–8003.
2. Vogel J, Luisi BF (2011) Hfq and its constellation of RNA. Nat Rev Microbiol 9: 578–589.
3. Waters LS, Storz G (2009) Regulatory RNAs in bacteria. Cell 136: 615–628.
4. Brennan RG, Link TM (2007) Hfq structure, function and ligand binding. Current Opinion in Microbiology 10: 125–133.
5. Moller T, Franch T, Hojrup P, Keene DR, Bachinger HP, et al. (2002) Hfq: a bacterial Sm-like protein that mediates RNA-RNA interaction. Mol Cell 9: 23–30.
6. Panja S, Woodson SA (2012) Hexamer to monomer equilibrium of *E. coli* Hfq in solution and its impact on RNA annealing. Journal of Molecular Biology 417: 406–412.
7. Tsui HC, Leung HC, Winkler ME (1994) Characterization of broadly pleiotropic phenotypes caused by an hfq insertion mutation in *Escherichia coli* K-12. Mol Microbiol 13: 35–49.
8. Ding Y, Davis BM, Waldor MK (2004) Hfq is essential for Vibrio cholerae virulence and downregulates sigma expression. Mol Microbiol 53: 345–354.
9. Muffler A, Traulsen DD, Fischer D, Lange R, Hengge-Aronis R (1997) The RNA-binding protein HF-I plays a global regulatory role which is largely, but not exclusively, due to its role in expression of the sigmaS subunit of RNA polymerase in *Escherichia coli*. J Bacteriol 179: 297–300.
10. Brennan CM, Keane ML, Hunt TM, Goulet MT, Mazzucca NQ, et al. (2013) *Shewanella oneidensis* Hfq promotes exponential phase growth, stationary phase culture density, and cell survival. BMC Microbiology 13: 33.
11. Myers CR, Nealson KH (1988) Bacterial manganese reduction and growth with manganese oxide as the sole electron acceptor. Science 240: 1319–1321.
12. Nealson KH, Saffarini D (1994) Iron and manganese in anaerobic respiration: environmental significance, physiology, and regulation. Annu Rev Microbiol 48: 311–343.
13. Lovley DR (2006) Bug juice: harvesting electricity with microorganisms. Nature Reviews Microbiology 4: 497–508.
14. Fredrickson JK, Romine MF, Beliaev AS, Auchtung JM, Driscoll ME, et al. (2008) Towards environmental systems biology of *Shewanella*. Nature Reviews Microbiology 6: 592–603.
15. Panek H, O'Brian MR (2002) A whole genome view of prokaryotic haem biosynthesis. Microbiology 148: 2273–2282.
16. Heidelberg JF, Paulsen IT, Nelson KE, Gaidos EJ, Nelson WC, et al. (2002) Genome sequence of the dissimilatory metal ion-reducing bacterium *Shewanella oneidensis*. Nat Biotechnol 20: 1118–1123.
17. Meyer TE, Tsapin AI, Vandenberghe I, de Smet L, Frishman D, et al. (2004) Identification of 42 possible cytochrome C genes in the *Shewanella oneidensis* genome and characterization of six soluble cytochromes. Omics: a journal of integrative biology 8: 57–77.
18. Myers CR, Myers JM (1992) Localization of cytochromes to the outer membrane of anaerobically grown *Shewanella putrefaciens* MR-1. Journal of Bacteriology 174: 3429–3438.
19. Bouhenni R, Gehrke A, Saffarini D (2005) Identification of genes involved in cytochrome c biogenesis in *Shewanella oneidensis*, using a modified mariner transposon. Applied and Environmental Microbiology 71: 4935–4937.
20. Schobert M, Jahn D (2002) Regulation of heme biosynthesis in non-phototrophic bacteria. Journal of Molecular Microbiology and Biotechnology 4: 287–294.
21. Wang L, Elliott M, Elliott T (1999) Conditional stability of the HemA protein (glutamyl-tRNA reductase) regulates heme biosynthesis in *Salmonella typhimurium*. Journal of Bacteriology 181: 1211–1219.
22. Viollier E, Inglett PW, Hunter K, Roychoudhury AN, Van Cappellen P (2000) The ferrozine method revisited: Fe(II)/Fe(III) determination in natural waters. Appl Geochem 15: 785–790.
23. Berry EA, Trumpower BL (1987) Simultaneous determination of hemes a, b, and c from pyridine hemochrome spectra. Analytical Biochemistry 161: 1–15.
24. Kovach ME, Elzer PH, Hill DS, Robertson GT, Farris MA, et al. (1995) Four new derivatives of the broad-host-range cloning vector pBBR1MCS, carrying different antibiotic-resistance cassettes. Gene 166: 175–176.
25. Guzman LM, Belin D, Carson MJ, Beckwith J (1995) Tight regulation, modulation, and high-level expression by vectors containing the arabinose PBAD promoter. Journal of Bacteriology 177: 4121–4130.
26. Simon R, Priefer U, Puhler A (1983) A Broad Host Range Mobilization System for In Vivo Genetic Engineering: Transposon Mutagenesis in Gram Negative Bacteria. Nat Biotech 1: 784–791.
27. Anzaldi LL, Skaar EP (2010) Overcoming the heme paradox: heme toxicity and tolerance in bacterial pathogens. Infection and Immunity 78: 4977–4989.
28. Abdul-Tehrani H, Hudson AJ, Chang YS, Timms AR, Hawkins C, et al. (1999) Ferritin mutants of *Escherichia coli* are iron deficient and growth impaired, and fur mutants are iron deficient. Journal of Bacteriology 181: 1415–1428.
29. Kane AL, Bond DR, Gralnick JA (2013) Electrochemical analysis of *Shewanella oneidensis* engineered to bind gold electrodes. ACS Synth Biol 2: 93–101.
30. Shi L, Deng S, Marshall MJ, Wang Z, Kennedy DW, et al. (2008) Direct involvement of type II secretion system in extracellular translocation of *Shewanella oneidensis* outer membrane cytochromes MtrC and OmcA. J Bacteriol 190: 5512–5516.
31. Nakahigashi K, Nishimura K, Miyamoto K, Inokuchi H (1991) Photosensitivity of a protoporphyrin-accumulating, light-sensitive mutant (*visA*) of *Escherichia coli* K-12. Proceedings of the National Academy of Sciences of the United States of America 88: 10520–10524.

17

Screening the Expression of ABCB6 in Erythrocytes Reveals an Unexpectedly High Frequency of Lan Mutations in Healthy Individuals

Magdalena Koszarska[1]☯, Nora Kucsma[2]☯, Katalin Kiss[2], Gyorgy Varady[2], Melinda Gera[2], Geza Antalffy[2], Hajnalka Andrikovics[1], Attila Tordai[1], Maciej Studzian[4], Dominik Strapagiel[5], Lukasz Pulaski[4], Yoshihiko Tani[6], Balazs Sarkadi[1,2,3], Gergely Szakacs[2]*

1 Hungarian National Blood Transfusion Service, Budapest, Hungary, **2** Institute of Enzymology, Research Centre for Natural Sciences, Hungarian Academy of Sciences, Budapest, Hungary, **3** Molecular Biophysics Research Group of the Hungarian Academy of Sciences, Semmelweis University, Budapest, Hungary, **4** Department of Molecular Biophysics, University of Lodz, Lodz, Poland, **5** Biobank Lab, Department of Molecular Biophysics, University of Lodz, Lodz, Poland, **6** Japanese Red Cross Kinki Block Blood Center, Osaka, Japan

Abstract

Lan is a high-incidence blood group antigen expressed in more than 99.9% of the population. Identification of the human ABC transporter ABCB6 as the molecular basis of Lan has opened the way for studies assessing the relation of ABCB6 function and expression to health and disease. To date, 34 ABCB6 sequence variants have been described in association with reduced ABCB6 expression based on the genotyping of stored blood showing weak or no reactivity with anti-Lan antibodies. In the present study we examined the red blood cell (RBC) surface expression of ABCB6 by quantitative flow cytometry in a cohort of 47 healthy individuals. Sequencing of the entire coding region of the *ABCB6* gene in low RBC ABCB6 expressors identified a new allele (IVS9+1G>A, affecting a putative splice site at the boundary of exon 9) and two nonsynonymous SNPs listed in the SNP database (R192Q (rs150221689) and G588 S (rs145526996)). The R192Q mutation showed co-segregation with reduced RBC ABCB6 expression in a family, and we found the G588 S mutation in a compound heterozygous individual with undetectable ABCB6 expression, suggesting that both mutations result in weak or no expression of ABCB6 on RBCs. Analysis of the intracellular expression pattern in HeLa cells by confocal microscopy indicated that these mutations do not compromise overall expression or the endolysosomal localization of ABCB6. Genotyping of two large cohorts, containing 235 and 1039 unrelated volunteers, confirmed the high allele frequency of Lan-mutations. Our results suggest that genetic variants linked to lower or absent cell surface expression of ABCB6/Langereis may be more common than previously thought.

Editor: Szabolcs Semsey, Niels Bohr Institute, Denmark

Funding: This work was supported by the Lendulet Program of the Hungarian Academy of Sciences (GS), OTKA 83533 and by the Polish POIG grant 01.01.02-10-005/08 TESTOPLEK, supported by the EU through the European Regional Development Fund. Hajnalka Andrikovics is a recipient of the Janos Bolyai Research Scholarship from the Hungarian Academy of Sciences. The funders had no role in study design, data collection and analysis, decision to publish, or preparation of the manuscript.

* Email: szakacs.gergely@ttk.mta.hu

☯ These authors contributed equally to this work.

Introduction

ATP-binding cassette (ABC) transporters make up one of the largest protein families from bacteria to man [1]. ABC proteins are essential for many physiological processes, and mutations in these genes have been linked to several human genetic disorders including cystic fibrosis, connective tissue mineralization, neurological disease, retinal degeneration, cholesterol and bile transport defects, anemia and gout [2]. Human ABC transporters transport a large variety of endogenous substrates and xenobiotic compounds. Despite extensive studies, the physiological function of several ABC transporters remains unknown.

ABC proteins are divided into seven subfamilies, based on domain organization and sequence homology. ABCB6 belongs to the ABCB subfamily, which includes P-glycoprotein (ABCB1/MDR1) causing multidrug resistance of cancer cells [3]; the TAP1/2 complex (ABCB2-3) mediating the translocation of immunogenic peptides from the cytosol into the endoplasmic reticulum [4]; ABCB4-MDR3 influencing the translocation of phosphatidylcholine [5], and ABCB11 involved in the secretion of bile acids [6].

ABCB6 is one of the four ABC transporters that were assigned to the mitochondria. Initially, ABCB6 was reported to be a regulator of de novo porphyrin biosynthesis by promoting the ATP-dependent mitochondrial uptake of porphyrins [7]. Although initial findings suggested that loss of one Abcb6 allele in embryonic stem (ES) cells impairs porphyrin synthesis, mice derived from these stem cells were phenotypically normal [8]. Recent studies have challenged the paradigm linking the function of ABCB6 to mitochondria, and suggested that ABCB6 is localized in the endolysosomal continuum including the plasma membrane [9], the Golgi apparatus [10], and organelles of the vesicular system [11,12,13,14]. ABCB6 is upregulated during erythroid differentiation, and although a proportion is lost during reticulocyte maturation through secreted exosomes, ABCB6 is expressed in mature red blood cells at relatively high levels [15]. In 2012, ABCB6 was revealed as the molecular basis of the Lan blood group antigen [16]. Lan is a high frequency blood group, expressed in more than 99.9% of most populations. Consequently, Lan-negativity is extremely rare, estimated to appear in approximately 0.005% of the Caucasian population [17]. Consistent with the knock-out mouse study, Lan-negative individuals lack an overt phenotype, arguing against a vital role of ABCB6 in porphyrin synthesis. Still, the Lan antigen is medically relevant since individuals with Lan(−) blood group may develop anti-Lan antibodies, which can cause transfusion reactions or hemolytic disease of the fetus or newborn.

The NCBI SNP database lists 417 ABCB6 variants/SNPs, of which 34 have been associated with the Lan-negative phenotype. All the Lan-negeive individuals genotyped so far have inherited two recessive null mutations. Heterozygous mutations result in reduced erythrocytic protein levels, indicating bi-allelic expression of ABCB6. Based on the Phase 1 publication of the 1000 Genome genotype data [18], the global minor allele frequency (MAF) of the Lan-associated SNPs is low, indicating that individual variations are relatively rare. Recent studies have associated mutations in ABCB6 with various hereditary diseases including ocular coloboma [19], dominant familial pseudohyperkalemia [20] and dyschromatosis universalis hereditaria (DUH) [21]. The pathophysiological role of ABCB6 in these conditions is not known since it is not possible to directly correlate sequence variations to ABCB6 function or expression. This is partly due to the lack of our understanding of the physiological function and the structure-activity relationships within ABCB6, and also to the complex regulation of protein synthesis, maturation, trafficking and posttranslational modifications of membrane proteins.

Recently, we have characterized the quantitative expression of the ABCG2 multidrug transporter corresponding to the Jr^a blood group in human erythrocytes and have shown that pharmacologically relevant polymorphisms are associated with significantly reduced ABCG2 protein expression [22]. Here we show that RBC ABCB6 expression levels display a large variation in healthy individuals, with an unexpectedly high frequency of low expressors. Genotype screening of two large cohorts (containing 235 and 1039 unrelated volunteers) confirmed that genetic variations underlying low surface ABCB6 expression are more common than previously inferred based on the frequency of Lan-negative blood type.

Methods

Probands

The "discovery cohort" consisted of 47 healthy, Hungarian unrelated individuals [(12 males and 35 females; median age: 37 (26–66)]. Family members (n = 4) of 2 healthy volunteers with low ABCB6 expression and two Lan-negative (Lan−) individuals with a previous history of hemolytic disease of the newborn caused by anti-Lan antibody were investigated additionally [23]. The Hungarian genetic screening cohort consisted of 184 healthy, unrelated first or second time Hungarian blood donors ((94 males, 90 females; median age 37 (22–76)). The Polish genetic screening cohort included 1039 healthy, unrelated subjects (555 males, 484 females, median age 39 (19–76)). This sample was randomly selected within the "normal Polish population" genetic collection at the Biobank, Department of Molecular Biophysics, University of Lodz. Genetic material for this collection was sampled in 2011–2012 within the EU-funded TESTOPLEK research project. A professional public opinion polling and survey-taking company (SMG/KRC Poland, a Millward Brown subsidiary) was subcontracted to select a cross-sectional sample of >10000 individuals from the population at large, with representation from each geographical region of Poland (number of samples from each powiat/county proportional to the population of the county). The individuals were selected from public records, visited in their domiciles by SMG/KRC pollsters and asked to provide genetic material (saliva, see below) and to fill out a general anthropological and medical questionnaire. Since proband selection was random from the overall population, the probands were not necessarily healthy individuals, although the sample excluded hospitalized patients and those unable to give informed consent. All subjects gave their written informed consent to participate in the study. This study was approved by the respective regional ethical committees (The University Committee on Bioethics Research (University of Lodz); Scientific and Research Ethics Committee of the Healthcare Scientific Council of Hungary), and all procedures were performed in accordance with the Declaration of Helsinki.

One patient's sample was obtained through the NIH Undiagnosed Diseases Program (UDP) in the United States [24]. The patient was enrolled in clinical protocol 76-HG-0238, approved by the Institutional Review Board of the National Human Genome Research Institute. The parents gave written, informed consent.

Genotyping

In the Hungarian cohort, genomic DNA was isolated from EDTA anticoagulated peripheral blood by Gentra Purege Blood Kit (Qiagen, Hamburg, Germany). Sanger sequencing of the ABCB6 coding region and exon-intron boundaries (exons 1–19, NCBI Reference Sequence: NT_005403.18) was performed by Applied Biosystems 310 Genetic Analyzer (Life Technologies, Carlsbad, USA). Screening for ABCB6 variants at R192 (rs150221689) or G588 (rs145526996) was performed by the PCR restriction fragment length polymorphism method using SsiI and Sau96I, respectively. Digested PCR products were size-separated by electrophoresis on 2% agarose gels and visualized by ethidium bromide staining. For the detection of ABCB6 R192 codon variants the primer pair for amplification of exons 1–2 (ABCB6-2 and ABCB6-4) was used according to Helias et al. [16], while for the detection of ABCB6 G588 S variants the following primers were used ABCB6-37 [16] and ABCB6-13R (5′-GGAGGCTGCACCATTCAATC-3′).

For the Polish population study, saliva was collected into Oragene OG-500 DNA collection/storage receptacles (DNA Genotek, Kanata, Canada) and genomic DNA was subsequently isolated by the MagNA Pure LC DNA Isolation Kit - Large Volume (Roche, Basel, Switzerland) with its final concentration normalized to 0.2 μg/ml. Screening for expected ABCB6 SNP variants at R192, G588, R276 as well as the exon 9 boundary splice site was performed by High Resolution Melting (HRM) analysis of PCR products amplified and subsequently melted on a BioRad C1000/CFX384 thermocycler. The reaction used 500 pg genomic DNA as template, 2xGoTaq polymerase master mix (Promega, Madison, USA) and LCGreen dye (BioFire Defence, Salt Lake City, USA). HRM curves were interpreted using the

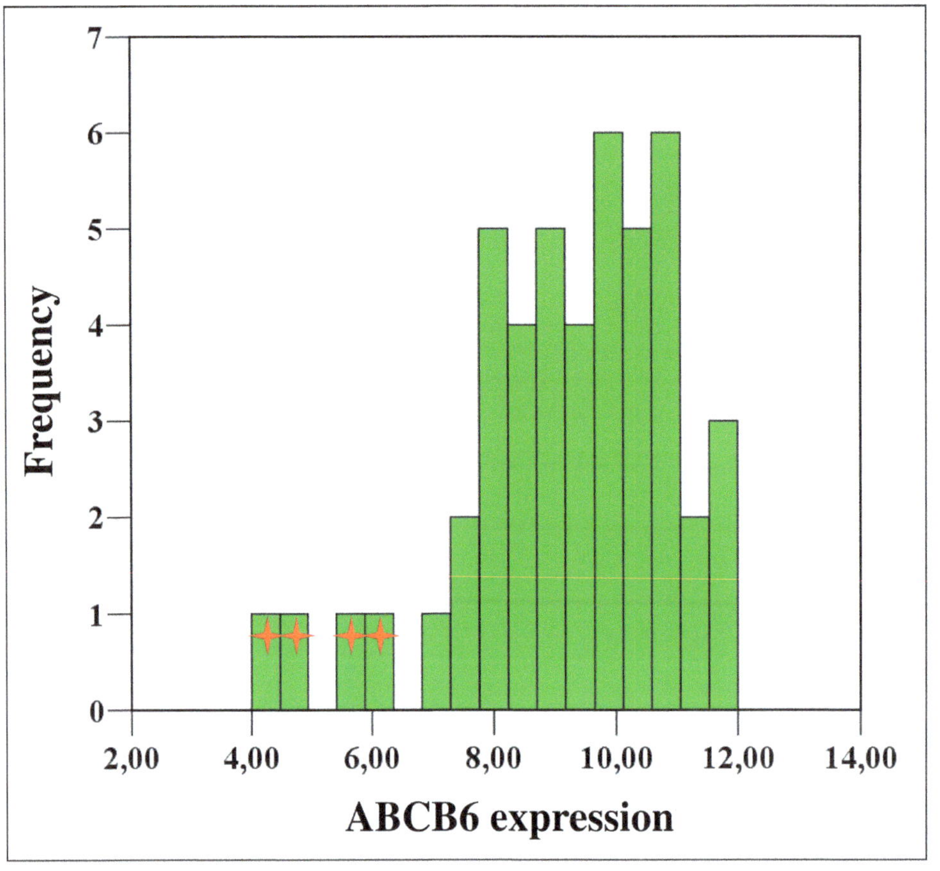

Figure 1. Erythrocytic ABCB6 expression in 47 healthy individuals. Histogram illustrating the distribution of erythrocytic ABCB6 expression in 47 unrelated healthy individuals, as measured by a quantitative FACS assay using the OSK43 monoclonal antibody specifically recognizing a surface epitope of ABCB6 (see Methods). The four individuals exhibiting significantly lower ABCB6 levels (below the 10th percentile) are labeled by asterisks.

Precision Melt Analysis Software from BioRad. Samples with divergent melting curves were selected for re-amplification, cloning and Sanger sequencing to confirm the presence of respective SNPs.

The following primers were used for HRM analysis (all at 59°C annealing temperature):

ABCB6-HRM-R192-F 5′-GTTCAGTTTAGCCTGTGGGTG-3′

ABCB6-HRM-R192-R 5′-CAAACAGCCCTCCAGAGACC-3′

ABCB6-HRM-R276-F 5′-CTGGGGCTCATGGGTTTG-3′

ABCB6-HRM-R276-R 5′-GGCACCAACACATTGAGTG-3′

ABCB6-HRM-G588-F 5′-TGGAGCAGGGCCCCTTC-3′

ABCB6-HRM-G588-R 5′-CATCGGCATAGCTGAAGTGC-3′

ABCB6-HRM-IVS9-F 5′-GCGCATACTTTGTCACTGAG-CAG-3′

ABCB6-HRM-IVS9-R 5′-CCCACTCTCTCATCCAAGATCC-3′

Quantitative analysis of ABCB6 expression by flow cytometry

Freshly drawn human blood (25 μl) was diluted in 4 ml of phosphate buffered saline (PBS), the cells were centrifuged at 3,000×g for 10 min. Samples were processed within 3 hours, or stored for a maximum of 2 days after fixation in 1% PFA for 60 min at 25°C. Antibody staining was performed for 40 min at 37°C by using the Human monoclonal anti-Lan (Clone OSK43; IgG1κ) (0.7 μl/tubes) specifically recognizing ABCB6 protein [16], or without primary antibody (negative staining). Antibody concentrations for ABCB6 labeling in red cells were carefully calibrated to provide maximum labeling in a full range of protein expression. After washing out the primary antibodies, secondary antibodies corresponding to the IgG type and labeled with phycoerythrin (PE) were added to the cells (Goat F(ab')2 fragment anti-human IgG-PE (Beckman Coulter, PNI 1626)), in 50× dilution, incubated for 30 min at 37oC, washed and resuspended in PBS. The labeled samples were subjected to flow cytometry (FACS); intact red cells were gated based on the forward scatter (FSC) and side scatter (SSC) parameters. Intact cells were analyzed for antibody staining by a FACSCalibur flow cytometer (excitation wavelength: 488 nm (Argon ion laser) emission filters: 585/42 nm for PE). RBC ABCB6 was measured 4 times in each individual (Figure S1); relative ABCB6 expression was calculated by dividing the median values obtained with the primary and secondary antibodies with the weighted average of the median values obtained with secondary antibody only. The weighted average (WA) was calculated as follows: WA = (average secondary fluorescence of all measured samples*2+individually measured secondary fluorescence)/3. Surface expression of ABCB6 variants expressed in K562 cells was performed as described previously [15].

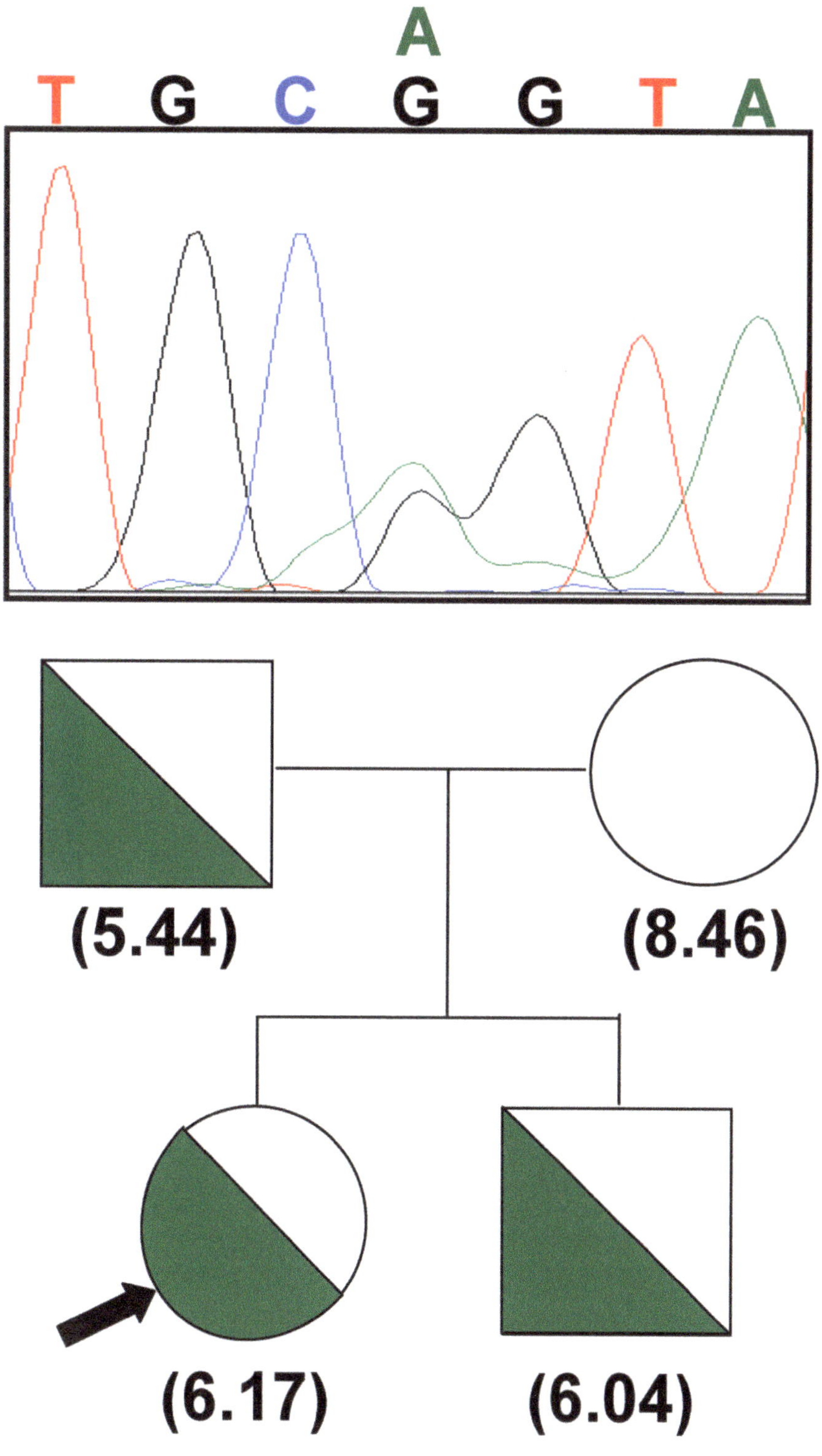

Figure 2. Pedigree of a family carrying the ABCB6 R192Q mutation– co-segregation of the heterozygous mutation with reduced erythrocytic ABCB6 expression levels. Blood samples obtained from the family members of the healthy volunteer proband carrying the R192Q ABCB6 mutation (indicated with black arrow) were analyzed for ABCB6 expression and the presence of the mutation. The upper panel represents a heterozygous R192Q (c.575G>A) sequence. The lower panel shows the segregation of R192Q heterozygosity (marked with green half circles and squares for females and males, respectively) with reduced ABCB6 expression in erythrocytes (values in parentheses).

Mutagenesis

cDNA encoding wild-type human ABCB6 (NM_005689) bearing an HA-tag at its C-terminus [9,15] was mutated using the QuikChange site-directed mutagenesis kit (Stratagene) using the following primers:

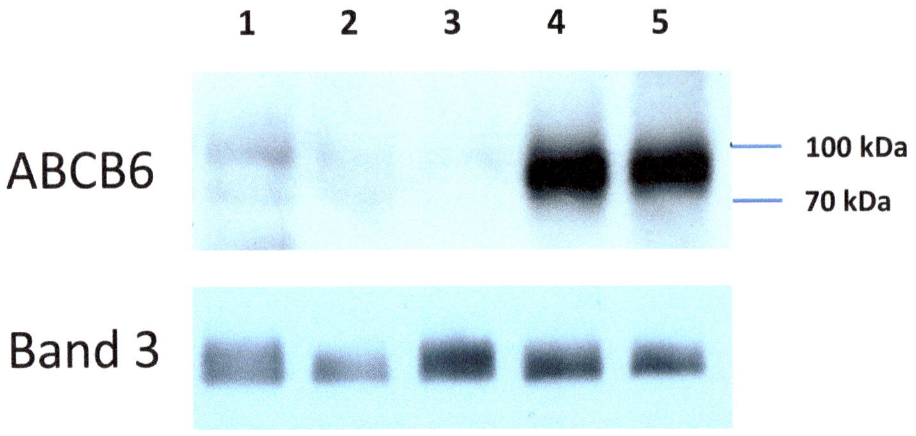

Figure 3. Characterization of ABCB6 mutations responsible for the Lan- blood type. RBC membrane lysates (80 ug/lane) were prepared from a compound heterozygote individual carrying the R276W and the G588S mutations (lane 1); homozygotes carrying the R192W mutation (c.574C>T, p.Arg192Trp); lanes 2, 3); or individuals carrying two wild-type alleles (lanes 4, 5). ABCB6 expression is revealed by the ABCB6-567 monoclonal antibody [9], Band III is shown as loading control.

ABCB6-R192W-F 5′-CCTGTGGGTGCTGtGGTATGTGGTCTCTGG-3′

ABCB6-R192W-R 5′-CCAGAGACCACATACCaCAGCACC-CACAGG-3′

ABCB6-R192Q-F 5′-CCTGTGGGTGCTGCaG-TATGTGGTCTCTGG-3′

ABCB6-R192Q-R 5′-CCAGAGACCACATACtGCAGCACC-CACAGG-3′

ABCB6-G588S-F 5′-CCCCTTCGCTTTCAGAAGaGCCG-TATTGAGTTTGAG-3′

ABCB6-G588S-R 5′-CTCAAACTCAATACGGCtCTTCT-GAAAGCGAAGGGG-3′

Mutations were confirmed by sequencing.

Cell lines

The HA-tagged ABCB6 and its variants (ABCB6-G588S-HA, ABCB6-R192Q-HA or ABCB6-R192W-HA, respectively) were cloned into a pSEW lentiviral vector and stably expressed in K562 and HeLa cells by lentiviral transduction. Lentiviral particles were produced in HEK293T cells transfected by the calcium phosphate co-precipitation method according to manufacturer's protocol [25]. Viral titers of the supernatants were estimated by flow cytometric measurement of HEK cells infected with a dilution series of the supernatants; transduced cells were selected with 2 ug/ml puromycin for 2 weeks.

The K562 cell line (ATCC) was grown in RPMI 1640 medium without nucleosides, supplemented with 10% (v/v) fetal bovine serum (Invitrogen Cat.No. 10106-169) and with 2 mM glutamine, 100 units/mL penicillin, and 100 units/mL streptomycin (Invitrogen-Gibco, Carlsbad, CA, USA) at 37°C in humidified air/CO2 (19:1) atmosphere. The HeLa cell line (ATCC) was grown in DMEM, supplemented with 10% (v/v) fetal bovine serum (Invitrogen Cat.No. 10106-169) and with 2 mM glutamine, 100 units/mL penicillin, and 100 units/mL streptomycin (Invitrogen-Gibco, Carlsbad, CA, USA) at 37°C in humidified air/CO2 (19:1) atmosphere. Cell lines were regularly screened with the Mycoplasm Detection Kit (Lonza), and the assays were carried out in mycoplasma-negative cells.

Confocal Microscopy

Cells at 70%–80% confluency were gently washed with Dulbecco's modified phosphate-buffered saline (DPBS), fixed with 4% paraformaldehyde (PFA) in DPBS for 10 minutes at room temperature, and permeabilized in methanol for 90 seconds at room temperature. The samples were then blocked for 1 h at room temperature in DPBS containing 2 mg/mL BSA (Sigma, A7030), 1% fish gelatin from cold water fish skin (Sigma, G7765), 0.1% Triton-X 100 and 5% goat serum (Sigma, G9023). After blocking, the cells were incubated for 1 h at room temperature with the primary antibody diluted in blocking buffer. After washing with DPBS, the cells were incubated for 1 hour at room temperature with the respective Alexa Fluor-conjugated secondary antibody diluted at 1:250 in blocking buffer. Where indicated, DAPI was diluted in DPBS and added to the cells after the incubation with the secondary antibody, for 10 minutes at room temperature. Wheat Germ Agglutinin and LysoTracker were added to living cells before the immunostaining procedure and incubated for 10 min or 30 min at 37C, respectively. To label cellular organelles, the following dyes and antibodies were used: LysoTracker Red DND-99 (Invitrogen, L7528), DAPI (49,6-diamidino-2-phenylindole, dihydrochloride, Sigma D9564), Alexa Fluor 633 conjugate of WGA (Invitrogen, W21404), anti-COX IV (3E11) Rabbit mAb #4850 (Cellular Localization IF Antibody Sampler Kit, Cell Signaling, #4753), anti-Calnexin (Rabbit, Cell Signaling, #4753), anti-ABCB6-567 [9], anti-HA. As secondary antibodies we used Alexa Fluor 488 Goat Anti-Mouse IgG (H+L) (Invitrogen, A11001), Alexa Fluor 594 Goat Anti-Rabbit IgG (H+ L) (Invitrogen, A11012) and Alexa Fluor 594 Goat Anti-Mouse IgG (H+L) (Invitrogen, A11005). As isotype controls reagent grade IgG from mouse and rabbit serum were used (Sigma). Samples were studied with an Olympus IX-81/FV500 laser scanning confocal microscope, using an Olympus PLAPO 606 (1.4 NA) oil immersion objective (Olympus Europa GmbH). Dual channel colocalization analysis was performed by the ImageJ software with the Colocalization Threshold and Colocalization Test plugins. Averaged Pearson's coefficients are reported for each subcellular marker from 5 random pictures [26,27].

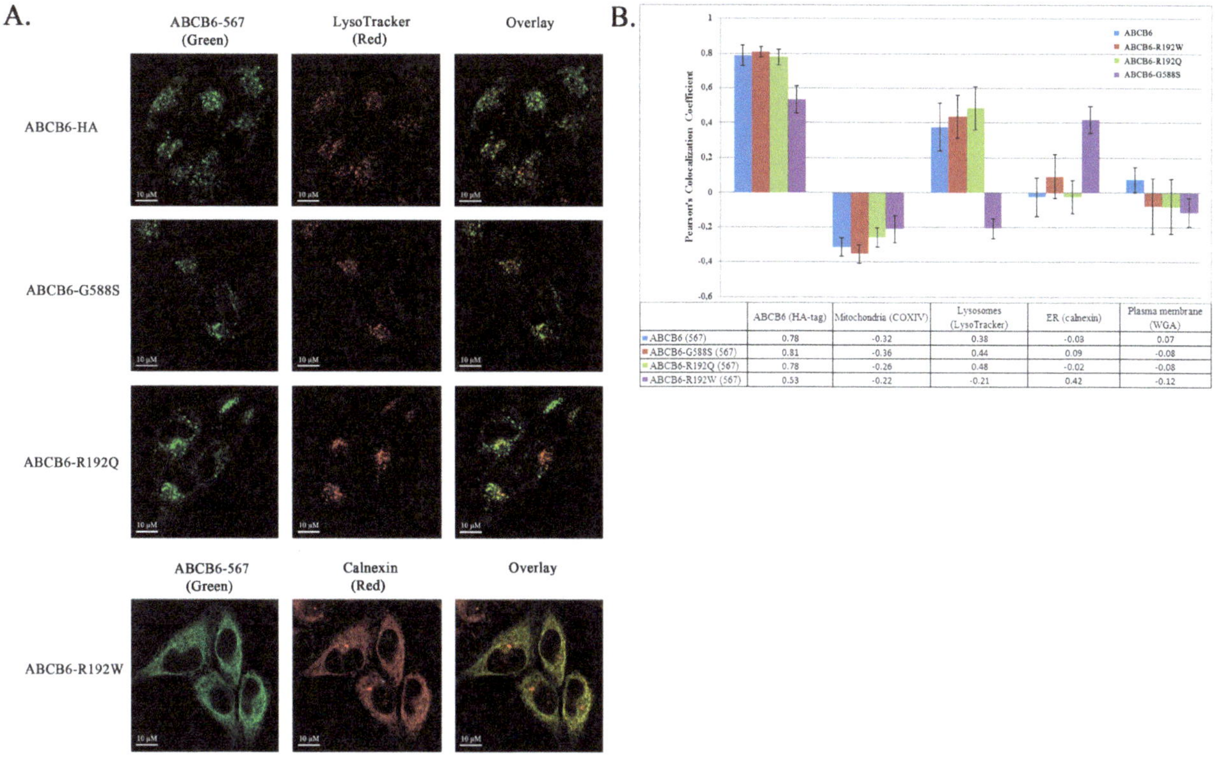

	ABCB6 (HA-tag)	Mitochondria (COXIV)	Lysosomes (LysoTracker)	ER (calnexin)	Plasma membrane (WGA)
ABCB6 (567)	0.78	-0.32	0.38	-0.03	0.07
ABCB6-G588S (567)	0.81	-0.36	0.44	0.09	-0.08
ABCB6-R192Q (567)	0.78	-0.26	0.48	-0.02	-0.08
ABCB6-R192W (567)	0.53	-0.22	-0.21	0.42	-0.12

Figure 4. Determination of the subcellular localization of ABCB6 variants. A. Double immunofluorescence labeling and laser-scanning confocal microscopy images of HeLa cells overexpressing ABCB6-HA, ABCB6-HA-G588S, ABCB6-HA-R192Q or ABCB6-HA-R192W, probed with the ABCB6-567 antibody (green) [9] in the context of LysoTracker (red) or Calnexin (red). B. Colocalization of ABCB6-variants with various intracellular markers. Bars represesent averaged Pearson's coefficients +/− standard deviation for each subcellular marker from 5 random pictures. Blue: ABCB6-HA; red: ABCB6-HA-G588S; green: ABCB6-HA-R192Q; purple: ABCB6-HA-R192W.

Results and Discussion

Population analysis of gene expression is typically achieved by quantifying levels of mRNA; however, gene expression is also a function of protein translation and turnover [28]. We used a flow cytometry-based assay for the quantitative determination of red blood cell ABCB6 expression in 47 unrelated, healthy individuals. ABCB6 expression was measured with the OSK43 monoclonal antibody specifically recognizing the Lan blood group antigen that is carried by ABCB6 [16]. Significant ABCB6 levels, encompassing a wide range of expression were detected in all but four individuals, who showed significantly lower ABCB6 levels (below the 10th percentile, Figure 1, Figure S1). Differences in RBC ABCB6 expression could not be attributed to age or sex. Since mutations in the *ABCB6* gene were shown to result in the rare Lan- blood type, which is characterized by the absence of ABCB6 in red blood cells [16], we sequenced the entire coding region of the *ABCB6* gene of the four individuals exhibiting reduced RBC ABCB6 expression. Sequencing revealed alterations in each subject: two unrelated subjects were heterozygous for the missense mutation c.1762G>A, p.Gly588Ser (G588 S) encoded by the minor allele of SNP rs145526996; one subject was heterozygous for a mutation affecting the splice donor site of intron 9 (IVS9+1G>A); and a fourth subject was heterozygous for the missense mutation c.574G>A,p.Arg192Gln (R192Q) encoded by the minor allele of SNP rs150221689. The G588 S mutation was previously reported to be associated with lower RBC ABCB6 levels [28], the putative splice site mutation has not been described. Mutation of arginine to tryptophan at position 192 (R192W) was shown to be a null mutation that is responsible for the Lan-negative phenotype [28] but the presence of a glutamine at the same position has not been linked to low RBC ABCB6 expression.

In order to clarify if a direct relationship exists between the mutation R192Q and the RBC ABCB6 expression levels, we obtained blood samples from the family members of the proband carrying this mutation. We found co-segregation of the reduced RBC ABCB6 expression and the R192Q mutation, confirming the direct genotype-phenotype correlation (Figure 2). Segregation of the mutation with reduced expression indicates that the missense mutation R192Q defines a novel ABCB6 allele related to weak or no expression of ABCB6 on RBCs.

The G588S (rs145526996) mutation was reported to result in a significant drop in RBC ABCB6 expression in heterozygous individuals in a previous study that also found decreased RBC ABCB6 levels in heterozygous individuals carrying the p.Arg276Trp mutation [28]. Our study confirms the association of both of these mutations with reduced RBC ABCB6 levels. We were unable to detect ABCB6 expression in the erythrocyte of a compound heterozygote patient referred to us carrying both the R276W and the G588S mutations (c. 826C>T, p.Arg276Trp/c.1762G>A, p.Gly588Ser), corroborating the conclusion that these mutations correspond to weak or no expression of ABCB6 on RBCs (Figure 3).

Next, we wanted to further analyze the apparent deleterious effect of the mutations identified in low RBC ABCB6 expressors using Hela cells stably expressing the wild-type or the mutant ABCB6 proteins. Since the mutations did not compromise overall

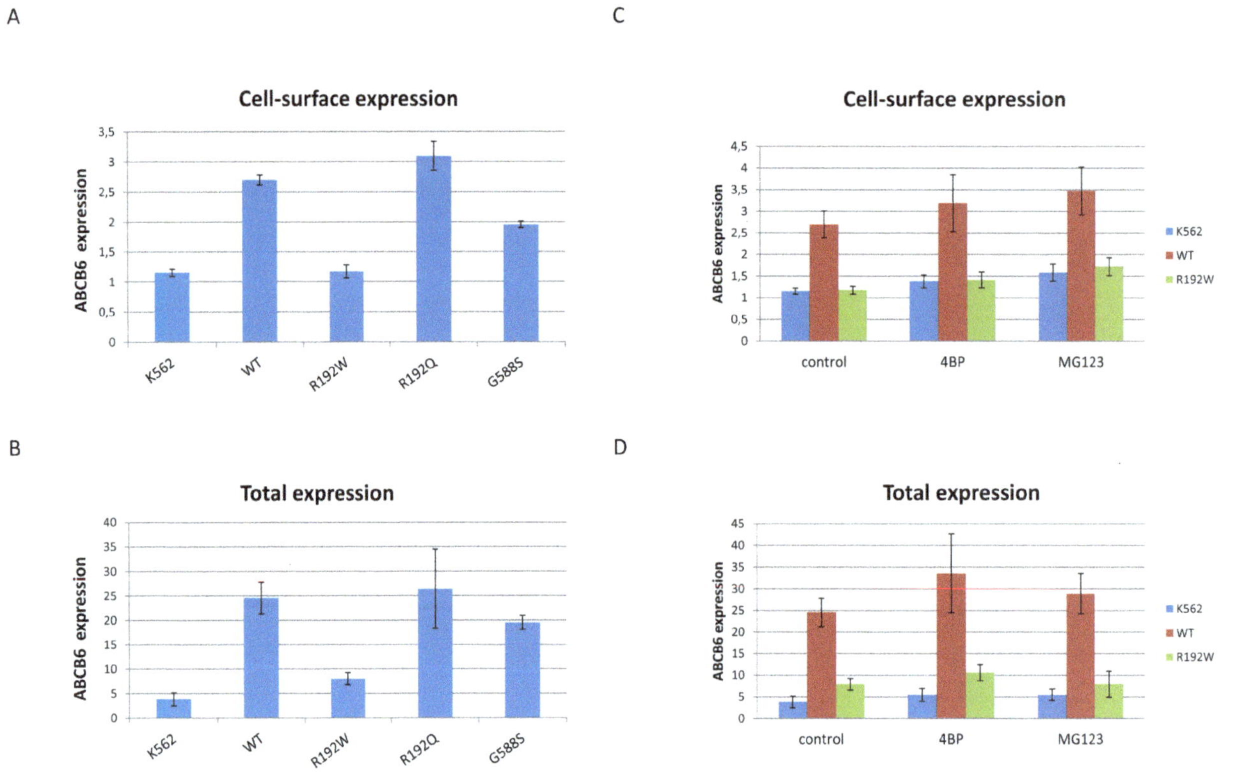

Figure 5. Detection of relative plasma membrane ABCB6 levels by flow cytometry. K562 cells were stably transduced with retroviral constructs encoding wild-type (WT), or mutated ABCB6 variants (R192W, R192Q, G588S). Cell surface (A, C) and total (B, D) ABCB6 expression was analyzed by flow cytometry using the monoclonal anti-Lan OSK43 antibody [16] in intact and permeabilized cells, respectively. The effect of pharmacological chaperoning and the inhibition of the proteasome (C, D) was studied by culturing the cells in the presence of 2 mM 4-PBA or 0.5 uM MG132, respectively. Bars represent average ABCB6 expression +/− standard deviation of at least 3 independent experiments.

expression levels, we analyzed the localization of ABCB6 variants in intracellular compartments using confocal microscopy. While initial reports indicated localization of ABCB6 in the outer mitochondrial membrane [7,9], more recent studies detected ABCB6 in the plasma membrane [9], the Golgi apparatus [10], and in organelles of the vesicular system [11,12,13,14,15]. In line with the reports demonstrating the endolysosomal localization of ABCB6, our HA-tagged ABCB6 construct appeared in the lysosomal compartment of Hela cells, and not in the mitochondria (Figure 4). As opposed to the distinct endolysosomal pattern of the wild-type protein, the R192W variant showed ER localization, supporting the conclusion that the R192W mutation results in the ER-retention of the protein [28]. Although both the R192Q and R192W mutations are predicted to be potentially damaging by the PolyPhen-2 algorithm [29], the R192Q mutation did not change the expression pattern of ABCB6 in Hela cells. Similarly, the intracellular expression pattern of the G588 S variant did not differ from that of wild-type ABCB6 (Figure 4A, B).

Low RBC ABCB6 expression may be the result of a general folding defect, or may be linked to a yet unknown, erythrocyte-specific trafficking event. Red blood cells undergo significant membrane remodeling during the late stages of differentiation. During this process proteins residing in intracellular membrane compartments are redistributed to the plasma membrane of mature erythrocytes. Regulation of the intracellular trafficking and the molecular details of targeting of the ABCB6 protein are not known. In our experiments, endogenous ABCB6 is confined to the endolysosomal compartment in most cell lines, including the HeLa cells used in this study. We have also shown that C-terminal tags do not influence intracellular localization of ABCB6 [15] –still, there are numerous reasons why epithelial HeLa cells may not be an ideal model for membrane expression in erythrocytes. Therefore, we turned to K562 human erythroleukemia cells that are frequently used as a model system for erythroid cells [30]. Surface expression of the ABCB6 variants was monitored in intact cells, using the OSK43 antibody that recognizes an extracellular epitope (i.e., the Lan antigen) while global expression was monitored after permeabilizing the cells. Expression of the wild-type protein resulted in significant surface labeling, showing that 2–5% of the total protein population resides in the plasma membrane when ABCB6 is overexpressed in K562 cells. The R192Q and G588S mutations did not impede expression levels. The R192W variant did not reach the plasma membrane of K562 cells, in line with its ER retention in HeLa cells (Figure 5A, B). Disease-causing mutations of medically relevant ABC proteins (such as ABCC7-CFTR and ABCC6) often result in deficient folding, altered trafficking and a consequent degradation mediated by the proteasome [31,32]. Treatment of K562 cells with the chemical chaperone 4-phenylbutyrate (4-PBA) or the proteasome inhibitor MG132 did not restore the expression of the R192W-ABCB6 variant, indicating that the folding defect could not be overcome (Figure 5C, D).

The function of ABCB6 in red blood cells is unknown. The medical relevance of RBC ABCB6 expression is based on its association with severe haemolytic transfusion reactions or the mild haemolytic disease of the foetus and newborn. The Lan-negative blood type is believed to be very rare (1:20000 random individuals are Lan-negative) [17], and is usually identified

Table 1. Molecular genetics of the *ABCB6* gene.

NUCLEOTIDE CHANGE	AMINO ACID CHANGE	rs#	AF (%) (NCBI/this study)	EFFECT OF THE SNP	SOURCE
1A>C				Lan (−) blood type	[41]
55A>T	M19L			Lan (−) blood type	[41]
85_87del	F29del			Lan (−) blood type	[28]
197_198insG	A66fs			Lan (−) blood type	[16]
296_301insG	A101fs			Lan (−) blood type	[42]
376delG	V126fs	rs377591749	N.D.	Lan (−) blood type	[17]
459del	L154fs			Lan (−) blood type	[42]
574C>T	R192W	rs149202834	0.09/0.86	Lan (−) blood type	[17] [28] this study
717G>A	Q239X	rs148458820	0.05	Lan (−) blood type	[16]
718C>T	R240X			Lan (−) blood type	[42]
827G>A	R276Q	rs200125320	N.D./0.27	Lan (−) blood type	[41] this study
881_884del	T294fs			Lan (−) blood type	[42]
953_956del	G318fs			Lan (−) blood type	[16]
971−1G>A	splice variant			Lan (−) blood type	[41]
1236G>A	W412X			Lan (−) blood type	[17]
1533_1543dup	L515fs			Lan (−) blood type	[16]
1558_1559insT	V520fs			Lan (−) blood type	[17]
1617delG	G539del			Lan (−) blood type	[42]
1690_1691del	M564fs			Lan (−) blood type	[16]
1709_1710del	Q570fs			Lan (−) blood type	[16]
1825G>A	V609M	rs374541748	N.D.	Lan (−) blood type	[41]
1867delins	G623fs			Lan (−) blood type	[16]
1912C>T	R638C			Lan (−) blood type	[41]
1942C>T	R648X	rs376664522	N.D.	Lan (−) blood type	[16]
1985_1986del	L662fs			Lan (−) blood type	[16] [17]
2155C>T	Q719X			Lan (−) blood type	[41]
2256+2T>G	splice variant			Lan (−) blood type	[16]
2351+1G>A	splice variant	rs150574070	N.D.	Lan (−) blood type	[41]
575G>A	R192Q	rs150221689	0.14/0.51	lower ABCB6 expression	this study
826C>T	R276W	rs57467915	0.6/1.18	lower ABCB6 expression	[17] [28] this study
1028G>A	R343Q	rs60322991	3.99	lower ABCB6 expression	[17]
1762G>A	G588S	rs145526996	0.23/0.98	lower ABCB6 expression	[17] [28] this study
1766G>A	R589H	rs483352876	N.D./0.04		this study
2216G>A	R739H	rs192931087	0.05	lower ABCB6 expression	[17]
1578+1G>A	splice variant		N.D./0.04	lower ABCB6 expression	this study
169G>A	A57T			coloboma	[19]
2431C>G	L811V			coloboma	[19]
508A>G	S170G			DUH	[21]
964A>C	S322L			DUH	[43]
1067T>C	L356P			DUH	[21]
1358C>T	A453V	rs373246472	N.D.	DUH	[43]
459delC				DUH	[44]
1663C>A	G555K			DUH	[44]
1736G>A	G579E			DUH	[21]
1123C>T	R375W			pseudohyperkalemia	[20]
1124G>A	R375Q			pseudohyperkalemia	[20]

Abbreviations: DUH: dyschromatosis universalis hereditaria; del: deletion; dup: duplication; fs: frameshift; ins: insertion; N.D.:not determined; rs: RefSNP.

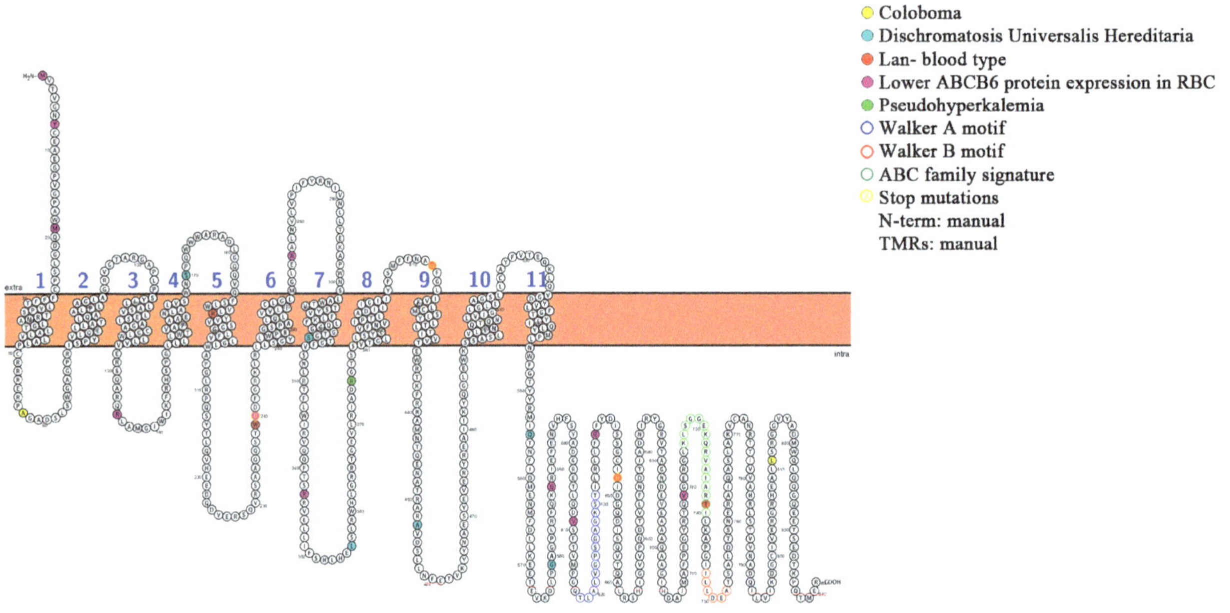

Figure 6. Topology model of ABC6 showing mutations and SNPs [39,40].

through the presence of anti-Lan antibodies stimulated by transfusion or pregnancy [33]. In this study we use a quantitative FACs assay and immunoblotting to associate genetic variations with reduced ABCB6 expression in red blood cells. Since weak expression of the ABCB6 protein may be sufficient to suppress the production of anti-Lan antibodies, further serological tests, based on the reactivity of anti-Lan containing sera, are needed to confirm the association of these mutations with Lan-negativity or the Lan-weak phenotype [34]. The Lan-phenotype is not screened routinely – in view of the genetic heterogeneity and the variable expression levels, genetic and serologic screening of the population is challenging and may be unrealistic [17]. To date, 34 alleles have been described in association with reduced ABCB6 expression in erythrocytes (a complete inventory is shown in Figure 6 and Table 1). Currently, there is no information available on the distribution of ABCB6 expression levels across the general population, healthy subpopulations, and disease-diagnosed individuals. Screening of our cohort revealed a surprisingly high frequency of mutations associated with reduced ABCB6 expression. To obtain carrier frequency data, we screened remaining individuals from the discovery cohort (n = 43) and a control cohort of 184 Hungarian blood donors for the presence of R192Q and G588 S mutations. Further individuals carrying the R192Q allele were not identified (suggesting an allele frequency (AF) of 0.2±0.2% (1/462)). The c.1762G>A, p.Gly588Ser mutation was present in 3 additional unrelated individuals, indicating an AF of 1.1±0.5% (5/462).

In order to corroborate this finding, we analyzed a library of genetic material from 1039 healthy Polish individuals. This analysis (based on High Resolution Melting (HRM) screening followed by detailed sequencing analysis of variant individuals) also led to identification of a surprisingly high number of probands carrying mutations at the studied alleles (Table 1). At the R192 position, our analysis established the following frequencies: for the c.574C>T variant (p.R192W, rs149202834), we found 20 heterozygous and 1 homozygous individual, with an AF of 1.06±0.22%; for the c.575G>A variant (p.R192Q, rs150221689), we found 12 heterozygous individuals, with an AF of 0.58±0.17% (these polymorphisms are not allelomorphic as they concern separate, adjacent nucleotides within codon 192). At the codon 276, we also identified two non-allelomorphic variants: the c.826C>T (p.R276W, rs57467915) with 28 heterozygous and 1 homozygous individual, for an AF of 1.40±0.26%; and the c.827G>A (p.R276Q, rs200125320) with 7 heterozygous individuals, with an AF of 0.34±0.13%. Screening of the G588 position yielded 20 heterozygous individuals with the c.1762G>A (p.G588S, rs145526996) polymorphic variant, for an AF of 0.96±0.21%. In the same screen, we also identified an individual with a divergent HRM curve revealing a heterozygous carrier of a novel, hitherto unreported polymorphic variant in an adjacent codon: c.1766G>A (p.R589H), which we registered as rs483352876. No carriers of the splice site mutation (IVS9+1G>A) allele were identified in the Polish cohort. Interestingly, all 7 heterozygous carriers of the R276Q polymorphism also carried the G588S polymorphism (presumably on the same chromosome), suggesting a one-sided linkage between the two variants in the Polish population, perhaps due to a founder effect. The large size of the Polish cohort allowed us to confirm with relatively high certainty the high allele frequencies of the variants linked to weak or no expression of ABCB6 on RBCs.

Protein levels are heritable molecular phenotypes that exhibit considerable variation between individuals, populations and sexes [35]. Difference in gene expression levels is thought to be a major determinant of phenotypic variation. However, correlation between protein and mRNA levels is generally modest; variation in messenger RNA expression levels is not a perfect surrogate especially for membrane protein expression because the latter is influenced by an array of post-transcriptional regulatory mechanisms. Population proteomics is the protein-level equivalent to population genomics, where individuals are interrogated with the aim of cataloging common genetic variants and determining how they are distributed among people, within populations, and among populations in different parts of the world [36]. The quantitative analysis of the RBC membrane proteins may provide a new biomarker platform for this type of analysis. The red cell plasma membrane contains more than 200 proteins, mostly with unknown function in the mature erythrocyte, but with key physiological and/or pathological roles in other cell types [37,38]. Interestingly, the RBC membrane protein levels in many cases reflect both the genetic alterations and the cellular regulation of the expression of these proteins [22,38]. In the present work we show that the analysis of the ABCB6 expression in the RBC membrane allows the combined estimation of the expression and trafficking of this protein to the plasma membrane, as well as the discovery of heritable mutations related to the Lan-negative phenotype.

Supporting Information

Figure S1 RBC ABCB6 expression in 47 individuals.

Acknowledgments

We thank Dr. Camilo Toro and Dr. William Gahl of the NIH Undiagnosed Diseases Program for an affected patient specimen; that work was supported by the Intramural Research Program of the National Human Genome Research Institute and the Office of the Director of the NIH. We thank Lionel Arnaud (National Institute of Blood Transfusion (INTS), Paris, France) for helpful discussions.

Author Contributions

Conceived and designed the experiments: LP BS GS. Performed the experiments: MK NK KK GV MG GA MS DS. Analyzed the data: MK HA LP BS GS. Contributed reagents/materials/analysis tools: HA AT YT. Contributed to the writing of the manuscript: LP GS.

References

1. Higgins CF (1992) ABC transporters: from microorganisms to man. Annu Rev Cell Biol 8: 67–113.
2. Dean M, Rzhetsky A, Allikmets R (2001) The human ATP-binding cassette (ABC) transporter superfamily. Genome Res 11: 1156–1166.
3. Türk D, Szakács G (2009) Relevance of multidrug resistance in the age of targeted therapy. Curr Opin Drug Discov Devel 12: 246–252.
4. Parcej D, Tampé R (2010) ABC proteins in antigen translocation and viral inhibition. Nat Chem Biol 6: 572–580. doi:10.1038/nchembio.410.
5. Van Helvoort A, Smith AJ, Sprong H, Fritzsche I, Schinkel AH, et al. (1996) MDR1 P-glycoprotein is a lipid translocase of broad specificity, while MDR3 P-glycoprotein specifically translocates phosphatidylcholine. Cell 87: 507–517.
6. Stieger B, Meier Y, Meier PJ (2007) The bile salt export pump. Pflüg Arch Eur J Physiol 453: 611–620. doi:10.1007/s00424-006-0152-8.
7. Krishnamurthy PC, Du G, Fukuda Y, Sun D, Sampath J, et al. (2006) Identification of a mammalian mitochondrial porphyrin transporter. Nature 443: 586–589. doi:10.1038/nature05125.
8. Ulrich DL, Lynch J, Wang Y, Fukuda Y, Nachagari D, et al. (2012) ATP-dependent mitochondrial porphyrin importer ABCB6 protects against phenylhydrazine toxicity. J Biol Chem 287: 12679–12690. doi:10.1074/jbc.M111.336180.
9. Paterson JK, Shukla S, Black CM, Tachiwada T, Garfield S, et al. (2007) Human ABCB6 localizes to both the outer mitochondrial membrane and the plasma membrane. Biochemistry (Mosc) 46: 9443–9452. doi:10.1021/bi700015 m.
10. Tsuchida M, Emi Y, Kida Y, Sakaguchi M (2008) Human ABC transporter isoform B6 (ABCB6) localizes primarily in the Golgi apparatus. Biochem Biophys Res Commun 369: 369–375. doi:10.1016/j.bbrc.2008.02.027.
11. Bagshaw RD, Mahuran DJ, Callahan JW (2005) A proteomic analysis of lysosomal integral membrane proteins reveals the diverse composition of the organelle. Mol Cell Proteomics 4: 133–143. doi:10.1074/mcp.M400128-MCP200.
12. Schroder B, Wrocklage C, Pan C, Jager R, Kosters B, et al. (2007) Integral and associated lysosomal membrane proteins. Traffic 8: 1676–1686. doi:10.1111/j.1600-0854.2007.00643.x.
13. Della Valle MC, Sleat DE, Zheng H, Moore DF, Jadot M, et al. Classification of subcellular location by comparative proteomic analysis of native and density-shifted lysosomes. Mol Cell Proteomics 10: M110 006403. doi:10.1074/mcp.M110.006403.
14. Jalil YA, Ritz V, Jakimenko A, Schmitz-Salue C, Siebert H, et al. (2008) Vesicular localization of the rat ATP-binding cassette half-transporter rAbcb6. Am J Physiol Cell Physiol 294: C579–C590. doi:10.1152/ajpcell.00612.2006.
15. Kiss K, Brozik A, Kucsma N, Toth A, Gera M, et al. (2012) Shifting the Paradigm: The Putative Mitochondrial Protein ABCB6 Resides in the Lysosomes of Cells and in the Plasma Membrane of Erythrocytes. PLoS ONE 7: e37378. doi:10.1371/journal.pone.0037378.
16. Helias V, Saison C, Ballif BA, Peyrard T, Takahashi J, et al. (2012) ABCB6 is dispensable for erythropoiesis and specifies the new blood group system Langereis. Nat Genet advance online publication. Available: http://dx.doi.org/10.1038/ng.1069. Accessed 20 January 2012.
17. Reid ME, Hue-Roye K, Huang A, Velliquette RW, Tani Y, et al. (2014) Alleles of the LAN blood group system: molecular and serologic investigations. Transfusion (Paris) 54: 398–404. doi:10.1111/trf.12285.
18. 1000 Genomes Project Consortium, Abecasis GR, Auton A, Brooks LD, DePristo MA, et al. (2012) An integrated map of genetic variation from 1,092 human genomes. Nature 491: 56–65. doi:10.1038/nature11632.
19. Wang L, He F, Bu J, Liu X, Du W, et al. (2012) ABCB6 Mutations Cause Ocular Coloboma. Am J Hum Genet. Available: http://www.ncbi.nlm.nih.gov/pubmed/22226084. Accessed 11 January 2012.
20. Andolfo I, Alper SL, Delaunay J, Auriemma C, Russo R, et al. (2013) Missense mutations in the ABCB6 transporter cause dominant familialpseudohyperkalemia. Am J Hematol 88: 66–72. doi:10.1002/ajh.23357.
21. Zhang C, Li D, Zhang J, Chen X, Huang M, et al. (2013) Mutations in ABCB6 Cause Dyschromatosis Universalis Hereditaria. J Invest Dermatol. doi:10.1038/jid.2013.145.
22. Kasza I, Várady G, Andrikovics H, Koszarska M, Tordai A, et al. (2012) Expression Levels of the ABCG2 Multidrug Transporter in Human Erythrocytes Correspond to Pharmacologically Relevant Genetic Variations. PLoS ONE 7: e48423. doi:10.1371/journal.pone.0048423.
23. Kuśnierz-Alejska G, Wiecek B (1993) [Lan antigen of erythrocytes and clinical significance of anti-Lan antibody]. Acta Haematol Pol 24: 169–175.
24. Gahl WA, Markello TC, Toro C, Fajardo KF, Sincan M, et al. (2012) The National Institutes of Health Undiagnosed Diseases Program: insights into rare diseases. Genet Med Off J Am Coll Med Genet 14: 51–59. doi:10.1038/gim.0b013e318232a005.
25. Tátrai P, Szepesi Á, Matula Z, Szigeti A, Buchan G, et al. (2012) Combined introduction of Bmi-1 and hTERT immortalizes human adipose tissue-derived stromal cells with low risk of transformation. Biochem Biophys Res Commun 422: 28–35. doi:10.1016/j.bbrc.2012.04.088.
26. Manders EM, Stap J, Brakenhoff GJ, van Driel R, Aten JA (1992) Dynamics of three-dimensional replication patterns during the S-phase, analysed by double labelling of DNA and confocal microscopy. J Cell Sci 103 (Pt 3): 857–862.
27. Costes SV, Daelemans D, Cho EH, Dobbin Z, Pavlakis G, et al. (2004) Automatic and quantitative measurement of protein-protein colocalization in live cells. Biophys J 86: 3993–4003. doi:10.1529/biophysj.103.038422.
28. Saison C, Helias V, Peyrard T, Merad L, Cartron J-P, et al. (2013) The ABCB6 mutation p.Arg192Trp is a recessive mutation causing the Lan- blood type. Vox Sang 104: 159–165. doi:10.1111/j.1423-0410.2012.01650.x.
29. Adzhubei IA, Schmidt S, Peshkin L, Ramensky VE, Gerasimova A, et al. (2010) A method and server for predicting damaging missense mutations. Nat Methods 7: 248–249. doi:10.1038/nmeth0410-248.
30. Fader CM, Colombo MI (2006) Addenda Multivesicular Bodies and Autophagy in Erythrocyte Maturation. Autophagy 2: 122–125.
31. Pomozi V, Brampton C, Fülöp K, Chen L-H, Apana A, et al. (2014) Analysis of Pseudoxanthoma Elasticum-Causing Missense Mutants of ABCC6 In Vivo; Pharmacological Correction of the Mislocalized Proteins. J Invest Dermatol 134: 946–953. doi:10.1038/jid.2013.482.
32. Lukacs GL, Verkman AS (2012) CFTR: folding, misfolding and correcting the ΔF508 conformational defect. Trends Mol Med 18: 81–91. doi:10.1016/j.molmed.2011.10.003.
33. Daniels G (2009) The molecular genetics of blood group polymorphism. Hum Genet 126: 729–742. doi:10.1007/s00439-009-0738-2.
34. Daniels G (2013) Human Blood Groups. John Wiley & Sons. 763 p.
35. Wu L, Candille SI, Choi Y, Xie D, Jiang L, et al. (2013) Variation and genetic control of protein abundance in humans. Nature advance online publication. Available: http://www.nature.com/nature/journal/vaop/ncurrent/full/nature12223.html?WT.ec_id=NATURE-20130516. Accessed 1 June 2013.
36. Nedelkov D (2008) Population proteomics: Investigation of protein diversity in human populations. PROTEOMICS 8: 779–786. doi:10.1002/pmic.200700501.
37. D'Alessandro A, Righetti PG, Zolla L (2010) The Red Blood Cell Proteome and Interactome: An Update. J Proteome Res 9: 144–163. doi:10.1021/pr900831f.
38. Várady G, Cserepes J, Németh A, Szabó E, Sarkadi B (2013) Cell surface membrane proteins as personalized biomarkers: where we stand and where we are headed. Biomark Med 7: 803–819. doi:10.2217/bmm.13.90.
39. Tusnády GE, Sarkadi B, Simon I, Váradi A (2006) Membrane topology of human ABC proteins. FEBS Lett 580: 1017–1022. doi:10.1016/j.febslet.2005.11.040.
40. Omasits U, Ahrens CH, Müller S, Wollscheid B (2013) Protter: interactive protein feature visualization and integration with experimental proteomic data. Bioinformatics: btt607. doi:10.1093/bioinformatics/btt607.
41. Haer-Wigman L, Ait Soussan A, Ligthart P, de Haas M, van der Schoot CE (2014) Molecular analysis of immunized Jr(a-) or Lan- patients and validation of a high-throughput genotyping assay to screen blood donors for Jr(a-) and Lan-

phenotypes: Genotyping of the Jr(a-) and Lan- Phenotype. Transfusion (Paris): n/a – n/a. doi:10.1111/trf.12544.
42. Tanaka M, Yamamuro Y, Takahashi J, Ogasawara K, Osabe T, et al. (2014) Novel alleles of Lan− in Japanese populations: Removal of BRMs in PCs by columns. Transfusion (Paris) 54: 1438–1439. doi:10.1111/trf.12540.
43. Liu H, Li Y, Hung KKH, Wang N, Wang C, et al. (2014) Genome-Wide Linkage, Exome Sequencing and Functional Analyses Identify ABCB6 as the Pathogenic Gene of Dyschromatosis Universalis Hereditaria. PLoS ONE 9: e87250. doi:10.1371/journal.pone.0087250.
44. Cui Y-X, Xia X-Y, Zhou Y, Gao L, Shang X-J, et al. (2013) Novel Mutations of ABCB6 Associated with Autosomal Dominant Dyschromatosis Universalis Hereditaria. PLoS ONE 8: e79808. doi:10.1371/journal.pone.0079808.

18

The Sodium-Glucose Co-Transporter 2 Inhibitor Empagliflozin Improves Diabetes-Induced Vascular Dysfunction in the Streptozotocin Diabetes Rat Model by Interfering with Oxidative Stress and Glucotoxicity

Matthias Oelze[1,♋,¶], Swenja Kröller-Schön[1,♋,¶], Philipp Welschof[1], Thomas Jansen[1], Michael Hausding[1], Yuliya Mikhed[1], Paul Stamm[1], Michael Mader[1], Elena Zinßius[1], Saule Agdauletova[1], Anna Gottschlich[1], Sebastian Steven[1], Eberhard Schulz[1], Serge P. Bottari[2], Eric Mayoux[3], Thomas Münzel[1], Andreas Daiber[1]*

1 2nd Medical Clinic, Department of Cardiology, Medical Center of the Johannes Gutenberg University, Mainz, Germany, **2** Laboratory of Fundamental and Applied, Bioenergetics, INSERM U1055, Grenoble-Alpes Université et Pôle de Biologie, CHU, Grenoble, France, **3** Boehringer Ingelheim Pharma GmbH & Co. KG, Ingelheim, Germany

Abstract

Objective: In diabetes, vascular dysfunction is characterized by impaired endothelial function due to increased oxidative stress. Empagliflozin, as a selective sodium-glucose co-transporter 2 inhibitor (SGLT2i), offers a novel approach for the treatment of type 2 diabetes by enhancing urinary glucose excretion. The aim of the present study was to test whether treatment with empagliflozin improves endothelial dysfunction in type I diabetic rats via reduction of glucotoxicity and associated vascular oxidative stress.

Methods: Type I diabetes in Wistar rats was induced by an intravenous injection of streptozotocin (60 mg/kg). One week after injection empagliflozin (10 and 30 mg/kg/d) was administered via drinking water for 7 weeks. Vascular function was assessed by isometric tension recording, oxidative stress parameters by chemiluminescence and fluorescence techniques, protein expression by Western blot, mRNA expression by RT-PCR, and islet function by insulin ELISA in serum and immunohistochemical staining of pancreatic tissue. Advanced glycation end products (AGE) signaling was assessed by dot blot analysis and mRNA expression of the AGE-receptor (RAGE).

Results: Treatment with empagliflozin reduced blood glucose levels, normalized endothelial function (aortic rings) and reduced oxidative stress in aortic vessels (dihydroethidium staining) and in blood (phorbol ester/zymosan A-stimulated chemiluminescence) of diabetic rats. Additionally, the pro-inflammatory phenotype and glucotoxicity (AGE/RAGE signaling) in diabetic animals was reversed by SGLT2i therapy.

Conclusions: Empagliflozin improves hyperglycemia and prevents the development of endothelial dysfunction, reduces oxidative stress and improves the metabolic situation in type 1 diabetic rats. These preclinical observations illustrate the therapeutic potential of this new class of antidiabetic drugs.

Editor: Andrea Cignarella, University of Padova, Italy

Funding: The present work was supported by a vascular biology research grant from Boehringer Ingelheim Pharma GmbH & Co. KG (A.D. and T.M.) and by the Centre of Translational Vascular Biology (CTVB). Yuliya Miked holds a stipend from the International PhD Programme on the "Dynamics of Gene Regulation, Epigenetics and DNA Damage Response" from the Institute of Molecular Biology gGmbH, (Mainz, Germany) funded by the Boehringer Ingelheim Foundation. This paper contains results that are part of the doctoral thesis of Philipp Welschof. The funders had no role in data collection and analysis, decision to publish, or preparation of the manuscript. E.M. (Boehringer Ingelheim Pharma GmbH & Co. KG) was involved in the study design.

Competing Interests: T.M. and A.D. received research grants from Boehringer Ingelheim Pharma GmbH & Co. KG. E.M. is an employee of Boehringer Ingelheim Pharma GmbH & Co. KG. The remaining authors declare that they have no competing interests in connection with this manuscript.

* Email: andreas.daiber@bioredox.com

♋ These authors contributed equally to this work.

¶ MO and SKS should both be considered as first author.

Introduction

Diabetes mellitus is one of the major risk factors for the development of cardiovascular disease [1]. Several studies have demonstrated that endothelial dysfunction due to increased oxidative stress is frequently encountered in the diabetic state (for review see [2]). The vascular NADPH oxidase and an uncoupled endothelial nitric oxide synthase (eNOS, type 3) have been identified as enzymatic sources of increased vascular production of reactive oxygen species (ROS) [3]. Pharmacological treatment of diabetic animals with HMG-CoA-reductase inhibitors, AT_1-receptor blockers or heme oxygenase-1 induction by NO donor therapy with pentaerithrityl tetranitrate have been demonstrated to prevent the activation of the NADPH oxidase and to recouple the dysfunctional eNOS [4–6]. The mechanisms underlying eNOS uncoupling in vessels from diabetic animals include increased functional depletion of BH_4 due to the oxidation to the $^{\bullet}BH_3$ radical, oxidation of the zinc-sulfur-complex and S-glutathionylation of the enzyme [4,6]. Adverse phosphorylation of eNOS at Thr495 and Tyr657 may potentially play a significant role as well [7,8]. Another major concept of diabetic pathology is based on direct glucotoxicity, including increased formation of advanced glycation end products (AGE) and their signaling via specific receptors (RAGE) leading to vascular dysfunction and end organ damage [9,10]. Most importantly, oxidative stress and AGE/RAGE components interact with each other in a cross-talk fashion, wherein AGE/RAGE signaling can activate sources of reactive oxygen species (ROS) [11,12] and normalization of mitochondrial ROS formation in turn normalizes hyperglycemic damage by decreasing AGE/RAGE signaling [13]. In addition, increased vascular oxidative stress can lead to immune cell activation [14,15] or is even mediated by inflammatory cells, as was recently demonstrated in the angiotensin II infusion model [16].

A new class of anti-diabetic drugs targets the sodium-glucose co-transporter 2 (SGLT2), which is the main glucose transporter of the kidney, located in the S1 and S2 segments of the proximal tubule and is responsible for the reabsorption of >90% of the glucose from primary urine [17]. SGLT2 inhibition (SGLT2i) reduces the reabsorption of glucose and therefore enhances urinary glucose excretion, consequently decreasing both fasting and postprandial hyperglycemia. Since conventional anti-diabetic therapies rely on insulin secretion, their efficacy may get lost over time due to progressing β-cell dysfunction and desensitization to insulin signaling (especially with increasing age) [18]. Therapy with SGLT2i does not share these drawbacks, since its action is independent of insulin secretion and signaling. Likewise, in contrast to conventional anti-diabetics, SGLT2i removes excessive glucose from the body and thereby prevents glucotoxicity, which should represent a straight-forward strategy to prevent hyperglycemia-induced damage. Empagliflozin is a SGLT2i that was recently approved for clinical use in the United States of America and Europe. According to randomized, placebo-controlled, double-blind clinical studies, empagliflozin had a good safety and tolerability profile in healthy Japanese male subjects [19,20].

With the present study we sought to test whether treatment of diabetic animals with the SGLT2i empagliflozin improves endothelial dysfunction, oxidative stress, AGE/RAGE signaling and inflammation in a well-characterized rat model of type 1 diabetes mellitus [3].

Materials and Methods

Materials

The High-Capacity cDNA Reverse Transcription Kit was purchased from Applied Biosystems, Darmstadt, Germany. All oligonucleotides and dual labeled probes were purchased from MWG Biotech, Ebersberg, Germany. The Bradford reagent was obtained from BioRad, Munich, Germany. For isometric tension studies, nitroglycerin (GTN) was used from a Nitrolingual infusion solution (1 mg/ml) from G.Pohl-Boskamp (Hohenlockstedt, Germany). SGLT2-inhibitor (SGLT2i, empagliflozin) was a kind gift from Boehringer Ingelheim Pharma GmbH & Co KG (Biberach, Germany). For induction of diabetes we used streptozotocin (STZ) from Fluka (Steinheim, Germany). L-012 (8-amino-5-chloro-7-phenylpyrido[3,4-d]pyridazine-1,4-(2H,3H)dione sodium salt) was purchased from Wako Pure Chemical Industries (Osaka, Japan). All other chemicals were of analytical grade and were obtained from Sigma-Aldrich, Fluka or Merck.

Animals and in vivo treatment

All animals were treated in accordance with the Guide for the Care and Use of Laboratory Animals as adopted by the U.S. National Institutes of Health and approval was granted by the Ethics Committee of the University Hospital Mainz and the Landesuntersuchungsamt Rheinland-Pfalz (Koblenz, Germany; permit number: 23 177-07/G 12-1-025). All surgery was performed under isoflurane or ketamine/xylazine anesthesia, and all efforts were made to minimize suffering. A total number of 48 male Wistar Rats (6 weeks old, 300 g, Charles River Laboratories, Sulzfeld, Germany) were divided into 4 treatment groups: untreated controls (Ctr), streptozotocin-induced diabetes mellitus type 1 with placebo (STZ), SGLT2i low dose (10 mg/kg/d p.o.) or SGLT2i high dose (30 mg/kg/d p.o.) therapy. Given the maximal acute glucosuric effect of empagliflozin, the dose of 10 mg/kg/d was chosen according to previous animal studies [21–23]. Moreover, considering the higher metabolism of rats, the dose of 30 mg/kg/d allowed a higher 24 h drug exposure as already observed in previous study with chronic treatment [24]. The study was performed as 3 sub-studies with 4, 5 and 3 animals per group. Not all animals were used for all assays. For induction of diabetes mellitus type 1, rats were injected with a single dose of STZ into the vena dorsalis penis (60 mg/kg s.c., in 5 mM pH 4.5 citrate buffer). Control animals were injected with the solvent. SGLT2i treatment by drinking water, containing the requested concentrations of the drug to reach the desired doses of 10 and 30 mg/kg/d, was started 1 week after STZ-injection and continued for 7 weeks. After 8 weeks of total treatment duration, animals were killed under isoflurane anesthesia by transection of the diaphragm and removal of the heart and thoracic aorta. For protein and mRNA expression also the abdominal part and the arch of the aorta were used as well. Diabetes was diagnosed by measuring glucose levels and glycosylated hemoglobin (HbA1c) in whole blood (for STZ-treated rats it was diluted 1:5 with NaCl solution) using the ACCU-CHEK Sensor system from Roche Diagnostics GmbH (Mannheim, Germany) and A1C Now$^+$ system from Bayer HealthCare Diabetes Care (Basel, Switzerland), respectively. STZ treatment was previously shown to be a valid type 1 diabetes model and hyperglycemic complications such as vascular dysfunction and oxidative stress were completely reversed by insulin administration [25].

Detection of serum cholesterol, triglyceride and interferon-γ levels

Serum cholesterol, triglyceride and interferon-γ levels were analysed in the Department of Clinical Chemistry, University Hospital Mainz, Germany, using the daily routine facilities for in-patient care. Total cholesterol in serum was also assessed by HF5 (Superon GmbH, Dernbach, Germany). More detailed information on determination of cholesterol by Field-Flow Fractionation (FFF) can be found in the online supplemental data in File S1.

Immunohistochemistry of pancreatic tissue

Pancreatic segments were fixed in paraformaldehyde (4%), paraffin-embedded and stained with primary antibodies against glucagon (1:4000, Abcam, UK) and insulin (1:200, LifeSpan BioSciences, Seattle, USA); depending upon the species of primary antibodies, appropriate biotinylated secondary antibodies were used at dilutions according to the manufacturer's instructions. For immunochemical detection ABC reagent (Vector) and then DAB reagent (peroxidase substrate Kit, Vector) were used as substrates.

Detection of insulin serum levels by ELISA and by RIA

Venous blood was transferred into serum-vials, left on ice for 30 min and centrifuged for 10 min at 2000 g. The supernatant (serum) was stored at −80°C. Quantitative measurement of serum insulin levels was performed using a rat insulin ELISA (DRG Instruments GmbH, Marburg, Germany) and a rat insulin RIA (Cat. # SRI-13K, Millipore, St. Charles, Missouri, USA) according to the manufacturer's instructions.

Histological staining of aortic rings and pancreatic tissue

Sirius red staining for vascular fibrosis and trichrom staining was performed with paraffin-embedded samples of aortic tissue upon deparaffination [26]. The nuclei were prestained with hemalum prior to staining for 1 hour in 0.1% with Sirius red solution in saturated picric acid (1.2%) [26]. Finally, tissue samples were dehydrated with 70%, 96% and 100% isopropanol and coverslipped with Entellan. Trichrom staining (according to Goldner et al.) was performed with paraffin-embedded samples of pancreatic tissue upon deparaffination [26]. After prestaining of the nuclei with haematoxylin (according to Harris et al.), the samples were stained for 5 minutes with mallory red in 100% acetic acid, fuchsin acid and Orange G (Merck, Darmstadt, Germany), followed by 15 minutes in 1% molybdatophosphoric acid hydrate (VWR, Darmstadt, Germany) and 5 minutes in acid light green. Finally tissue samples were dehydrated in glacial acetic acid and 100% ethanol and coverslipped in Entellan.

Isometric tension studies

Vasodilator responses to acetylcholine (ACh) and nitroglycerin (GTN) and vasoconstrictor responses to KCl were assessed with endothelium-intact isolated rat aortic rings mounted for isometric tension recordings in organ chambers, preconstricted with phenylephrine (PheE), as described previously [5,27].

Detection of oxidative stress in whole blood, cardiac membrane fractions and aorta

Whole blood leukocyte-dependent ROS formation was measured in fresh blood (in citrate tubes) which was diluted 1:50 in PBS with Ca^{2+}/Mg^{2+} (each 1 mM) and L-012. The oxidative burst (activation of the phagocytic NADPH oxidase) was triggered by the phorbol ester PDBu (10 µM) or the fungal endotoxin zymosan A (50 µg/ml) and assessed with L-012 (100 µM) enhanced chemiluminescence (ECL) [28]. NADPH oxidase activity in cardiac membrane fractions was determined by lucigenin (5 µM) ECL in the presence of NADPH (200 µM) using a Lumat LB9507 single photon counter as described [5,29]. Vascular ROS formation was determined using dihydroethidium (DHE, 1 µM)-dependent fluorescence microtopography in aortic cryo-sections as described [5,29]. To investigate involvement of eNOS uncoupling in ROS production and endothelial dysfunction within the endothelial monolayer, aortic rings were preincubated with the NOS inhibitor L-NAME [5,25,29]. ROS-derived red fluorescence was detected using a Zeiss Axiovert 40 CFL microscope, Zeiss lenses and Axiocam MRm camera. Intensity of the DHE oxidation products' fluorescence was evaluated by densitometry.

Western blot and dot blot analysis

Protein expression and modification was assessed by standard Western and dot blot analysis using established protocols [5,25,29]. Isolated aortic tissue was frozen and homogenized in liquid nitrogen. Proteins were separated by SDS-Page and blotted onto nitrocellulose membranes. After blocking, immunoblotting was performed with the following antibodies: monoclonal mouse α-actinin (100 kDa) as a control for loading and transfer, polyclonal rabbit NADPH oxidase isoform 1 (Nox1) (1:500, Abcam, UK) and monoclonal mouse NADPH oxidase isoform 2 (Nox2) ($gp91^{phox}$, 1:1000, BD Biosciences, USA), monoclonal mouse eNOS (1:1000, BD Biosciences, USA), polyclonal rabbit phospho-Ser1177-eNOS (1:1000, Upstate Biotechnology, MA, USA), monoclonal mouse dihydrofolate reductase (1 µg/ml, Abnova Corp., Germany), monoclonal mouse heme oxygenase-1 (HO-1) (4 µg/ml, Stressgen, San Diego, CA), polyclonal goat cGMP-dependent protein kinase (cGK-I, 1:200, Santa Cruz Biotechnologies, USA), vasodilator stimulated phosphoprotein (VASP) phosphorylated on serine239 (P-VASP, clone 16C2, 1.5 µg/ml, Calbiochem, UK), polyclonal rabbit monocyte-chemoattractant-protein-1 (MCP-1 or CCL-2, Serotec, UK), polyclonal rabbit receptor for advanced glycation end products (RAGE, 1:1000, Cell Signaling Technology, Danvers, MA). Detection and quantification were performed by ECL with peroxidase conjugated anti–rabbit/mouse (1:10000, Vector Lab., Burlingame, CA) and anti-goat (1:5000, Santa Cruz Biotechnologies, USA) secondary antibodies. Densitometric quantification of antibody-specific bands was performed with a ChemiLux Imager (CsX-1400 M, Intas, Göttingen, Germany) and Gel-Pro Analyzer software (Media Cybernetics, Bethesda, MD).

Advanced glycation end products (AGE) positive proteins were assessed by dot blot analysis of aortic protein homogenate, which was transferred to a Protran BA85 (0.45 µm) nitrocellulose membrane (Schleicher & Schuell, Dassel, Germany) by a Minifold I vacuum dot-blot system (Schleicher&Schuell, Dassel, Germany). Each slot was washed with 250 µl PBS and the membrane was dried for 15 min at 60°C. For detection of AGE's, a mouse monoclonal AGE antibody (Antibodies-online GmbH, Aachen, Germany) was used at a dilution of 1:1000. Positive dots were detected by enhanced chemiluminescence after incubation with a peroxidase-coupled secondary antibody (1:10000, Vector Lab., Burlingame, CA). All incubation and washing steps were performed according to the manufacturer's instructions. Densitometric quantification of the dots was performed as described in the Western blot section.

Detection of serum methylglyoxal levels and liver ALDH-2 activity by HPLC-based quantification

Methylglyoxal serum levels were quantified by an HPLC-based method upon derivatization of the reactive aldehyde as adapted from a previously described protocol [30]. Briefly, 500 µl serum was filtrated by size exclusion centrifugation in a 30 kDa filter device (Millipore, Billierica, MA, USA) for 60 min at 17000 g. The eluate (350 µl) was mixed with 70 µl 7M $HClO_4$, 10 µl 100 µM 2,3-dimethylquinoxaline (internal standard) and 70 µl 9.2 mM 1,2-diaminobenzene (derivatization reagent) for 30 min at 25°C. 50 µl of each sample were subjected to HPLC analysis. The system consisted of a Jasco HPLC system and a C_{18}-Nucleosil 125×4 100-3 reversed phase column from Macherey & Nagel (Düren, Germany). The mobile phase consisted of solvent A (50 mM citric acid pH 2.2) and solvent B (acetonitrile (90 v/v%) and water (10 v/v%)). The substrate and its products were eluted at a flow rate of 1 ml/min using a gradient (0 min: 37% B; 12 min: 60% B; 12.5 min: 90% B; 13 min: 37% B; 15 min: 37% B), detected by their absorption at 315 nm, and quantified using internal and external standards (methylglyoxal derivatization product served as external standard and 2,3-dimethylquinoxaline was the internal standard). The typical retention times were 3.9 and 4.4 min, respectively.

The activity of ALDH-2 in isolated mitochondria was determined by measuring the conversion of 2-hydroxy-3-nitro-benzaldehyde to 2-hydroxy-3-nitro-benzoic acid as described previously [31]. Briefly, liver samples were homogenized in HEPES buffer (composition in mM: 50 HEPES, 70 sucrose, 220 mannitol, 1 EGTA and 0.033 BSA) and centrifuged at 1500 g (10 min at 4°C) and 2000 g for 5 min (the pellets were discarded). The supernatant was then centrifuged at 20000 g for 20 min, and the pellet resuspended in 1 ml of HEPES buffer. The latter step was repeated and the pellet resuspended in 1 ml of Tris buffer (composition in mM: 10 Tris, 340 sucrose, 100 KCl and 1 EDTA). The mitochondrial fraction (total protein approximately 5–10 mg/ml) was kept on ice and diluted to approximately 1 mg/ml protein in 0.25 ml of PBS and preincubated for 10 min at room temperature. For measurement of ALDH-2 dehydrogenase activity, 2-hydroxy-3-nitro-benzaldehyde (100 µM) was added and the samples were incubated for another 30 min at 37°C. Samples were sonicated, centrifuged at 20000 g (4°C) for 20 min, and the supernatant was purified by size exclusion centrifugation in a 10 kDa filter device (Millipore). 50 µl of each sample were subjected to HPLC analysis. The system consisted of a Jasco HPLC system and a C_{18}-Nucleosil 125×4 100-3 reversed phase column from Macherey & Nagel (Düren, Germany). The mobile phase consisted of solvent A (50 mM citric acid pH 2.2) and solvent B (acetonitrile (90 v/v%) and water (10 v/v%)). The substrate and its products were eluted at a flow rate of 1 ml/min using a gradient (0 min: 25% B; 7 min: 50% B; 8 min: 100% B; 9 min: 25% B; 11 min: 25% B), detected by their absorption at 360 nm, and quantified using internal and external standards (2-hydroxy-3-nitro-benzoic acid and 2-hydroxy-3-nitro-benzaldehyde). The typical retention times were 2.4 and 3.7 min, respectively.

Quantitative reverse transcription real-time PCR (qRT-PCR)

mRNA expression was analyzed with quantitative reverse transcription real-time PCR (qRT-PCR) as previously described [32]. Briefly, total RNA from rat aorta was isolated (RNeasy Fibrous Tissue Mini Kit; Qiagen, Hilden, Germany), and 50 ng of total RNA was used for real-time RT-PCR analysis with the QuantiTect Probe RT-PCR kit (Qiagen). TaqMan Gene Expression assays for monocyte chemoattractant protein-1 (MCP-1 or CCL-2), monocyte/macrophage-specific protein CD68, cytokine interleukin-6 (IL-6), immune-signaling proteins interferon-γ (IFN-γ) and tumor necrosis factor-α (TNF-α), intercellular adhesion molecule-1 (ICAM-1), cyclooxygenase-2 (COX-2) and the receptor for advanced glycation end products (RAGE) as well as TBP were purchased as probe-and-primer sets (Applied Biosystems, Foster City, CA). The comparative Ct method was used for relative mRNA quantification. Gene expression was normalized to the endogenous control, TATA box binding protein (TBP) mRNA, and the amount of target gene mRNA expression in each sample was expressed relative to the control.

Statistical analysis

Results are expressed as the means ±SEM. Two-way ANOVA (with Bonferroni's correction for comparison of multiple means) was used for comparisons of concentration-relaxation curves. In addition, one-way ANOVA (with Bonferroni's or Dunn's correction for comparison of multiple means) was used for comparisons of vasodilator potency (EC_{50}, pD_2 see Table 1) and efficacy (max. relaxation see Table 1). One-way ANOVA (with Bonferroni's or Dunn's correction for comparison of multiple means) was used for comparisons of weight gain, blood glucose, HbA1c levels, other serum parameters, such as insulin, triglycerides and methylglyoxal levels, histological data, aortic and cardiac ROS formation, protein and mRNA expression, vasoconstriction and hepatic ALDH-2 activity. p values <0.05 were considered as statistically significant. The number of replicates in the different assays may vary due to the death of some rats in the different sub-studies and since some values were excluded when they exceeded a deviation of 2xSD from the means.

Results

Diabetes-related parameters (Table 2)

During the treatment period 3 (STZ), 1 (SGLT2i low dose) and 1 (SGLT2i high dose) rats died. The weight gain was significantly decreased in the STZ-treated diabetic rats and not significantly affected by a low dose but increased by a high dose SGLT2i therapy. Diabetic animals had higher triglyceride and total cholesterol levels compared to controls and to diabetic animals treated with SGLTi. Blood glucose was higher in all STZ-treated groups (approximately 4-fold as compared to the control group) when measured 3 days after STZ injection, clearly excluding any interference of the drug therapy (which was started 7 days after STZ injection) with the induction of diabetes. Blood glucose levels were determined 8 weeks after STZ injection and the untreated STZ rats showed an almost 5-fold increase in this parameter, which was dose-dependently decreased by SGLT2i therapy in non-fasting rats. In fasting rats, blood glucose levels were increased almost 4-fold in the untreated STZ rats and were reduced by low and high dose SGLT2i therapy to near control levels. The parameter for long-term glycemic conditions, HbA1c, was increased more than 4-fold by STZ injection and was dose-dependently decreased by SGLT2i therapy. Trichrome staining of pancreatic tissue revealed morphological changes in the islet cells in untreated diabetic rats (Figure S1 in File S1). Glucagon production as detected by immunohistochemical staining of pancreatic tissue, showed no obvious change in control, diabetic and SGLT2i treated groups (if at all a moderate increase in staining in the STZ group) (Figure 1A). In contrast, immunohistochemical staining for insulin showed a clear decrease in the STZ group as compared to the controls with only minor part of the islets producing any insulin at all (not shown) and even in these "active" islets only few β-cells were producing insulin. Low dose SGLT2i therapy showed some improvement of islet insulin production which was clearly increased by high dose SGLT2i therapy (Figure 1B). In accordance with these observations, the

Table 1. Potencies and efficacies of the endothelium-dependent vasodilator acetylcholine and the endothelium-independent vasodilator nitroglycerin in rat aorta.

	In vivo treatment group			
Parameter[a]	**Ctr**	**STZ**	**STZ+low SGLT2i**	**STZ+high SGLT2i**
Potency (pD2), ACh	7.52±0.07 (n = 12)	7.12±0.06 (n = 9)*	7.33±0.06 (n = 10)#	7.28±0.05 (n = 9)*#
Efficacy (%), ACh	90.3±1.4 (n = 12)	80.3±2.3 (n = 9)*	91.5±0.7 (n = 10)#	85.5±2.4 (n = 9)§
Potency (pD2), GTN	7.81±0.07 (n = 12)	7.62±0.11 (n = 9)*	7.73±0.08 (n = 10)	7.70±0.12 (n = 9)
Efficacy (%), GTN	99.4±0.2 (n = 12)	96.7±1.6 (n = 9)*	99.2±0.1 (n = 10)	98.8±0.3 (n = 9)

[a]Potency is –log EC_{50} and EC_{50} is the concentration that induces half-maximal relaxation with respect to the maximal relaxation achieved with the highest concentration of the vasodilator used. Efficacy is defined as maximal relaxation obtained with the highest concentration of the vasodilator used. The data are the means ± SEM of the indicated number of animals/group.
*, $p<0.05$ vs. control and #, $p<0.05$ vs. STZ-injected and §, $p<0.05$ vs. low dose SGLT2i treated.

serum insulin levels were significantly decreased to background concentrations (measured both by ELISA and RIA) in the STZ group and dose-dependently normalized by SGLT2i therapy (Figure 1C and D). Interferon-γ levels showed no significant changes (Table 2).

Vascular parameters

Histological staining for collagen (sirius red) and aortic wall (media) thickness revealed no significant increase in thickening (remodeling) in the STZ group but substantial reduction of these parameters by both doses of SGLT2i (Figure 2A). STZ injection caused endothelial dysfunction (acetylcholine [ACh]-dependent relaxation), which was improved by both SGLT2i doses (Figure 2B). The effects on endothelium-independent (nitroglycerin [GTN]) relaxation were less pronounced (Figure 2C). Vasodilator potency (EC_{50}, pD_2) and efficacy (max. relaxation) are presented in Table 1. KCl-induced vasoconstriction did not change in any group but the phenylephrine-induced constriction was increased in almost all STZ groups and interestingly not corrected by SGLT2i therapy (Figure S2 in File S1).

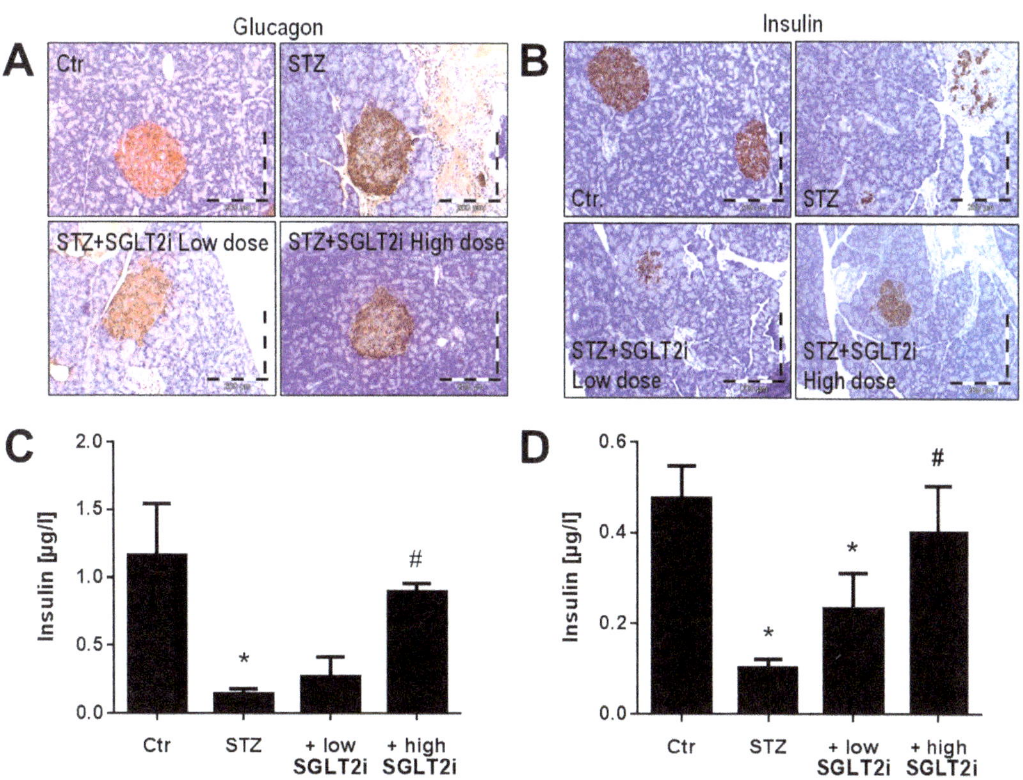

Figure 1. Glucagon and insulin measurements in controls and diabetic rats 8 weeks after STZ injection and 7 weeks of SGLT2i (low and high dose) treatment. Representative immunohistochemical stainings of pancreatic tissue for glucagon (**A**), insulin (**B**) and ELISA (**C**) or RIA (**D**) based determination of insulin serum levels. The data are the means ±SEM of 3–4 (**A,B**), 3–5 (**C**) or 9–11 (**D**) animals/group. *, $p<0.05$ vs. control and #, $p<0.05$ vs. STZ-injected group.

Table 2. Weight gain, and blood and serum parameters in controls and diabetic rats.

Parameter[a]	In vivo treatment group Ctr	STZ	STZ+low SGLT2i	STZ+high SGLT2i
Weight gain [g]	137±10 (n=12)	27±19 (n=8)*	43±19 (n=9)*	97±14 (n=10)#§
Blood glucose [mg/dl], 3d post STZ, non-fasting, before SGLT2i treatment	120±6 (n=7)	441±22 (n=9)*	457±22 (n=11)*	447±26 (n=11)*
Blood glucose [mg/dl], 8w post STZ, non-fasting	132±8 (n=11)	509±20 (n=9)*#	336±49 (n=10)*#	230±30(n=10)*#§
Blood glucose [mg/dl], 8w post STZ, fasting	117±4 (n=11)	395±42 (n=9)*	185±15 (n=10)#	168±19 (n=10)#
HbA1c [mmol/mol]	24±2 (n=10)	99±12 (n=8)*	68±8 (n=8)*#	40±6 (n=8)*#§
HbA1c [%]	4.3±2.3	11.2±3.2	8.4±2.9	5.8±2.7
Cholesterol [mg/dl], ELISA	83±6 (n=9)	105±8 (n=7)*	93±4(n=7)	83±5 (n=7)#
Cholesterol [mg/dl], HF5[b]	102±5(n=11)	125±4 (n=9)*	108±4 (n=9)#	105±3 (n=9)#
Triglycerides [mg/dl]	87±7(n=7)	273±79 (n=5)*	178±31 (n=6)	95±15 (n=7)#
Interferon-γ [pg/dl]	n.d.(n=5)	6±3 (n=4)	2±2 (n=4)	n.d. (n=3)

[a]Weight gain was calculated from the difference of values prior and 8 weeks post STZ injection. Blood glucose was determined three days after STZ injection without SGLT2i treatment; fasting and non-fasting blood glucose as well as HbA1c levels were measured 8 weeks post STZ injection. The data are the means ± SEM of the indicated number of animals/group; n.d. means not detectable.
*, $p<0.05$ vs. control and #, $p<0.05$ vs. STZ-injected and §, $p<0.05$ vs. low dose SGLT2i treated.
[b]Separation of HDL and LDL using HF5 (Hollow Fiber Flow Field Flow Fractionation).

Oxidative stress parameters

Oxidative burst in whole blood in response to zymosan A was increased in the diabetic rats and normalized by both SGLT2i doses and a similar pattern was observed in response to the synthetic phorbol ester analogue PDBu (mainly reflecting leukocyte NADPH oxidase activity) without displaying significant changes (Figure 3A and C). The signal in the STZ group was largely suppressed by the NADPH oxidase inhibitor VAS2870 (highest affinity for Nox2 isoform) and the intracellular calcium chelator BAPTA-AM, indicating the involvement of the phagocytic NADPH oxidase and $[Ca^{2+}]_i$ in this process (Figure 3B). NADPH oxidase activity from heart membranes was increased in the STZ group and dose-dependently inhibited by SGLT2i therapy (Figure 3D). In line with this, activity of the redox-sensitive enzyme mitochondrial aldehyde dehydrogenase (ALDH-2) was decreased in diabetic rats but not significantly impaired under SGLT2i therapy (Figure S3 in File S1).

Aortic reactive oxygen species formation was increased in the STZ group and reduced by high dose of SGLT2i, although still increased as compared to the control (Figure 3E). An almost similar pattern was observed for endothelial dihydroethidium staining of aortic cryo-sections, however, without significant reduction in the endothelial dihydroethidium fluorescence signal by either SGLT2i dose (Figure 3F). Experiments with the eNOS inhibitor L-NAME reduced the superoxide signal in the endothelial cell layer of vessels from the STZ group, compatible with eNOS uncoupling. SGLT2i treatment showed a mixed effect suggesting that eNOS uncoupling is not completely prevented. The dihydroethidium staining signal was sensitive to low concentration SOD treatment and high concentration catalase pre-incubation (Figure S4 in File S1).

Protein expression

We have shown previously that eNOS and dihydrofolate reductase (DHFR) expression was increased in aorta from diabetic animals suggesting compensatory up-regulation of these enzymes due to the dysfunction/uncoupling of eNOS and oxidative depletion of its co-factor tetrahydrobiopterin (BH_4) with subsequent induction of dihydrofolate reductase, the BH_2 recycling enzyme. STZ treatment significantly increased eNOS and dihydrofolate reductase expression and SGLT2i therapy decreased it dose-dependently suggesting that SGLT2i therapy normalized these adverse effects of hyperglycemia, thereby preventing the compensatory up-regulation of these enzymes (Figure 4 A and C). It should be noted that eNOS up-regulation per se is a beneficial event but if overexpressed in an oxidized environment (with depleted BH_4 levels or in S-glutathionylated state) the enzyme might be uncoupled and might further aggravate the phenotype. Phosphorylation of eNOS at Ser1177, which increases eNOS activity, was impaired in STZ-treated rats and dose-dependently improved with SGLT2i therapy (Figure 4B). The expression of cGMP-dependent kinase was slightly increased in the STZ group and reduced to control levels by high dose SGLT2i therapy (Figure 4D, Figure S6D in File S1). Likewise, the phosphorylation of VASP at Ser239 (as a read-out of activation of the cGMP-dependent kinase) was decreased in the STZ-treated rats and normalized by high dose SGLT2i therapy (Figure 4D, Figure S6D in File S1). As a consequence, the ratio of P-VASP/cGK-I was significantly decreased in diabetic rats and improved dose-dependently by SGLT2i therapy with no significant impairment as compared to controls under low dose SGLT2i therapy and significant improvement as compared to STZ group under high dose SGLT2i therapy (Figure 4D). The expression of NADPH oxidase isoforms Nox1 and Nox2 was increased in diabetes and significantly reduced by high dose SGLT2i therapy (Figure 4E and F). As a general stress response, the antioxidant enzyme heme oxygenase-1 (HO-1) was up-regulated in diabetic rats without therapy and significantly reduced by high dose SGLT2i therapy (Figure 4G). The inflammatory protein monocyte chemoattractant protein-1 (MCP-1 or CCL-2) was up-regulated in untreated STZ rats, and normalized by high dose SGLT2i therapy (Figure 4H).

AGE/RAGE signaling

Quantification of advanced glycation end products (AGE)-positive proteins by dot blot analysis (Figure 5A) and AGE signaling was assessed by expression levels of their receptor

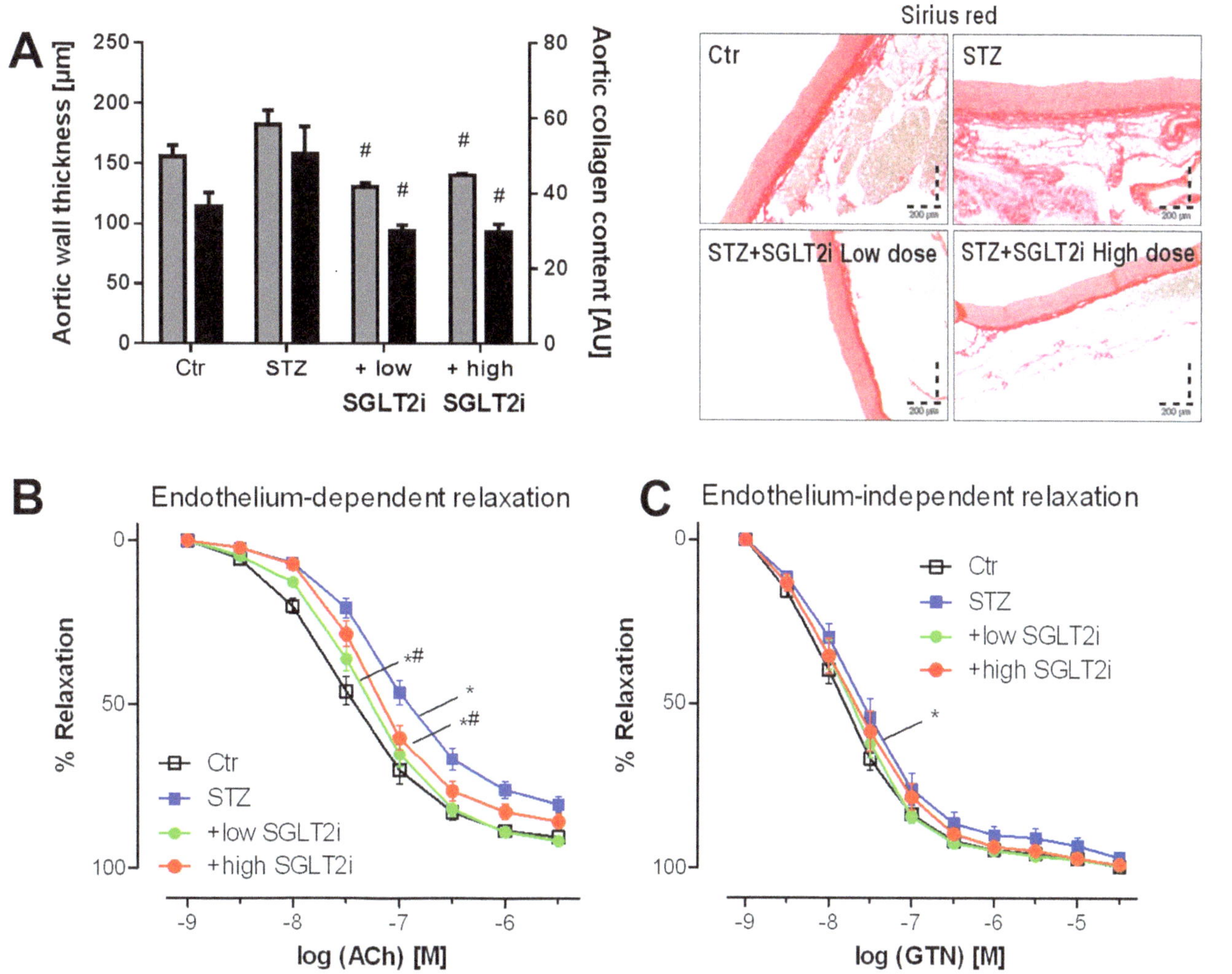

Figure 2. Effects of SGLT2i treatment on vascular parameters in diabetic rats. Microscopic determination of wall thickness (grey) and collagen content (black) by sirius red staining of paraffinated aortic sections (**A**). Representative microscope images are shown along with the densitometric quantification. Effects of SGLT2i therapy on endothelium-dependent and independent vascular relaxation by the vasodilators acetylcholine (ACh, **B**) and nitroglycerin (GTN, **C**), respectively. Data are the means±SEM from 6–7 (**A**) and 9–12 (**B,C**) animals/group. Each single value for an animal corresponds to the means of 4 individual aortic rings from this animal. *, $p<0.05$ vs. control and #, $p<0.05$ vs. STZ-injected group. For the vascular function data the significance levels were determined by two-way-ANOVA and significances for the entire curves are indicated when at least one compared concentration condition showed significant differences. Vasodilator potency (EC_{50}, pD_2) and efficacy (max. relaxation) were also calculated and subjected to statistical analysis using one-way-ANOVA. The data and results are presented in Table 1.

(RAGE) at mRNA and protein level (Figure 5B and C). Aortic RAGE protein expression and levels of AGE-positive proteins was increased in the STZ group and normalized by a high dose SGLT2i therapy. Aortic RAGE mRNA expression showed similar results. In agreement with this, serum levels of the AGE precursor methylglyoxal were significantly increased in the STZ group and improved by high dose SGLT2i therapy (Figure 5D).

mRNA expression

We also determined a number of inflammation markers by RT-PCR-based measurement of mRNA levels. The already mentioned monocyte chemoattractant protein-1 (MCP-1 or CCL-2, Figure 6A), the monocyte/macrophage-specific protein CD68 (Figure 6B) and the cytokine interleukin-6 (IL-6, Figure 6C) were up-regulated at the mRNA level in the aorta and significantly reduced by at least one SGLT2i dose. Likewise, the immune-signaling protein tumor necrosis factor-α (TNF-α, Figure 6E) was up-regulated in STZ-treated rats and reduced by both doses of SGLT2i, a pattern that was mirrored for interferon-γ (IFN-γ) and intercellular adhesion molecule-1 (ICAM-1) expression without reaching significant differences (Figure 6D and 6F). The general marker of inflammation, cyclooxygenase-2 (COX-2, Figure S5 in File S1) was increased in diabetic rats without treatment and normalized by both doses of SGLT2i.

Discussion

With the present study we demonstrate that chronic treatment of STZ-treated rats with the SGLT2i empagliflozin prevents the development of endothelial dysfunction, oxidative stress, AGE/RAGE signaling and inflammation in a well characterized animal model of type I diabetes mellitus. These beneficial effects are mainly due to antioxidant and anti-inflammatory effects of this compound, such as an inhibition of the activity of NADPH oxidase

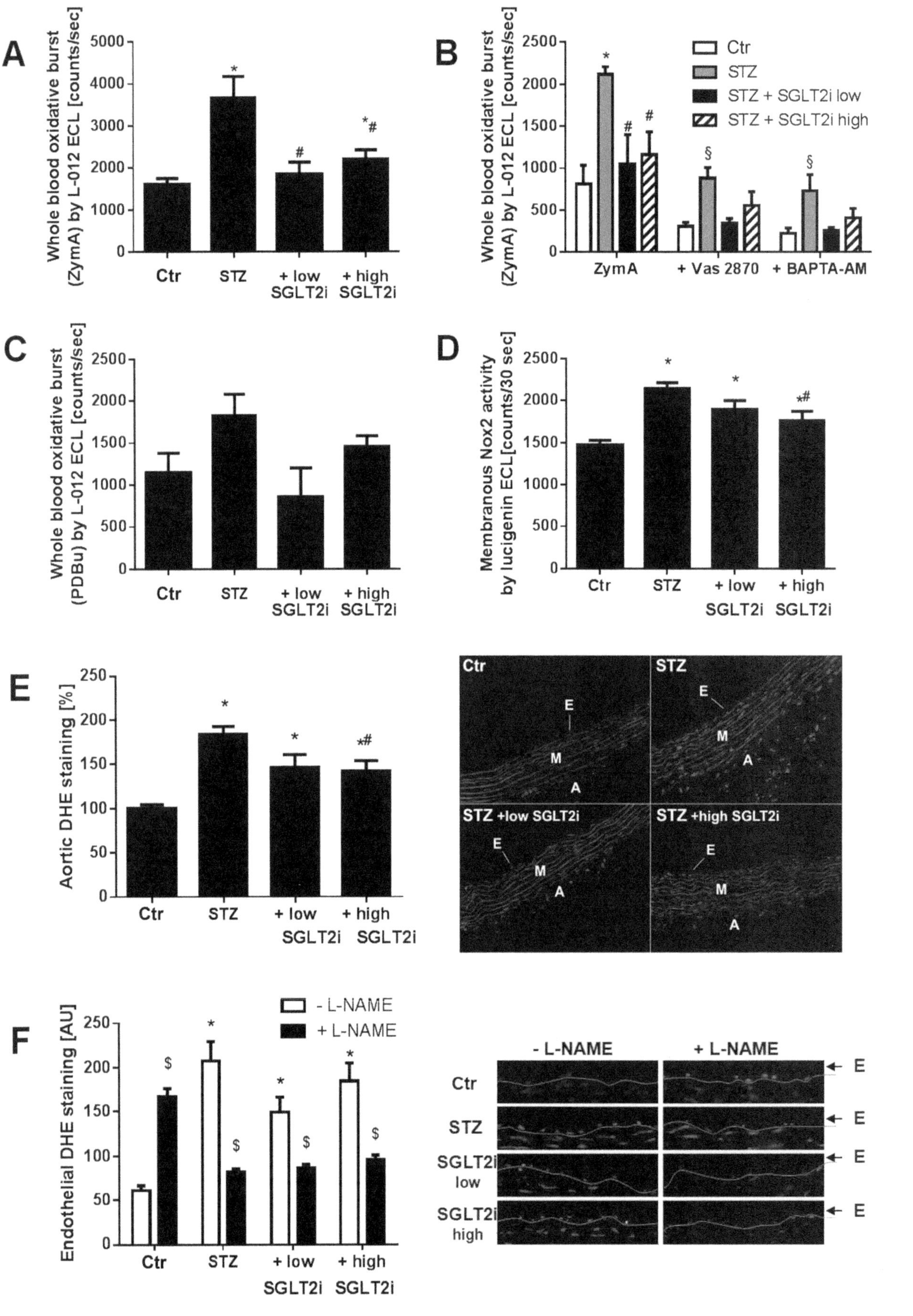
A
Whole blood oxidative burst (ZymA) by L-012 ECL [counts/sec]
Ctr
STZ
+ low SGLT2i
+ high SGLT2i
B
Whole blood oxidative burst (ZymA) by L-012 ECL [counts/sec]
Ctr
STZ
STZ + SGLT2i low
STZ + SGLT2i high
ZymA
+ Vas 2870
+ BAPTA-AM
C
Whole blood oxidative burst (PDBu) by L-012 ECL [counts/sec]
D
Membranous Nox2 activity by lucigenin ECL[counts/30 sec]
E
Aortic DHE staining [%]
STZ +low SGLT2i
STZ +high SGLT2i
F
Endothelial DHE staining [AU]
- L-NAME
+ L-NAME
SGLT2i low
SGLT2i high

Figure 3. Effects of SGLT2i treatment on oxidative stress parameters in diabetic rats. Leukocyte-derived ROS (oxidative burst) in whole blood at 30 min upon zymosan A (**A**) stimulation along with the effects of the NADPH oxidase isoform 2 (Nox2) inhibitor VAS2870 and the intracellular calcium chelator BAPTA-AM (**B**) and upon PDBu stimulation (**C**). (**D**) Quantification of cardiac NADPH oxidase activity in membrane preparations by lucigenin (5 μM)-derived chemiluminescence. Dihydroethidium (DHE, 1 μM)-fluorescence microtopography was used to assess the effects of SGLT2i treatment on vascular (**E**) and endothelial (**F**) ROS production with and without incubation with the eNOS inhibitor L-NAME. Representative microscope images are shown along with the densitometric quantification. Red fluorescence indicates ROS formation whereas green fluorescence represents basal laminae autofluorescence. Data are the means±SEM from 6–7 (**A,B**), 5 (**C**), 7–8 (**D**), 9 (**E**) or 5–6 (**F**) animals/group. *, $p<0.05$ vs. control and $^{\#}$, $p<0.05$ vs. STZ-injected and §, $p<0.05$ vs. low dose SGLT2i treated and $^{\$}$, $p<0.05$ vs. w/o L-NAME.

and decreased serum levels of the AGE precursor methylglyoxal. These antioxidant and anti-inflammatory effects are likely due to glucose lowering effects. Glucose lowering is likely due to removal of glucose by the kidney via SGLT2 inhibition but may also be secondary to improved glucose utilization by restored insulin production and signaling, all of which prevent AGE formation, AGE/RAGE signaling, metabolic dysfunction, oxidative stress and impairment of vascular function. As expected, SGLT2i-dependent glucose lowering decreases cellular glucotoxicity and thereby contributes to the survival of pancreatic islet cells and preserves insulin production (Figure 7).

Diabetes is the most common cause of blindness, non-traumatic amputations and end-stage renal disease and the sixth most common cause of death. Yet only limited knowledge exists about the pathogenesis, the cardiovascular consequences and the prevention of this disease. Previous data suggests that the cardiovascular consequences of diabetes mellitus are secondary to oxidative stress [3,6,25], as previously shown for hypercholesterolemia, hypertension or established atherosclerosis. NADPH oxidases, mitochondria, xanthine oxidase, as well as uncoupled eNOS have been identified as major sources of these reactive oxygen and nitrogen species [4,5,33,34]. Importantly, the efficacy of the current anti-diabetic treatments vanishes over time, leading to a progression of the disease [18]. This phenomenon is mostly explained by the reduction of the ß-cells' capacity to secrete insulin and by a desensitization of the insulin signalling pathways, while most of the treatments aim to induce insulin release or to improve insulin sensitivity. Mode of action of SGLT2 inhibitors is insulin independent, thus efficacy of empagliflozin should be preserved independently of the advancement of the ß-cell failure. Along these lines SGLT2 inhibitors have been demonstrated to be effective in diabetes mellitus type II [35] and are anticipated to be also effective in type 1 diabetic patients. The proof of concept that empagliflozin is effective in lowering glucose and sparing insulin has been recently demonstrated in a preclinical model of STZ-induced type 1 diabetes [22] but also in human studies [36,37].

In contrast to the classical anti-diabetic therapies, SGLT2i treatment removes the glucose from the body and is thereby highly efficient in preventing so-called glucotoxicity, increased methylglyoxal levels, formation of AGE and induction of RAGE. Importantly, methylglyoxal has recently been demonstrated to play an essential role in the development and progression of diabetic neuropathy in diabetic mice and patients and therefore represents a target of special interest for pharmacological modulation [38]. Increased AGE/RAGE signaling in STZ rats has been established [39] and its contribution to increased oxidative stress and vascular complications under hyperglycemic conditions was identified [40]. In 2001, it was demonstrated that macrophages from gp91phox deficient mice responded less to AGE stimulation providing a direct link between AGE/RAGE signaling and NADPH oxidase expression/activity [12]. The same authors also demonstrated a connection between AGE/RAGE signaling and inflammation by increased VCAM-1 and tissue factor expression in human endothelial cells in response to AGE treatment. Increased tissue levels of macrophages were identified by MCP-1 and CD68 staining in STZ rats [41]. Increased TNF-α, IFN-γ expression as well as ROS producing enzymes in STZ rats were normalized by multiple antioxidant therapy [42]. Therefore, hyperglycemia via increased AGE/RAGE signaling leads to oxidative stress from NADPH oxidases, impaired NO/cGMP

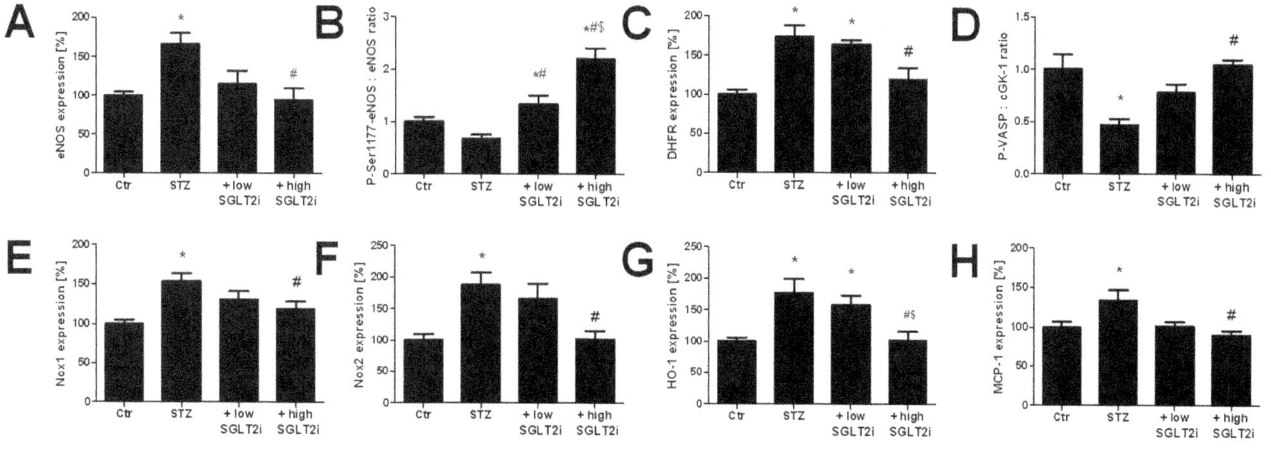

Figure 4. Effects of SGLT2i treatment on aortic protein expression of the NO/cGMP signaling cascade as well as oxidative stress and inflammatory pathways in diabetic rats. Expression of endothelial nitric oxide synthase (eNOS, **A**), serine1177 phosphorylated eNOS (**B**), dihydrofolate reductase (DHFR, **C**), ratio of cGK-I and serine239 phosphorylated VASP (**D**) were assessed by Western blotting analysis and specific antibodies. Expression of NADPH oxidases Nox1 (**E**) and Nox2 (**F**), heme oxygenase-1 (HO-1) (**G**) and monocyte-chemoattractant-protein-1 (MCP-1 or CCL-2, **H**) were assessed by Western blotting analysis and specific antibodies. Representative blots for all proteins are shown in supplemental Figure S6 in File S1. The data are expressed as % of control and are the means ± SEM from 8–9 (**A**), 5–6 (**B**), 7 (**C**), 4 (**D**), 6–7 (**E**), 7–9 (**F**), 7–9 (**G**) and 4–6 (**H**) animals/group. *, $p<0.05$ vs. control and $^{\#}$, $p<0.05$ vs. STZ-injected and $^{\$}$, $p<0.05$ vs. low dose SGLT2i treated.

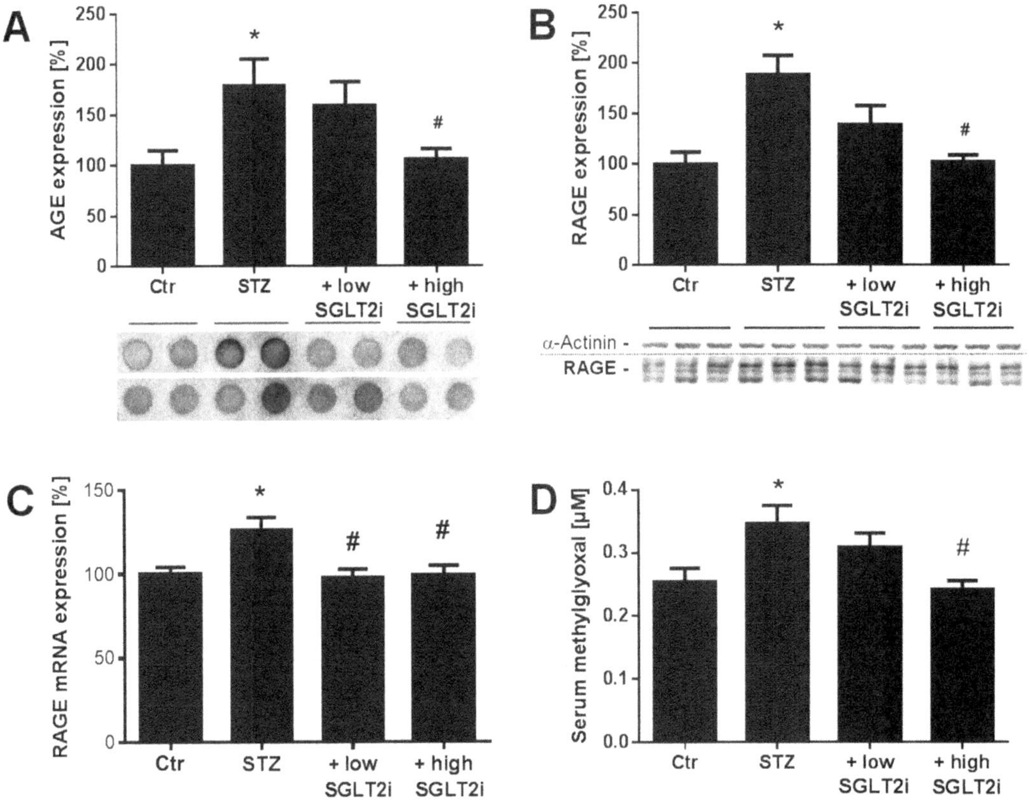

Figure 5. Effects of SGLT2i treatment on AGE/RAGE signaling in diabetic rats. Quantification of AGE-positive proteins by dot blot analysis (**A**) and RAGE expression was assessed by Western blotting analysis with specific antibodies (**B**) and quantitative RT-PCR analysis (**C**). Representative blots are shown at the bottom of the densitometric quantifications. Serum methylglyoxal levels were assessed by HPLC-based quantification (**D**). Representative chromatograms are shown in supplemental Figure S7 in File S1. The data are expressed as % of control and are the means ±SEM from 7 (**A**), 6–7 (**B**) and 8–11 (**C,D**) animals/group. *, $p<0.05$ vs. control and #, $p<0.05$ vs. STZ-injected.

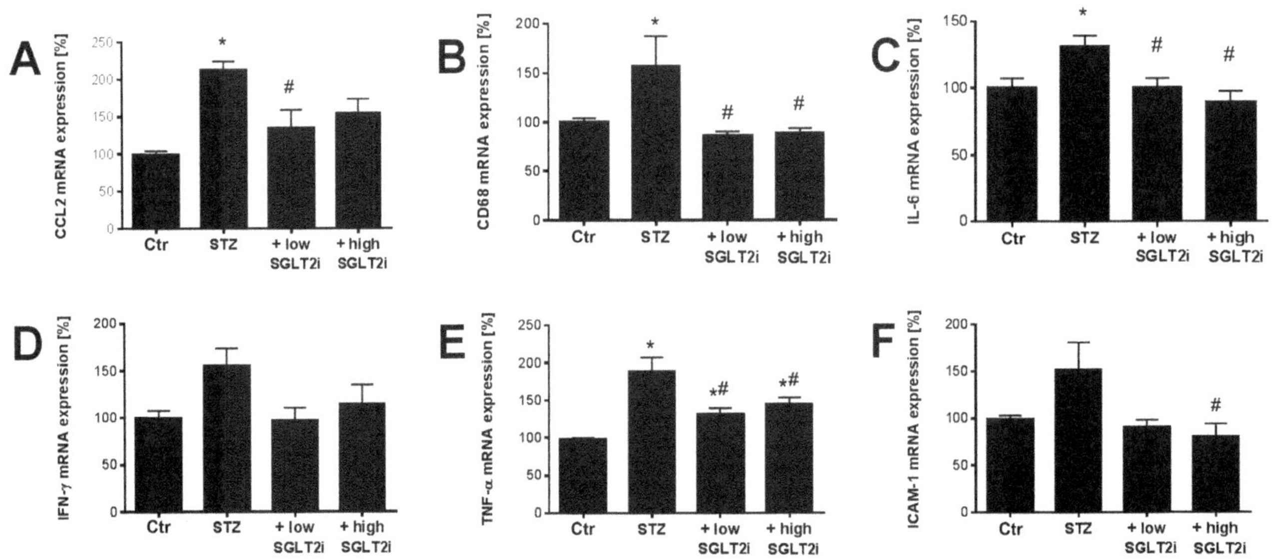

Figure 6. Effects of SGLT2i treatment on aortic mRNA expression of pro-inflammatory genes in diabetic rats. Expression of the monocyte chemoattractant protein-1 (CCL-2, **A**), the monocyte/macrophage-specific protein CD68 (**B**), the cytokine interleukin-6 (IL-6, **C**), the immune-signaling proteins interferon-γ (IFN-γ, **D**) and tumor necrosis factor-α (TNF-α, **E**) and the intercellular adhesion molecule-1 (ICAM-1, **F**) was assessed by quantitative RT-PCR. The data are expressed as % of control and are the means ±SEM from 7–9 (**A–C**), 9–10 (**D–E**) and 6–7 animals/group. *, $p<0.05$ vs. control and #, $p<0.05$ vs. STZ-injected.

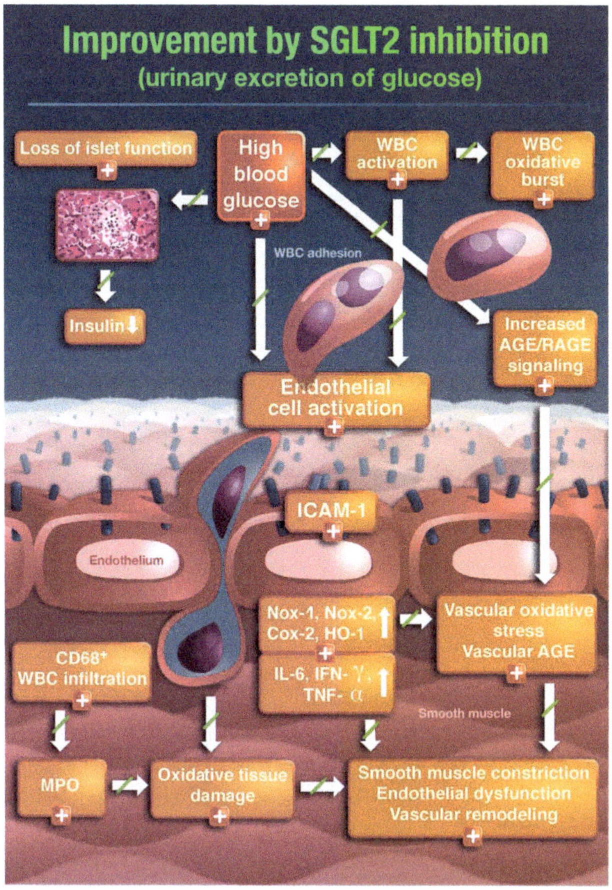

Figure 7. Summary of beneficial effects of SGLT2i treatment on diabetes induced vascular dysfunction and other adverse effects of hyperglycemia in rats.

signaling and low-grade inflammation as supported by the present protein and mRNA expression data and oxidative stress measurements. All of these adverse effects were normalized by SGLT2i treatment.

In line with this, the burden of oxidative stress was decreased by SGLT2i at all levels (whole blood, aorta, heart) supporting the concept of a cross-talk between AGE/RAGE signaling and ROS formation in diabetes mellitus. The contribution of calcium signaling in this process was demonstrated by the inhibitory effect of intracellular calcium chelation in the present work and the overall importance of calcium for the interaction of mitochondrial ROS with the activation of NADPH oxidases (Nox1 and Nox2) was demonstrated recently [15]. Related to the oxidative stress concept, the redox regulated mitochondrial aldehyde dehydrogenase (ALDH-2) is not only important as a nitroglycerin bioactivating enzyme [43,44] but also is an important antioxidant enzyme by degrading toxic aldehydes such as acetaldehyde, malondialdehyde and 4-hydroxynonenal [45,46]. More recently it has been shown that ALDH-2 plays an important role for the reduction of myocardial damage during ischemia/reperfusion by reducing the infarct size [47] and conferring cardio-protection in an experimental diabetes/MI model [48]. Therefore, the inactivation of ALDH-2 in the STZ group substantially supports the cardio-toxic phenotype of hyperglycemia and improved activity of this redox-sensitive enzyme by a high dose SGLT2i therapy clearly points to cardio-protective and anti-oxidant properties of this drug.

Limitations of the study

There are some limitations in the present study. We used not all animals for all assays. Therefore, to ensure that the treatment with STZ and other drugs was comparable among all rats, some parameters were measured in all of them (e.g. blood glucose, HbA1c, cholesterol, insulin by RIA, vascular function and oxidative stress (dihydroethidium staining)). The here observed increase in leukocyte activity (oxidative burst) in diabetic rats, which also nicely correlates with all other measured markers of inflammation, is at variance with previous reports indicating impaired oxidative burst in neutrophils [49] and monocytes [50] in diabetic individuals, which correlates with the impaired phagocytic clearance of bacterial pathogens in these individuals. The major limitation of the study is that STZ treatment kills only some part of the islet cells directly. The remaining β-cells probably die due to glucotoxicity within the first 2 weeks after the injection of STZ. This represents a clear difference as compared to human T1DM where all islet cells are lost due to autoimmune-driven killing of these cells. This limitation will complicate the translation of our findings to the clinical situation. It is also unclear, whether the present results from T1DM can be translated to T2DM, which is the much more frequent form of diabetes in humans. Therefore, our future studies will address whether 1) much later onset of SGLT2i therapy (6 weeks after STZ for weeks 7 and 8 after STZ) will improve the diabetic complications even when all islet cells have died and 2) early onset of SGLT2i therapy (only the first 2 weeks after STZ, w/o treatment for weeks 3-8 after STZ) will still have a beneficial effect by preserving islet cell function. Finally, similar studies on SGLT2i therapy in a T2DM model (e.g. ZDF rats) and assessment of parameters of diabetic complications at all levels are highly recommended.

Conclusions and clinical implications

The results of the present study confirm previous findings that vascular dysfunction in the setting of diabetes is associated with increased vascular oxidative stress, AGE/RAGE signaling and low-grade inflammation (Figure 7). The clinical implications of the present findings originate from the complex interaction of redox and inflammatory pathways in cardiovascular pathogenesis [15,16] requiring multi-targeted therapy to improve the disease progression at all levels. The presented data clearly shows that SGLT2i therapy leading to enhanced glucose excretion improves glucose-induced vascular dysfunction by reducing glucotoxicity, oxidative stress, low-grade inflammation and restoring insulin signaling, ultimately improving endothelial dysfunction as an important determinant of future cardiovascular events.

Supporting Information

File S1 Online supplemental data.

Acknowledgments

We thank Philip Wenzel (University Medical Center Mainz, 55101 Mainz, Germany) for helpful discussions. We are also indebted to Angelica Karpi (University Medical Center Mainz, 55101 Mainz, Germany), Jörg Schreiner (University Medical Center Mainz, 55101 Mainz, Germany), Jessica Rudolph (University Medical Center Mainz, 55101 Mainz, Germany) and Bettina Mros (University Medical Center Mainz, 55101 Mainz, Germany) for expert technical assistance. The graphical assistance of Thilo Weckmüller is gratefully acknowledged. We thank Dr. Ulrich Rösch (Superon GmbH, Dernbach, Germany) for the Field-Flow Fractionation (FFF) measurements. This work contains data that are part of the thesis of Philipp Welschof.

Author Contributions

Conceived and designed the experiments: MO EM AD. Performed the experiments: MO SKS PW MH YM PS MM EZ SA AG SS SPB AD. Analyzed the data: MO SKS PW MH YM SPB AD. Contributed reagents/materials/analysis tools: EM. Wrote the paper: MO TJ YM ES SPB TM AD.

References

1. Nathan DM, Cleary PA, Backlund JY, Genuth SM, Lachin JM, et al. (2005) Intensive diabetes treatment and cardiovascular disease in patients with type 1 diabetes. N Engl J Med 353: 2643–2653.
2. Jay D, Hitomi H, Griendling KK (2006) Oxidative stress and diabetic cardiovascular complications. Free Radic Biol Med 40: 183–192.
3. Hink U, Li H, Mollnau H, Oelze M, Matheis E, et al. (2001) Mechanisms Underlying Endothelial Dysfunction in Diabetes Mellitus. Circ Res 88: E14–E22.
4. Wenzel P, Daiber A, Oelze M, Brandt M, Closs E, et al. (2008) Mechanisms underlying recoupling of eNOS by HMG-CoA reductase inhibition in a rat model of streptozotocin-induced diabetes mellitus. Atherosclerosis 198: 65–76.
5. Wenzel P, Schulz E, Oelze M, Muller J, Schuhmacher S, et al. (2008) AT1-receptor blockade by telmisartan upregulates GTP-cyclohydrolase I and protects eNOS in diabetic rats. Free Radic Biol Med 45: 619–626.
6. Schuhmacher S, Oelze M, Bollmann F, Kleinert H, Otto C, et al. (2011) Vascular Dysfunction in Experimental Diabetes Is Improved by Pentaerithrityl Tetranitrate but not Isosorbide-5-Mononitrate Therapy. Diabetes 60: 2608–2616.
7. Lin MI, Fulton D, Babbitt R, Fleming I, Busse R, et al. (2003) Phosphorylation of threonine 497 in endothelial nitric-oxide synthase coordinates the coupling of L-arginine metabolism to efficient nitric oxide production. J Biol Chem 278: 44719–44726.
8. Loot AE, Schreiber JG, Fisslthaler B, Fleming I (2009) Angiotensin II impairs endothelial function via tyrosine phosphorylation of the endothelial nitric oxide synthase. J Exp Med 206: 2889–2896.
9. Forbes JM, Cooper ME, Thallas V, Burns WC, Thomas MC, et al. (2002) Reduction of the accumulation of advanced glycation end products by ACE inhibition in experimental diabetic nephropathy. Diabetes 51: 3274–3282.
10. Yamamoto Y, Yamagishi S, Yonekura H, Doi T, Tsuji H, et al. (2000) Roles of the AGE-RAGE system in vascular injury in diabetes. Ann N Y Acad Sci 902: 163-170; discussion 170–162.
11. Coughlan MT, Thorburn DR, Penfold SA, Laskowski A, Harcourt BE, et al. (2009) RAGE-induced cytosolic ROS promote mitochondrial superoxide generation in diabetes. J Am Soc Nephrol 20: 742–752.
12. Wautier MP, Chappey O, Corda S, Stern DM, Schmidt AM, et al. (2001) Activation of NADPH oxidase by AGE links oxidant stress to altered gene expression via RAGE. Am J Physiol Endocrinol Metab 280: E685–694.
13. Nishikawa T, Edelstein D, Du XL, Yamagishi S, Matsumura T, et al. (2000) Normalizing mitochondrial superoxide production blocks three pathways of hyperglycaemic damage. Nature 404: 787–790.
14. Schulz E, Wenzel P, Munzel T, Daiber A (2014) Mitochondrial redox signaling: Interaction of mitochondrial reactive oxygen species with other sources of oxidative stress. Antioxid Redox Signal 20: 308–324.
15. Kroller-Schon S, Steven S, Kossmann S, Scholz A, Daub S, et al. (2014) Molecular mechanisms of the crosstalk between mitochondria and NADPH oxidase through reactive oxygen species-studies in white blood cells and in animal models. Antioxid Redox Signal 20: 247–266.
16. Wenzel P, Knorr M, Kossmann S, Stratmann J, Hausding M, et al. (2011) Lysozyme M-positive monocytes mediate angiotensin II-induced arterial hypertension and vascular dysfunction. Circulation 124: 1370–1381.
17. Rieg T, Masuda T, Gerasimova M, Mayoux E, Platt K, et al. (2014) Increase in SGLT1-mediated transport explains renal glucose reabsorption during genetic and pharmacological SGLT2 inhibition in euglycemia. Am J Physiol Renal Physiol 306: F188–193.
18. Evans JL, Goldfine ID (2013) Aging and insulin resistance: just say iNOS. Diabetes 62: 346–348.
19. Sarashina A, Koiwai K, Seman LJ, Yamamura N, Taniguchi A, et al. (2013) Safety, tolerability, pharmacokinetics and pharmacodynamics of single doses of empagliflozin, a sodium glucose cotransporter 2 (SGLT2) inhibitor, in healthy Japanese subjects. Drug Metab Pharmacokinet 28: 213–219.
20. Ferrannini E, Seman L, Seewaldt-Becker E, Hantel S, Pinnetti S, et al. (2013) A Phase IIb, randomized, placebo-controlled study of the SGLT2 inhibitor empagliflozin in patients with type 2 diabetes. Diabetes Obes Metab 15: 721–728.
21. Hansen HH, Jelsing J, Hansen CF, Hansen G, Vrang N, et al. (2014) The sodium glucose cotransporter type 2 inhibitor empagliflozin preserves beta-cell mass and restores glucose homeostasis in the male zucker diabetic fatty rat. J Pharmacol Exp Ther 350: 657–664.
22. Luippold G, Klein T, Mark M, Grempler R (2012) Empagliflozin, a novel potent and selective SGLT-2 inhibitor, improves glycaemic control alone and in combination with insulin in streptozotocin-induced diabetic rats, a model of type 1 diabetes mellitus. Diabetes Obes Metab 14: 601–607.
23. Grempler R, Thomas L, Eckhardt M, Himmelsbach F, Sauer A, et al. (2012) Empagliflozin, a novel selective sodium glucose cotransporter-2 (SGLT-2) inhibitor: characterisation and comparison with other SGLT-2 inhibitors. Diabetes Obes Metab 14: 83–90.
24. Vickers SP, Cheetham SC, Headland KR, Dickinson K, Grempler R, et al. (2014) Combination of the sodium-glucose cotransporter-2 inhibitor empagliflozin with orlistat or sibutramine further improves the body-weight reduction and glucose homeostasis of obese rats fed a cafeteria diet. Diabetes Metab Syndr Obes 7: 265–275.
25. Oelze M, Knorr M, Schuhmacher S, Heeren T, Otto C, et al. (2011) Vascular dysfunction in streptozotocin-induced experimental diabetes strictly depends on insulin deficiency. J Vasc Res 48: 275–284.
26. Oelze M, Kroller-Schon S, Steven S, Lubos E, Doppler C, et al. (2013) Glutathione Peroxidase-1 Deficiency Potentiates Dysregulatory Modifications of Endothelial Nitric Oxide Synthase and Vascular Dysfunction in Aging. Hypertension.
27. Daiber A, Oelze M, Coldewey M, Bachschmid M, Wenzel P, et al. (2004) Oxidative stress and mitochondrial aldehyde dehydrogenase activity: a comparison of pentaerythritol tetranitrate with other organic nitrates. Mol Pharmacol 66: 1372–1382.
28. Kroller-Schon S, Knorr M, Hausding M, Oelze M, Schuff A, et al. (2012) Glucose-independent improvement of vascular dysfunction in experimental sepsis by dipeptidyl-peptidase 4 inhibition. Cardiovasc Res 96: 140–149.
29. Oelze M, Daiber A, Brandes RP, Hortmann M, Wenzel P, et al. (2006) Nebivolol inhibits superoxide formation by NADPH oxidase and endothelial dysfunction in angiotensin II-treated rats. Hypertension 48: 677–684.
30. Shiryaeva YK, Krylin VV, Titov VN (2012) Chromatographic determination of methyl glyoxal in blood plasma as the test for glycotoxicity and accumulation of glycation end-products. Bull Exp Biol Med 153: 114–117.
31. Wenzel P, Hink U, Oelze M, Seeling A, Isse T, et al. (2007) Number of nitrate groups determines reactivity and potency of organic nitrates: a proof of concept study in ALDH-2-/- mice. Brit J Pharmacol 150: 526–533.
32. Hausding M, Jurk K, Daub S, Kroller-Schon S, Stein J, et al. (2013) CD40L contributes to angiotensin II-induced pro-thrombotic state, vascular inflammation, oxidative stress and endothelial dysfunction. Basic Res Cardiol 108: 386.
33. Pricci F, Leto G, Amadio L, Iacobini C, Cordone S, et al. (2003) Oxidative stress in diabetes-induced endothelial dysfunction involvement of nitric oxide and protein kinase C. Free Radic Biol Med 35: 683–694.
34. Yu Y, Lyons TJ (2005) A lethal tetrad in diabetes: hyperglycemia, dyslipidemia, oxidative stress, and endothelial dysfunction. Am J Med Sci 330: 227–232.
35. Ferrannini E, Muscelli E, Frascerra S, Baldi S, Mari A, et al. (2014) Metabolic response to sodium-glucose cotransporter 2 inhibition in type 2 diabetic patients. J Clin Invest 124: 499–508.
36. Perkins BA, Cherney DZ, Partridge H, Soleymanlou N, Tschirhart H, et al. (2014) Sodium-Glucose Cotransporter 2 Inhibition and Glycemic Control in Type 1 Diabetes: Results of an 8-Week Open-Label Proof-of-Concept Trial. Diabetes Care 37: 1480–1483.
37. Cherney DZ, Perkins BA, Soleymanlou N, Har R, Fagan N, et al. (2014) The effect of empagliflozin on arterial stiffness and heart rate variability in subjects with uncomplicated type 1 diabetes mellitus. Cardiovasc Diabetol 13: 28.
38. Bierhaus A, Fleming T, Stoyanov S, Leffler A, Babes A, et al. (2012) Methylglyoxal modification of Nav1.8 facilitates nociceptive neuron firing and causes hyperalgesia in diabetic neuropathy. Nat Med 18: 926–933.
39. Sun M, Yokoyama M, Ishiwata T, Asano G (1998) Deposition of advanced glycation end products (AGE) and expression of the receptor for AGE in cardiovascular tissue of the diabetic rat. Int J Exp Pathol 79: 207–222.
40. Wautier JL, Wautier MP, Schmidt AM, Anderson GM, Hori O, et al. (1994) Advanced glycation end products (AGEs) on the surface of diabetic erythrocytes bind to the vessel wall via a specific receptor inducing oxidant stress in the vasculature: a link between surface-associated AGEs and diabetic complications. Proc Natl Acad Sci U S A 91: 7742–7746.
41. Jeong KH, Lee TW, Ihm CG, Lee SH, Moon JY, et al. (2009) Effects of sildenafil on oxidative and inflammatory injuries of the kidney in streptozotocin-induced diabetic rats. Am J Nephrol 29: 274–282.
42. Kumar S, Prasad S, Sitasawad SL (2013) Multiple antioxidants improve cardiac complications and inhibit cardiac cell death in streptozotocin-induced diabetic rats. PLoS One 8: e67009.
43. Chen Z, Zhang J, Stamler JS (2002) Identification of the enzymatic mechanism of nitroglycerin bioactivation. Proc Natl Acad Sci U S A 99: 8306–8311.
44. Sydow K, Daiber A, Oelze M, Chen Z, August M, et al. (2004) Central role of mitochondrial aldehyde dehydrogenase and reactive oxygen species in nitroglycerin tolerance and cross-tolerance. J Clin Invest 113: 482–489.
45. Oelze M, Knorr M, Schell R, Kamuf J, Pautz A, et al. (2011) Regulation of human mitochondrial aldehyde dehydrogenase (ALDH-2) activity by electrophiles in vitro. J Biol Chem 286: 8893–8900.
46. Wenzel P, Hink U, Oelze M, Schuppan S, Schaeuble K, et al. (2007) Role of reduced lipoic acid in the redox regulation of mitochondrial aldehyde dehydrogenase (ALDH-2) activity. Implications for mitochondrial oxidative stress and nitrate tolerance. J Biol Chem 282: 792–799.

47. Chen CH, Budas GR, Churchill EN, Disatnik MH, Hurley TD, et al. (2008) Activation of aldehyde dehydrogenase-2 reduces ischemic damage to the heart. Science 321: 1493–1495.
48. Wang J, Wang H, Hao P, Xue L, Wei S, et al. (2011) Inhibition of aldehyde dehydrogenase 2 by oxidative stress is associated with cardiac dysfunction in diabetic rats. Mol Med 17: 172–179.
49. Osar Z, Samanci T, Demirel GY, Damci T, Ilkova H (2004) Nicotinamide effects oxidative burst activity of neutrophils in patients with poorly controlled type 2 diabetes mellitus. Exp Diabesity Res 5: 155–162.
50. Chang FY, Shaio MF (1995) Respiratory burst activity of monocytes from patients with non-insulin-dependent diabetes mellitus. Diabetes Res Clin Pract 29: 121–127.

Effects of Radiofrequency Catheter Ablation of Atrial Fibrillation on Soluble P-Selectin, Von Willebrand Factor and IL-6 in the Peripheral and Cardiac Circulation

Jelena Kornej[1,2]*, Borislav Dinov[1], Andrew D. Blann[2], Sascha Rolf[1], Arash Arya[1], Josephine Schmidl[1], Daniela Husser[1], Gerhard Hindricks[1], Andreas Bollmann[1¶], Gregory Y. H. Lip[2¶]

1 University of Leipzig, Heart Center, Department of Electrophysiology, Leipzig, Germany, **2** University of Birmingham Centre for Cardiovascular Sciences, City Hospital, Birmingham, United Kingdom

Abstract

Background: Catheter ablation (CA) of atrial fibrillation (AF) is associated with inflammatory response, endothelial damage and with increased risk of thrombosis. However, whether these processes differ in peripheral *and* cardiac circulation is unknown.

Methods: Plasma markers (von Willebrand factor (vWf), soluble P-selectin (sPsel) and interleukin-6 (IL-6)) were measured by ELISA at three time points in 80 patients (62±10 years, 63% males, 41% paroxysmal AF) undergoing CA. These were at baseline – from femoral vein (FV) and left atrium (LA) before ablation; directly after ablation – from the pulmonary vein (PV), LA and FV; and 24 hours after procedure – from a cubital vein (CV).

Results: The levels of vWF and IL6 – but not sP-sel – increased significantly 24h after procedure ($p<0.001$). Baseline vWF was significantly associated with persistent AF (Beta = .303, p = 0.006 and Beta = .300, p = 0.006 for peripheral and cardiac levels, respectively), while persistent AF (Beta = .250, p = 0.031) and LAA flow pattern (Beta = .386, $p<0.001$) remained associated with vWF in cardiac blood after ablation. Advanced age was significantly associated with IL6 levels at baseline and after ablation in peripheral and cardiac blood. There were no clinical, procedural or anti-coagulation characteristics associated with sP-sel levels in cardiac blood, while peripheral sP-sel levels were associated with hypertension before (Beta = −.307, p = 0.007) and with persistent AF after ablation (Beta = −.262, p = 0.020).

Conclusions: vWF levels are higher in persistent AF and are associated with LAA rheological pattern after AF ablation. Increase of peripheral vWF and IL6 levels after procedure supports current AF ablation management with careful control of post-procedural anticoagulation to avoid ablation-related thromboembolism.

Editor: Carmine Pizzi, University of Bologna, Italy

Funding: JK was supported by the German Cardiac Society St. Jude Medical Stipend. The funders had no role in study design, data collection and analysis, decision to publish, or preparation of the manuscript.

Competing Interests: The authors have declared that no competing interests exist.

* Email: jelena.kornej@gmx.de

¶ AB and GYHL are joint senior authors on this work.

Introduction

Atrial fibrillation (AF) is a major public health problem and its incidence increases as the population ages. AF is a pro-thrombotic and pro-inflammatory disorder leading to substantial mortality and morbidity due to severe cardio- and cerebrovascular complications. Catheter ablation has become a frequently performed procedure for symptomatic relief of this condition multiple procedures are required to achieve acceptable success rates [1].

An association between rhythm outcomes after catheter ablation and markers of inflammation is known [2,3,4]. Recently, we demonstrated that AF ablation leads to changes in inflammatory biomarkers that had an impact on AF recurrences during 6 months follow-up after procedure [3,5]. Some studies analyzed acute changes in biomarker levels related to ablation itself. For example, soluble P-selectin (sP-sel, implying platelet activation) increased in cardiac circulation within minutes of AF onset [6,7]. Furthermore, catheter ablation demonstrated effects on pro-coagulant state and endothelial dysfunction, with increased concentrations of tissue plasminogen activator and von Willebrand factor (vWF, implying endothelial damage) at 24 h after procedure [8]. However, immediate effects on biomarkers of endothelial function, pro-thrombotic and pro-inflammatory changes in patients with AF in peripheral *and* cardiac blood are still unexplored. Furthermore, recent studies have failed to compare directly responses in paroxysmal (PAF) versus persistent AF (PersAF).

While the changes in plasma marker profiles in *peripheral* blood are associated with ablation – that partly might be explained by a 'wash-out' phenomenon – and this association in cardiac blood is understudied. Therefore, we hypothesized that AF ablation leads to increase of pro-inflammatory, pro-thrombotic and markers of endothelial damage that is more presentable in cardiac than in peripheral blood. Furthermore, we hypothesized that these markers correlate significantly in both peripheral and cardiac circulation.

Methods

Study population

We recruited 80 patients with symptomatic AF who underwent AF catheter ablation at Heart Center Leipzig, Germany in October 2012 and January 2013. The study was approved by the local ethics committee (Medical Faculty, University Leipzig) and patients provided written informed consent for participation. Paroxysmal (PAF) and persistent AF (PersAF) were defined according to the current guidelines [9]. PAF was defined as self-terminating within 7 days after onset documented by previous ECG or Holter-ECG. PersAF was defined as an AF episode either lasting longer than 7 days or requiring drug or direct current cardioversion for termination. In all patients, transthoracic and transesophageal echocardiography were performed prior to the ablation. All class I or III antiarrhythmic medications with exception of amiodarone were discontinued for at least 5 half-lives before the AF ablation.

Catheter ablation

Patients presenting with AF at the beginning of the procedure were electrically cardioverted and ablation was performed during sinus rhythm (i.e. AF termination with ablation was not attempted). Pulmonary vein (PV) isolation was performed by sequential application of radiofrequency energy at the antrum of the pulmonary veins. End-point was isolation of the PV with proof of both exit and entrance block. After the isolation of the pulmonary veins, electoanatomical voltage maps of the LA body in sinus rhythm were created in each patient using ablation catheter as a roving catheter. Potentials with amplitudes over 0.5 mV were defined as normal, and potentials under 0.2 mV as low-voltage. According to the underlying substrate and induced left atrial macro reentry tachycardias (LAMRT) additional lines transecting the scar areas to connect with healthy tissue or anatomical obstacles were ablated. Linear ablation of cavotricuspid isthmus was performed in cases of induction of typical atrial flutter after obtaining the blood samples from left atrium. Detailed ablation protocol is provided as **File S1**.

Blood samples

Blood samples were obtained during catheter ablation and 24-(48) hours after procedure. All plasma markers were serially measured at three defined time points: baseline samples (blood from femoral vein (FV) and left atrium (LA) before first radiofrequency pulse) were taken immediately after obtaining the first access to the FV and immediately after trans-septal puncture (T1); at the end of the procedure further blood samples (left superior pulmonary vein (PV), LA and FV) were taken before the catheter and sheath removal (T2); the last sample was taken at the day after procedure from cubital vein (CV) (T3; 24 h). The blood from LSPV (in 41 patients, 51% study population) was taken to investigate the differences in plasma markers up- and downstream regarding the ablation place (LA). Because the patients were usually discharged 24 h after ablation, only in small part of study population (10 patients) the blood was taken 48 h after procedure (cubital vein, T4; 48 h).

All blood samples were centrifuged within 1 h of collection (3500×g for 10 min at 20°C) and plasma aliquots were stored at −70°C for subsequent analysis. Plasma levels of soluble P-selectin (sP-sel), interleukin-6 (IL-6, using a high-sensitivity kit) and von Willebrand factor (vWF) were quantified using commercially available specific enzyme-linked immunoabsorbent assays (ELISA) according to manufacturers protocols (R&D Systems (Abingdon, UK) for sP-sel and IL-6 (high sensitivity); Dako-Patts (Ely, UK) for vWF). The unit for vWF is IU/dL and was standardized with reference vWF from National Institute for Biological Standards and Controls (Potters Bar, Hertfordshire, UK). Intra-assay coefficients of variation for all ELISA assays were <5%, and inter-assay variances were <10%. Results were compared with standard curves and the lower detection limits were as follows: P-Selectin 125 pg/ml; high-sensitive IL-6 0.132 pg/ml; von Willebrand factor −5 IU/ml.

Statistical analysis

Data are presented as mean and standard deviation (SD) for normally distributed or median [interquartile range] for skewed continuous variables and as proportions for categorical variables. Continuous variables were tested for distribution using the Kolmogorov-Smirnov test. The differences between continuous values were assessed using an unpaired t-test or the Mann–Whitney, and a chi-square test for categorical variables. Paired data was analysed by paired t-test or Wilcoxon's method. Comparison of markers from different sites was performed using repeated measures ANOVA test or by Friedman's method. Correlations were performed using Spearman's rank correlation method. Linear regression analysis was used to identify factors associated with plasma marker changes related to ablation. Multivariable analysis, which included variables with a p-value <0.2 found on univariable analysis, was performed to identify independent predictors of plasma marker changes.

A p-value <0.05 was considered as statistically significant, and all analyses were performed with SPSS statistical software version 17.

Results

Baseline plasma marker profiles

Baseline, echocardiographic and procedural characteristics of the study population are presented in **Table 1**. Transesophageal echocardiography was performed in sinus rhythm (40%) and AF (60%). Although patients with SR had better LAA blood flow than those with AF but these differences were not significant (0.61 [0.5–0.8] m/s versus 0.5 [0.4–0.7] m/s, p = 0.524).

Using multivariable analysis, baseline vWF levels were significantly associated with persistent AF (Beta = .303, p = 0.006 and Beta = .300, p = 0.006 for peripheral and cardiac levels, respectively, **Table 2**), while advanced age was significantly associated with IL6 levels at baseline in peripheral and cardiac blood (**Table 3**). There were no clinical characteristics associated with sP-sel levels in cardiac blood, but peripheral sP-sel levels at baseline were associated with hypertension (Beta = −.307, p = 0.007) before ablation (**Table 4**). There were significant correlations between vWF and IL6 levels in peripheral (r^2 = .251, p = 0.026) but not cardiac blood (r^2 = .147, p = 0.196) before AF ablation.

Table 1. Clinical, echocardiographic and procedural characteristic of the study population.

	Study population	PAF	PersAF
	n = 80	n = 34	n = 46
Age, years	62±10	60±11	63±10
Males, %	62	62	65
Paroxysmal AF, %	41		
Re-do, %	35	38	35
RR systolic, mmHg	144±22	141±33	141±18
RR diastolic, mmHg	84±13	82±10	84±14
Heart rate, bpm	79±22	71±20	86±20
BMI, (kg/m^2)	30±6	29±7	30±5
eGFR, ml/min/1.73 m^2	97±31	96±28	99±34
Medical history, %			
Hypertension	85	77	89
Diabetes mellitus	19	9	26
Vascular disease	29	18	37
Previous TE	8	9	7
$CHADS_2$ score	1 [1–2]	1 [1–2]	1 [1–2]
CHA_2DS_2-VASc score	2 [1–3]	2 [1–3]	3 [2–4]
Medical treatment, %			
Beta blockers	85	82	87
ACEI/ARB	63	50	74
Statins	34	21	41
Anticoagulation, %			
VKA	58	50	65
NOACs	28	24	33
Echocardiographic data			
LAD, mm	44±6	41±6	46±6
LV-EDd, mm	51±6	49±6	52±8
EF, %	56±10	59±8	54±10
Procedural data			
Substrate modification, %	32	18	46
CTI, %	27	21	28
Low voltage areals, %	34	27	41
CV during procedure, %	61	38	78
Heparin, total, IU	13,253±3,152	12,382±3,257	13,957±3,049
First ACT	268±60	259±56	271±67
ACT at the end of procedure	285±49	282±54	287±45
Ablation time, s	1,688 [1103–2,704]	1,278 [962–2,004]	2,109 [1,398–2,843]
Total ablation power, J	56,616 [39,009–90,262]	45,414 [35,061–61,952]	72,769 [44,587–93,872]
Procedure time, min	150 [120–213]	120 [106–175]	180 [148–233]

Abbreviations: BMI – body mass index; TE - thromboembolic events, VKA – vitamin K antagonists; ACEI – angiotensin converting enzyme inhibitors; ARB – angiotensin receptor blockers; non-OAC – anticoagulation with aspirin, clopidogrel or low molecular weight heparins, LAD – left atrial diameter, IVSd – interventricular septum end-diatolic, LV-EDd – left ventricular end-diastolic diameter, EF – ejection fraction, LAA – left atrial appendage, SR – sinus rhythm, CV – electrical cardioversion, ACT – activated clotting time.
Data mean ± SD, median [interquartile range], or actual numbers/%.

Effects of catheter ablation on plasma markers

The levels of vWF and IL6 – but not sP-sel – increased significantly 24 h after procedure (vWF_{pre} 32 [20–61] vs vWF_{post} 36 [19–55] vs vWF_{post_24h} 44 [29–87], $p<0.001$, and $IL6_{pre}$ 1.6 [0.9–2.8] vs $IL6_{post}$ 4.3 [1.9–5.9] vs $IL6_{post\_24\ h}$ 11.3 [6.0–16.5], $p<0.001$, Figure 1, Figure 2, Figure 3). Persistent AF (Beta = .250, $p = 0.031$) and LAA flow velocity (Beta = .386, $p<0.001$) were associated with vWF in cardiac blood after ablation (**Table 5**). Similar as with baseline IL6 levels, advanced age was significantly associated with IL6 levels after ablation in both peripheral and cardiac blood (**Table 6**). In contrast to baseline plasma marker levels, there was significant correlation between vWF and IL6

Table 2. Association between clinical parameters and baseline (pre-ablation) von Willebrandt factor levels.

Variables	vWF $_{FV\_pre}$				vWF $_{LA\_pre}$			
	UV		MV		UV		MV	
	Beta	*p*-value	Beta	*p*-value	Beta	*p*-value	Beta	*p*-value
Age	−.099	0.386			.031	0.788		
Persistent AF	.317	0.004	.303	0.006	.323	0.004	.300	0.006
Female gender	.062	0.586			.069	0.547		
Hypertension	.043	0.708			.092	0.421		
Diabetes	.102	0.373			.029	0.796		
CAD/PAD	.004	0.971			.104	0.363		
BMI	.216	0.056	.163	0.162	.176	0.120	.156	0.147
eGFR	.148	0.192	.079	0.497	−.004	0.971		
LA diameter	.067	0.557			.074	0.518		
EF	−.141	0.216			.028	0.808		
Spontaneous contrast	.135	0.236			.176	0.121	.157	0.145
Oral anticoagulation	−.064	0.235			−.093	0.415		

Table 3. Association between clinical parameters and baseline (pre-ablation) interleukin-6 levels.

Variables	$IL6_{FV\_pre}$				$IL6_{LA\_pre}$			
	UV		MV		UV		MV	
	Beta	*p*-value	Beta	*p*-value	Beta	*p*-value	Beta	*p*-value
Age	.211	0.062	.241	0.029	.252	0.025	.279	0.011
Persistent AF	.134	0.239			.058	0.609		
Female gender	.101	0.376			.101	0.374		
Hypertension	.021	0.852			.083	0.469		
Diabetes	.065	0.568			.056	0.624		
CAD/PAD	−.055	0.632			−.057	0.618		
BMI	.201	0.075	.207	0.059	.201	0.076	.213	0.052
eGFR	−.042	0.714			−.059	0.606		
LA diameter	.133	0.243			.080	0.482		
EF	−.195	0.085	−.197	0.073	−.151	0.184	−.155	0.154
Spontaneous contrast	−.062	0.585			−.092	0.422		
Oral anticoagulation	−.018	0.872			.012	0.913		

Table 4. Association between clinical parameters and baseline (pre-ablation) soluble p-Selectin levels.

Variables	sP-sel $_{FV\_pre}$				sP-sel $_{LA\_pre}$			
	UV		MV		UV		MV	
	Beta	*p*-value	Beta	*p*-value	Beta	*p*-value	Beta	*p*-value
Age	−.153	0.179	−.077	0.487	−.120	0.293		
Persistent AF	−.124	0.278			−.236	0.036	−.209	0.063
Female gender	−.137	0.229			−.029	0.800		
Hypertension	−.315	0.005	−.307	0.007	−.206	0.068	−.174	0.121
Diabetes	.039	0.731			.034	0.768		
CAD/PAD	.035	0.758			.043	0.709		
BMI	−.090	0.429			.046	0.690		
eGFR	.128	0.261			.118	0.301		
LA diameter	.007	0.949			−.119	0.298		
EF	−.090	0.431			−.019	0.866		
Spontaneous contrast	−.166	0.143	−.186	0.086	.044	0.703		
Oral anticoagulation	.020	0.858			−.069	0.545		

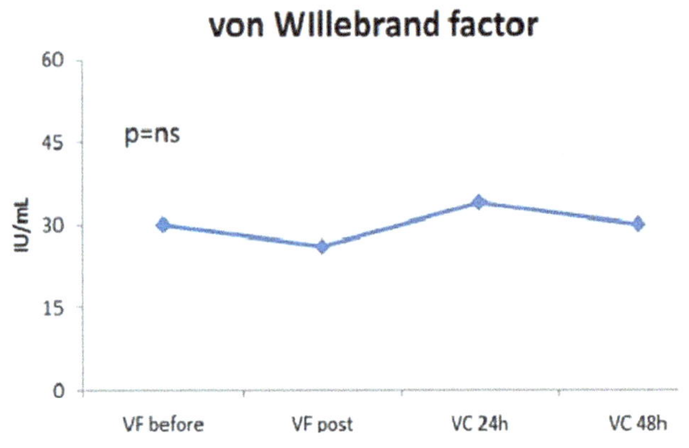

Figure 1. Changes in von Willebrand factor levels after catheter ablation.

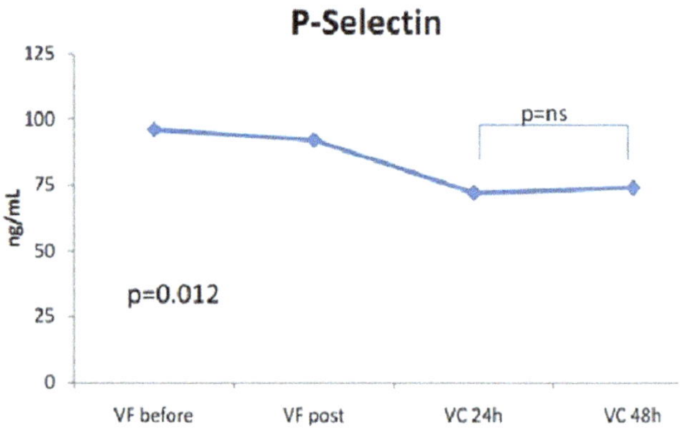

Figure 3. Changes in soluble P-selectin levels after catheter ablation.

levels in cardiac blood ($r^2=.341$, $p=0.002$) directly after AF ablation while the correlation in peripheral blood did not reach significance ($r^2=.199$, $p=0.079$).

There were no clinical, procedural or anti-coagulation characteristics associated with post-procedural sP-sel levels in cardiac blood, but only persistent AF remained significantly associated with sP-sel levels in peripheral blood (Beta $= -.262$, $p=0.020$; **Table 7**).

Ablation effects on trans-pulmonary and intra-cardiac gradients in PAF and PersAF are presented in supplemental files (**Tables S1, Figure S1-S3 in File S1**).

Sub-acute changes in plasma marker levels

In sub-group of 10 patients (age 57±13 years, 70% females) dynamic changes in plasma marker levels were measured in peripheral blood within 2 days after procedure (FV pre-ablation and post-ablation, CV 24 h and 48 h after procedure). Compared to sP-sel and vWF levels 24 h after procedure, the biomarker levels taken 48 h after procedure remained unchanged (**Figure 1**). In contrast, IL-6 levels decreased significantly at 48 h post-procedure compared to levels at 24 h and reached the levels seen directly after procedure.

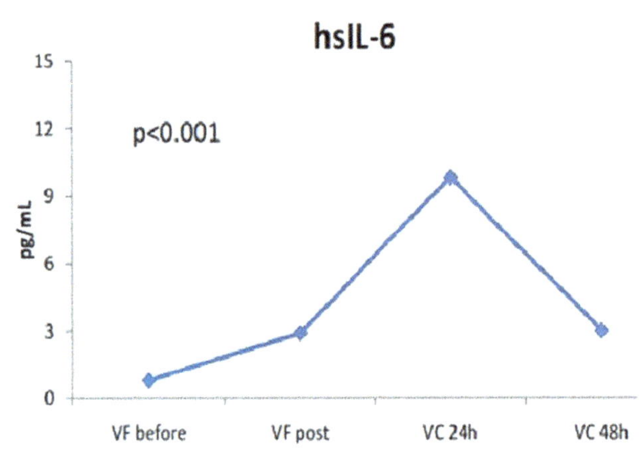

Figure 2. Changes in interleukin-6 levels after catheter ablation.

Discussion

In this study we hypothesized increase of pro- inflammatory, pro-thrombotic and markers of endothelial damage in peripheral *and* cardiac blood after AF ablation and analyzed the association between clinical, echocardiographic and procedural parameters with these markers. We found that the levels of vWF and IL6 correlated and increased significantly immediately after catheter ablation. Second, vWF levels in cardiac blood were associated with persistent AF and rheological LAA pattern after AF ablation. Finally, while sub-acute vWF levels remained constantly increased, IL6 significantly decreased already 2 days after procedure.

Catheter ablation and inflammation

Several lines of evidence support a strong association between inflammation and the pathogenesis of AF. Furthermore, inflammatory markers have been investigated in different settings, focusing on their role in prediction of AF occurrence after CABG [10], success of cardioversion [11] or catheter ablation [3].

Several studies suggest that the complement system may serve as a link between inflammation and thrombosis and reveal specific interactions between complement proteins and platelets. Pro-inflammatory cytokines, as IL6, promote thrombosis by increasing expression of different pro-thrombotic markers (e.g. tissue factor, factor VIII and vWF) [12]. These have been linked to increased platelet aggregation, endothelial activation and endothelial cell damage. Moreover, increased IL6 levels lower the concentration of the natural inhibitors of hemostasis as antithrombin and protein S [13]. In this study we demonstrate a 2-fold increase of IL6 levels in both cardiac and peripheral blood directly after procedure followed by 10-fold increase of this marker in peripheral circulation 24 h after procedure. Thus, this might contribute to modulation of later outcomes, e.g. occurrence of thromboembolic complications.

Indeed, we found significant correlations between vWF and IL-6 levels in cardiac circulation after ablation. In contrast to previous study [14], where prolonged inflammatory response for several weeks after ablation was described, we found significant IL6 reduction 48 h after procedure ($p<0.001$), but still reaching the post-ablative IL6 levels. This dynamic change within 2 days after AF ablation might be partly explained by short half-life of IL6 since it is considered as acute phase protein.

Table 5. Association between clinical and procedural characteristics with von Willebrandt factor levels after ablation.

Variables	vWF $_{FV\_post}$				vWF $_{LA\_post}$			
	UV		MV		UV		MV	
	Beta	*P*-value	Beta	*P*-value	Beta	*P*-value	Beta	*P*-value
Age	−.057	0.620			.116	0.307		
Females	−.198	0.081	−.170	0.128	−.028	0.805		
Persistent AF	.274	0.015	.228	0.056	.343	0.002	.250	0.031
LA diameter	.177	0.119	.090	0.463	.192	0.089	.173	0.134
Spontaneous contrast	.151	0.184	.142	0.210	.371	0.001	.386	<0.001
Heparin*	−.060	0.599			−.079	0.492		
Low voltage areas	.013	0.911			.090	0.431		
Cardioversion	.102	0.372			.150	0.188	.006	0.957
Ablation time	.084	0.471			.047	0.690		
Ablation power	.119	0.304			.050	0.670		

Abbreviations: UV – univariable analysis, MV – multivariable analysis, CAD – coronary artery disease, PAD – peripheral artery disease, LA – left atrial, EF – ejection fraction, LAA – left atrial appendage, SC – spontaneous contrast, Heparin* - peri-procedural anticoagulation.

Table 6. Association between clinical and procedural characteristics with interleukin-6 levels after ablation.

Variables	hsIL6 $_{FV\_post}$				hsIL6 $_{LA\_post}$			
	UV		MV		UV		MV	
	Beta	*P*-value	Beta	*P*-value	Beta	*P*-value	Beta	*P*-value
Age	.240	0.033	.282	0.021	.241	0.032	.249	0.046
Females	−.013	0.910			.122	0.285		
Persistent AF	.207	0.067	.021	0.867	.229	0.042	.052	0.690
BMI	.157	0.167	.122	0.286	.208	0.066	.182	0.125
LA diameter	.315	0.005	.260	0.069	.214	0.059	.149	0.308
Spontaneous contrast	−.128	0.261			−.110	0.334		
Low voltage areas	.194	0.086	.052	0.686	.152	0.181	.063	0.633
Cardioversion	.202	0.074	−.039	0.757	.226	0.046	.061	0.643
Ablation time	.265	0.021	.266	0.530	.166	0.152	.199	0.647
Ablation power	.254	0.027	−.101	0.804	.154	0.184	−.150	0.720

Table 7. Association between clinical and procedural characteristics with soluble p-Selectin levels after ablation.

Variables	sP-sel $_{FV\_post}$				sP-sel $_{LA\_post}$			
	UV		MV		UV		MV	
	Beta	P-value	Beta	P-value	Beta	P-value	Beta	P-value
Age	−.117	0.306			−.131	0.251		
Females	−.043	0.705			−.060	0.600		
Persistent AF	−.295	0.008	−.262	0.020	−.152	0.182	−.141	0.264
LA diameter	−.116	0.310			−.193	0.089	−.238	0.068
Spontaneous contrast	−.192	0.090	.175	0.180	−.018	0.872		
Heparin*	−.149	0.189	−.102	0.359	−.072	0.527		
Low voltage areas	.029	0.801			.161	0.156		
Cardioversion	−.084	0.460			−.040	0.728		
Ablation time	−.073	0.533			.154	0.185	.275	0.510
Ablation power	−.070	0.547			.154	0.184	.009	0.983

Abbreviations: as in Tables 5–6.

Endothelial damage/dysfunction

Endothelial damage/dysfunction is one of the pro-thrombotic mechanisms of Virchow's triad [15]. Previous studies have reported increased endocardial expression of vWF in association with thrombus formation in the left atrial appendage (LAA) in patients with AF [16]. This supports the importance of endothelial damage/dysfunction as a plausible mechanism of increased thrombus formation. Although we did not find any association between baseline vWF levels and spontaneous contrast, for the first time we demonstrate that in therapeutically anticoagulated patients LAA flow pattern relates to cardiac vWF levels directly after AF ablation. This finding implicates the necessity of careful anticoagulation during procedure and continuous control thereafter in such group of patients.

The impact on endothelial damage caused by AF catheter ablation is well known [2,4]. Bulava et al [8] showed changes after catheter ablation on pro-thrombotic and endothelial damage markers, and we confirm their finding showing significantly increased vWF directly after procedure. In contrast to previous study, vWF levels in our study reached their maximum after 24 h, and remained unchanged 48 h after procedure suggesting prolonged endothelial dysfunction and increased risk for early thromboembolic events within first 48 h. In a recent study [17] we demonstrated that majority of post-interventional thromboembolic complications occurred within 2 days after catheter ablation. Prolonged increase of vWF levels 48 h after procedure found in our study indicates possible pathophysiologic relationship between endothelial damage with TE occurrence directly after catheter ablation. Of note, there were no peri-procedural TE in current study, however, this might be related to relatively small patient numbers in the current study.

Platelet activation

AF is associated with pro-thrombotic state as demonstrated by higher levels of different hemostatic indices [18,19,20]. Despite known multiple links between thrombogenesis and inflammation [12] there were no significant correlations between sP-sel and other plasma markers as demonstrated by other studies [20]. As already demonstrated in the SPAF III trial, where several atherosclerotic factors, e.g. male gender, hypertension, peripheral artery disease and diabetes were associated with elevated sP-sel levels [16], in our study baseline sP-sel levels in peripheral blood were significantly associated with hypertension. However, we failed to demonstrate an association between LAA flow pattern and sP-sel levels, as has been shown previously [13].

In contrast to other studies [21] the sP-sel levels were very low in our study population. As possible explanation would be continuous oral anticoagulation before and after procedure (each procedure was performed without cessation of vitamin K antagonists or NOACs) as well as peri-procedural ACT-driven anticoagulation with heparin during ablation. Although we did not find any differences between oral anticoagulation regimes (NOACs/VKA before procedure or with peri-procedural heparin) and sP-sel this might be biased by initially low sP-sel levels.

Clinical implications

In current study we demonstrated significant increase of vWF and IL6 in peripheral blood within 2 days after procedure which might be partly explained by wash-out phenomenon. Interestingly, while IL6 decreased significantly already 48 h after procedure, vWF remained constant at that time. Our findings support the hypothesis that post-procedural inflammatory response might be a driver of pro-thrombotic reactions facilitating the increased occurrence of peri-interventional thromboembolic events [17].

Although continuous monitoring of anticoagulation before, during and directly after procedure is a standard in current AF ablation management, for the first time our study demonstrates that changes in plasma marker profiles support this clinical approach.

Limitations

Because of continuous anticoagulation of our study population we found very low sP-sel levels and failed to demonstrate significant sP-sel changes with catheter ablation.

The time of dynamic changes related to catheter ablation was limited by 24 h and in a smaller part by 48 hours. Whether the pattern of these changes is different during longer period after ablation should be investigated in further larger studies. All patients in current study underwent *radiofrequency* catheter ablation. Thus, although some studies demonstrated similar levels of plasma marker changes due to cryoablation or duty-cycled bipolar and unipolar radiofrequency pulmonary vein ablation catheter (PVAC), our findings cannot be directly compared with other AF ablation modalities [22,23].

Conclusions

Increase of peripheral vWF and IL6 levels after catheter ablation supports the necessity of continuous and careful control of post-procedural anticoagulation to avoid ablation-related thromboembolic complications.

Supporting Information

File S1 File includes Methods, Table S1, and Figures S1-S3. Figure S1: Effects of catheter ablation on sP-sel levels. A: Peripheral circulation. B: Cardiac circulation. Figure S2: Effect of catheter ablation on hsIL-6 levels. A: Peripheral circulation. B: Cardiac circulation. Figure S3: Effect of catheter ablation on vWF levels. A: Peripheral circulation. B: Cardiac circulation. Methods: Radiofrequency catheter ablation. Table S1: Effects of catheter ablation on plasma markers in different AF types. A: sP-selectin. B: Von Willebrand factor. C: IL-6.

Author Contributions

Conceived and designed the experiments: JK AB GYHL. Performed the experiments: JK. Analyzed the data: JK BD ADB AB GYHL. Contributed reagents/materials/analysis tools: JK ADB. Wrote the paper: JK BD ADB AB GYHL. Patient inclusion, critical revision of manuscript: SR AA GH. Data collection: JS DH.

References

1. Calkins H, Kuck KH, Cappato R, Brugada J, Camm AJ, et al. (2012) 2012 HRS/EHRA/ECAS Expert Consensus Statement on Catheter and Surgical Ablation of Atrial Fibrillation: recommendations for patient selection, procedural techniques, patient management and follow-up, definitions, endpoints, and research trial design. Europace 14: 528–606.
2. Davlouros PA, Simeonidou E, Tsakas S, Vlachojannis I, Alexopoulos D, et al. (2005) Release of endothelin-1 from human endocardium after radiofrequency catheter ablation and coronary angioplasty: comparative results. Int J Cardiol 102: 187–193.
3. Kornej J, Reinhardt C, Kosiuk J, Arya A, Hindricks G, et al. (2012) Response of high-sensitive C-reactive protein to catheter ablation of atrial fibrillation and its relation with rhythm outcome. PLoS One 7: e44165.
4. Ma J, Cheng G, Xu G, Lu X (2006) Effect of radiofrequency catheter ablation on endothelial function and oxidative stress. Acta Cardiol 61: 339–342.
5. Kornej J, Reinhardt C, Kosiuk J, Arya A, Hindricks G, et al. (2013) Response of circulating heat shock protein 70 and anti-heat shock protein 70 antibodies to catheter ablation of atrial fibrillation. J Transl Med 11: 49.
6. Akar JG, Jeske W, Wilber DJ (2008) Acute onset human atrial fibrillation is associated with lokal cardiac platelet activation and endothelial dysfunction. J Am Coll Cardiol 51: 1790–1793.
7. Lim HS, Willoughby SR, Schultz C, Gan C, Alasady M, et al. (2013) Effect of atrial fibrillation on atrial thrombogenesis in humans: impact of rate and rhythm. J Am Coll Cardiol 61: 852–860.
8. Bulava A, Slavik L, Fiala M, Heinc P, Skvarilova M, et al. (2004) Endothelial damage and activation of the hemostatic system during radiofrequency catheter isolation of pulmonary veins. J Interv Card Electrophysiol 10: 271–279.
9. Camm AJ, Kirchhof P, Lip GY, Schotten U, Savelieva I, et al. (2010) Guidelines for the management of atrial fibrillation: the Task Force for the Management of Atrial Fibrillation of the European Society of Cardiology (ESC). Europace 12: 1360–1420.
10. Kaireviciute D, Blann AD, Balakrishnan B, Lane DA, Patel JV, et al. (2010) Characterisation and validity of inflammatory biomarkers in the prediction of post-operative atrial fibrillation in coronary artery disease patients. Thromb Haemost 104: 122–127.
11. Vizzardi E, Nodari S, Zanini G, Manerba A, Frattini S, et al. (2009) High sensitivity C-reactive protein: a predictor for recurrence of atrial fibrillation after successful cardioversion. Intern Emerg Med 4: 309–313.
12. Kerr R, Stirling D, Ludlam CA (2001) Interleukin 6 and haemostasis. Br J Haematol 115: 3–12.
13. Conway DS, Buggins P, Hughes E, Lip GY (2004) Relation of interleukin-6, C-reactive protein, and the prothrombotic state to transesophageal echocardiographic findings in atrial fibrillation. Am J Cardiol 93: 1368–1373, A6.
14. McCabe JM, Smith LM, Tseng ZH, Badhwar N, Lee BK, et al. (2008) Protracted CRP elevation after atrial fibrillation ablation. Pacing Clin Electrophysiol 31: 1146–1151.
15. Lip GY (1995) Does atrial fibrillation confer a hypercoagulable state? Lancet 346: 1313–1314.
16. Conway DS, Pearce LA, Chin BS, Hart RG, Lip GY (2002) Plasma von Willebrand factor and soluble p-selectin as indices of endothelial damage and platelet activation in 1321 patients with nonvalvular atrial fibrillation: relationship to stroke risk factors. Circulation 106: 1962–1967.
17. Kosiuk J, Kornej J, Bollmann A, Piorkowski C, Myrda K, et al. (2014) Early Cerebral Thromboembolic Complications following Radiofrequency Catheter Ablation of Atrial Fibrillation: Incidence, Characteristics and Risk Factors. Heart Rhythm doi: 10.1016/j.hrthm.2014.07.039.
18. Kannel WB, Wolf PA, Benjamin EJ, Levy D (1998) Prevalence, incidence, prognosis, and predisposing conditions for atrial fibrillation: population-based estimates. Am J Cardiol 82: 2N–9N.
19. Li-Saw-Hee FL, Blann AD, Lip GY (2000) Effects of fixed low-dose warfarin, aspirin-warfarin combination therapy, and dose-adjusted warfarin on thrombogenesis in chronic atrial fibrillation. Stroke 31: 828–833.
20. Roldan V, Marin F, Blann AD, Garcia A, Marco P, et al. (2003) Interleukin-6, endothelial activation and thrombogenesis in chronic atrial fibrillation. Eur Heart J 24: 1373–1380.
21. Kaireviciute D, Lip GY, Balakrishnan B, Uzdavinys G, Norkunas G, et al. (2011) Intracardiac expression of markers of endothelial damage/dysfunction, inflammation, thrombosis, and tissue remodeling, and the development of postoperative atrial fibrillation. J Thromb Haemost 9: 2345–2352.
22. Herrera Siklody C, Arentz T, Minners J, Jesel L, Stratz C, et al. (2012) Cellular damage, platelet activation, and inflammatory response after pulmonary vein isolation: a randomized study comparing radiofrequency ablation with cryoablation. Heart Rhythm 9: 189–196.
23. Malmborg H, Lonnerholm S, Blomstrom P, Blomstrom-Lundqvist C (2013) Ablation of atrial fibrillation with cryoballoon or duty-cycled radiofrequency pulmonary vein ablation catheter: a randomized controlled study comparing the clinical outcome and safety; the AF-COR study. Europace 15: 1567–1573.

Efficient Uptake of Blood-Borne BK and JC Polyomavirus-Like Particles in Endothelial Cells of Liver Sinusoids and Renal Vasa Recta

Jaione Simon-Santamaria[1], Christine Hanssen Rinaldo[2,3], Piotr Kardas[4], Ruomei Li[1], Ivana Malovic[1], Kjetil Elvevold[1], Peter McCourt[1], Bård Smedsrød[1], Hans H. Hirsch[4,5]❾, Karen Kristine Sørensen[1]*❾

1 Department of Medical Biology, UiT – The Arctic University of Norway, Tromsø, Norway, **2** Department of Microbiology and Infection Control, University Hospital of North Norway, Tromsø, Norway, **3** Department of Clinical Medicine, UiT - The Arctic University of Norway, Tromsø, Norway, **4** Department of Biomedicine, University of Basel, Basel, Switzerland, **5** Divisions of Infectious Diseases and Hospital Epidemiology, University Hospital of Basel, Basel, Switzerland

Abstract

Liver sinusoidal endothelial cells (LSECs) are specialized scavenger cells that mediate high-capacity clearance of soluble waste macromolecules and colloid material, including blood-borne adenovirus. To explore if LSECs function as a sink for other viruses in blood, we studied the fate of virus-like particles (VLPs) of two ubiquitous human DNA viruses, BK and JC polyomavirus, in mice. Like complete virions, VLPs specifically bind to receptors and enter cells, but unlike complete virions, they cannot replicate. ^{125}I-labeled VLPs were used to assess blood decay, organ-, and hepatocellular distribution of ligand, and non-labeled VLPs to examine cellular uptake by immunohisto- and -cytochemistry. BK- and JC-VLPs rapidly distributed to liver, with lesser uptake in kidney and spleen. Liver uptake was predominantly in LSECs. Blood half-life (~1 min), and tissue distribution of JC-VLPs and two JC-VLP-mutants (L55F and S269F) that lack sialic acid binding affinity, were similar, indicating involvement of non-sialic acid receptors in cellular uptake. Liver uptake was not mediated by scavenger receptors. In spleen, the VLPs localized to the red pulp marginal zone reticuloendothelium, and in kidney to the endothelial lining of vasa recta segments, and the transitional epithelium of renal pelvis. Most VLP-positive vessels in renal medulla did not express PV-1/Meca 32, suggesting location to the non-fenestrated part of vasa recta. The endothelial cells of these vessels also efficiently endocytosed a scavenger receptor ligand, formaldehyde-denatured albumin, suggesting high endocytic activity compared to other renal endothelia. We conclude that LSECs very effectively cleared a large fraction of blood-borne BK- and JC-VLPs, indicating a central role of these cells in early removal of polyomavirus from the circulation. In addition, we report the novel finding that a subpopulation of endothelial cells in kidney, the main organ of polyomavirus persistence, showed selective and rapid uptake of VLPs, suggesting a role in viremic organ tropism.

Editor: Jianming Qiu, University of Kansas Medical Center, United States of America

Funding: The work was supported by a grant from The Tromsø Research Foundation (Tromsø, Norway) to BS, and an institutional grant of the University of Basel (Basel, Switzerland) to HHH. The funders had no role in study design, data collection and analysis, decision to publish, or preparation of the manuscript.

Competing Interests: The authors have declared that no competing interests exist.

* Email: karen.sorensen@uit.no

❾ These authors contributed equally to this work.

Introduction

The mucosal surfaces of the respiratory, oral-pharyngeal and gastrointestinal tracts are constantly exposed to a multitude of different viruses, only some of which eventually cause infection and disease [1]. Similarly to bacteria, viruses are likely to leak from the gut to the portal vein, and many of these viruses end up in the liver [2–8]. Some picornaviruses such as hepatitis A virus initially replicate in the intestinal mucosal surface and cause acute hepatitis when reaching the liver. Other viruses such as cytomegalovirus, Epstein-Barr virus, adenovirus, parvovirus B19, and polyomavirus cause only limited liver damage, if at all.

The liver has a critical role in pathogen detection and host defense, and contains the single largest number of macrophages, the highest concentration of natural killer cells and natural killer T cells, and the largest reticuloendothelial network in the body [9]. Of the various liver cells involved in host defense, liver sinusoidal endothelial cells (LSECs), which line the numerous sinusoids of this organ, are the least known. However, studies over the last three decades have revealed that these cells are highly active scavenger cells, removing large amounts of soluble waste macromolecules and nanoparticulate material from blood each day [10]. Thus, LSECS clearly play an important role as sentinel cells of the immune system due to: **1**) their location exposing them to 25–30% of cardiac output; **2**) their expression of several molecules involved in innate immunity such as various scavenger receptors [11–13]), the mannose receptor [14,15], toll-like receptors 2–4, 7 and 9 [16–19], and **3**) their capacity to produce cytokines and other molecules to alert their environment [16,19]. Furthermore, LSECs express Fc gamma-receptor IIb2 [20,21], which mediates endocytosis of soluble immune complexes, and other receptors involved in virus uptake such as L-SIGN [22] and LSECtin [23]. Ligands eliminated from blood mainly by LSECs, and to a lesser by Kupffer cells (resident liver macrophages), include connective tissue turnover products, lysosomal enzymes [13,15,24–26]), modified plasma proteins and lipoproteins [27–30], soluble IgG immune complexes [31], yeast mannan [32], and adenovirus/adenoviral vectors [7,33]. Differently to macrophages, LSECs operate essentially via clathrin-mediated endocytosis, and not by phagocytosis, and the cells are equipped with an endocytic machinery capable of super-efficient uptake and degradation of the internalized ligands [10,34]. We have previously shown that this high scavenging activity of LSECs is conserved among all land-based vertebrates (amphibians, reptiles, birds, mammals) suggesting that this is a general mechanism for how soluble macromolecular waste material, and small colloidal particles, such as viruses, are cleared from blood [10,35].

Cellular uptake of virus has traditionally been studied in the context of productive infection with disease-forming virus in permissive cells. Apart from the recently reported central role of LSECs in clearing blood-borne adenovirus and adenoviral vectors [7,33], little is actually known about the role of LSECs in the uptake of virus. To explore the hypothesis that these cells act as general virus scavengers, we have studied the circulatory fate of virus-like particles (VLPs) of two non-enveloped, human DNA viruses; polyomavirus BK and JC (BKV and JCV), in mice. These viruses are approximately 40–45 nm in diameter, and are taken up in their permissive host cells via caveolin-mediated and clathrin-mediated endocytosis, respectively [36]. The VLPs represent a well-established model for endocytosis studies [37,38]. These particles are empty virus capsids consisting of 72 capsomers of polyoma viral protein 1 (VP1), which mediate the virus binding to sialic acid receptors during infection of susceptible cells [39].

BKV and JCV infect most people early in life and establish lifelong persistent infections in the renourinary tract with asymptomatic episodes of viral reactivation and shedding in urine. While reactivation of BKV may result in severe diseases in the kidney graft and bladder of kidney- and hematopoietic stem cell transplant patients [40], JCV may lead to severe demyelinating brain disease, progressive multifocal leukoencephalopathy (PML) in immunocompromised individuals, and in patients treated with novel immunomodulatory or depleting therapies for autoimmune diseases [41]. Following respiratory or gastrointestinal transmission, BKV and JCV colonize the renourinary tract as the major site of persistence. To reach the renourinary tract, a viremic phase has been postulated, but the fate of BKV and JCV when they first appear in the circulation is currently unknown. Like most polyomavirus, BKV and JCV replication is highly specific to the human host, which hampered studies of replicative disease in animal models. However, the alpha(2,3)-linked and alpha(2,6)-linked sialic acid receptors used by BKV and JCV, respectively, are widespread in vertebrates, including mice. This encouraged us to study the fate of BK- and JC-VLPs in the blood and their cellular site of uptake in a mouse model similar to other recent studies [37,42].

Here we present evidence for a central role of LSECs in the initial uptake of polyomavirus from blood. Despite the fact that mouse is not a permissive host for BKV and JCV, LSEC endocytic functions and receptor expression are highly similar between mammalian species, including humans [10,11,15,43–45], arguing that human LSECs are likely to also take up these virus particles when they first appear in the circulation. In addition, we found that the BK- and JC-VLPs rapidly distributed to a distinct population of endothelial cells in kidney medulla. These endothelial cells also avidly endocytosed a scavenger receptor ligand, suggesting that they represent a subpopulation of endothelial cells with extraordinarily high endocytic activity.

Materials and Methods

Ethics statement

All animal experiments were approved by the Norwegian National Animal Research Authority (NARA) (approval IDs: ID-1912, ID-2775, ID-4720, ID-4894). The substances used for mouse anesthesia were either 1) a combination of tiletamine hydrochloride (Zoletil forte vet, Virbac) and xylazine (Narcoxyl vet, Intervet), or 2) a combination of fentanyl/fluanisone (Hypnorm, VetaPharma) and midazolam (Dormicum, Roche). The mice were euthanized in 100% CO_2, while anesthetized as described above.

Animals

Wild-type C57BL/6 male mice were obtained from Charles River laboratory (France). Mannose-receptor knock-out ($MR^{-/-}$) C57BL/6 mice [46] were kindly provided by Professor Michel Nussenzweig, The Rockefeller University, New York, NY. The $MR^{-/-}$ status was tested by polymerase chain reaction [46]. The animals were housed in rooms specially designed for mice, with 12 h/12 h day-night cycle, and free access to water and food (standard chow, Scanbur BK, Nittedal, Norway).

Chemicals and reagents

Liberase TM (collagenase) was from Roche Applied Science (Oslo, Norway), Iodogen™ from Pierce Chemicals (Rockford, IL), and carrier-free Na125I from PerkinElmer Norge AS (Oslo, Norway). Bovine serum albumin was from MP Biomedicals (Solon, OH), bovine collagen type I (Vitrogen 100) from Cohesion Technologies (Palo Alto, CA), and Percoll™ and PD-10 columns (Sephadex G-25) from GE Healthcare (Uppsala, Sweden). Roswell Park Memorial Institute (RPMI) 1640 cell culture medium (supplemented with 20 mM sodium bicarbonate, 0.006% penicillin, and 0.01% streptomycin) was from Sigma-Aldrich (St Louis, MO), and Falcon cell culture plates from BD Biosciences (San Jose, CA). Draq5 was from Biostatus limited (Leicestershire, UK). Antibodies and suppliers are listed in Table 1.

Cells

Hepatic non-parenchymal liver cells (NPCs) were prepared by collagenase (Liberase) perfusion of mouse livers, followed by low-speed differential centrifugation to remove hepatocytes, and density sedimentation of the NPCs on 25%–45% Percoll gradients to collect LSEC and Kupffer cells, as described in [47]. Purified LSECs (>90% purity) were obtained after a panning step (8 min, 37°C), to remove Kupffer cells. Primary cell cultures were established on glass cover slides (mixed LSEC and Kupffer cells), and in Falcon plates (LSECs), pre-coated with 2.7 µg/ml collagen type I and maintained in serum-free RPMI-1640 medium at 37°C at 5% CO_2. The cultures were washed 40 min after seeding, and allowed to continue spreading for approximately 1 h before use. Seeding of 3×10^5 LSEC/cm^2 gave confluent monolayers, with approximately 1.5×10^5 cells per cm^2.

Virus-like particles (VLPs)

BK- and JC-VLPs were prepared as described previously [48]. Briefly, BK- and JC-VLPs were isolated from Sf9 insect cells infected with recombinant baculovirus encoding Dunlop BK-VP1 or Mad-1 JC-VP1 capsid protein. Recombinant baculoviruses containing PML variants of JC VP1 sequences L55F or S269F

Table 1. Antibodies and lectins used in the study.

Antigen	Host	Clone	Isotype	Source	Dilution
BK-VP1	Rabbit	Antiserum	-	[53]	1:1600
Mannose receptor (CD206)	Goat	Polyclonal	IgG	R&D Systems, AF2534	1 µg/ml
F4/80	Rat	Cl:A31	IgG2b	AbD Serotec, MCA497G	10 µg/ml
CD31	Rat	MEC13.3	IgG2a	Biolegend, 102502	5 µg/ml
CD68	Rat	FA-11	IgG2a	Abcam, ab53444	10 µg/ml
CD163	Rat	ED2	IgG1	AbD Serotec, MCA342GA	10 µg/ml
Meca 32	Rat	-	IgG2a	Antibodies online ABIN298904	10 µg/ml
Biotinylated *Sambucus nigra* agglutinin	-	-	-	Vector Laboratories B-1305	10 µg/ml
Biotinylated *Maackia amurensis II* hemagglutinin	-	-	-	Vector Laboratories B-1265	10 µg/ml

Secondary antibodies: Alexa488-, Alexa546-, or Alexa555- anti-rat, anti-rabbit or anti-goat IgG (H+L), raised in donkey, goat, or rabbit, all diluted 1:500 (Life Technologies; Catalog No: A11006, A11008, A11055, A11081, A11010, A21431, A21434, A21428).
Positive lectin labeling was visualized by Alexa555-streptavidin, diluted 1:200 (Life Technologies; Catalog No S-21381).

were obtained by site specific mutagenesis PCR using the following primers: L55F-Fwd (5′-ACC CAG ATG AGC ATT TTA GGG GTT TTA G-3′) and L55F-Rev (5′-CTA AAA CCC CTA AAA TGC TCA TCT GGG T-3′), S269F-Fwd (5′-TAA CAG ATC TGG TTT CCA GCA GTG GAG A-3′) and S269F-Rev (5′-TCT CCA CTG CTG GAA ACC AGA TCT GTT A-3′), respectively. Infected Sf9 cells were disrupted by sonication and glass mortar and pestle treatment. VLPs were purified from cellular lysate by CsCl gradient and stored in buffer consisting of 150 mM NaCl, 10 mM Tris-HCl pH 7.4 and 1.0 mM $CaCl_2$. The 3-dimensional structure and integrity of VLPs was confirmed by transmission electron microscopy (**Figure 1**). In short, JC-VLPs or BK-VLPs in 0.9% NaCl were placed on discharged pallodium coated mesh grids for 2 min; then washed twice with double distilled water, and once with freshly made 2% uranyl acetate. Another drop of 2% uranyl acetate was added for 10 sec. The grids were gently washed on drops of double distilled water and air dried before electron microscopy. The images were recorded in a FEI CM100 TEM transmission electron microscope (FEI, OR, USA), operating at 80 kV, and equipped with Veleta digital CCD camera (Olympus, Germany).

Ligand labeling procedures

VLPs in phosphate buffered saline (PBS) were labeled with carrier-free $Na^{125}I$, using Iodogen as described by the manufacturer (Pierce Chemicals), and separated from unbound ^{125}I on a PD-10 column. The resulting specific radioactivity was approximately $4-7\times10^6$ cpm per µg protein. ^{125}I-VLPs for injections were mixed with 0.9% NaCl to a final concentration of approximately 0.5 µg protein/100 µl (= dose injected per mouse).

Fluorescein isothiocyanate-labeled formaldehyde-denatured bovine serum albumin (FITC-FSA) was prepared by incubating FSA and FITC in sodium carbonate buffer (0.5 mol/L, pH 9.5) at a protein-dye ratio of 4:1 at 4°C overnight, and dialyzed against PBS.

Blood clearance and organ distribution of radiolabeled VLPs

^{125}I-BK-VLP, ^{125}I-JC-VLP, ^{125}I-JC-VLP_{L55F}, or ^{125}I-JC-VLP_{S269F} (approximately 0.5 µg protein) were injected into the tail vein of anaesthetized mice (n = 3–5 per group). Immediately thereafter blood samples (5 µl) were collected over short time intervals from the tail tip, mixed with 0.3 ml of 13 mM citric acid, after which 0.3 ml 2% bovine serum albumin in water and 0.6 mL of 20% (wt/vol) trichloroacetic acid were added to the samples to precipitate non-degraded protein. Acid-soluble radioactivity represented degraded ligand [25]. To test if the higher doses of VLPs injected for immunohistochemistry would influence blood clearance and organ distribution, non-labeled JC-VLPs (15 µg = dose used for immunohistochemistry) were injected simultaneously with ^{125}I-JC-VLPs (0.5 µg). This did not change the blood clearance or organ distribution pattern of the radiolabeled ligand. In some

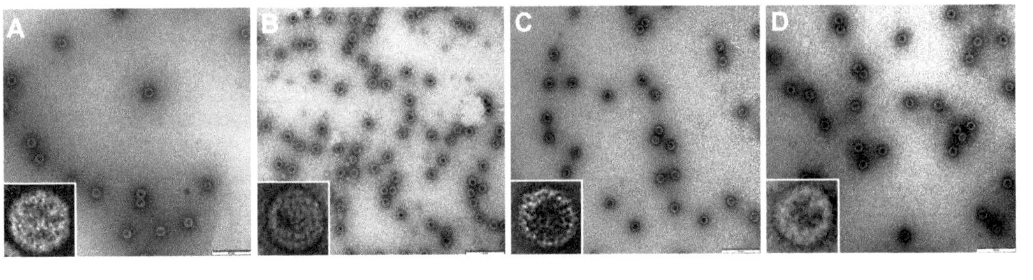

Figure 1. Electron microscopy of BK- and JC-virus like particles (VLPs). The figure show transmission electron micrographs of negatively stained BK- and JC-VLPs constructed from BK-VP1 or JC-VP1 proteins: A) BK-VP1 VLPs (Dunlop strain); B) JC-VP1-Mad-1 VLPs; C) JC-VP1-L55F VLPs; D) JC-VP1-S269F VLPs. Scale bars: 200 nm.

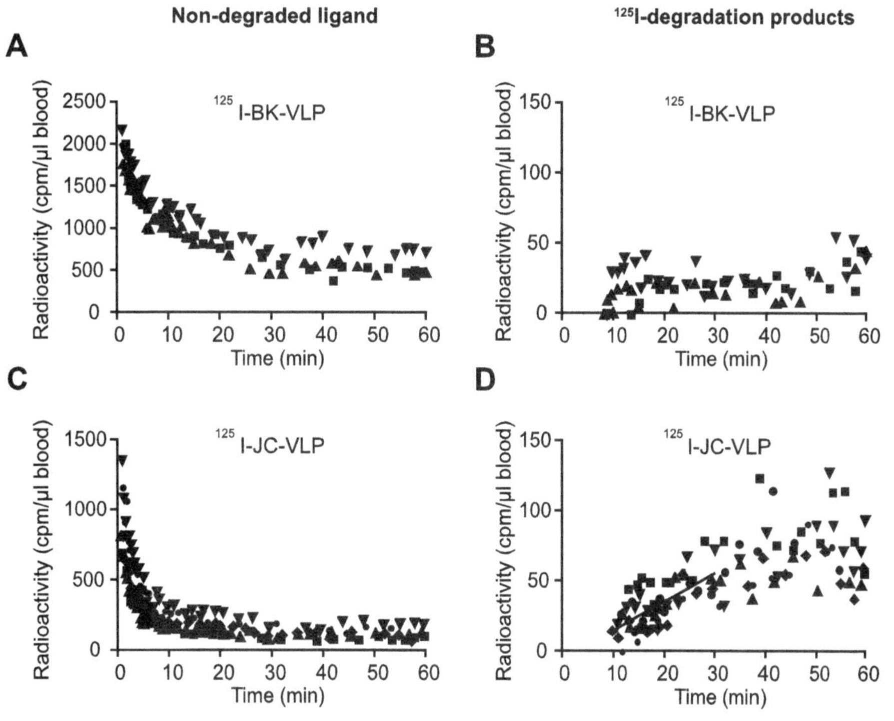

Figure 2. Blood clearance and subsequent in vivo degradation of BK- and JC-virus like particles (VLPs). Mice were injected intravenously with approximately 0.5 µg of ^{125}I-BK-VLPs (n = 3; A, B), or ^{125}I-JC-VLPs (n = 5; C, D), and blood samples taken at the indicated time points and analyzed for ^{125}I-labeled degradation products and intact ligand [15]. Panels A and C show decrease of intact ligand in blood as a function of time. Panels B and D show increase in degradation products released into the blood with time. Results are given as cpm per µl blood. Different symbols refer to separate animals. cpm, counts per minute. The slope of line drawn in panel D represents the average rate of release of degradation products in the 10–30 min period after ligand injection where this release followed approximate first order kinetics.

animals FSA (0.8 mg protein in100 µl 0.9% NaCl) was injected immediately before the administration of radiolabeled ligand to check for inhibition of blood clearance.

At the end of the monitoring period (10 min or 60 min) the anaesthetized animals were euthanized with 100% CO_2. The abdomens and thoraces were opened, and the animals were perfused via the left cardiac ventricle (outlet via the right atrium) with PBS to remove free tracer from the vasculature before the organs were excised and analyzed for radioactivity. The amount of tracer recovered was considered the sum of radioactivity of individual organs and carcass without organs.

Hepatocellular distribution of ^{125}I-VLPs

^{125}I-BK-VLP, ^{125}I-JC-VLP, ^{125}I-JC-VLP$_{L55F}$, or ^{125}I-JC-VLP$_{S269F}$ (approximately 0.5 µg protein) was injected into the tail vein of anaesthetized mice (n = 3 per group). Ten minutes after the injection the animals were euthanized with 100% CO_2 and liver cells isolated by collagenase perfusion of liver via the portal vein, before separating the dispersed liver cells into hepatocytes and NPCs [47]. All steps during cell isolation and separation, except the liver perfusion step, were carried out on ice/below 4°C. Radioactivity in the hepatocyte and NPC fractions was measured in a Packard Gamma Counter. Cell numbers were assessed by cell counting in a hemocytometer.

Table 2. Rate of blood clearance of BK- or JC virus-like particles (VLPs) in mouse.

Ligand	$t_{1/2}$ α (min)*	$t_{1/2}$ β (min)*	Fraction (%) eliminated in α phase	Fraction (%) eliminated in β phase
^{125}I-BK-VLP	2.06±0.90	42.85±9.51	39.18±6.30	60.82±6.30
^{125}I-JC-VLP	1.17±0.11	46.08±37.20	75.70±3.84	24.30±3.84
^{125}I-JC-VLP$_{L55F}$	1.28±0.26	25.16±12.76	79.21±2.75	20.80±2.75
^{125}I-JC-VLP$_{S269F}$	1.06±0.30	41.81±7.62	70.92±11.60	29.08±11.60
^{125}I-BK-VLP+FSA	0.91±0.71	33.5±7.69	56.17±26.73	43.89±26.73
^{125}I-JC-VLP+FSA	1.04±0.11	31.13±8.50	85.62±2.78	14.37±2.78

N = 3 in all groups except ^{125}I-JC-VLP where n = 5. Results are given as mean ± SD.
*$t_{1/2}$ α and $t_{1/2}$ β were calculated as described in [52].

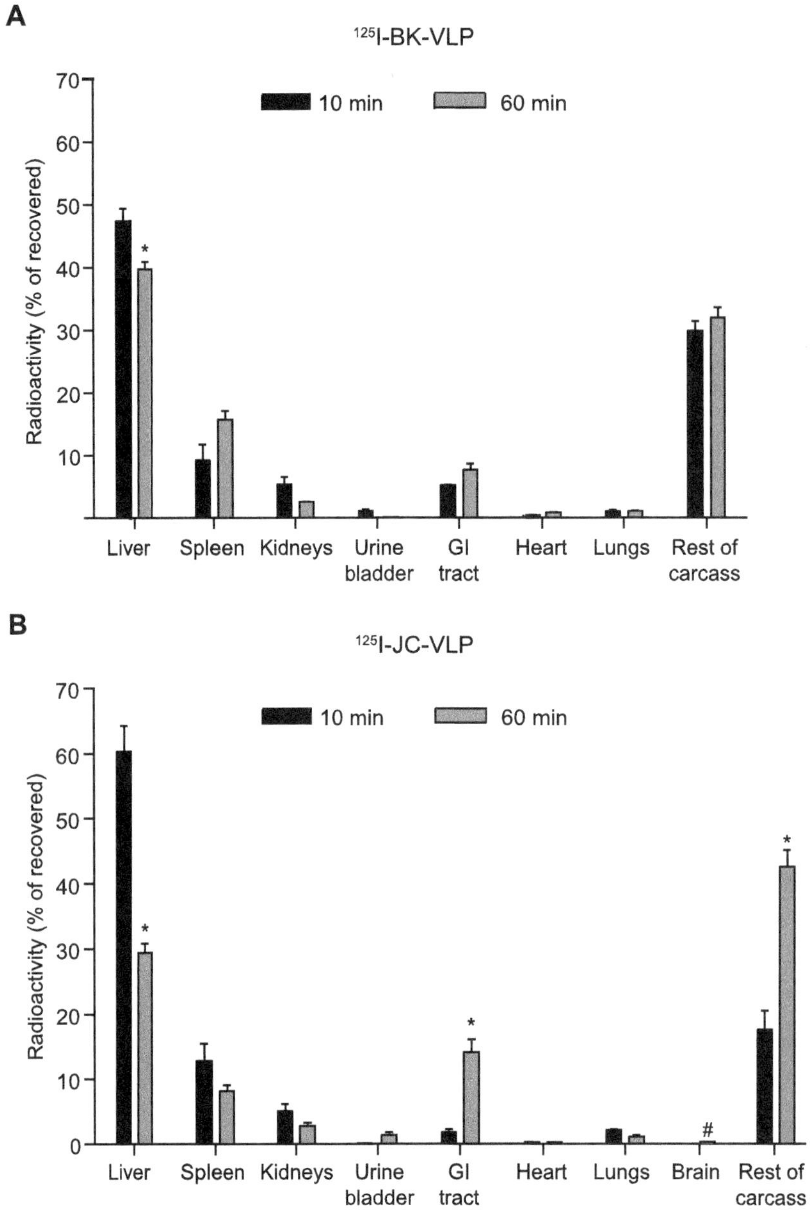

Figure 3. Anatomical distribution of ^{125}I-labelled BK- and JC-VLPs. Mice were injected intravenously with ^{125}I-labelled BK-VLPs (A) or JC-VLPs (B), euthanized after 10 min (black bars; n = 3) or 60 min (grey bars; n = 3 in A; n = 5 in B), and organs and tissues analyzed for radioactivity. The mice used in the circulatory half-life study (Figure 2) were included in this anatomical distribution study (60 min values). Total recovered radioactivity in all tissues at the given time points was taken as 100%. Error bars represent SEM. *Statistically significant difference ($p<0.01$) between tissue radioactivity at 10 min versus 60 min. # Brain radioactivity was measured at 60 min, only. GI tract, gastrointestinal tract (stomach and intestines including mesenterium).

Immunohistochemistry and lectin histochemistry

Non-labeled BK-VLPs or JC-VLPs (13–18 μg protein per mouse) was injected into the tail vein of anaesthetized mice (n = 3–5 per ligand). The animals were euthanized after 7–15 min, then perfused with PBS through the left cardiac ventricle to remove blood and thereafter with 4% paraformaldehyde (PFA) in PBS with 0.02 M sucrose. The perfusion fixed tissues were dehydrated, paraffin embedded and sectioned. In some animals, FITC-FSA (50 μg protein per mouse) was injected into the tail vein 5 min after injection of 10 μg JC-VLP, JC-VLP$_{L55F}$, or JC-VLP$_{S269F}$, and the mice euthanized 10 min thereafter, before perfusion fixation and tissue preparation for immunohistochemistry as described above. Antigen retrieval was achieved by 30 min microwaving in citrate buffer, pH 6. Blocking buffer was 5% goat serum or 1% BSA in TBS and 0.05 M Tween 20, pH 8.4. Sections were incubated overnight (37°C) with primary antibodies (**Table 1**) or non-immune IgG diluted in blocking buffer, washed and incubated with secondary antibody in blocking buffer for 1 h at room temperature. Nuclear stain was Draq5 (diluted 1:1000 in PBS). Sections were analysed in a Zeiss LSM 510 confocal laser scanning microscope (Carl Zeiss, Germany).

Lectin histochemistry on tissue sections. Biotinylated lectins, *Sambuccus nigra* agglutinin (SNA), and *Maackia amurensis* hemagglutinin (MAH), were purchased from Vector Labo-

Table 3. Liver uptake of BK- and JC-VLPs from blood takes place in NPCs.

	Ratio of radioactivity in NPCs versus hepatocytes after injection of ^{125}I-BK-VLPs		Ratio of radioactivity in NPCs versus hepatocytes after injection of ^{125}I-JC-VLPs
Mouse 1	6.5: 1	Mouse 1	22.1: 1
Mouse 2	6.3: 1	Mouse 2	29.8: 1
Mouse 3	26.5: 1	Mouse 3	22.3: 1
Average	13.1: 1	Average	24.8: 1

The mice were injected intravenously with ^{125}I-labelled VLPs, approximately 0.5 µg per animal, and euthanized after 10 min. Liver cells were then isolated by *in situ* perfusion with collagenase, and separated by low-speed differential centrifugation and subsequent density centrifugation on a Percoll gradient [47]. Radioactivity (counts per minute) was measured in the purified hepatocyte fraction, and in the NPC fraction enriched in LSECs and Kupffer cells.

ratories (Vector Laboratories Inc, CA, USA), and Alexa555-streptavidin from Life Technologies (**Table 1**). SNA recognizes alpha(2,6)-linked sialic acids, and MAH recognizes alpha(2,3)-linked sialic acids [49]. Lectin labeling of paraffin tissue sections of liver, kidney and spleen were done according to the instructions from Vector Laboratories.

Endocytosis experiments in isolated liver cells

Confocal microscopy. Primary NPC cultures, enriched in LSECs with approximately 10–20% Kupffer cells, were established on collagen coated glass cover slides. Since LSECs rapidly lose their *in vivo* uptake functions after isolation [50] endocytosis experiments were performed under serum-free conditions within 4 h of plating. Antibody markers for LSECs and Kupffer cells are listed in **Table 1**. The cells were incubated with BK-VLP, JC-VLP, or BKV for 30 min-1 h, washed, fixed in 4% PFA in PBS/ 0.02 M sucrose for 15 min, immune labeled, and subjected to confocal laser scanning microscopy.

Immune EM. Purified LSECs (approximately 1.5 million cells in 8 cm^2 Falcon wells) were incubated with 2.06E+10 genomic equivalents of CsCl gradient purified BKV in 1 ml serum-free RPMI 1640 medium for 2 h, washed in PBS and fixed in 4% formaldehyde in 200 mM Hepes buffer, pH 7.5, overnight, embedded in gelatin and 2.3 M sucrose, and snap frozen in liquid nitrogen. Immune labeling of ultrathin cryosections was performed as described [51]. Positive BK-VP1 labeling was detected by protein A-conjugated 10 nm gold complexes. The dried sections were examined in a JOEL JEM 1010 transmission electron microscope (JOEL, Tokyo, Japan) operating at 80 kV. Control experiments were included in parallel by omission of the primary antibody.

Statistics and pharmacokinetic analyses

The statistical calculations (Mann-Whitney U test, ANOVA two-way analysis of variance) were performed with GraphPad Prism (GraphPad Software Inc. San Diego, CA). Clearance kinetics were analyzed as described [52].

Results

Removal of blood-borne BK- and JC-virus like particles (VLPs) was rapid, with JC-VLPs being cleared more efficiently than BK-VLPs

BK-VLPs and JC-VLPs were radiolabeled and injected via the tail vein. The rate of blood clearance of ^{125}I-BK-VLP and ^{125}I-JC-VLP is shown in **Figure 2A, C**. Semi-logarithmic decay plots revealed a biphasic pattern of elimination from blood, with an initial rapid $t_{1/2}\,\alpha$ of 1–2 min for both ligands (**Table 2**). During this early phase the uptake from blood of ^{125}I-BK-VLP and ^{125}I-JC-VLP were 39% and 76%, respectively, revealing a considerably more effective initial blood clearance of JC-VLP than BK-VLP. After 60 min approximately 30% of the BK-VLP associated radioactivity was still in the circulation (**Figure 2A**), suggesting that BK-VLPs may interact with some unknown blood factor(s) protecting them from being taken up. In contrast, only 10% of JC-VLP associated radioactivity was left in blood after 30 min (**Figure 2C**).

Intracellular degradation of ^{125}I-labeled proteins normally generates ^{125}I-tagged low molecular mass degradation products that are released from the cells, and can be measured in blood following trichloroacetic precipitation of intact proteins [25]. Acid soluble ^{125}I-degradation products appeared in blood 10 min after injection of the radiolabeled VLPs (**Figure 2B, D**). In agreement with the more efficient blood clearance of JC-VLPs, more degradation products were released to blood after injection of ^{125}I-JC-VLPs than after ^{125}I-BK-VLP injection in the 60 min monitoring period.

BK- and JC-VLPs distributed to liver, with a minor uptake in spleen and kidney

To minimize the escape of label from the site of uptake due to intracellular ligand degradation, organ distribution of radiolabeled ligands was measured already 10 min after injection. At this point, the majority of the ^{125}I-BK-VLP (48%) and ^{125}I-JC-VLP (60%) associated radioactivity was found in liver, whereas spleen and kidneys contained 9% and 5% of the ^{125}I-BK-VLPs, and 12% and 5% of the ^{125}I-JC-VLPs, respectively (**Figure 3**).

To investigate the kinetics of organ distribution the VLPs following administration, the liver-associated radioactivity was followed from 10 to 60 min after injection. For ^{125}I-BK-VLP, liver-associated radioactivity decreased only slightly (**Figure 3A**), which may reflect that cellular uptake and degradation overlap due to the slower blood clearance of BK-VLP. In contrast, for ^{125}I-JC-VLP, the liver-associated radioactivity decreased from 60% to 30% of total recovered radioactivity during the same time period (**Figure 3B**), indicating effective hepatocellular degradation of JC-VLP. A corresponding increase of radioactivity in the gastrointestinal tract (including mesenterium and lymph nodes) and the rest of carcass in the same period was judged to be caused by redistribution of degradation products, which is commonly noted following administration of ^{125}I-labeled ligands [26].

To measure the relative contribution of different liver cells in the VLP uptake mice injected intravenously with ^{125}I-labelled BK- or JC-VLPs were sacrificed after 10 min for liver cell isolation and separation into hepatocytes and NPCs, the latter consisting mainly of LSECs and some Kupffer cells, as described in Materials and

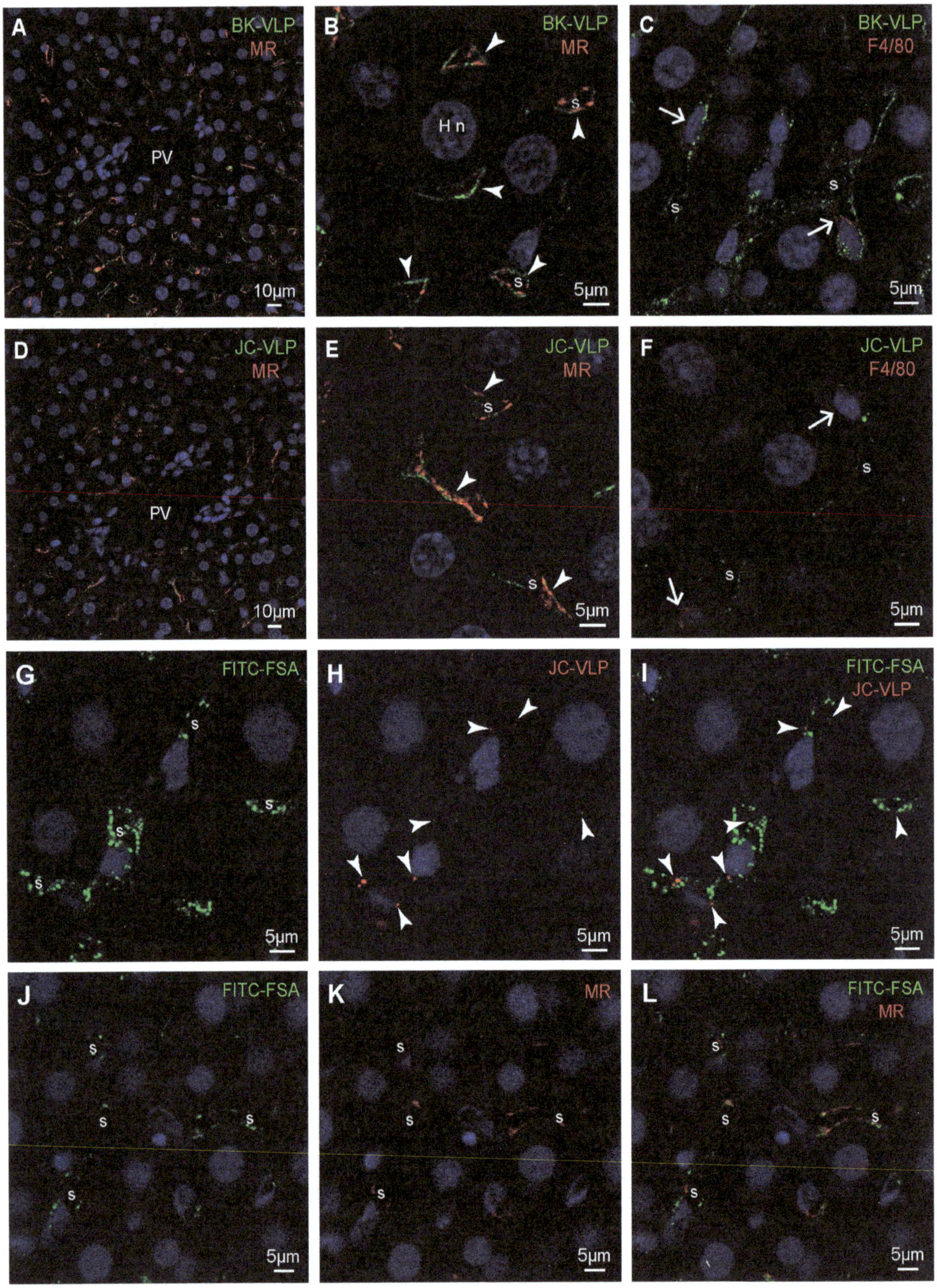

Figure 4. Liver cell distribution of BK- and JC-VLPs after uptake from blood. Panels A–F: Mouse livers were perfusion fixed 15 min after intravenous injection of BK-VLPs (A–C), or JC-VLPs (D–F). Paraffin embedded tissue sections were double immune labeled using a rabbit antiserum against BK-VP1 [53], and antibodies against the mannose receptor (MR), which is an LSEC marker in mouse liver [26], or F4/80 (Kupffer cell marker). Antibodies are listed in Table 1. The VP1 staining (green), indicative of BK-/JC-VLP uptake, showed a typical LSEC pattern (A, D, overview; B, E, close ups), as evidenced by similar localization of green VP1 and red MR staining along the sinusoids (arrowheads in B, E; overlap of red and green fluorescence is shown in yellow). Some BK- and JC-VLP uptake was also observed in F4/80 positive (red) Kupffer cells (arrows in C, F). PV, portal vein; S, sinusoid; Hn, nucleus of hepatocyte. Panels G–L: In G–L, FITC-labeled formaldehyde-denatured serum albumin (FITC-FSA) was injected into the tail vein 5 min after intravenous injection of JC-VLPs to functionally label the endothelium of the liver sinusoids [54,62]. Ten min thereafter the animals were euthanized, tissues perfusion fixed, paraffin embedded and prepared for immune histochemistry. Panels G-I show the distribution of FITC-FSA (green) and JC-VLP (red, arrowheads) in liver sinusoids (s). Panels J–L show similar distribution of FITC-FSA (green) and MR expression (red) in the sinusoids, s.

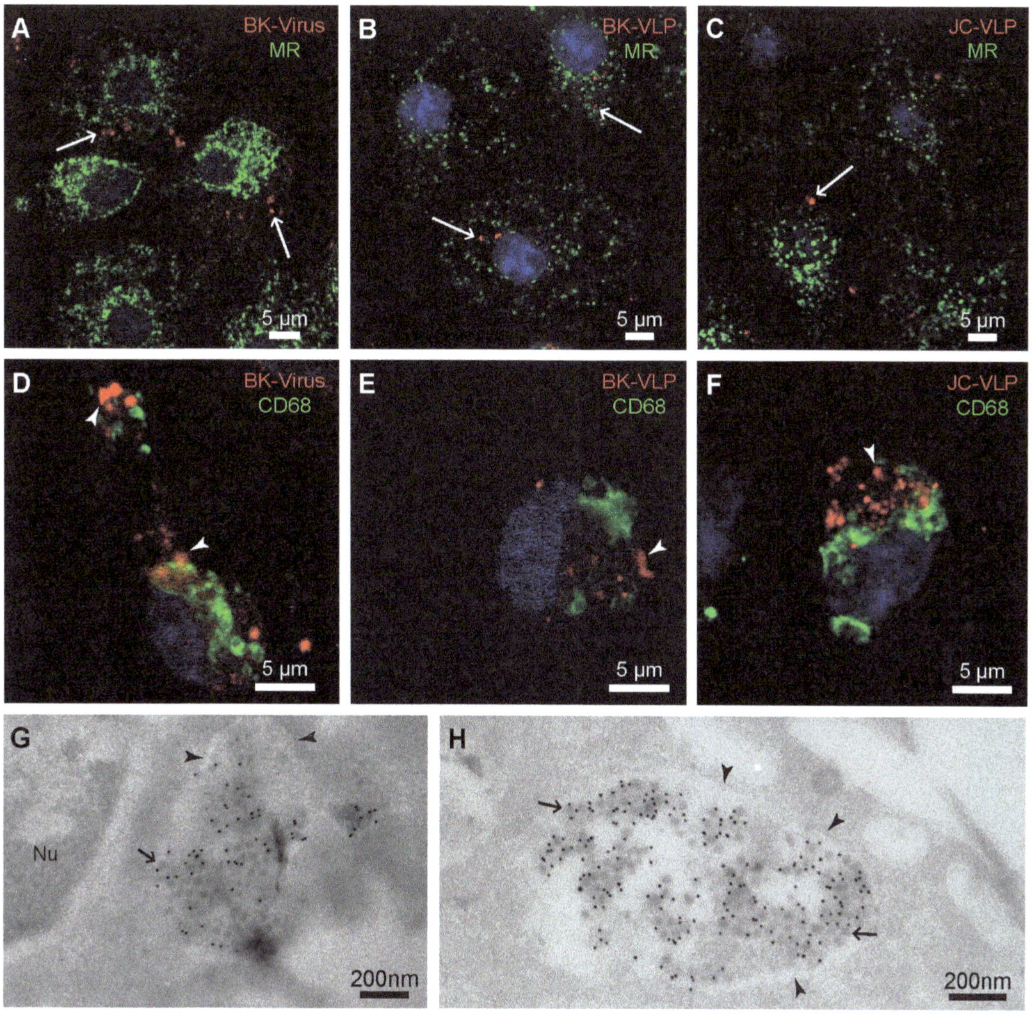

Figure 5. In vitro endocytosis of BK- and JC-VLPs, and BK virions in liver sinusoidal cells. Freshly isolated non-parenchymal liver cells (mixed LSEC and Kupffer cell cultures) were incubated at 37°C for 30 min with BK virions (A, D), or for 1 h with 10 µg/ml BK-VLPs (B, E), or JC-VLPs (C, F), fixed, and double immune labeled with a rabbit anti-BK-VP1 antiserum (red fluorescence) and antibodies against the mannose receptor (MR; LSEC marker; shown in green), or CD68 (Kupffer cell marker; green). Antibodies are listed in Table 1. Uptake of BK virions and BK-/JC-VLPs was observed both in isolated LSECs (arrows, A–C) and Kupffer cells (arrow heads, D–F). Panels G–H: Cryo-immune electron microscopy of BK virion uptake in LSEC membrane-bound vesicles. Purified LSEC cultures were incubated with BK virions for 2 h at 37°C. Positive BK-VP1 staining was visualized by protein-A-10 nm gold particles (black dots). Arrowheads points to vesicular membranes, and arrows to virus particles. Nu, nucleus.

Methods. The liver radioactivity was mainly associated with the NPC fraction (**Table 3**).

The liver uptake of BK- and JC-VLPs took place mainly in the sinusoidal endothelium

To identify the cellular distribution of VLPs in liver, non-labeled BK-VLPs or JC-VLPs were injected intravenously, and organs harvested after 7–15 min, fixed, paraffin embedded, and processed for immunohistochemistry using a rabbit antiserum against BK-VP1 [53] (**Table 1**) that cross-reacts with JC-VP1.

In liver, BK- and JC-VLP staining was observed along the hepatic sinusoids, colocalizing with cells expressing the mannose receptor (LSEC marker) (**Figure 4A, B, D, E; Figure S1**), or in cells that had endocytosed the scavenger receptor ligand FITC-FSA, a functional LSEC marker [30,54] (**Figure 4G–I**). In C57BL/6 mouse liver, the mannose receptor is expressed in LSECs but not in Kupffer cells [26]. Some uptake of BK- and JC-VLPs was also seen in F4/80 positive Kupffer cells (**Figure 4C, F**), whereas no BK- or JC-VLP positive staining was observed in hepatocytes, endothelial cells of portal venules or arteries, bile ducts or other liver structures.

To characterize in greater detail the cells involved in the hepatic uptake of polyomavirus, freshly isolated liver NPCs were incubated with infectious BKV, non-labeled BK-VLPs, or JC-VLPs for various time periods (30 min–1 h), immune labeled and subjected to confocal microscopy (**Figure 5A–F**). Both LSECs and Kupffer cells took up BK- and JC-VLPs, and BKV *in vitro*. Results were confirmed by double labeling with anti-BK-VP1 antiserum and antibodies against the mannose receptor (LSEC marker in liver [26]; **Figure 5A–C; Figure S2**) or CD68 (Kupffer cell marker; **Figure 5D–F**). Cryo-immune electron microscopy of purified LSEC cultures incubated with infectious BKV for 2 h showed virus accumulation in membrane-bound compartments (**Figure 5G, H**).

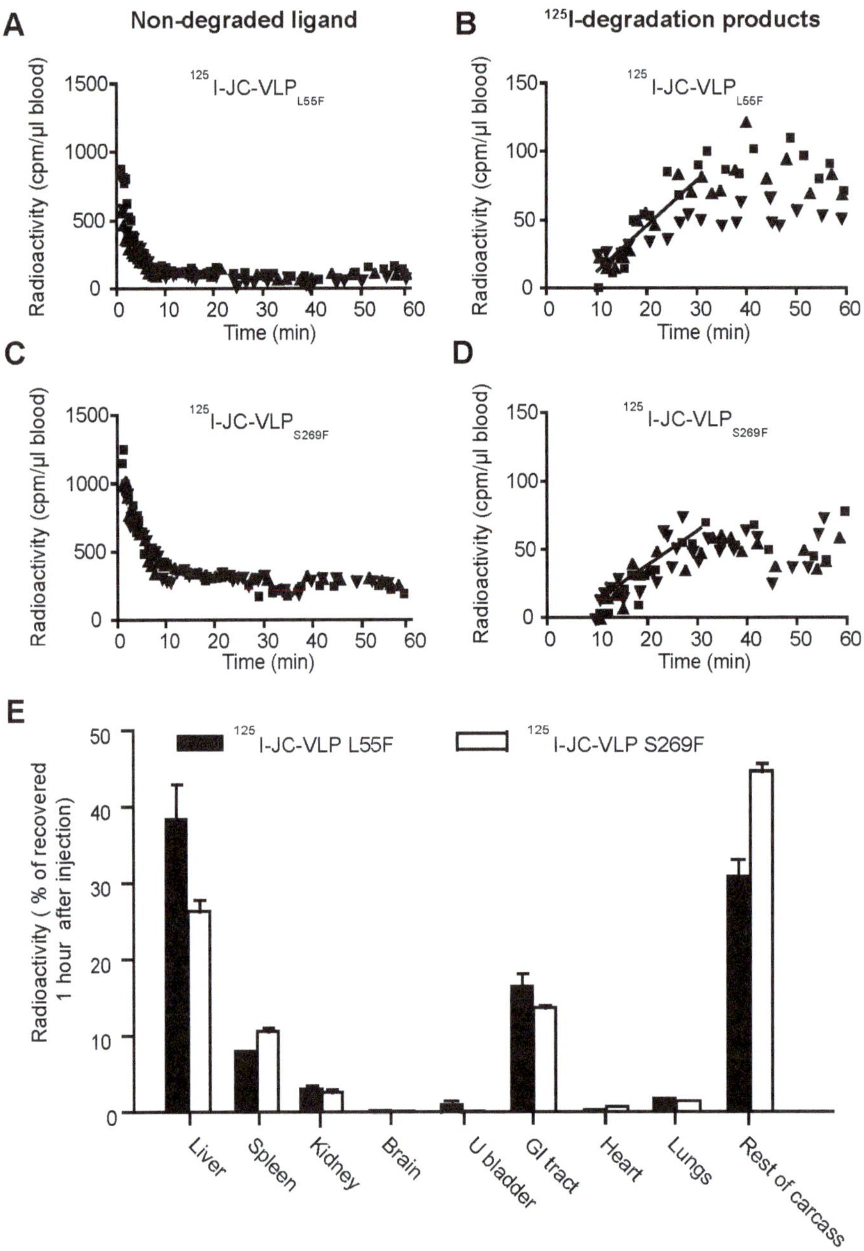

F

Ratio of radioactivity (cpm per million cells) in NPCs versus hepatocytes 10 min after intravenous injection of 125I-labelled VLPs	
^{125}I-JC-VLP$_{L55F}$	7 ± 4.9 (n=3)
^{125}I-JC-VLP$_{S269F}$	6.3 ± 1.3 (n=3)

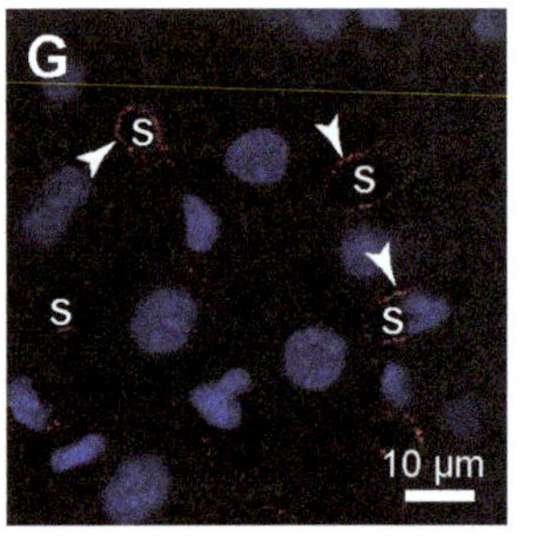

Figure 6. Blood clearance and organ distribution of mutant JC-VLPs. Mice were injected intravenously with ^{125}I-JC-VLP$_{L55F}$ (n = 3, A–B), or ^{125}I-JC-VLP$_{S269F}$ (n = 3, C–D), and blood samples taken at the indicated time points and analyzed for ^{125}I-labeled degradation products and intact ligand [15]. Panels A and C show the decrease of intact ligand in blood as a function of time. Panels B and D show the increase in degradation products released into the blood with time. Different symbols refer to separate animals, and cpm to counts per minute. The slopes of the lines drawn in B and D represent the average release rate of degradation products in the 10–30 min period after ligand injection where this release followed approximate first order kinetics. E) Tissue distribution 60 min post injection. The animals in A–D were sacrificed after 60 min, and organs and tissues

analyzed for radioactivity. Recovered radioactivity in all tissues at this time point was taken as 100%. Error bars represent SEM. GI tract, gastrointestinal tract (stomach and intestines including mesenterium); U bladder, urine bladder. F) Hepatocellular distribution (±SD) of ^{125}I-labeled JC-VLP mutants 10 min after intravenous injection; liver tissue was dispersed by collagenase perfusion, and radioactivity was measured in hepatocyte and non-parenchymal cell (NPC) fractions, respectively. G) Cellular distribution of JC-VLP$_{S269F}$ (anti-VP1 staining) 15 min after VLP injection. Uptake of JC-VLP$_{S269F}$ (red fluorescence; arrowheads) is seen along the sinusoids (s).

Liver uptake of blood-borne VLPs was not dependent on sialic acids

It is reported that BKV and JCV enter their natural host cells via carbohydrate receptors [55]. While BKV binds to alpha(2,3)-linked sialic acids on (for instance) gangliosides [56], JCV binds to alpha(2,6)-linked glycan lactoseries tetrasaccharide c (LSTc) [57]. To test whether blood clearance of JCV in mice is dependent on alpha(2,6)-linked sialic acids, we examined the elimination from blood of two JC-VLP variants occurring frequently in PML patients, namely JC-VLP$_{L55F}$ and JC-VLP$_{S269F}$ (**Figure 6A–D, Table 2**), which had been shown to no longer hemagglutinate red blood cells and to have lost their respective sialic acid receptor binding properties [58]. These VLPs were constructed from mutant forms of the JCV capsid protein VP1, in which one amino acid in the sialic acid binding loop of VP1 had been substituted. The data show that ^{125}I-JC-VLP$_{L55F}$ and ^{125}I-JC-VLP$_{S269F}$ were removed from the circulation in a similar manner as the JC-VLPs made from Mad-1 JC-VP1 (named here as JC-VLP) (**Table 2**). After 60 min nearly all ^{125}I-JC-VLP$_{L55F}$, and 80% of the ^{125}I-JC-VLP$_{S269F}$ were eliminated from blood (**Figure 6A, C**). Similarly to the JC-VLPs, acid soluble ^{125}I-degradation products appeared in the circulation already after 10 min (**Figure 6B, D**).

Organ distribution of ^{125}I-JC-VLP$_{L55F}$ and ^{125}I-JC-VLP$_{S269F}$ 60 min post injection (**Figure 6E**) was similar to that of JC-VLP (**Figure 3B**), with the highest radioactivity measured in liver. Notably, radioactivity in the brain was negligible. Hepatocellular distribution studies, monitoring radioactivity in hepatocytes and NPCs separated10 min after injection of radiolabeled ligands, showed that the uptake of ^{125}I-JC-VLP$_{L55F}$ and ^{125}I-JC-VLP$_{S269F}$ was predominantly in the NPC fraction (**Figure 6F**). Immunohistochemistry revealed an LSEC-like pattern of distribution along the sinusoids (**Figure 6G**), as with JC-VLP (**Figure 4**). Of note, lectin histochemistry for SNA and MAH revealed that all hepatic endothelia expressed alpha(2,6)-linked-sialic acids and alpha(2,3)-linked sialic acids (**Figure S3**), whereas BK-VLPs and JC-VLPs (Mad-1 and mutants) distributed only to sinusoids (**Figures 4, and 6**), suggesting that these sialic acids are not essential for liver uptake.

The scavenger receptor ligand formaldehyde-denatured serum albumin (FSA) reduced the rate of intracellular degradation of JC-VLP, but did not interfere with VLP uptake in liver

LSECs mediate their effective blood clearance of most known ligands via a limited set of endocytosis receptors of broad ligand specificity [10]. To study if LSEC scavenger receptors were involved in the uptake of circulating BK-VLPs or JC-VLPs, a high dose of FSA (0.8 mg/mouse) was injected immediately prior to the injection of ^{125}I-labeled VLPs. FSA is a soluble scavenger receptor ligand and is reported to distribute mainly to the LSEC after intravenous administration [59]. No effect was observed on the blood clearance kinetics of ^{125}I-BK-VLP (**Table 2**) or ^{125}I-JC-VLP (**Figure S4, Table 2**). However, the release of ^{125}I-JC-VLP degradation products to the blood (**Figure S4-B**) was slightly reduced by simultaneous FSA injection compared to injection of only ^{125}I-JC-VLP (**Figure 2D**). This resulted in significantly more liver-associated radioactivity after 60 min (**Figure S4-C**) compared to injection of ^{125}I-JC-VLP alone (**Figure 3B**), suggesting that metabolic turnover, but not uptake was rate limiting following targeting of the same cell by FSA and JC-VLP.

To investigate if the clearance of the VLPs was mediated by the mannose receptor, a C-type lectin with broad ligand binding properties and highly expressed in mouse, rat and human LSECs [15,26,43], mannose receptor deficient mice [46] were injected with ^{125}I-JC-VLPs (**Figure S5**). These mice showed similar clearance and organ distribution of JC-VLPs as wild type mice (**Figures 2B, 3B**), indicating that the rapid JC-VLP blood clearance was not mediated by the mannose receptor pathway.

Extrahepatic clearance of blood-borne BK- and JC-VLPs took place in endothelial cells of kidney vasa recta segments, and in reticuloendothelial cells of spleen red pulp marginal zone

The organ distribution studies of radiolabelled ligands showed a minor, but significant uptake in kidney and spleen. This prompted us to examine the VLP uptake in these organs by immunohistochemistry.

In kidney, BK- and JC-VLP uptake was specifically associated with microvessels of renal medulla (**Figure 7A–D**). Staining intensity of positive vessels was distinct and strong. However, VLP uptake was not seen in all medullary vessels, suggesting discrimination between different segments of vasa recta. Most of the VLP staining did not overlap with staining for Meca 32 (syn. PV-1, a component of fenestral diaphragms) (**Figure 8A–F**), which label endothelial cells of fenestrated segments of vasa recta [60,61]. This suggests that the BK- and JC-VLP uptake took place in non-fenestrated endothelial cells, which are located in descending segments of the vasa recta. Endothelial cells that took up VLPs also rapidly and selectively endocytosed FITC-FSA (**Figure 8G–I**), which in liver is a functional marker for LSECs [30,54,59,62]. FITC-FSA uptake in kidney was seen in medullary vessels only, and the uptake showed little overlap with Meca 32 staining (**Figure 8J–L**). The distribution pattern of JC-VLP and FITC-FSA in kidney medullary vessels almost completely overlapped, suggesting the presence of a highly endocytically active endothelium in these vessels.

BK- and JC-VLPs also distributed to the transitional epithelium of the renal pelvis (**Figure 7G, H**), whereas glomeruli and tubular structures of the nephron were negative in all mice (**Figure 7E, F**) except for one animal injected with BK-VLP, which showed positive staining of a few glomeruli (not shown). Lectin histochemistry for SNA and MAH showed positive labeling of all endothelia in kidney (**Figure S3**).

In spleen, the BK- and JC-VLPs distributed to the marginal zone that separates the lymphocyte rich white pulp from the red pulp (**Figure 9, and Figure S6**). The VP1 labeling showed a net-like staining pattern in this region. Double immune labeling for VP1 and the macrophage marker F4/80 (**Figure 9A–C**), or CD31 (**Figure 9D–F**), which is expressed by many endothelial cells, revealed scattered co-localisation of VLPs with CD31 and F4/80 positive cells, suggesting that the marginal zone reticulo-endothelial network of macrophages and endothelial cells are involved in VLP uptake in the spleen. Staining for the macrophage

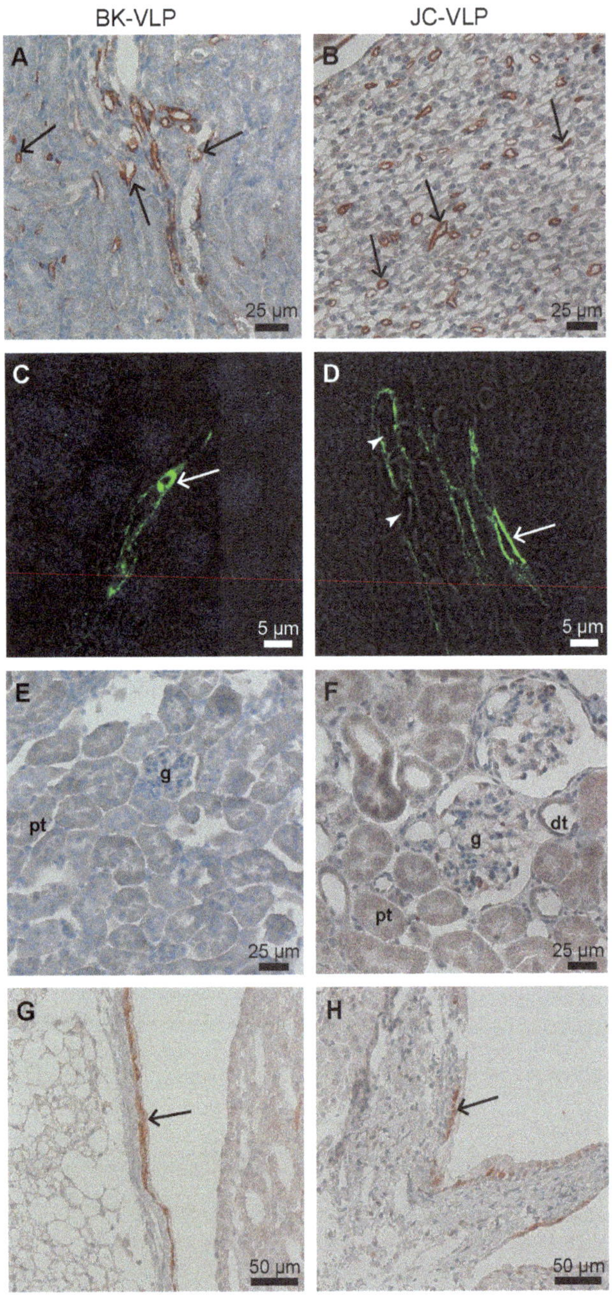

Figure 7. Kidney distribution of intravenously administered BK- and JC-VLPs. Mouse tissues were perfusion fixed 7 or 15 min after injection of BK-VLPs (A, C, E, G), or JC-VLPs (B, D, F, H). Paraffin sections were labeled using a rabbit anti-BK-VP1 antiserum [53]. VP1-labeling was visualized using HRP polymer/DAB reaction (brown color), or Alexa488-goat-anti-rabbit (green fluorescence). Specific uptake of VLPs was seen in the endothelial lining of microvessels in kidney medulla (arrows in A–D; with arrowheads in D pointing to blood filled medullary capillaries), whereas glomeruli (E, F), and tubular structures were negative (A–F). Epithelial cells in the transitional epithelium of renal pelvis also showed positive VP1 staining (arrows in G, H). g, glomerulus; pt, proximal tubulus; dt, distal tubulus.

antigen CD163 [63] did not co-localize with VP1 staining (**Figure 9G–I**), indicating VLP uptake only in subsets of spleen red pulp macrophages. Some of the JC-VLP uptake in spleen co-localized with FITC-FSA which also distributed to the reticulo-endothelium of the spleen red pulp marginal zone (**Figure 9J–L**).

Discussion

Clinical models of BKV and JCV infection demonstrating replicative pathologies with close correlation to nephropathy, cystitis or multifocal leukoencephalopathy are currently lacking. However, these viruses are recognized and taken up by cells from non-permissive hosts, including mice [37,42], allowing us to study their cellular site of uptake in a mouse model. Primary infection with these viruses is believed to occur during early childhood, but their initial infection route or organ distribution is not well known. Using well characterized VLPs, we present evidence that LSECs are highly effective in clearing a large fraction of blood-borne BKV and JCV particles. Moreover, we observed that BK and JC VLPs are efficiently taken up in some microvessels of renal medulla and the spleen marginal zone reticuloendothelium. By effectively acting as a virion sink in the absence of specific antibodies, LSECs may play a key role in the mostly asymptomatic course of primary BKV and JCV infection, leaving only little virus to escape and reach the renal medulla (and possibly the spleen), an important site of BKV and JCV persistence [40,41]. LSECs represent a highly specialized type of scavenger endothelium preserved across different vertebrate species including rodents and humans [10,45]. Several signature characteristics are the same in LSECs across mammals: Cell morphology and endocytosis receptor expression in human LSECs are identical to that of rodents and pig [10,11,15,43,44], and the scavenger function of rat, mouse, and pig LSECs is strikingly similar [64]. It is therefore likely that our present findings on the efficient LSEC endocytosis of polyoma VLPs in mice reflect the fate of these viruses also in human livers.

The observed biphasic pattern of polyoma VLP clearance from blood, with a rapid α-phase and a slower β-phase is comparable to the clearance kinetics of many macromolecules and colloids that are efficiently eliminated via receptor-mediated endocytosis in the LSECs [15,25,26]. There were, nevertheless, some interesting differences between the BK-VLP and JC-VLP clearance patterns. While JC-VLPs were almost completely removed from the circulation within 10 minutes, the α-phase was less dominant in the elimination of BK-VLPs, suggesting a rapid saturation of BK binding/uptake receptors or interaction of BK-VLPs with blood factors (proteins or cells), delaying the blood clearance. Interestingly, in their natural host cells BKV is reported to be internalized via caveolin-mediated endocytosis whereas JCV enters via clathrin-mediated endocytosis [36]. This could also be an explanation of our results, because LSECs have well-developed clathrin-mediated endocytosis machinery, and rely heavily on this type of endocytosis to maintain their signature scavenging activity [34,65].

Our hypothesis is that LSECs protect against virus infections, due to their very efficient endocytosis and high catabolic activity which rapidly destroy internalized material [10]. Our *in vivo* data indicate that at least JC-VLPs are rapidly degraded in the liver, as reported for other macromolecules taken up by the LSECs [10,26]. In this context, it is of interest to note that BKV viremia is readily detectable in transplant patients with BKV-associated diseases, while JCV viremia is only rarely detected in patients with JCV-associated diseases [66] [67].

However, degradation of VLPs is not a proof of cellular destruction of infective virus, and to establish whether BKV or JCV uptake in LSECs will lead to destruction of all internalized virus particles, or allow for endosomal escape and intracellular

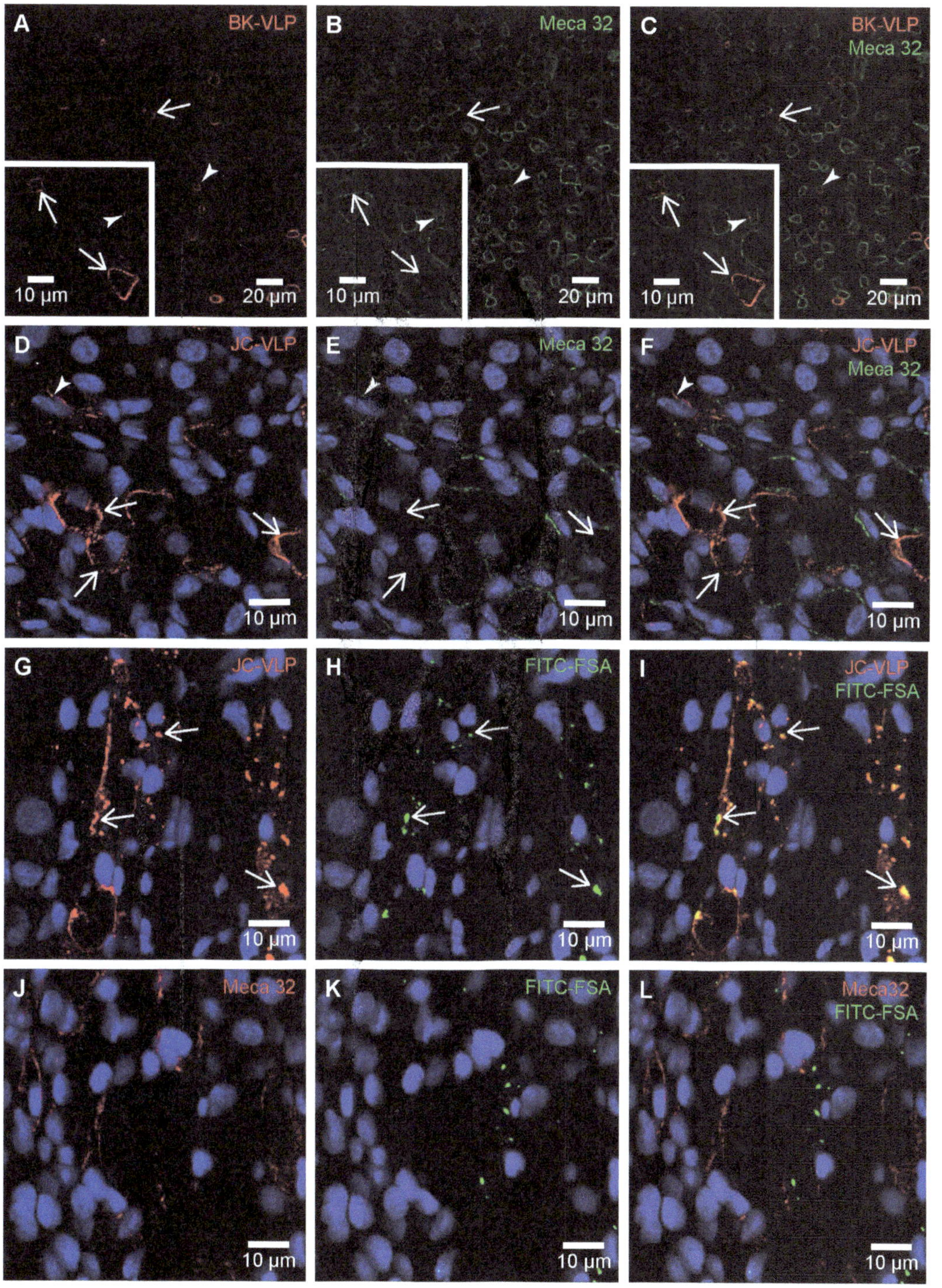

Figure 8. Polyoma VLP and FITC-FSA uptake in renal medullary endothelial cells. Panels A–F: Mouse tissues were perfusion fixed 7 min after intravenous injection of BK-VLP (A–C), or JC-VLP (D–F), and paraffin sections double immune labeled with anti-BK-VP1 (red) and anti-Meca 32 (green). Panels A–C: Arrows indicate endothelial uptake of BK-VLPs in Meca 32 negative vessels, and arrow heads to BK-VLP uptake in Meca 32 positive vessels. Panels D–F: Arrows indicate endothelial uptake of JC-VLPs in Meca 32 negative vessels, and arrow heads to JC-VLP uptake in Meca 32 positive vessels. Most BK-VLP or JC-VLP-positive vessels were Meca 32 negative or showed only weak Meca32 staining. Panels G–L: Tail vein injection of JC-VLPs was followed by injection of the scavenger receptor ligand FITC-FSA in the opposite tail vein and tissues perfusion fixed 15 min after the VLP administration. Paraffin sections were immune labeled with either anti-BK-VP1 (red; G–I) or anti-Meca 32 (red; J–L). G–I) The JC-VLP uptake in medullary vessel endothelia totally overlapped with FITC-FSA uptake (arrows). J–L) FITC-FSA uptake occurred mainly in Meca 32 negative vessels.

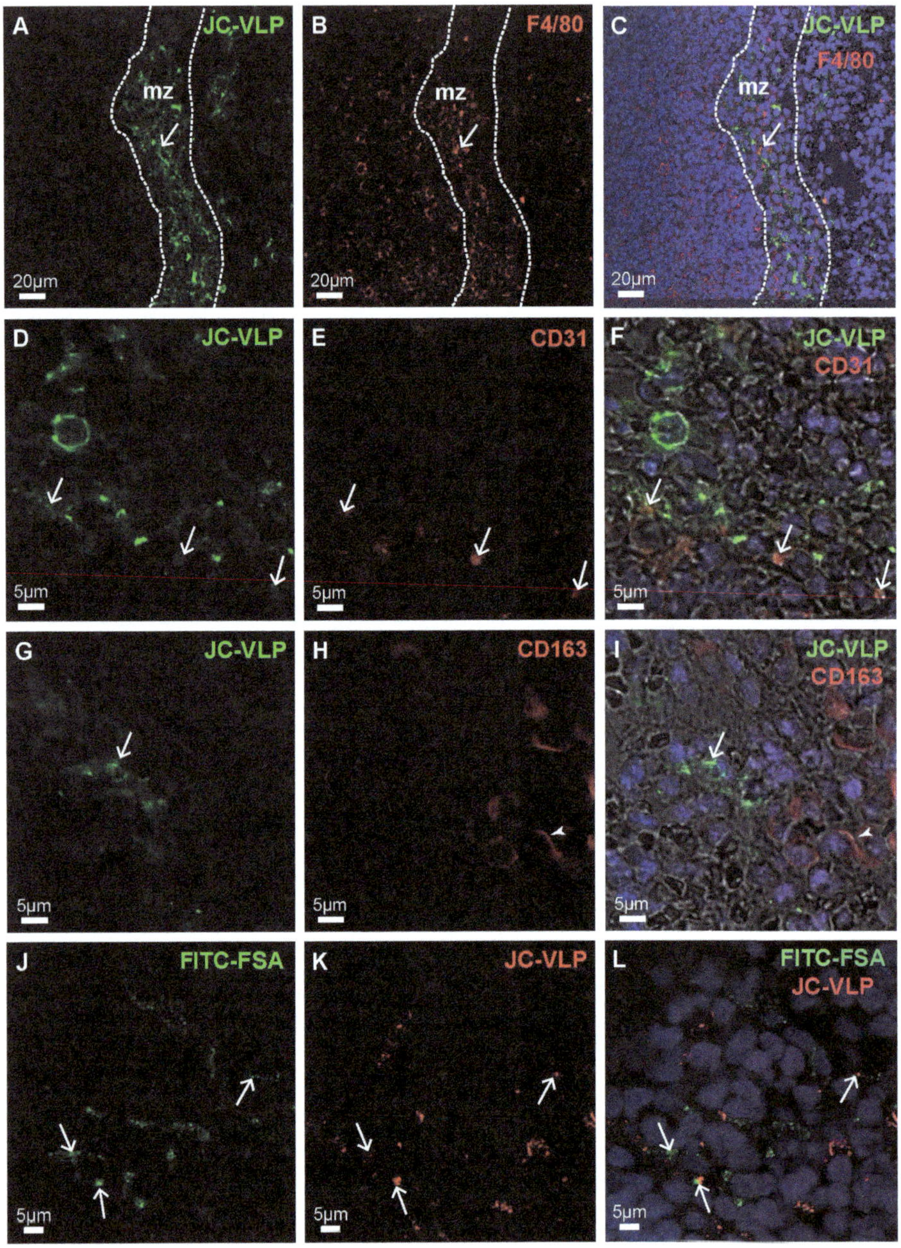

Figure 9. JC-VLP uptake in spleen. Panels A–I: Mouse tissues were perfusion fixed 7 min after intravenous injection of JC-VLPs. Paraffin sections of spleen were double immune labeled using a rabbit antiserum against BK-VP1 [53] (reacts also with JC-VP1), and antibodies against F4/80 (A–C), CD31 (D–F) or CD163 (G–I). Antibodies are listed in Table 1. The VP1 staining pattern (green) showed that the uptake of VLPs was concentrated in the red pulp marginal zone, mz (A), and here partly co-localized with F4/80 (C, arrow), and CD31 (F, arrows), but not with CD163 (I; arrow indicates VP1, and arrow head to CD163 staining). The F4/80 (B, C), CD31 (E, F), and CD163 (H, I) staining patterns are all shown in red. Panels J–L: In J–L, tail vein injection of JC-VLPs was followed by injection of FITC-FSA in the opposite tail vein and tissues perfusion fixed 15 min after the VLP administration. Both JC-VLP (K; red fluorescence) and FITC-FSA (J; green fluorescence) distributed to the reticuloendothelial network of the spleen red pulp marginal zone (L; arrows point to overlap of JC-VLP staining and FITC-FSA uptake).

replication of a fraction of the internalized virions would require further studies. However, *in vitro* model systems are currently lacking that recapitulate the known *in vivo* physiological activity of human LSECs, hence impeding such studies.

In addition to a major hepatic uptake, a minor, but significant BK-/JC-VLP uptake was also measured in spleen red pulp and kidney medulla. The spleen red pulp is known to harbor scavenger type of endothelia [10] and could thereby serve as a secondary site of BKV and JCV clearance. Of note, the rapid and specific uptake of polyoma virus or VLPs in kidney medullary vessels has to our knowledge not been reported before, and may reveal novel insights into the infection route of BKV and JCV. It is notable, however, that clinical recommendations emphasize the importance of medullary tissue for a sensitive tissue diagnosis of BK polyomavirus-associated nephropathy in kidney transplant recipients [68]. Moreover, BKV infection of endothelial cells has been reported in a patient with AIDS and a renal transplant recipient [69,70]. The kidney uptake reported in the present study was associated with the endothelial lining of distinct vasa recta segments. Most of the VLP-positive vessels did not express PV-1/Meca32, suggesting location of VLPs in the non-fenestrated, or descending part of vasa recta [61]. The VLP positive endothelial cells also efficiently endocytosed a functional LSEC marker and scavenger receptor ligand, FITC-FSA, suggesting high endocytic activity of these cells compared to other renal endothelia. Whether this uptake will aid in persistence or clearance of the infectious virus remains to be revealed.

The brain, which is the main site for JCV pathology (PML) [41], was not readily identified by the intravenously injected VLPs, as judged by the extremely low levels of radioactivity accumulating in this organ. This apparent lack of uptake in brain may be explained partly by the intact blood-brain and blood-cerebrospinal fluid barrier of adult mammals. However, the steps in colonization of the brain by JCV are not well characterized and it is still unclear if this occurs during primary viremia or during reactivation [41], if it requires replication competent JCV as opposed to VLPs, or access via other cell types including B-lymphocytes and/or hematopoietic progenitor cells [71]. In addition to the usually distinct VP1 amino acid mutations found [58], virus causing PML bear a rearranged non-coding control region that increases the replication potential [72].

We tested the *in vivo* fate of VLPs of the two of the most frequently identified JCV mutants, namely JC-VLP_{L55F} and JC-VLP_{S269F}, both of which have lost their ability to bind alpha(2,6)-linked sialic acid residues on gangliosides, used by JCV for cellular entry [41,58]. The rate of blood clearance was rapid, and organ distribution after 60 min was almost similar for Mad-1 and mutant JC-VLPs, suggesting that their blood clearance by scavenger cells did not depend on binding to alpha(2,6)-linked sialic acid receptors.

The high scavenging capacity of LSECs for most ligands is mediated by a limited set of high affinity endocytosis receptors [10]. Together with the mannose receptor, the scavenger receptors stabilin-1 and stabilin-2 are considered the main endocytic workhorses of these cells [10,65], and are responsible for the uptake of a wide range of macromolecules, including oxidized LDLs, hyaluronan, chondroitin sulphate, procollagen propeptides, and advanced glycation end products [13,30,65]. Many serum proteins that are phosphorylated as a consequence of platelet activation and blood coagulation are also recognized by the LSEC scavenger receptors [73]. Recent data suggest that the VP1 molecules of BKV contain posttranslational modifications including phosphate groups [74]. FSA, a well-known ligand for the scavenger/stabilin receptors [30,59] was unable to alter the clearance kinetics of blood-borne VLPs, suggesting that the LSEC scavenger receptors were not involved in the hepatic uptake of the particles. However, intracellular degradation of JC-VLPs in liver was significantly impaired. Together, these data suggest traffic of FSA and JC-VLP to the same degradation compartments, but via different receptors. However, we cannot exclude binding to different sites of the same endocytosis receptor, as non-reciprocal cross-competition is described for binding of FSA and hyaluronan to scavenger receptors/stabilin-2 in LSECs [11,13,25]. Mice deficient in the mannose receptor [46] showed similar clearance and organ distribution of BK/JC-VLPs as wild-type mice with normal expression of mannose receptor in LSECs. Although this is consistent with the fact that polyomavirus VLPs including BKV and JCV are not glycosylated [74], it should be noted that the mannose receptor has binding sites for non-glycosylated residues in addition to acting as a lectin [10,75].

Conclusions

Mouse LSECs were identified as efficient scavengers of BK- and JC-VLPs. Despite this efficient clearance mechanism, the VLPs still reached the kidney which is a key organ of BKV and JCV persistence in humans. Of note, the kidney was targeted by VLPs, i.e. in the absence of virus replication. Here we identified uptake predominantly in endothelial cells of the non-fenestrated segments of vasa recta, which also possessed high endocytic activity towards the scavenger receptor ligand FITC-FSA, a hitherto unknown function of these renal endothelial cells. A better understanding of LSEC-mediated polyomavirus clearance may shed light into the role of these cells in the development of polyomavirus-associated diseases. Moreover, this may permit the development of strategies to harness this process for immunocompromised subjects at risk of polyoma virus replication.

Supporting Information

Figure S1 Liver distribution of BK- and JC-VLPs – details of Figure 4B and 4E. The figure shows the green and red channels, white field (WF) image, and merged image of immune labeled paraffin sections of liver from mice injected with BK-VLPs (A–D), or JC-VLPs (E–H). The livers were perfusion fixed 15 min after intravenous injection, and sections labeled with rabbit antiserum to BK-VP1 (cross-reacts with JC-VP1), and an antibody to the mannose receptor (MR; LSEC marker [26]). The staining patterns of VLPs (A, E; green) and MR (B, F; red) were similar (overlay in D, H), and localized exclusively to sinusoids (s; arrowheads), whereas hepatocytes (outlined in C, D, G, H) were negative. Hn, hepatocyte nucleus.

Figure S2 Uptake of JC-VLPs in LSECs in vitro – Z-stack. Freshly isolated LSECs were incubated at 37°C for 1 h with 10 µg/ml JC-VLPs, fixed, and double immune labeled with rabbit anti-serum to BK-VP1 (red), and an antibody to an LSEC marker (the mannose receptor, MR; green). Draq5 was used to stain the cell nucleus. The panel shows the images of a Z-stack recorded by confocal laser scanning microscopy. Every image shows the same cell at different depth (Z axis) with 0.3 µm distance from the previous optical image, recorded from a given 0 µm (A) to 1.2 µm depth (E). The intensity of the Draq5 staining increased gradually from A to D, meaning that the images were taken from a layer close to the cell plasma membrane in A, towards the center of the cell in D. Positive VP1 staining (red) can be seen in all images, indicating cellular uptake of VLPs. The MR is a constitutively recycling endocytosis receptor in LSECs [14] and MR staining is strongest towards the periphery of the cell.

Figure S3 Lectin histochemistry of liver, kidney and spleen. Panels A–H: Paraffin sections of liver (A, B), kidney medulla (C, D), kidney cortex (E, F), and spleen (G, H) were labeled with biotinylated agglutinins: *Maackia amurensis II* (MAH; A, C, E, G) that binds to alpha(2,3)-linked sialic acid, and *Sambucus nigra* (SNA; B, D, F, H) that binds to alpha(2,6)-linked sialic acid. Lectin binding to sialic acids was visualized by Alexa555-streptavidin. Both type of lectins bound to all endothelia in liver (A, B), and kidney (C–F). In spleen (G–H), the lectin staining pattern was more diffuse than in the two other organs. PV, portal vein; CV, central vein; g, glomerulus.

Figure S4 Effects of the scavenger receptor ligand FSA on uptake and intracellular degradation of JC-VLP. Panels A–C: Rate of blood clearance, and subsequent organ distribution of ^{125}I-JC-VLP in mice injected with a saturating dose (0.8 mg/mouse) of the scavenger receptor ligand FSA immediately prior to the injection of ^{125}I-JC-VLP (dose: 0.5 µg/mouse). Blood samples were taken at the indicated time points in A, B and analyzed for ^{125}I-labeled degradation products and intact ligand [15]. A, B) The graph in A shows decrease of intact ligand in blood as a function of time, whereas the graph in B shows increase in degradation products released into the blood with time. Results are given in cpm per µl blood. Different symbols refer to separate animals (n = 3). cpm, counts per minute. The slope of the line drawn in B represents the average release rate of degradation products in the 10–30 min period after ligand injection where this release followed approximate first order kinetics. C) Organ distribution of radioactivity 60 min after the intravenous administration of ^{125}I-JC-VLP and FSA. *Significantly more radioactivity (p-value <0.01) was recovered in liver after 60 min following competitive inhibition with FSA (Figure S4-C; 44%), than after injection with ^{125}I-JC-VLP alone (Figure 3B; 30%). U bladder, urine bladder; GI tract, gastrointestinal tract; FSA, formaldehyde denatured serum albumin.

Figure S5 Blood clearance and tissue distribution of ^{125}I-JC-VLPs in MR$^{-/-}$ mice. C57BL/6 MR$^{-/-}$ mice (n = 2) were injected intravenously with approximately 0.5 µg of ^{125}I-JC-VLP, and blood samples taken at the time points indicated in A and B and analyzed for ^{125}I-labeled degradation products and intact ligand [15]. After 60 min, the animals were euthanized, then perfused free of blood, and radioactivity measured in tissues and organs. A) Kinetics of decrease of intact ^{125}I-labeled ligand in blood. B) Increase in ^{125}I-degradation products released into the blood with time. Results in A and B are given in counts per minute (cpm) per µl blood. C) Organ distribution of radioactivity 60 min after injection of ligand. Recovered radioactivity in organs and tissues at this time point was taken as 100%.

Figure S6 Uptake of blood-borne BK-VLPs in spleen. The figure shows the distribution of BK-VLPs in spleen 15 min after intravenous injection. Paraffin sections were stained with anti-BK-VP1 (Table 1) and Alexa488-goat-anti-rabbit antibody (green fluorescence). The VLPs were taken up in the reticuloendothelial network in the spleen red pulp marginal zone (mz, arrowheads). rp, red pulp; wp, white pulp.

Acknowledgments

We thank Wenche Helen Bakkelund, Randi Olsen and Helga-Marie Bye, Department of Medical Biology, University of Tromsø, for skilled technical assistance with histology sectioning and immune electron microscopy.

Author Contributions

Conceived and designed the experiments: JSS CHR RL IM KE PM BS HHH KKS. Performed the experiments: JSS RL PK IM KKS. Analyzed the data: JSS CHR RL IM BS HHH KKS. Contributed reagents/materials/analysis tools: CHR PK BS HHH KKS. Wrote the paper: JSS CHR HHH KKS. Provided critical evaluation of the manuscript, and read and approved the final version of the manuscript: JSS CHR PK RL IM KE PM BS HHH KKS.

References

1. Virgin HW (2014) The Virome in Mammalian Physiology and Disease. Cell 157: 142–150.
2. Zhang L, Dailey PJ, He T, Gettie A, Bonhoeffer S, et al. (1999) Rapid clearance of simian immunodeficiency virus particles from plasma of rhesus macaques. J Virol 73: 855–860.
3. Mims CA (1959) The response of mice to large intravenous injections of ectromelia virus. II. The growth of virus in the liver. Br J Exp Pathol 40: 543–550.
4. Alemany R, Suzuki K, Curiel DT (2000) Blood clearance rates of adenovirus type 5 in mice. J Gen Virol 81: 2605–2609.
5. Inchley CJ (1969) The activity of mouse Kupffer cells following intravenous injection of T4 bacteriophage. Clin Exp Immunol 5: 173–187.
6. Green NK, Herbert CW, Hale SJ, Hale AB, Mautner V, et al. (2004) Extended plasma circulation time and decreased toxicity of polymer-coated adenovirus. Gene Ther 11: 1256–1263.
7. Ganesan LP, Mohanty S, Kim J, Clark KR, Robinson JM, et al. (2011) Rapid and Efficient Clearance of Blood-borne Virus by Liver Sinusoidal Endothelium. PLoS Pathog 7: e1002281.
8. Funk GA, Gosert R, Hirsch HH (2007) Viral dynamics in transplant patients: implications for disease. Lancet Infect Dis 7: 460–472.
9. Jenne CN, Kubes P (2013) Immune surveillance by the liver. Nat Immunol 14: 996–1006.
10. Sorensen KK, McCourt P, Berg T, Crossley C, Couteur DL, et al. (2012) The scavenger endothelial cell: a new player in homeostasis and immunity. Am J Physiol Regul Integr Comp Physiol 303: R1217–1230.
11. Politz O, Gratchev A, McCourt PA, Schledzewski K, Guillot P, et al. (2002) Stabilin-1 and -2 constitute a novel family of fasciclin-like hyaluronan receptor homologues. Biochem J 362: 155–164.
12. Malerod L, Juvet K, Gjoen T, Berg T (2002) The expression of scavenger receptor class B, type I (SR-BI) and caveolin-1 in parenchymal and nonparenchymal liver cells. Cell Tissue Res 307: 173–180.
13. McCourt PA, Smedsrod BH, Melkko J, Johansson S (1999) Characterization of a hyaluronan receptor on rat sinusoidal liver endothelial cells and its functional relationship to scavenger receptors. Hepatology 30: 1276–1286.
14. Magnusson S, Berg T (1989) Extremely rapid endocytosis mediated by the mannose receptor of sinusoidal endothelial rat liver cells. Biochem J 257: 651–656.
15. Malovic I, Sorensen KK, Elvevold KH, Nedredal GI, Paulsen S, et al. (2007) The mannose receptor on murine liver sinusoidal endothelial cells is the main denatured collagen clearance receptor. Hepatology 45: 1454–1461.
16. Martin-Armas M, Simon-Santamaria J, Pettersen I, Moens U, Smedsrod B, et al. (2006) Toll-like receptor 9 (TLR9) is present in murine liver sinusoidal endothelial cells (LSECs) and mediates the effect of CpG-oligonucleotides. J Hepatol 44: 939–946.
17. Uhrig A, Banafsche R, Kremer M, Hegenbarth S, Hamann A, et al. (2005) Development and functional consequences of LPS tolerance in sinusoidal endothelial cells of the liver. J Leukoc Biol 77: 626–633.
18. Hosel M, Broxtermann M, Janicki H, Esser K, Arzberger S, et al. (2012) Toll-like receptor 2-mediated innate immune response in human nonparenchymal liver cells toward adeno-associated viral vectors. Hepatology 55: 287–297.
19. Wu J, Meng Z, Jiang M, Zhang E, Trippler M, et al. (2010) Toll-like receptor-induced innate immune responses in non-parenchymal liver cells are cell type-specific. Immunology 129: 363–374.
20. Mousavi SA, Sporstol M, Fladeby C, Kjeken R, Barois N, et al. (2007) Receptor-mediated endocytosis of immune complexes in rat liver sinusoidal endothelial cells is mediated by FcgammaRIIb2. Hepatology 46: 871–884.
21. Ganesan LP, Kim J, Wu Y, Mohanty S, Phillips GS, et al. (2012) FcgammaRIIb on liver sinusoidal endothelium clears small immune complexes. J Immunol 189: 4981–4988.
22. Seckert CK, Renzaho A, Tervo HM, Krause C, Deegen P, et al. (2009) Liver sinusoidal endothelial cells are a site of murine cytomegalovirus latency and reactivation. J Virol 83: 8869–8884.
23. Li Y, Hao B, Kuai X, Xing G, Yang J, et al. (2009) C-type lectin LSECtin interacts with DC-SIGNR and is involved in hepatitis C virus binding. Mol Cell Biochem 327: 183–190.
24. Smedsrod B, Melkko J, Risteli L, Risteli J (1990) Circulating C-terminal propeptide of type I procollagen is cleared mainly via the mannose receptor in liver endothelial cells. Biochem J 271: 345–350.
25. Melkko J, Hellevik T, Risteli L, Risteli J, Smedsrod B (1994) Clearance of NH2-terminal propeptides of types I and III procollagen is a physiological function of the scavenger receptor in liver endothelial cells. J Exp Med 179: 405–412.
26. Elvevold K, Simon-Santamaria J, Hasvold H, McCourt P, Smedsrod B, et al. (2008) Liver sinusoidal endothelial cells depend on mannose receptor-mediated recruitment of lysosomal enzymes for normal degradation capacity. Hepatology 48: 2007–2015.
27. Smedsrod B, Melkko J, Araki N, Sano H, Horiuchi S (1997) Advanced glycation end products are eliminated by scavenger-receptor-mediated endocytosis in hepatic sinusoidal Kupffer and endothelial cells. Biochem J 322 (Pt 2): 567–573.
28. Svistounov D, Oteiza A, Zykova SN, Sorensen KK, McCourt P, et al. (2013) Hepatic disposal of advanced glycation end products during maturation and aging. Exp Gerontol 48: 549–556.
29. Van Berkel TJ, De Rijke YB, Kruijt JK (1991) Different fate in vivo of oxidatively modified low density lipoprotein and acetylated low density

lipoprotein in rats. Recognition by various scavenger receptors on Kupffer and endothelial liver cells. J Biol Chem 266: 2282–2289.
30. Li R, Oteiza A, Sorensen KK, McCourt P, Olsen R, et al. (2011) Role of liver sinusoidal endothelial cells and stabilins in elimination of oxidized low-density lipoproteins. Am J Physiol Gastrointest Liver Physiol 300: G71–81.
31. Skogh T, Blomhoff R, Eskild W, Berg T (1985) Hepatic uptake of circulating IgG immune complexes. Immunology 55: 585–594.
32. Asumendi A, Alvarez A, Martinez I, Smedsrod B, Vidal-Vanaclocha F (1996) Hepatic sinusoidal endothelium heterogeneity with respect to mannose receptor activity is interleukin-1 dependent. Hepatology 23: 1521–1529.
33. Jacobs F, Wisse E, De Geest B (2010) The role of liver sinusoidal cells in hepatocyte-directed gene transfer. Am J Pathol 176: 14–21.
34. Kjeken R, Mousavi SA, Brech A, Gjoen T, Berg T (2001) Fluid phase endocytosis of [125I]iodixanol in rat liver parenchymal, endothelial and Kupffer cells. Cell Tissue Res 304: 221–230.
35. Seternes T, Sorensen K, Smedsrod B (2002) Scavenger endothelial cells of vertebrates: a nonperipheral leukocyte system for high-capacity elimination of waste macromolecules. Proc Natl Acad Sci U S A 99: 7594–7597.
36. Neu U, Stehle T, Atwood WJ (2009) The Polyomaviridae: Contributions of virus structure to our understanding of virus receptors and infectious entry. Virology 384: 389–399.
37. Suzuki S, Sawa H, Komagome R, Orba Y, Yamada M, et al. (2001) Broad distribution of the JC virus receptor contrasts with a marked cellular restriction of virus replication. Virology 286: 100–112.
38. Goldmann C, Petry H, Frye S, Ast O, Ebitsch S, et al. (1999) Molecular cloning and expression of major structural protein VP1 of the human polyomavirus JC virus: formation of virus-like particles useful for immunological and therapeutic studies. J Virol 73: 4465–4469.
39. Tsai B, Qian M (2010) Cellular entry of polyomaviruses. Curr Top Microbiol Immunol 343: 177–194.
40. Hirsch HH (2005) BK virus: opportunity makes a pathogen. Clin Infect Dis 41: 354–360.
41. Hirsch HH, Kardas P, Kranz D, Leboeuf C (2013) The human JC polyomavirus (JCPyV): virological background and clinical implications. APMIS 121: 685–727.
42. Tan CS, Broge TA Jr, Seung E, Vrbanac V, Viscidi R, et al. (2013) Detection of JC virus-specific immune responses in a novel humanized mouse model. PLoS One 8: e64313.
43. Martens JH, Kzhyshkowska J, Falkowski-Hansen M, Schledzewski K, Gratchev A, et al. (2006) Differential expression of a gene signature for scavenger/lectin receptors by endothelial cells and macrophages in human lymph node sinuses, the primary sites of regional metastasis. J Pathol 208: 574–589.
44. Lalor PF, Lai WK, Curbishley SM, Shetty S, Adams DH (2006) Human hepatic sinusoidal endothelial cells can be distinguished by expression of phenotypic markers related to their specialised functions in vivo. World J Gastroenterol 12: 5429–5439.
45. Esbach S, Pieters MN, van der Boom J, Schouten D, van der Heyde MN, et al. (1993) Visualization of the uptake and processing of oxidized low-density lipoproteins in human and rat liver. Hepatology 18: 537–545.
46. Lee SJ, Evers S, Roeder D, Parlow AF, Risteli J, et al. (2002) Mannose receptor-mediated regulation of serum glycoprotein homeostasis. Science 295: 1898–1901.
47. Smedsrod B (2012) Protocol for the preparation of mouse liver Kupffer cells and liver sinusoidal endothelial cells. Munin open research archive: University of Tromsø, Tromsø, Norway. pp. Available: http://hdl.handle.net/10037/14575.
48. Bodaghi S, Comoli P, Bosch R, Azzi A, Gosert R, et al. (2009) Antibody responses to recombinant polyomavirus BK large T and VP1 proteins in young kidney transplant patients. J Clin Microbiol 47: 2577–2585.
49. Brinkman-Van der Linden EC, Sonnenburg JL, Varki A (2002) Effects of sialic acid substitutions on recognition by Sambucus nigra agglutinin and Maackia amurensis hemagglutinin. Anal Biochem 303: 98–104.
50. Martinez I, Nedredal GI, Oie CI, Warren A, Johansen O, et al. (2008) The influence of oxygen tension on the structure and function of isolated liver sinusoidal endothelial cells. Comp Hepatol 7: 4.
51. Slot JW, Geuze HJ (2007) Cryosectioning and immunolabeling. Nat Protoc 2: 2480–2491.
52. Hellevik T, Bondevik A, Smedsrod B (1996) Intracellular fate of endocytosed collagen in rat liver endothelial cells. Exp Cell Res 223: 39–49.
53. Rinaldo CH, Myhre MR, Alstad H, Nilssen O, Traavik T (2003) Human polyomavirus BK (BKV) transiently transforms and persistently infects cultured osteosarcoma cells. Virus Res 93: 181–187.
54. Xie G, Wang L, Wang X, DeLeve LD (2010) Isolation of periportal, midlobular, and centrilobular rat liver sinusoidal endothelial cells enables study of zonated drug toxicity. Am J Physiol Gastrointest Liver Physiol 299: G1204–1210.
55. Olofsson S, Bergstrom T (2005) Glycoconjugate glycans as viral receptors. Ann Med 37: 154–172.
56. Neu U, Allen SA, Blaum BS, Liu Y, Frank M, et al. (2013) A structure-guided mutation in the major capsid protein retargets BK polyomavirus. PLoS Pathog 9: e1003688.
57. Neu U, Maginnis MS, Palma AS, Stroh LJ, Nelson CD, et al. (2010) Structure-function analysis of the human JC polyomavirus establishes the LSTc pentasaccharide as a functional receptor motif. Cell Host Microbe 8: 309–319.
58. Gorelik L, Reid C, Testa M, Brickelmaier M, Bossolasco S, et al. (2011) Progressive multifocal leukoencephalopathy (PML) development is associated with mutations in JC virus capsid protein VP1 that change its receptor specificity. J Infect Dis 204: 103–114.
59. Blomhoff R, Eskild W, Berg T (1984) Endocytosis of formaldehyde-treated serum albumin via scavenger pathway in liver endothelial cells. Biochem J 218: 81–86.
60. Stan RV, Kubitza M, Palade GE (1999) PV-1 is a component of the fenestral and stomatal diaphragms in fenestrated endothelia. Proc Natl Acad Sci U S A 96: 13203–13207.
61. Pannabecker TL, Dantzler WH (2007) Three-dimensional architecture of collecting ducts, loops of Henle, and blood vessels in the renal papilla. Am J Physiol Renal Physiol 293: F696–704.
62. Elvevold K, Smedsrod B, Martinez I (2008) The liver sinusoidal endothelial cell: a cell type of controversial and confusing identity. Am J Physiol Gastrointest Liver Physiol 294: G391–400.
63. Lau SK, Chu PG, Weiss LM (2004) CD163: a specific marker of macrophages in paraffin-embedded tissue samples. Am J Clin Pathol 122: 794–801.
64. Elvevold KH, Nedredal GI, Revhaug A, Smedsrod B (2004) Scavenger properties of cultivated pig liver endothelial cells. Comp Hepatol 3: 4.
65. Hansen B, Longati P, Elvevold K, Nedredal GI, Schledzewski K, et al. (2005) Stabilin-1 and stabilin-2 are both directed into the early endocytic pathway in hepatic sinusoidal endothelium via interactions with clathrin/AP-2, independent of ligand binding. Exp Cell Res 303: 160–173.
66. Egli A, Infanti L, Dumoulin A, Buser A, Samaridis J, et al. (2009) Prevalence of polyomavirus BK and JC infection and replication in 400 healthy blood donors. J Infect Dis 199: 837–846.
67. Drachenberg CB, Hirsch HH, Papadimitriou JC, Gosert R, Wali RK, et al. (2007) Polyomavirus BK versus JC replication and nephropathy in renal transplant recipients: a prospective evaluation. Transplantation 84: 323–330.
68. Hirsch HH, Randhawa P, Practice ASTIDCo (2013) BK polyomavirus in solid organ transplantation. Am J Transplant 13 Suppl 4: 179–188.
69. Petrogiannis-Haliotis T, Sakoulas G, Kirby J, Koralnik IJ, Dvorak AM, et al. (2001) BK-related polyomavirus vasculopathy in a renal-transplant recipient. N Engl J Med 345: 1250–1255.
70. Vallbracht A, Lohler J, Gossmann J, Gluck T, Petersen D, et al. (1993) Disseminated BK type polyomavirus infection in an AIDS patient associated with central nervous system disease. Am J Pathol 143: 29–39.
71. Ferenczy MW, Marshall LJ, Nelson CD, Atwood WJ, Nath A, et al. (2012) Molecular biology, epidemiology, and pathogenesis of progressive multifocal leukoencephalopathy, the JC virus-induced demyelinating disease of the human brain. Clin Microbiol Rev 25: 471–506.
72. Gosert R, Kardas P, Major EO, Hirsch HH (2010) Rearranged JC virus noncoding control regions found in progressive multifocal leukoencephalopathy patient samples increase virus early gene expression and replication rate. J Virol 84: 10448–10456.
73. Hansen B, Melkko J, Smedsrod B (2002) Serum is a rich source of ligands for the scavenger receptor of hepatic sinusoidal endothelial cells. Mol Cell Biochem 229: 63–72.
74. Fang CY, Chen HY, Wang M, Chen PL, Chang CF, et al. (2010) Global analysis of modifications of the human BK virus structural proteins by LC-MS/MS. Virology 402: 164–176.
75. Napper CE, Drickamer K, Taylor ME (2006) Collagen binding by the mannose receptor mediated through the fibronectin type II domain. Biochem J 395: 579–586.

Effects of Sex, Age, and Fasting Conditions on Plasma Lipidomic Profiles of Fasted Sprague-Dawley Rats

Kosuke Saito[1], Masaki Ishikawa[1], Mayumi Murayama[1], Masayo Urata[1], Yuya Senoo[1], Katsuko Toyoshima[1], Yuji Kumagai[2], Keiko Maekawa[1]*, Yoshiro Saito[1]

1 Division of Medical Safety Science, National Institute of Health Sciences, 1-18-1 Kamiyoga, Setagaya, Tokyo, Japan, **2** Clinical Research Center, Kitasato University School of Medicine, 1-15-1 Kitasato, Minami, Sagamihara, Kanagawa, Japan

Abstract

Circulating lipid molecules reflect biological processes in the body and, thus, are useful tools for preclinical estimation of the efficacy and safety of newly developed drugs. However, background information on profiles of circulating lipid molecules in preclinical animal models is limited. Therefore, we examined the effects of multiple factors such as sex (fasted male vs. female), age (fasted 10 vs. 30 weeks old), and feeding conditions (feeding vs. fasting, 16 vs. 22 hr fasting, 10 AM vs. 4 PM blood collection), on the global profiles of lipid molecules in plasma from Sprague-Dawley rats by using a lipidomic approach. Our assay platform determined 262 lipid molecules (68 phospholipids, 20 sphingolipids, 138 neutral lipids, and 36 polyunsaturated fatty acids and their metabolites) in rat plasma. Multivariate discriminant analysis (orthogonal partial least squares discriminant analysis) and heat maps of statistically significant lipid molecules revealed that the plasma lipid profiles in rats are predominantly influenced by feeding conditions, followed by sex and age. In addition, the fasting duration (16 vs. 22 hr fasting) or the time of blood collection (10 AM vs. 4 PM blood collection) has limited or no contribution on the profiles of lipid molecules in rat plasma. Our results provide useful, fundamental information for exploring and validating biomarkers in future preclinical studies and may help to establish regulatory standards for such studies.

Editor: Yvette Tache, University of California, Los Angeles, United States of America

Funding: This work was supported by the Health Labour Sciences Research Grants (grant number 028) from the Ministry of Health, Labour and Welfare (http://www.mhlw.go.jp/), and by the Advanced Research for Products Mining Program (grant number 10-45) from the National Institute of Biomedical Innovation of Japan (http://www.nibio.go.jp/). YS received the fundings. The funders had no role in study design, data collection and analysis, decision to publish, or preparation of the manuscript.

Competing Interests: The authors have declared that no competing interests exist.

* Email: maekawa@nihs.go.jp

Introduction

Circulating metabolites are useful tools to diagnose diseases such as lung and gastrointestinal cancer [1–3]. The advantages of diagnostic applications using circulating metabolites are non- or low-invasiveness, as well as homogeneity between humans and experimental animal models. These advantages are also shared with the application of circulating metabolites as biomarkers for estimation of the efficacy and safety of newly developed drugs. The rat is a useful and essential animal model for preclinical studies investigating drug metabolism, pharmacokinetics, and toxicological tests [4,5]. Therefore, background data of circulating metabolites in rats are useful in designing such studies.

Lipids, including fatty acids and their metabolites, phospholipids, sphingolipids, and neutral lipids, are one major class of circulating metabolites, and their hydrophobicity could allow their levels in blood to substantially reflect their levels in tissues (e.g., liver and brain tissues) [6,7]. Phospholipids and sphingolipids are major components of cell membranes, and neutral lipids serve as energy sources for the cells. The phospholipid 18:0/18:1 phosphatidylcholine (PC) acts as a circulating regulator of fatty acid uptake in muscle [8], and ceramides (Cer), a class of sphingolipids, mediate saturated fatty acid-induced insulin resistance [9]. Fatty acid metabolites such as arachidonate metabolites are signaling molecules of inflammatory response [10]. Therefore, lipids are potential biomarkers to predict the efficacy and toxicity of newly developed drugs.

Circulating lipids in human have been reported to vary with blood matrices and subjects' backgrounds, including sex and age, as well as sample collection and storage conditions. Our previous reports demonstrated that plasma and serum, two matrices obtained from blood, presented different profiles of circulating lipids [11,12]. For example, the levels of more than 100 lipid molecules showed differences between plasma and serum samples from aged women [12]. Sphingolipids are present at higher concentration in blood in female than in male individuals [12–14]. Storage temperature and freezing-thawing cycles affect the levels of many lipid species, including diacylglycerols (DGs) [12,15]. In addition, of 80 lipids circulating in the plasma, majorities were present at varying levels among different anticoagulant supplements (citrate, EDTA, and heparin) [16]. However, few comprehensive studies focusing on the factors affecting circulating lipids have been performed in preclinical animal models such as rats.

A lipidomic approach is a high-throughput measurement of a broad range of lipid molecules [17,18]. This method applies liquid chromatography for the separation of lipid molecules and mass spectrometry for their qualitative and quantitative analyses. Although the range of measurable lipid classes varies among assay platforms, a lipidomic approach usually can measure over 100 lipid molecules from plasma as well as from tissues (e.g., liver tissues) [19,20]. Recently, we characterized and measured 253 lipid molecules in our assay platforms by using human blood plasma [12]. In the present study, we employed the same platforms and examined the effects of multiple factors on circulating lipids, including sex, age, and feeding conditions (feeding, length of fasting period, and diurnal time of sample collection) in the plasma of rats, which is the most-frequently used animal model in preclinical studies. In total, we determined and examined 262 lipid molecules (68 phospholipids, 20 sphingolipids, 138 neutral lipids, and 36 polyunsaturated fatty acids [PUFAs] and their metabolites). Multivariate statistical analysis, i.e., orthogonal partial least squares discriminant analysis (OPLS-DA), demonstrated that the plasma lipid profiles of rats are predominantly affected by feeding conditions, followed by sex and age. No component separating length of fasting period or diurnal time of sample collection was observed. In addition, we also addressed the effects of multiple factors on individual circulating lipid molecules.

Materials and Methods

Animals

Male and female Sprague-Dawley rats (8 weeks old) were purchased from Charles River Japan (Kanagawa, Japan) and housed until they were 10 or 30 weeks old. The animals were housed in a 12-hr light/dark cycle and were allowed food (CRF-1, nutrient composition were described in Table S1; Oriental Yeast, Tokyo, Japan) and water ad libitum. The plasma samples were obtained in the presence of EDTA-Na from rats after the indicated fasting periods and were collected at the indicated times (Fig. 1A and Table S2). The plasma samples were frozen immediately and stored at −80°C. The use of animal specimens was approved by the Ethics Review Committee for Animal Experimentation of the National Institute of Health Sciences (Tokyo, Japan).

Lipid extraction

Lipid extraction was performed as described previously [12]. In brief, lipids were extracted from 90 μL of plasma by using the Bligh and Dyer's method with a few modifications. The lower organic phase was used for measurement of phospholipids, sphingolipids, and neutral lipids. The upper aqueous phase was subjected to solid extraction and was used for measurement of PUFAs and their metabolites. Hexadeuterated 16:0/16:0 PC (16:0/16:0-d6 PC; Larodan Fine Chemicals, Malmo, Sweden) and tetradeuterated leukotriene B4 (LTB4-d4; Cayman Chemical, Ann Arbor, MI) were added as internal standards before extraction.

Measurement of phospholipids, sphingolipids, and neutral lipids

Phospholipids, sphingolipids, and neutral lipids were measured using liquid chromatography-time-of-flight mass spectrometry (LC-TOFMS; ACQUITY UPLC System [Waters, Milford]-LCT Premier XE [Waters, Milford]), as described previously [12]. The samples from each experimental group were random-

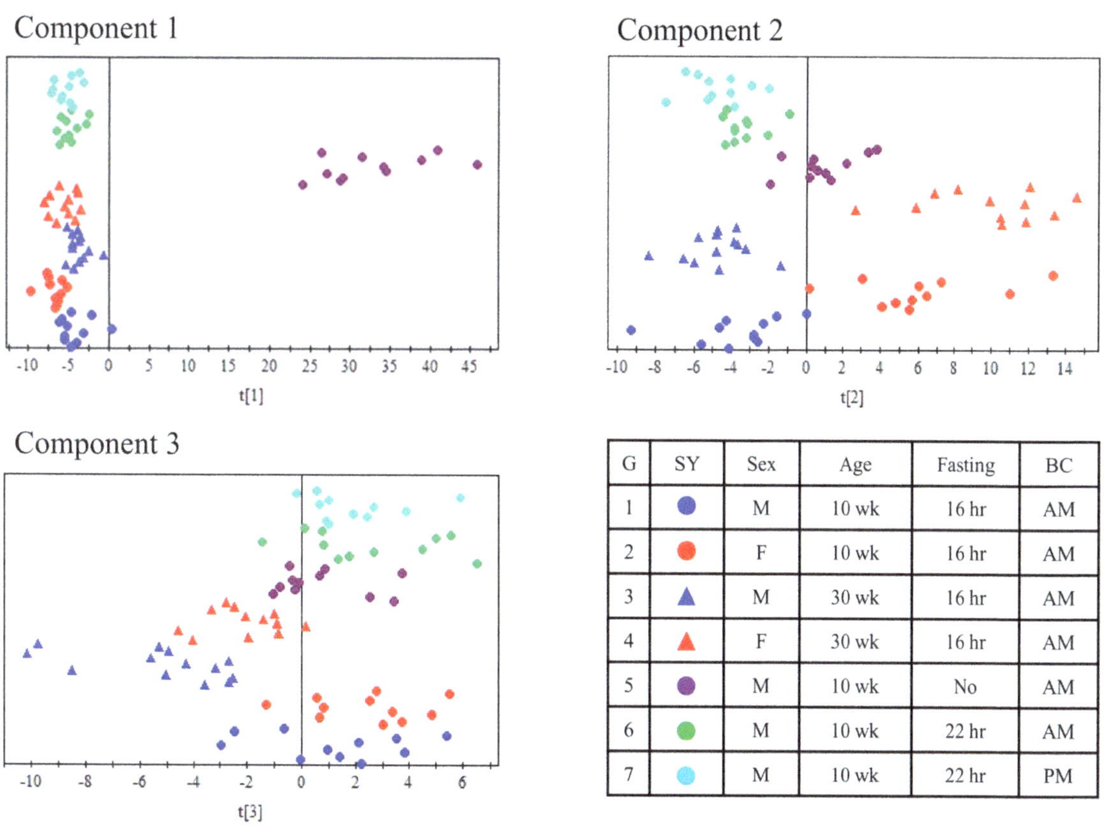

G	SY	Sex	Age	Fasting	BC
1	● (blue)	M	10 wk	16 hr	AM
2	● (red)	F	10 wk	16 hr	AM
3	▲ (blue)	M	30 wk	16 hr	AM
4	▲ (red)	F	30 wk	16 hr	AM
5	● (purple)	M	10 wk	No	AM
6	● (green)	M	10 wk	22 hr	AM
7	● (cyan)	M	10 wk	22 hr	PM

Figure 1. OPLS-DA model of overall profiles of lipid molecules. The goodness-of-fit parameters R2X, R2Y, and Q2 values are as follows; 0.469, 0.159, and 0.149 for component 1, 0.094, 0.143, and 0.127 for component 2, and 0.034, 0.107, and 0.088 for component 3. M, male; F, female; wk, week; SY, symbol; BC, time of blood collection.

Table 1. Lipid classes identified and numbers of individual lipid molecules in rat plasma.

Lipid types	Detected ion mode	Lipid classes	Number of molecules
		lysophosphatidylcholine (LPC)	9
		lysophosphatidylethanolamine (LPE)	1
		phosphatidylcholine (PC)	40
Phospholipid	Negative	ether-type PC (ePC)	4
		phosphatidylethanolamine (PE)	4
		ether-type PE (ePE)	3
		phosphatidylinositol (PI)	7
		sphingomyelin (SM)	14
Sphingolipid	Negative	ceramide (Cer)	5
		hexosylceramide (HexCer)	1
		cholesterol/cholesterolester (Ch/ChE)	26
Neutral lipid	Positive	diacylglycerol (DG)	10
		triacylglycerol (TG)	101
		coenzyme Q (CoQ)	1
poly unsaturated fatty		arachidonic acid (AA) and its metabolites	18
acids (PUFAs)	Negative	eicosapentaenoic acid (EPA) and its metabolites	8
and their metabolites		docosahexaenoic acid (DHA) and its metabolites	10
		total	262

ized across the run. Raw data obtained by LC-TOFMS were processed using the 2DICAL software (Mitsui Knowledge Industry, Tokyo, Japan), which allows detection and alignment of the ion peaks of each ionized biomolecule obtained at the specific m/z and column retention time (RT). The main parameter of 2DICAL was set as described previously with a few modifications [12]. To extract the ion peaks of phospholipids (lysophosphatidylcholine [LPC], lysophosphatidylethanolamine [LPE], PC, ether-type PC [ePC], PE, ePE, phosphatidylinositol [PI]) and sphingolipids (sphingomyelin [SM], Cer, hexosylceramide [HexCer]), the RT range was from 2.0 to 38.0 min in the negative ion mode; while for ion peaks of neutral lipids (cholesterol/cholesterol ester [Ch/ChE], DG, triacylglycerol [TG], coenzyme Q), the RT range was from 2.0 to 60.0 min in the positive ion mode. The intensities of each extracted ion peak were normalized to those of the internal standard (16:0/16:0-d6 PC). To monitor experimental quality throughout extraction, measurement, and data extraction, the relative standard deviation (RSD) of the internal standard (16:0/16:0-d6 PC) was calculated (7.34%). Extracted ion peaks were subjected to identification of lipid molecules by comparison of the ion features, including RT, m/z, preferred adducts, and in-source fragments, of the experimental samples with those of our reference library of lipid molecule entries, as described previously [12]. Processing of extracted ion peaks yielded 226 lipid molecules (88 and 138 lipid molecules from negative ion mode and positive ion mode, respectively; Table 1 and Table S3).

Measurements of PUFAs and their metabolites

PUFAs and their metabolites were measured by targeted approach using LC-MS/MS (ACQUITY UPLC System-5500QTRAP quadrupole-linear ion trap hybrid mass spectrometer [AB Sciex, Framingham, MA]), as described previously [12]. The samples from each experimental group were randomized across the run. Targeted lipid molecules were annotated by comparison of RT, parent ion, and MS/MS ion fragments with standard lipid molecules using MultiQuant Software (Version 2.1, AB Sciex). The intensities of each ion peak from targeted lipid molecules were normalized to those of the internal standard (LTB4-d4). To monitor experimental quality throughout extraction, measurement, and data processing, the RSD of the internal standard (LTB4-d4) was calculated (18.22%). Processing of targeted lipid molecules yielded 36 lipid molecules (Table 1 and Table S3).

Data processing

All data obtained of individual lipid molecules were normalized to the median values of all measured samples as 1. The average values ± standard deviations of the normalized levels of each lipid molecule in each study group are presented in Table S4. For overall comparison, data were loaded into SIMCA-P+12 (Umetrics, Umea, Sweden), pareto-scaled, and analyzed using OPLS-DA to visualize the variance among the groups in the present study. Comparison of individual metabolite levels among groups was performed by the Welch's t-test to assess statistical differences. In the present study, $p<0.05$ represents statistical significance.

Results

Effects of multiple factors on global profiles of lipid molecules in rat plasma

To compare the differences caused by multiple factors (sex, age, and feeding conditions) on the determined 262 lipid molecules, the OPLS-DA model was applied. In the present study, we employed

A

	Male/Female	
	10 week	30 week
16:0LPC	1.09	
16:1LPC		0.80
17:0LPC		0.50
18:0LPC	0.55	0.45
18:1LPC	1.17	0.72
18:2LPC		0.63
20:1LPC	1.24	0.56
20:4LPC		0.66
22:6LPC	0.61	0.29
32:0PC		
32:1PC	0.75	
33:2PC	1.24	
34:0PC	0.62	0.48
34:1PC		0.75
34:2PC		
34:3PC		
35:2PC		0.60
35:4PC		
36:0PC	0.30	0.18
36:1PC	0.46	0.36
36:2PCa		
36:2PCb	0.63	0.47
36:3PCa	1.24	
36:3PCb	1.35	0.69
36:4PCa	1.35	
36:4PCb		
36:5PCa		
36:5PCb	0.63	0.31
37:2PCa		0.61
37:2PCb		0.38
37:4PC	0.52	0.35
38:3PCa		0.45
38:3PCb	0.55	0.23
38:4PCa		0.56
38:4PCb	0.47	0.40
38:5PCa		0.60
38:5PCb	0.36	0.19
38:6PCa		0.73
38:6PCb	0.73	0.52
39:4PCa		0.53
39:4PCb	0.49	0.34
39:6PC	0.49	0.36
40:4PC	0.46	0.46
40:5PCa	0.66	0.36
40:5PCb	0.26	0.19
40:6PCa		0.53
40:6PCb	0.33	0.25
40:7PC		0.45
40:8PC	0.75	0.62
34:1ePC	0.60	0.56
36:4ePC	0.77	
36:5ePC	0.66	0.61
38:5ePC		

B

18:0LPE	0.57	0.54
36:2PE		
36:4PE	1.44	1.34
38:4PE		
40:6PE		0.52
36:5ePE		
38:5ePE	0.66	
38:6ePE		
34:2PI	0.77	0.62
36:2PI	0.60	
36:4PI		0.54
37:4PI		0.45
38:4PI	0.51	0.41
38:5PI		0.64
40:6PI		

C

	Male/Female	
	10 week	30 week
34:0SM	1.29	1.52
34:1SM		
34:2SM		0.74
36:1SM	0.42	0.39
36:2SM	0.53	0.40
38:1SM	0.52	0.41
40:1SM	0.49	0.42
41:1SM	0.57	0.43
41:2SM	0.50	0.30
42:1SMa	1.30	
42:1SMb	0.64	0.49
42:2SM	0.59	0.43
42:3SM	0.61	0.39
43:1SM	1.64	1.33
41:1Cer	0.46	0.49
42:1Cera		
42:1Cerb	0.56	0.52
42:2Cer	0.54	0.49
43:1Cer	1.29	
42:1HexCer	0.34	0.17

D

Ch	0.85	0.83
16:0ChE		
16:1ChE		
17:0ChE		
17:1ChE		0.74
18:0ChEa		0.65
18:0ChEb	0.68	0.56
18:1ChEa		
18:1ChEb		
18:2ChE		0.75
18:3ChE	0.68	0.46
19:1ChE	1.32	
19:2ChE		0.68
20:1ChE		0.60
20:2ChE		0.49
20:3ChEa	0.76	
20:3ChEb		0.44
20:4ChE	0.62	0.61
20:5ChE	0.46	0.20
21:4ChE	0.52	0.49
21:5ChEa	0.54	0.47
21:5ChEb	0.46	0.22
22:3ChE	0.35	0.23
22:5ChE	0.56	0.42
22:6ChE	0.44	0.29
24:6ChE	0.44	0.31

E

34:1DG		0.66
34:2DG	1.81	
36:2DG		0.60
36:3DG		0.60
36:4DG	1.75	0.69
38:5DG		0.45
38:6DG		0.67
40:7DG	1.99	
40:8DG	1.79	
44:10DG		0.78

F

	Male/Female	
	10 week	30 week
48:0TG	2.58	2.61
48:1TG		
48:2TG		
49:1TG	1.98	1.55
49:2TG	2.63	1.84
50:0TG	1.98	1.81
50:1TG		
50:2TG		
50:3TG		
50:4TG		
51:1TG		
51:2TG	2.81	1.62
51:3TG		
51:4TG	2.10	
52:0TG		
52:1TG		
52:2TG		
52:3TG		
52:4TG	2.08	2.65
52:5TGa		
52:5TGb		
52:6TGa		
52:6TGb		
52:6TGc		
52:7TG		
53:2TG		1.52
53:3TG		
53:4TG	1.78	
53:5TG		
53:6TG	1.93	1.67
54:0TG		
54:1TG	2.17	
54:2TG		
54:3TG		
54:4TGa		
54:4TGb		1.71
54:5TG		
54:6TGa	2.29	1.56
54:6TGb		
54:7TGa		
54:7TGb		
54:7TGc		
54:8TGa		
54:8TGb	1.90	1.48
55:2TG	2.32	2.28
55:7TG		
55:8TG	2.24	1.71
56:0TG		2.36
56:1TG	2.33	1.91
56:2TG	2.52	
56:3TG		
56:4TGa		
56:4TGb		
56:5TGa	2.22	
56:5TGb	2.34	
56:5TGc		
56:6TG		
56:7TGa		
56:7TGb		
56:8TGa		1.40
56:8TGb	3.47	2.13
56:9TGa		
56:9TGb		
56:10TG		
57:2TG	3.19	2.22
58:1TG		
58:2TG	2.45	
58:3TG	2.71	
58:4TG		
58:5TG		

	Male/Female	
	10 week	30 week
58:6TG		
58:7TGa	1.90	1.46
58:7TGb		
58:8TGa	2.82	2.03
58:8TGb		
58:9TGa	3.50	2.54
58:9TGb	2.16	1.46
58:10TGa		0.75
58:10TGb		
58:11TG	0.41	0.32
60:1TG		
60:2TG		
60:3TG		
60:4TG	2.55	
60:5TGa	2.40	1.56
60:5TGb		2.05
60:9TG	1.75	
60:11TGa		
60:11TGb	0.63	0.63
60:12TGa	1.93	
60:12TGb		
60:13TG		
62:2TG		
62:3TG		
62:4TG		
62:5TGa		
62:5TGb		
62:12TG	2.27	2.17
62:13TGa	2.91	1.64
62:13TGb		
62:14TG	1.90	1.58
CoQ9		0.62

G

AA	0.71	0.64
PGD2		
PGF2a		
TXB2		
12-HHT		
5-HETE		
8-HETE		
12-HETE	0.35	
15-HETE		
5,15-diHETE		0.53
16-HETE		0.77
17-HETE		0.78
18-HETE		
20-HETE		0.58
8,9-diHETrE		
5,6-diHETrE	1.86	1.42
11,12-diHETrE		
14,15-diHETrE		
EPA	0.65	0.30
5-HEPE		0.35
8-HEPE		0.39
12-HEPE		
15-HEPE		0.29
18-HEPE		0.38
14,15-diHETE		0.31
17,18-diHETE		0.39
DHA		0.46
4-HDoHE		0.50
7-HDoHE		0.57
10-HDoHE		0.31
13-HDoHE		0.34
14-HDoHE		
17-HDoHE		0.36
10,17-diHDoHE		0.61
20-HDoHE		0.53
19,20-diHDoPE		0.61

2-fold 0.5-fold

Figure 2. Heat maps of lipid molecules among fasted male and female rats. The heat maps were generated with statistically significant different lipid molecules ($p<0.05$) of lysophosphatidylcholines and phosphoatidylcholines (A), other phospholipids (B), sphingolipids (C), cholesterol/cholesterolesters (D), diacylglycerols (E), triacylglycerol and coenzyme Q9 (F), and arachidonic acid, eicosapentaenoic acid, docosahexaenoic acid, and their metabolites (G). The numbers indicate the fold change of levels of individual lipid molecules in male over female at 10 and 30 weeks old. The alphabet of the lipid class is used to distinguish 2 lipid species possessing the same formula. LPC, lysophosphatidylcholine; PC, phosphatidylcholine; ePC, ether-type PC; LPE, lysophosphatidylethanolamine; PE, phosphatidylethanolamine; ePE, ether-type PE; SM, sphingomyelin; Cer, ceramide; HexCer, hexosylceramide; Ch, cholesterol; ChE, cholesterolester; DG, diacylglycerol; TG, triacylglycerol; CoQ9, coenzyme Q9; AA, arachidonic acid; PG, prostaglandin; TX, thromboxane; HETE, hydroxyeicosatetraenoic aicd; diHETE, dihydroxyeicosatetraenoic acid; diHETrE, dihydroxyeicosatrienoic acid; EPA, eicosapentaenoic acid; HEPE, hydroxyeicosapentaenoic acid; DHA, docosahexaenoic acid; HDoHE, hydroxydocosahexaenoic acid; diHDoHE, dihydroxydocosahexaenoic acid; diHDoPE, dihydroxydocosapentaenoic acid.

Table 2. Sex-based differences in the number of lipid molecules at significantly higher levels.

Lipid classes	Total lipid molecules	10 week		30 week		Common	
		Male	Female	Male	Female	Male	Female
Phospholipids	68	8	28	1	46	1	24
Sphingolipids	20	4	13	2	14	2	13
Neutral lipids	138	38	15	27	30	22	2
PUFAs and metabolites	36	1	3	1	21	1	2
Total	262	51	59	31	111	26	41

fasted conditions to examine the effect of sexes and ages, because food intake affects lipidomic profiles and therefore fasted condition is prefer to identify biomarkers from lipid molecules in preclinical study. We used all 7 groups listed in Figure 1 and Table S2. As shown in Fig. 1, component 1 separated fed (purple circle) and fasted (all others) rats; component 2 separated female (red) and male (blue, purple, green, and light blue) rats,; and component 3 separated 10-week-old (dot) and 30-week-old (triangle) rats. There is no component separating fasting duration (16 hr [blue dot] vs. 22 [green dot]) or time of blood collection (10 AM [green dot] vs. 4 PM [light blue dot]).

Differences in the fasted levels of lipid molecules between sexes

To gain insight into sex-dependent differences in plasma lipid molecules, we next compared the levels of individual lipid molecules between fasted male and female rats. Of the 262 lipid molecules we determined, 110 and 142 lipid molecules were significantly different between male and female at 10 and 30 weeks old, respectively (Table 2). Of these lipid molecules, 67 lipid metabolites were commonly changed among 10- and 30-week-old rats (Fig. 2). Higher levels of most of the SMs (9/14 molecules), such as 36:1 and 36:2 SM, were consistent among 10- and 30-week-old female rats (Table 2 and Fig. 2C). In addition to the SMs, PUFAs containing ChEs are higher in both 10- and 30-week-old female rats (Fig. 2D). On the other hand, higher levels of PUFAs and their metabolites, such as eicosapentaenoic acid (EPA) and 5-hydroxyeicosatetraenoic acid, were almost specific for 30-week-old female rats. Furthermore, most of the PUFAs and their metabolites that showed higher levels in 30-week-old female rats are EPA, docosahexaenoic acid (DHA), and their metabolites (Fig. 2G).

Differences in the fasted levels of lipid molecules between ages

Subsequently, we compared the levels of individual lipid molecules between 10- and 30-week-old rats. In fasted male rats, 76 lipid molecules were significantly different, and the levels of 61 molecules were high in 10-week-old rats whereas the levels of 15 molecules were high in 30-week-old rats (Table 3). The phospholipids that presented higher levels at 10 weeks in male rats were LPCs and PCs (Fig. 3A and B). In addition, most of the PUFAs and their metabolites that showed higher levels at 10 weeks in male rats than those at 30 weeks were EPA, DHA, and their metabolites (Fig. 3G). In contrast, in fasted female rats, 101 lipid molecules were significantly different, and the levels of 98 were higher at 30 weeks than at 10 weeks (Table 3). Most of these lipid molecules are neutral lipids (72 out of 101). As shown in Fig. 3F, levels of relatively shorter and less unsaturated TGs, such as 48:0, 50:0, and 52:1 TGs, were higher at 30 weeks than at 10 weeks in female rats. In contrast, levels of relatively longer and highly unsaturated TGs, such as 56:10, 58:11, and 60:13 TGs, were lower at 30 weeks than at 10 weeks in male rats. Only 16 lipid molecules, such as 36:4 and 40:6 PE, showed significantly different levels between 10- and 30-week-olds in both male and female rats (Fig. 3).

Differences in the levels of lipid molecules among feeding conditions

To gain insight into the effects of feeding conditions on plasma lipid molecules, we next compared the levels of individual lipid molecules between rats that were fed and fasted, 16-hr fasted and 22-hr fasted, and from which blood was collected at 10 AM and 4

A

	10 week/30 week	
	Male	Female
16:0LPC		0.81
16:1LPC	1.24	
17:0LPC	1.30	
18:0LPC	1.20	
18:1LPC	1.25	0.77
18:2LPC	1.26	0.74
20:1LPC	1.64	0.75
20:4LPC		
22:6LPC		0.46
32:0PC		
32:1PC		
33:2PC		
34:0PC		0.73
34:1PC		
34:2PC		0.86
34:3PC		
35:2PC	1.28	
35:4PC		
36:0PC		
36:1PC	1.41	
36:2PCa		
36:2PCb	1.35	
36:3PCa	1.36	
36:3PCb	1.71	
36:4PCa		
36:4PCb		
36:5PCa		
36:5PCb	1.68	
37:2PCa	1.34	
37:2PCb	1.54	
37:4PC		
38:3PCa	1.87	
38:3PCb	2.49	
38:4PCa	1.80	
38:4PCb		
38:5PCa		0.66
38:5PCb	1.65	
38:6PCa		
38:6PCb	0.77	0.55
39:4PCa		0.65
39:4PCb		
39:6PC		0.66
40:4PC		
40:5PCa	1.54	
40:5PCb	1.64	
40:6PCa	1.98	
40:6PCb		0.78
40:7PC		0.55
40:8PC		
34:1ePC		
36:4ePC		
36:5ePC		
38:5ePC		

B

18:0LPE		
36:2PE		
36:4PE	0.77	0.72
38:4PE		
40:6PE	0.61	0.50
36:5ePE		
38:5ePE		
38:6ePE		
34:2PI		0.75
36:2PI		
36:4PI		0.59
37:4PI		0.73
38:4PI		
38:5PI		
40:6PI		

C

	10 week/30 week	
	Male	Female
34:0SM	0.69	0.81
34:1SM		0.76
34:2SM		0.73
36:1SM		0.77
36:2SM		0.78
38:1SM		
40:1SM		
41:1SM	1.29	
41:2SM	1.47	
42:1SMa		0.78
42:1SMb		
42:2SM	1.37	
42:3SM	1.32	
43:1SM		0.75
41:1Cer		
42:1Cera		
42:1Cerb	1.36	
42:2Cer	1.34	
43:1Cer		
42:1HexCer		0.78

D

Ch		
16:0ChE		
16:1ChE	1.71	1.36
17:0ChE		0.77
17:1ChE	1.70	
18:0ChEa		0.62
18:0ChEb	1.33	
18:1ChEa		0.67
18:1ChEb	1.63	
18:2ChE	1.27	
18:3ChE	1.58	
19:1ChE		
19:2ChE		0.71
20:1ChE		0.72
20:2ChE		0.70
20:3ChEa	0.56	0.63
20:3ChEb	2.19	
20:4ChE		
20:5ChE	2.12	
21:4ChE	0.60	0.57
21:5ChEa		
21:5ChEb	1.73	
22:3ChE		0.57
22:5ChE		0.71
22:6ChE		0.58
24:6ChE	0.71	0.51

E

34:1DG		0.57
34:2DG		0.54
36:2DG		0.55
36:3DG		0.51
36:4DG		0.45
38:5DG		
38:6DG		
40:7DG	1.75	
40:8DG	1.61	
44:10DG		

F

	10 week/30 week	
	Male	Female
48:0TG	0.42	0.43
48:1TG		0.59
48:2TG		0.58
49:1TG		0.62
49:2TG		0.53
50:0TG	0.59	0.54
50:1TG		0.47
50:2TG		0.45
50:3TG		
50:4TG		0.44
51:1TG		0.56
51:2TG		0.44
51:3TG		0.43
51:4TG		0.42
52:0TG		
52:1TG		0.50
52:2TG		0.35
52:3TG		0.38
52:4TG	0.43	0.55
52:5TGa		0.50
52:5TGb		
52:6TGa		0.60
52:6TGb		
52:6TGc		
52:7TG		
53:2TG		0.54
53:3TG		0.41
53:4TG		0.40
53:5TG		0.57
53:6TG	0.68	0.59
54:0TG		
54:1TG		0.58
54:2TG		0.57
54:3TG		0.59
54:4TGa		
54:4TGb	0.56	0.65
54:5TG		0.57
54:6TGa		0.53
54:6TGb	0.60	0.45
54:7TGa		0.52
54:7TGb		
54:7TGc		
54:8TGa		
54:8TGb		
55:2TG		0.59
55:7TG		
55:8TG		
56:0TG		
56:1TG		0.52
56:2TG		0.44
56:3TG		0.58
56:4TGa		0.51
56:4TGb		
56:5TGa		0.48
56:5TGb		0.40
56:5TGc		0.55
56:6TG		0.55
56:7TGa		0.54
56:7TGb		
56:8TGa	0.68	
56:8TGb		
56:9TGa		
56:9TGb		
56:10TG	1.88	
57:2TG		0.58
58:1TG		
58:2TG		0.48
58:3TG		0.50
58:4TG		0.37
58:5TG		

	10 week/30 week	
	Male	Female
58:6TG		0.64
58:7TGa		0.59
58:7TGb		
58:8TGa		
58:8TGb		
58:9TGa		0.56
58:9TGb		
58:10TGa		
58:10TGb	0.59	0.60
58:11TG	1.77	
60:1TG		
60:2TG		
60:3TG		
60:4TG		0.44
60:5TGa		0.52
60:5TGb		
60:9TG		0.52
60:11TGa		
60:11TGb		
60:12TGa		
60:12TGb		
60:13TG	2.19	
62:2TG		
62:3TG		
62:4TG		
62:5TGa		
62:5TGb		
62:12TG		
62:13TGa		0.61
62:13TGb	1.67	
62:14TG	1.50	
CoQ9		

G

AA		
PGD2		
PGF2a		
TXB2		
12-HHT		
5-HETE		0.83
8-HETE		
12-HETE		
15-HETE		
5,15-diHETE	1.68	
16-HETE		
17-HETE	1.42	
18-HETE	1.37	1.38
20-HETE	1.94	
8,9-diHETrE		
5,6-diHETrE		
11,12-diHETrE		
14,15-diHETrE		
EPA	2.20	
5-HEPE	1.70	
8-HEPE	4.28	
12-HEPE		
15-HEPE	5.17	
18-HEPE	3.43	1.63
14,15-diHETE	3.11	
17,18-diHETE	2.45	
DHA	1.56	
4-HDoHE	1.47	
7-HDoHE	1.61	
10-HDoHE		
13-HDoHE	1.56	
14-HDoHE		
17-HDoHE	1.54	
10,17-diHDoHE	1.81	
20-HDoHE	1.40	
19,20-diHDoPE		

2-fold 0.5-fold

Figure 3. Heat maps of lipid molecules among fasted rats of different age groups. The heat maps were generated with statistically significant different lipid molecules ($p<0.05$) of lysophosphatidylcholines and phosphoatidylcholines (A), other phospholipids (B), sphingolipids (C), cholesterol/cholesterolesters (D), diacylglycerols (E), triacylglycerol and coenzyme Q9 (F), and arachidonic acid, eicosapentaenoic acid, docosahexaenoic acid, and their metabolites (G). The numbers indicate the fold change of levels of individual lipid molecules in 10-week-old over 30-week-old male and female rats. The alphabet of the lipid class is used to distinguish the 2 lipid species possessing the same formula. LPC, lysophosphatidylcholine; PC, phosphatidylcholine; ePC, ether-type PC; LPE, lysophosphatidylethanolamine; PE, phosphatidylethanolamine; ePE, ether-type PE; SM, sphingomyelin; Cer, ceramide; HexCer, hexosylceramide; Ch, cholesterol; ChE, cholesterolester; DG, diacylglycerol; TG, triacylglycerol; CoQ9, coenzyme Q9; AA, arachidonic acid; PG, prostaglandin; TX, thromboxane; HETE, hydroxyeicosatetraenoic aicd; diHETE, dihydroxyeicosatetraenoic acid; diHETrE, dihydroxyeicosatrienoic acid; EPA, eicosapentaenoic acid; HEPE, hydroxyeicosapentaenoic acid; DHA, docosahexaenoic acid; HDoHE, hydroxydocosahexaenoic acid; diHDoHE, dihydroxydocosahexaenoic acid; diHDoPE, dihydroxydocosapentaenoic acid.

Table 3. Age-based differences in the number of lipid molecules at significantly higher levels.

		Male		Female		Common	
Lipid classes	**Total lipid molecules**	**10 week**	**30 week**	**10 week**	**30 week**	**10 week**	**30 week**
Phospholipids	68	21	3	0	18	0	3
Sphingolipids	20	6	1	0	8	0	1
Neutral lipids	138	16	11	1	71	1	10
PUFAs and metabolites	36	18	0	2	1	2	0
Total	262	61	15	3	98	2	14

Table 4. Differences in the number of lipid molecules at significantly higher levels among rats subjected to different feeding conditions.

		Fasting		Duration of fasting		Blood collection time	
Lipid classes	**Total lipid molecules**	**Fasted**	**Fed**	**16 hr**	**22 hr**	**10 AM**	**4 PM**
Phospholipids	68	2	44	0	0	6	0
Sphingolipids	20	4	3	0	0	1	0
Neutral lipids	138	13	96	0	0	4	6
PUFAs and metabolites	36	16	5	0	0	0	0
Total	262	35	148	0	0	11	6

A

	Feeding conditions		
	Ft/Fd	16 hr /22 hr	AM /PM
16:0LPC	0.78		
16:1LPC	0.40		
17:0LPC	0.77		
18:0LPC	0.88		
18:1LPC	0.54		
18:2LPC	0.39		1.21
20:1LPC	0.77		
20:4LPC			
22:6LPC	0.74		
32:0PC	0.77		
32:1PC	0.19		
33:2PC	0.33		
34:0PC	0.65		
34:1PC	0.47		
34:2PC	0.55		
34:3PC	0.26		
35:2PC	0.34		1.31
35:4PC			
36:0PC	0.74		
36:1PC	0.55		
36:2PCa	0.80		
36:2PCb	0.56		
36:3PCa	0.29		
36:3PCb	0.42		
36:4PCa	0.14		1.28
36:4PCb			
36:5PCa	0.58		
36:5PCb	0.17		
37:2PCa	0.52		1.41
37:2PCb	0.36		
37:4PC			
38:3PCa	0.50		
38:3PCb	0.53		
38:4PCa	0.29		
38:4PCb			
38:5PCa	0.76		
38:5PCb	0.34		
38:6PCa	0.52		
38:6PCb			
39:4PCa	1.34		
39:4PCb			
39:6PC			
40:4PC			
40:5PCa			
40:5PCb			
40:6PCa	0.66		
40:6PCb			
40:7PC	0.67		
40:8PC			
34:1ePC			
36:4ePC			
36:5ePC			
38:5ePC			

B

18:0LPE	0.62		
36:2PE	0.17		
36:4PE	0.48		
38:4PE	0.59		
40:6PE	0.46		
36:5ePE			
38:5ePE			
38:6ePE			
34:2PI	0.40		1.21
36:2PI	0.40		
36:4PI	0.74		
37:4PI			
38:4PI	1.43		
38:5PI	0.54		1.35
40:6PI			

C

	Feeding conditions		
	Ft/Fd	16 hr /22 hr	AM /PM
34:0SM			
34:1SM			
34:2SM			
36:1SM	1.42		
36:2SM	1.41		
38:1SM			
40:1SM			
41:1SM			
41:2SM			
42:1SMa	1.44		
42:1SMb			
42:2SM			
42:3SM			
43:1SM	1.32		1.27
41:1Cer	0.74		
42:1Cera			
42:1Cerb	0.67		
42:2Cer	0.75		
43:1Cer			
42:1HexCer			

D

Ch			
16:0ChE	0.74		
16:1ChE	0.38		
17:0ChE	0.75		1.30
17:1ChE	0.57		
18:0ChEa			1.33
18:0ChEb			
18:1ChEa	0.64		
18:1ChEb			
18:2ChE	0.64		
18:3ChE	0.74		
19:1ChE	0.68		
19:2ChE	0.64		1.39
20:1ChE			
20:2ChE	0.54		1.36
20:3ChEa			
20:3ChEb	0.63		
20:4ChE			
20:5ChE	0.28		
21:4ChE			
21:5ChEa			
21:5ChEb	0.39		
22:3ChE			
22:5ChE			
22:6ChE			
24:6ChE			

E

34:1DG	0.25		
34:2DG	0.43		
36:2DG	0.23		
36:3DG	0.41		
36:4DG	0.63		
38:5DG	1.38		
38:6DG	3.06		
40:7DG			
40:8DG	2.01		
44:10DG	0.77		

F

	Feeding conditions		
	Ft/Fd	16 hr /22 hr	AM /PM
48:0TG	0.11		0.63
48:1TG	0.02		
48:2TG	0.05		
49:1TG	0.10		
49:2TG	0.17		
50:0TG	0.34		0.68
50:1TG	0.04		
50:2TG	0.09		
50:3TG	0.05		
50:4TG	0.12		
51:1TG	0.16		
51:2TG	0.09		
51:3TG	0.12		
51:4TG	0.22		
52:0TG	0.59		
52:1TG	0.10		
52:2TG	0.07		
52:3TG	0.20		
52:4TG			0.53
52:5TGa	0.11		
52:5TGb	0.15		
52:6TGa	0.15		
52:6TGb	0.27		
52:6TGc	0.15		
52:7TG	0.33		
53:2TG	0.19		
53:3TG	0.15		
53:4TG	0.18		
53:5TG	0.16		
53:6TG	0.64		
54:0TG	0.43		
54:1TG	0.26		
54:2TG	0.08		
54:3TG	0.08		
54:4TGa	0.06		
54:4TGb			0.63
54:5TG	0.30		
54:6TGa	0.05		
54:6TGb			
54:7TGa	0.06		
54:7TGb	0.27		
54:7TGc			
54:8TGa	0.45		
54:8TGb	0.30		
55:2TG	0.41		
55:7TG	0.37		
55:8TG	0.47		
56:0TG	0.40		
56:1TG	0.31		
56:2TG	0.20		
56:3TG	0.13		
56:4TGa	0.16		
56:4TGb			
56:5TGa	0.25		
56:5TGb	0.11		
56:5TGc	0.44		
56:6TG	0.18		
56:7TGa	0.45		
56:7TGb	0.25		
56:8TGa	1.59		
56:8TGb			
56:9TGa	0.65		
56:9TGb	0.42		
56:10TG	0.47		
57:2TG	0.38		
58:1TG	0.44		
58:2TG	0.31		
58:3TG	0.20		
58:4TG	0.12		
58:5TG			
58:6TG	0.46		
58:7TGa	0.58		
58:7TGb	0.41		
58:8TGa	0.53		
58:8TGb			0.68
58:9TGa			
58:9TGb	0.66		
58:10TGa			
58:10TGb	1.50		0.71
58:11TG	2.59		
60:1TG	0.59		
60:2TG	0.50		
60:3TG	0.30		
60:4TG	0.19		
60:5TGa	0.17		
60:5TGb			
60:9TG	0.65		
60:11TGa	2.13		
60:11TGb	1.41		
60:12TGa	2.19		
60:12TGb	4.35		
60:13TG	3.59		
62:2TG			
62:3TG	0.48		
62:4TG	0.45		
62:5TGa	0.26		
62:5TGb	2.56		
62:12TG			
62:13TGa			
62:13TGb			
62:14TG	2.76		
CoQ9	0.78		

G

AA	2.40		
PGD2			
PGF2a			
TXB2			
12-HHT			
5-HETE	1.77		
8-HETE	2.38		
12-HETE	4.04		
15-HETE	1.95		
5,15-diHETE			
16-HETE	2.33		
17-HETE	2.27		
18-HETE	1.49		
20-HETE	4.00		
8,9-diHETrE			
5,6-diHETrE	1.63		
11,12-diHETrE			
14,15-diHETrE			
EPA	3.29		
5-HEPE	1.62		
8-HEPE	0.71		
12-HEPE	5.77		
15-HEPE	1.94		
18-HEPE	0.48		
14,15-diHETE			
17,18-diHETE			
DHA	4.44		
4-HDoHE	0.46		
7-HDoHE	0.73		
10-HDoHE			
13-HDoHE			
14-HDoHE	2.75		
17-HDoHE			
10,17-diHDoHE			
20-HDoHE	0.71		
19,20-diHDoPE			

2-fold 0.5-fold

Figure 4. Heat maps of lipid molecules among rats subjected to different feeding conditions. The heat maps were generated with statistically significant different lipid molecules ($p<0.05$) of lysophosphatidylcholines and phosphoatidylcholines (A), other phospholipids (B), sphingolipids (C), cholesterol/cholesterolesters (D), diacylglycerols (E), triacylglycerol and coenzyme Q9 (F), and arachidonic acid, eicosapentaenoic acid, docosahexaenoic acid, and their metabolites (G). The numbers indicate the fold change of levels of individual lipid molecules in fasted over fed male rats (Ft/Fd), 16-hr fasted over 22-hr fasted male rats (16 vs. 22 hr), and blood collected from male rats at 10 AM over at 4 PM (AM/PM). The alphabet of the lipid class is used to distinguish 2 lipid species possessing the same formula. LPC, lysophosphatidylcholine; PC, phosphatidylcholine; ePC, ether-type PC; LPE, lysophosphatidylethanolamine; PE, phosphatidylethanolamine; ePE, ether-type PE; SM, sphingomyelin; Cer, ceramide; HexCer, hexosylceramide; Ch, cholesterol; ChE, cholesterolester; DG, diacylglycerol; TG, triacylglycerol; CoQ9, coenzyme Q9; AA, arachidonic acid; PG, prostaglandin; TX, thromboxane; HETE, hydroxyeicosatetraenoic aicd; diHETE, dihydroxyeicosatetraenoic acid; diHETrE, dihydroxyeicosatrienoic acid; EPA, eicosapentaenoic acid; HEPE, hydroxyeicosapentaenoic acid; DHA, docosahexaenoic acid; HDoHE, hydroxydocosahexaenoic acid; diHDoHE, dihydroxydocosahexaenoic acid; diHDoPE, dihydroxydocosapentaenoic acid.

PM. The results of the comparative analysis showed that 183 lipid molecules were significantly different between fed and fasted male rats (Table 4). More than half of the lipid molecules in phospholipids, neutral lipids, and PUFAs and their metabolites were significantly different between fed and fasted male rats. Forty-four out of 46 significantly different phospholipids and 96 out of 109 significantly different neutral lipids were higher in fed rats than in fasted rats (Table 4). As shown in the heat map presented in Fig. 4E and F, levels of relatively longer and highly unsaturated DGs and TGs, such as 40:8 DG, 58:11, 60:13, and 62:14 TGs, were higher in fasted rats than in fed rats. On the other hand, 16 out of 21 significantly different PUFAs and their metabolites were higher in fasted rats than in fed rats (Fig. 4G). In contrast to the other lipid classes, only 7 out of 20 sphingolipids were statistically significant and their fold changes were less than 50% (Fig. 4C). No significantly different level of lipid molecules was observed between 16 hr-fasted and 22 hr-fasted male rats (Fig. 4). In addition, only 17 lipid molecules, such as 18:2 LPC and 35:2 PC, showed significantly different levels among different blood collection conditions (10 AM vs. 4 PM; Fig. 4).

Discussion

In the present study, we compared effects of multiple factors on the global profiles of lipid molecules in rat plasma. Based on overall comparison by OPLS-DA, feeding condition has a predominant role in the global profiles of lipid molecules, followed by sex and age. The number of statistically different levels in the lipid molecules between fasted and fed male rats reached 70% of the total lipid molecules determined, indicating a massive impact of feeding on lipid molecule levels. Sex-based differences in the levels of 42% of the lipid molecules tested were observed at 10 weeks of age and in 54% of the lipid molecules tested, at 30 weeks of age; whereas, age led to differences in the levels of 29% of the lipid molecules tested in male rats and 39% of lipid molecules in female rats. In contrast, overall comparison did not show any component contributing to separation among length of fasting period (16 hr vs. 22 hr) or diurnal time of sample collection (10 AM vs. 4 PM). In addition, there was no statistically significant difference in the levels of lipid molecules among the length of fasting period. Only 6.5% of the total lipid molecules determined showed significantly different levels among diurnal time of sample collection. These observations indicate that feeding or fasting condition, sex, and age are dominant factors influencing the global profiles of lipid molecules in rat plasma, while length of fasting period and diurnal time of sample collection has no or minor effects.

Sexual differences in hepatic gene expression, including cytochrome P450s, are well known in rodents [21,22]. In the present study, we demonstrated that profiles of lipid molecules in plasma also sexually vary in rats. Levels of SMs and PUFAs containing ChEs were higher in both 10- and 30-week-old female rats. In humans, the levels of SM are higher in female than in male subjects throughout their lifespan, suggesting the sex-based differences in the plasma levels of SMs are conserved among these species [12,14,23]. The reason for higher levels of SMs in female rats has been proposed to be due to the nutritional preferences of women, because there are strong associations between fruit and vegetable intake and the serum levels of d18:1/26:1 SM [23]. In the present study, however, we housed rats with same diet between male and female. Thus, in addition to nutritional preference, there could be alternative factors responsible for the sexually different levels of SMs in plasma. On the other hand, the present study demonstrated that cholesterol and PUFAs were present in higher levels in female than in male rats, although the difference in the levels of most PUFAs levels in 10-week-old rats was not significant. In addition, the expression levels of hepatic acyl-coenzyme A:cholesterol transferase 2 were approximately 3-fold higher in female than in male subjects [24]. Thus, the higher levels of PUFA-containing ChEs in female rats might be due to higher levels of their substrates, as well as their synthesizing enzymes.

Unlike SMs and PUFA-containing ChEs, the levels of EPA, DHA, and their metabolites were higher in 30-week-old female but not in 10-week-old female rats. It remains unclear why the higher levels of EPA, DHA, and their metabolites in female rats were specific for the 30-week-old age group. However, in a previous study, the serum estradiol level in female rats was elevated from an undetectable level at 3 months of age, to 90 pM at 18 months of age [25]. Estrogens have been demonstrated to induce the synthesis of DHA in rat [26]. Thus, one possible mechanism for higher levels of PUFAs and their metabolites in 30-week-old female rats is the estrogen effect.

In the present study, we employed 10-week-old (young adult) and 30-week-old (matured adult) rats for examining the profiles of lipid molecules in plasma. Our study demonstrated that levels of relatively shorter and less unsaturated TGs (48:0, 50:0, and 52:1 TGs) were higher in 30-week-old female rats than in 10-week-old rats, but that levels of relatively longer and highly unsaturated TGs (56:10, 58:11, and 60:13 TGs) were not higher. It has been reported that blood TG levels increase between 10 weeks and 30 weeks in rats and that this increase is much more drastic in female than male rats [27]. Thus, relatively shorter and less unsaturated TGs dominantly contribute to age-associated increases in TGs observed in female rats, but the physiological mechanism for this remains unclear. However, it has been reported that estrogen treatment in turkey liver resulted in increased levels of TGs with total carbon numbers of 53, but in decreased levels of TGs with total carbon numbers of 57 [28]. Thus, estrogen might regulate the synthetic ratio of acyl side chains in TGs through an unknown mechanism in the liver, possibly leading to an increase in shorter, less unsaturated TGs in female plasma.

We have demonstrated that feeding and fasting condition represented a major contribution on the profiles of lipid molecules in plasma. The majority of lipid molecules that are significantly different between fasted and fed rats are food derivatives, which are at lower levels in fasted rats. On the other hand, relatively longer and highly unsaturated DGs and TGs, such as 40:8 DG, 58:11, 60:13, and 62:14 TGs, increased in fasted rats. In addition, PUFAs also increased in fasted rats. Because DGs and TGs are synthesized from glycerol and fatty acids, increased levels of PUFAs might contribute to increased levels of relatively longer and highly unsaturated DGs and TGs.

Unlike other lipid classes, sphingolipids were relatively stable among fasted and fed rats. Feeding condition, as well as food preference, is major concern of clinical tests. Recently, sphingolipids have emerged as biomarker candidates for cardiovascular events, traumatic brain injury, and depression [29–31]. Thus, stability of the levels of sphingolipids throughout feeding and fasting might be advantageous in the application of sphingolipids as biomarkers in clinical tests, although, the effect of gender on the levels of sphingolipids should be considered.

In conclusion, we demonstrated the effects of multiple factors on lipidomic profiles in rat plasma. Our results demonstrated that feeding condition and subjects' sex and age are dominant factors modulating the levels of lipid molecules in rat plasma. The levels of most sphingolipids and PUFAs and their metabolites are sexually different. Age of female rats modulates differently the levels of relatively shorter and less unsaturated TGs and of relatively longer and highly unsaturated TGs. In addition, feeding and fasting condition also bi-directionally influenced the levels of relatively shorter and less unsaturated DGs and TGs and of relatively longer and highly unsaturated DGs and TGs. The effects of feeding condition are relatively smaller on the levels of sphingolipids than phospholipids, neutral lipids, and PUFAs and their metabolites. Taken together, our present study provides useful, fundamental information for exploring and validating lipid biomarkers in future preclinical studies and may also help to establish the regulatory standards for these studies.

Supporting Information

File S1 Supplemental tables. Table S1. Nutrient composition of CRF-1 in 100 g. **Table S2.** Sample information. **Table S3.** Identified lipid molecules in plasma. **Table S4.** Normalized levels of lipid molecules in each sample group.

Acknowledgments

The authors thank Dr. Yukio Kodama for providing technical support for conducting the animal experiments.

Author Contributions

Conceived and designed the experiments: KS YK KM Y. Saito. Performed the experiments: KS MI MU Y. Senoo KT. Analyzed the data: KS MI MM Y. Senoo. Contributed reagents/materials/analysis tools: MI KM. Contributed to the writing of the manuscript: KS Y. Saito.

References

1. Wedge DC, Allwood JW, Dunn W, Vaughan AA, Simpson K, et al. (2011) Is serum or plasma more appropriate for intersubject comparisons in metabolomic studies? An assessment in patients with small-cell lung cancer. Anal Chem 83: 6689–6697.
2. Hori S, Nishiumi S, Kobayashi K, Shinohara M, Hatakeyama Y, et al. (2011) A metabolomic approach to lung cancer. Lung Cancer 74: 284–292.
3. Ikeda A, Nishiumi S, Shinohara M, Yoshie T, Hatano N, et al. (2012) Serum metabolomics as a novel diagnostic approach for gastrointestinal cancer. Biomed Chromatogr 26: 548–558.
4. Singh SS (2006) Preclinical pharmacokinetics: an approach towards safer and efficacious drugs. Curr Drug Metab 7: 165–182.
5. Kamp H, Fabian E, Groeters S, Herold M, Krennrich G, et al. (2012) Application of in vivo metabolomics to preclinical/toxicological studies: case study on phenytoin-induced systemic toxicity. Bioanalysis 4: 2291–2301.
6. Kotronen A, Seppänen-Laakso T, Westerbacka J, Kiviluoto T, Arola J, et al. (2010) Comparison of lipid and fatty acid composition of the liver, subcutaneous and intra-abdominal adipose tissue, and serum. Obesity 18: 937–944.
7. Tajima Y, Ishikawa M, Maekawa K, Murayama M, Senoo Y, et al. (2013) Lipidomic analysis of brain tissues and plasma in a mouse model expressing mutated human amyloid precursor protein/tau for Alzheimer's disease. Lipids Health Dis 12: 68.
8. Liu S, Brown JD, Stanya KJ, Homan E, Leidl M, et al. (2013) A diurnal serum lipid integrates hepatic lipogenesis and peripheral fatty acid use. Nature 502: 550–554.
9. Holland WL, Summers SA (2008) Sphingolipids, insulin resistance, and metabolic disease: new insights from in vivo manipulation of sphingolipid metabolism. Endocr Rev 29: 381–402.
10. Serhan CN, Chiang N, Van Dyke TE (2008) Resolving inflammation: dual anti-inflammatory and pro-resolution lipid mediators. Nat Rev Immunol 8: 349–361.
11. Ishikawa M, Tajima Y, Murayama M, Senoo Y, Maekawa K, et al. (2013) Plasma and serum from nonfasting men and women differ in their lipidomic profiles. Bio Pharm Bull 36: 682–685.
12. Ishikawa M, Maekawa K, Saito K, Senoo Y, Urata M, et al. (2014) Plasma and serum lipidomics of healthy white adults shows characteristic profiles by subjects' gender and age. PLoS One 9: e91806.
13. Menni C, Zhai G, Macgregor A, Prehn C, Römisch-Margl W, et al. (2013) Targeted metabolomics profiles are strongly correlated with nutritional patterns in women. Metabolomics 9: 506–514.
14. Nikkilä J, Sysi-Aho M, Ermolov A, Seppänen-Laakso T, Simell O, et al. (2008) Gender-dependent progression of systemic metabolic states in early childhood. Mol Syst Biol 4: 197.
15. Zivkovic AM, Wiest MM, Nguyen UT, Davis R, Watkins SM, et al. (2009) Effects of sample handling and storage on quantitative lipid analysis in human serum. Metabolomics 5: 507–516.
16. Gonzalez-Covarrubias V, Dane A, Hankemeier T, Vreeken RJ (2013) The influence of citrate, EDTA, and heparin anticoagulants to human plasma LC–MS lipidomic profiling. Metabolomics 9: 337–348.
17. Han X, Gross RW (2005) Shotgun lipidomics: electrospray ionization mass spectrometric analysis and quantitation of cellular lipidomes directly from crude extracts of biological samples. Mass Spectrom Rev 24: 367–412.
18. Taguchi R, Nishijima M, Shimizu T (2007) Basic analytical systems for lipidomics by mass spectrometry in Japan. Methods Enzymol 432: 185–211.
19. Houjou T, Yamatani K, Imagawa M, Shimizu T, Taguchi R (2005) A shotgun tandem mass spectrometric analysis of phospholipids with normal-phase and/or reverse-phase liquid chromatography/electrospray ionization mass spectrometry. Rapid Commun Mass Spectrom 19: 654–666.
20. Graessler J, Schwudke D, Schwarz PE, Herzog R, Shevchenko A, et al. (2009) Top-down lipidomics reveals ether lipid deficiency in blood plasma of hypertensive patients. PLoS One 4: e6261.
21. Ahluwalia A, Clodfelter KH, Waxman DJ (2004) Sexual dimorphism of rat liver gene expression: regulatory role of growth hormone revealed by deoxyribonucleic acid microarray analysis. Mol Endocrinol 18: 747–760.
22. Waxman DJ, Holloway MG (2009) Sex differences in the expression of hepatic drug metabolizing enzymes. Mol Pharmacol 76: 215–228.
23. Menni C, Zhai G, Macgregor A, Prehn C, Romisch-Margl W, et al. (2013) Targeted metabolomics profiles are strongly correlated with nutritional patterns in women. Metabolomics 9: 506–515.
24. Hewitt KN, Boon WC, Murata Y, Jones ME, Simpson ER (2003) The aromatase knockout presents with a sexually dimorphic disruption to cholesterol homeostasis. Endocrinology 144: 3895–3903.
25. Pei W, Bellows CG, Jia Y, Heersche JN (2006) Effect of age on progesterone receptor expression, and osteoprogenitor proliferation and differentiation in female rat vertebral cell populations. J Endocrinol 190: 261–270.
26. Alessandri JM, Extier A, Al-Gubory KH, Harbeby E, Lallemand MS, et al. (2012) Influence of gender on DHA synthesis: the response of rat liver to low dietary α-linolenic acid evidences higher ω3 Δ4-desaturation index in females. Eur J Nutr 51: 199–209.
27. Tsuchiya N, Harada Y, Taki M, Minematsu S, Maemura S, et al. (1995) Age-related changes and sex differences on the serum chemistry values in Sprague-Dawley rats-I. 6–30 weeks of age. Exp Anim 43: 671–678.
28. Dashti N, Kelley JL, Thaver RH, Ontko JA (1983) Concurrent inductions of avian hepatic lipogenesis, plasma lipids, and plasma apolipoprotein B by estrogen. J Lipid Res 24: 368–380.
29. Liu JY, Li N, Yang J, Qiu H, Ai D, et al. (2010) Metabolic profiling of murine plasma reveals an unexpected biomarker in rofecoxib-mediated cardiovascular events. Proc Natl Acad Sci USA 107: 17017–17022.
30. Sparvero LJ, Amoscato AA, Kochanek PM, Pitt BR, Kagan VE, et al. (2010) Mass-spectrometry based oxidative lipidomics and lipid imaging: applications in traumatic brain injury. JNeurochem 115: 1322–1336.
31. Demirkan A, Isaacs A, Ugocsai P, Liebisch G, Struchalin M, et al. (2013) Plasma phosphatidylcholine and sphingomyelin concentrations are associated with depression and anxiety symptoms in a Dutch family-based lipidomic study. J Physhiatr Res 47: 357–362.

Permissions

All chapters in this book were first published in PLOS ONE, by The Public Library of Science; hereby published with permission under the Creative Commons Attribution License or equivalent. Every chapter published in this book has been scrutinized by our experts. Their significance has been extensively debated. The topics covered herein carry significant findings which will fuel the growth of the discipline. They may even be implemented as practical applications or may be referred to as a beginning point for another development.

The contributors of this book come from diverse backgrounds, making this book a truly international effort. This book will bring forth new frontiers with its revolutionizing research information and detailed analysis of the nascent developments around the world.

We would like to thank all the contributing authors for lending their expertise to make the book truly unique. They have played a crucial role in the development of this book. Without their invaluable contributions this book wouldn't have been possible. They have made vital efforts to compile up to date information on the varied aspects of this subject to make this book a valuable addition to the collection of many professionals and students.

This book was conceptualized with the vision of imparting up-to-date information and advanced data in this field. To ensure the same, a matchless editorial board was set up. Every individual on the board went through rigorous rounds of assessment to prove their worth. After which they invested a large part of their time researching and compiling the most relevant data for our readers.

The editorial board has been involved in producing this book since its inception. They have spent rigorous hours researching and exploring the diverse topics which have resulted in the successful publishing of this book. They have passed on their knowledge of decades through this book. To expedite this challenging task, the publisher supported the team at every step. A small team of assistant editors was also appointed to further simplify the editing procedure and attain best results for the readers.

Apart from the editorial board, the designing team has also invested a significant amount of their time in understanding the subject and creating the most relevant covers. They scrutinized every image to scout for the most suitable representation of the subject and create an appropriate cover for the book.

The publishing team has been an ardent support to the editorial, designing and production team. Their endless efforts to recruit the best for this project, has resulted in the accomplishment of this book. They are a veteran in the field of academics and their pool of knowledge is as vast as their experience in printing. Their expertise and guidance has proved useful at every step. Their uncompromising quality standards have made this book an exceptional effort. Their encouragement from time to time has been an inspiration for everyone.

The publisher and the editorial board hope that this book will prove to be a valuable piece of knowledge for researchers, students, practitioners and scholars across the globe.

List of Contributors

Kuo-Hsiung Yang and Angela D. M. Kashuba
Division of Pharmacotherapy and Experimental Therapeutics, UNC Eshelman School of Pharmacy, Chapel Hill, North Carolina, United States of America

Craig Hendrix and Namandje Bumpus
Departments of Medicine and Pharmacology, Johns Hopkins University School of Medicine, Baltimore, Maryland, United States of America

Julie Elliott and Peter A. Anton
Center for HIV Prevention Research, David Geffen School of Medicine at UCLA, Los Angeles, California, United States of America

Karen Tanner
Department of Biostatistics, UCLA School of Public Health, Los Angeles, California, United States of America

Christine Mauck
CONRAD, Arlington, Virginia, United States of America

Ross Cranston and Ian McGowan
Department of Medicine, University of Pittsburgh, Pittsburgh, Pennsylvania, United States of America

Nicola Richardson-Harman
Alpha StatConsult LLC, Damascus, Maryland, United States of America

Hiromichi Matsushita
Research Center for Cancer Stem Cell, Tokai University School of Medicine, Isehara, Kanagawa, Japan
Medical Research Institute, Tokai University, Isehara, Kanagawa, Japan
Department of Laboratory Medicine, Tokai University School of Medicine, Isehara, Kanagawa, Japan

Takashi Yahata
Research Center for Cancer Stem Cell, Tokai University School of Medicine, Isehara, Kanagawa, Japan
Medical Research Institute, Tokai University, Isehara, Kanagawa, Japan
Department of Cell Transplantation, Tokai University School of Medicine, Isehara, Kanagawa, Japan

Yin Sheng, Yoshihiko Nakamura and Yukari Muguruma
Research Center for Cancer Stem Cell, Tokai University School of Medicine, Isehara, Kanagawa, Japan

Hideyuki Matsuzawa
Research Center for Cancer Stem Cell, Tokai University School of Medicine, Isehara, Kanagawa, Japan
Support Center for Medical Research and Education, Tokai University, Isehara, Kanagawa, Japan

Masayuki Tanaka, Hideki Hayashi and Tadayuki Sato
Support Center for Medical Research and Education, Tokai University, Isehara, Kanagawa, Japan

Anar Damdinsuren and Hayato Miyachi
Department of Laboratory Medicine, Tokai University School of Medicine, Isehara, Kanagawa, Japan

Makoto Onizuka
Division of Hematology and Oncology, Department of Internal Medicine, Tokai University School of Medicine, Isehara, Kanagawa, Japan

Mamoru Ito
Central Institute for Experimental Animals, Kawasaki, Kanagawa, Japan

Pier Paolo Pandolfi
Cancer Research Institute, Beth Israel Deaconess Cancer Center, Departments of Medicine and Pathology, Beth Israel Deaconess Medical Center, Harvard Medical School, Boston, Massachusetts, United States of America

Kiyoshi Ando
Research Center for Cancer Stem Cell, Tokai University School of Medicine, Isehara, Kanagawa, Japan
Medical Research Institute, Tokai University, Isehara, Kanagawa, Japan

Division of Hematology and Oncology, Department of Internal Medicine, Tokai University School of Medicine, Isehara, Kanagawa, Japan

Chen Yu, Qing-Zhong Li and Hong-Juan Li
School of Pharmacy, Binzhou Medical University, Yantai, Shandong, China

Dong Qi
Department of Nephrology, Yantai Yu-Huang-Ding/Qingdao University Hospital, Yantai, Shandong, China

Wei Lian
Yantai Yan-Tai-Shan Hospital, Yantai, Shandong, China

Hua-Ying Fan
School of Pharmacy, Yantai University, Yantai, Shandong, China

Qingqing Wu, Jizhou Zhang, Jun Shi, Meili Ge, Xingxin Li, Yingqi Shao, Jianfeng Yao and Yizhou Zheng
Severe Aplastic Anemia Studying Program, State Key Laboratory of Experimental Hematology, Institute of Hematology & Blood Diseases Hospital, Chinese Academy of Medical Sciences & Peking Union Medical College, 288 Nanjing Road, Tianjin, 300020, P.R.CHINA

Jie Wu, Ling Qiu, Xiu-zhi Guo, Xin-qi Cheng, Lin Zhang, Peng-chang Li and Qian Di
Department of Clinical Laboratory, Peking Union Medical College Hospital, Peking Union Medical College & Chinese Academy of Medical Science, Beijing, China

Tao Xu
Department of Epidemiology and Statistics, Institute of Basic Medical Sciences, Chinese Academy of Medical Sciences & Peking Union Medical College, Beijing, China

Qing Wang and Lan Ni
Medical Experimental Center, General Hospital of Ningxia Medical University, Yinchuan, China

Guang-jin Zhu
Department of Pathophysiology, Institute of Basic Medical Sciences, Chinese Academy of Medical Sciences & Peking Union Medical College, Beijing, China

Erik van Kampen, Reeni B. Hildebrand, Bart Lammers, Theo J. C. Van Berkel and Miranda Van Eck
Div. of Biopharmaceutics, Cluster of BioTherapeutics, Leiden Academic Centre for Drug Research, Leiden, The Netherlands

Olivier Beaslas and Vesa M. Olkkonen
Dept. of Lipid Signalling and Homeostasis, Minerva Foundation Institute for Medical Research, Helsinki, Finland

Nizam Uddin, Md. Rakib Hasan, Md. Mahadi Hasan, Md. Monir Hossain, Md. Robiul Alam, Mohammad Raquibul Hasan, A. F. M. Mahmudul Islam, Tasmina Rahman and Md. Sohel Rana
Department of Pharmacy, Jahangirnagar University, Savar, Dhaka, 1342, Bangladesh

Ola Kally Magnusdottir, Ingibjorg Gunnarsdottir and Inga Thorsdottir
Unit for Nutrition Research, Landspitali -The National University Hospital of Iceland and Faculty of Food Science and Nutrition, School of Health Sciences, University of Iceland, Reykjavík, Iceland

Rikard Landberg
Department of Food Science, BioCenter, Swedish University of Agricultural Sciences, Uppsala, Sweden
Division of Nutritional Epidemiology, Institute of Environmental Medicine, Karolinska Institutet, Stockholm, Sweden

Lieselotte Cloetens
Biomedical Nutrition, Pure and Applied Biochemistry, Lund University, Lund, Sweden

Björn Åkesson
Biomedical Nutrition, Pure and Applied Biochemistry, Lund University, Lund, Sweden
Department of Clinical Nutrition, Skåne University Hospital, Lund, Sweden

Fredrik Rosqvist and Ulf Risérus
Department of Public Health and Caring Sciences, Clinical Nutrition and Metabolism, Uppsala University, Uppsala, Sweden

Ursula Schwab
Institute of Public Health and Clinical Nutrition, University of Eastern Finland, Kuopio, Finland
Institute of Clinical Medicine, Internal Medicine, Kuopio University Hospital, Kuopio, Finland

Karl-Heinz Herzig
Institute of Biomedicine, Department of Physiology and Biocenter, Oulu University, Oulu, Finland and Department of Psychiatry, Kuopio University Hospital, Kuopio, Finland

Janne Hukkanen and Markku J. Savolainen
Department of Internal Medicine and Biocenter, Institute of Clinical Medicine, University of Oulu, Oulu, Finland and Clinical Research Center, Oulu University Hospital, Oulu, Finland

Lea Brader and Kjeld Hermansen
Department of Endocrinology and Internal Medicine, Aarhus University Hospital, Aarhus, Denmark

Marjukka Kolehmainen and Kaisa Poutanen
Institute of Public Health and Clinical Nutrition, University of Eastern Finland, Kuopio, Finland
VTT Technical Research Centre of Finland, Espoo and Kuopio, Finland

Matti Uusitupa
Institute of Public Health and Clinical Nutrition, University of Eastern Finland, Kuopio, Finland
Research Unit, Kuopio University Hospital, Kuopio, Finland

Hsin-Hou Chang and Der-Shan Sun
Department of Molecular Biology and Human Genetics, Tzu-Chi University, Hualien, Taiwan
Institute of Medical Sciences, Tzu-Chi University, Hualien, Taiwan

Ya-Wen Chiang and Ting-Kai Lin
Department of Molecular Biology and Human Genetics, Tzu-Chi University, Hualien, Taiwan

Guan-Ling Lin and You-Yen Lin
Institute of Medical Sciences, Tzu-Chi University, Hualien, Taiwan

Jyh-Hwa Kau
Department of Microbiology and Immunology, National Defense Medical Center, Taipei, Taiwan

Hsin-Hsien Huang and Hui-Ling Hsu
Institute of Preventive Medicine, National Defense Medical Center, Taipei, Taiwan

Jen-Hung Wang
Department of Medical Research, Tzu Chi General Hospital, Hualien, Taiwan

Peter Gresner, Jolanta Gromadzinska, Ewa Jablonska, Maciej Stepnik, Ewa Twardowska and Wojciech Wasowicz
Department of Toxicology and Carcinogenesis, Nofer Institute of Occupational Medicine, Lodz, Poland

Oscar Zambrano Quispe
Department of Oncology, Herlev Hospital, Herlev, Denmark

Kosuke Minai, Takayuki Ogawa, Makoto Kawai, Kimiaki Komukai, Toshikazu Tanaka, Kazuo Ogawa, Tomohisa Nagoshi, Satoshi Arase, Satoshi Morimoto, Yasunori Inoue, Hiroshi Sekiyama, Akihiro Urabe, Seiichiro Matsuo, Kenichi Hongo and Michihiro Yoshimura
Division of Cardiology, Department of Internal Medicine, The Jikei University School of Medicine, Tokyo, Japan

Preston E. Bratcher
Department of Medicine and Division of Pulmonary, Allergy, and Critical Care Medicine, University of Alabama at Birmingham, Birmingham, Alabama, United States of America
Program in Protease and Matrix Biology, University of Alabama at Birmingham, Birmingham, Alabama, United States of America

Amit Gaggar
Department of Medicine and Division of Pulmonary, Allergy, and Critical Care Medicine, University of Alabama at Birmingham, Birmingham, Alabama, United States of America
Gregory Fleming James Cystic Fibrosis Research Center, University of Alabama at Birmingham, Birmingham, Alabama, United States of America
University of Alabama at Birmingham, UAB Lung Health Center, Birmingham, Alabama, United States of America
Medicine Service, United States Department of Veterans Affairs Medical Center, Birmingham, Alabama, United States of America
Program in Protease and Matrix Biology, University of Alabama at Birmingham, Birmingham, Alabama, United States of America

Vivien A. Sheehan and Jonathan M. Flanagan
Hematology Center, Department of Pediatrics, Baylor College of Medicine, Houston, Texas, United States of America

Jacy R. Crosby
The University of Texas Graduate School of Biomedical Sciences at Houston, Department of Biostatistics, Bioinformatics, and Systems Biology, University of Texas, Houston, Texas, United States of America
Human Genetics Center, University of Texas, Houston, Texas, United States of America

Aniko Sabo, Donna M. Muzny, Shannon Dugan-Perez and Richard A. Gibbs
Human Genome Sequencing Center, Baylor College of Medicine, Houston, Texas, United States of America

Nicole A. Mortier, Thad A. Howard and Russell E. Ware
Division of Hematology, Cincinnati Children's Hospital Medical Center, Cincinnati, Ohio, United States of America

Banu Aygun
Steven and Alexandra Cohen Children's Medical Center of New York, New Hyde Park, New York, United States of America

Kerri A. Nottage
Department of Hematology, St. Jude Children's Research Hospital, Memphis, Tennessee, United States of America

Eric Boerwinkle
Human Genetics Center, University of Texas, Houston, Texas, United States of America
Human Genome Sequencing Center, Baylor College of Medicine, Houston, Texas, United States of America

Yoshikuni Kawaguchi, Yasuhiko Sugawara, Nobuhisa Akamatsu, Junichi Kaneko, Takeaki Ishizawa, Sumihito Tamura, Taku Aoki, Yoshihiro Sakamoto, Kiyoshi Hasegawa and Norihiro Kokudo
Artificial Organ and Transplantation Surgery Division, Department of Surgery, Graduate School of Medicine, University of Tokyo, Tokyo, Japan

Tsuyoshi Hamada
Department of Gastroenterology, Graduate School of Medicine, University of Tokyo, Tokyo, Japan

Tomohiro Tanaka
Organ Transplantation Service, University of Tokyo, Tokyo, Japan

Vesna Borovnik-Lesjak, Kasen Whitehouse, Alvin Baetiong, Yang Miao, Brian M. Currie and Sathya Velmurugan
Resuscitation Institute at Rosalind Franklin University of Medicine and Science, North Chicago, Illinois, United States of America

Jeejabai Radhakrishnan
Department of Medicine and Resuscitation Institute at Rosalind Franklin University of Medicine and Science, North Chicago, Illinois, United States of America

Raúl J. Gazmuri
Department of Medicine, Department of Physiology and Biophysics, and Resuscitation Institute at Rosalind Franklin University of Medicine and Science, and Critical Care Medicine at the Captain James A. Lovell Federal Health Care Center, North Chicago, Illinois, United States of America

Christopher M. Brennan, Nicholas Q. Mazzucca, Taylor Mezoian, Taylor M. Hunt, Meaghan L. Keane, Jessica N. Leonard, Emma N. Beer, Sarah Perdue and Brett J. Pellock
Department of Biology, Providence College, Providence, Rhode Island, United States of America

Shelby E. Scola
Department of Chemistry and Biochemistry, Providence College, Providence, Rhode Island, United States of America

Magdalena Koszarska, Hajnalka Andrikovics and Attila Tordai
Hungarian National Blood Transfusion Service, Budapest, Hungary

Nora Kucsma, Katalin Kiss, Gyorgy Varady, Melinda Gera, Geza Antalffy and Gergely Szakacs
Institute of Enzymology, Research Centre for Natural Sciences, Hungarian Academy of Sciences, Budapest, Hungary

Maciej Studzian4, Lukasz Pulaski
Department of Molecular Biophysics, University of Lodz, Lodz, Poland

Dominik Strapagiel
Biobank Lab, Department of Molecular Biophysics, University of Lodz, Lodz, Poland

Yoshihiko Tani
Japanese Red Cross Kinki Block Blood Center, Osaka, Japan

Balazs Sarkadi
Hungarian National Blood Transfusion Service, Budapest, Hungary
Institute of Enzymology, Research Centre for Natural Sciences, Hungarian Academy of Sciences, Budapest, Hungary
Molecular Biophysics Research Group of the Hungarian Academy of Sciences, Semmelweis University, Budapest, Hungary

Matthias Oelze, Swenja Kröller-Schön, Philipp Welschof, Thomas Jansen, Michael Hausding, Yuliya Mikhed, Paul Stamm, Michael Mader, Elena Zinßius, Saule Agdauletova, Anna Gottschlich, Sebastian Steven, Eberhard Schulz, Thomas Münzel and Andreas Daiber
2nd Medical Clinic, Department of Cardiology, Medical Center of the Johannes Gutenberg University, Mainz, Germany

Serge P. Bottari
Laboratory of Fundamental and Applied, Bioenergetics, INSERM U1055, Grenoble-Alpes Universitéet Pôle de Biologie, CHU, Grenoble, France

Eric Mayoux
Boehringer Ingelheim Pharma GmbH & Co. KG, Ingelheim, Germany

Jelena Kornej
University of Leipzig, Heart Center, Department of Electrophysiology, Leipzig, Germany
University of Birmingham Centre for Cardiovascular Sciences, City Hospital, Birmingham, United Kingdom

Borislav Dinov, Sascha Rolf, Arash Arya, Josephine Schmidl, Daniela Husser, Gerhard Hindricks and Andreas Bollmann
University of Leipzig, Heart Center, Department of Electrophysiology, Leipzig, Germany

Gregory Y. H. Lip and Andrew D. Blann
University of Birmingham Centre for Cardiovascular Sciences, City Hospital, Birmingham, United Kingdom

Jaione Simon-Santamaria, Ruomei Li, Ivana Malovic, Kjetil Elvevold, Peter McCourt, Bård Smedsrød and Karen Kristine Sørensen
Department of Medical Biology, UiT - The Arctic University of Norway, Tromsø, Norway

Christine Hanssen Rinaldo
Department of Microbiology and Infection Control, University Hospital of North Norway, Tromsø, Norway
Department of Clinical Medicine, UiT - The Arctic University of Norway, Tromsø, Norway

Piotr Kardas
Department of Biomedicine, University of Basel, Basel, Switzerland

Hans H. Hirsch
Department of Biomedicine, University of Basel, Basel, Switzerland
Divisions of Infectious Diseases and Hospital Epidemiology, University Hospital of Basel, Basel, Switzerland
Kosuke Saito, Masaki Ishikawa, Mayumi Murayama, Masayo Urata, Yuya Senoo, Katsuko Toyoshima, Keiko Maekawa and Yoshiro Saito
Division of Medical Safety Science, National Institute of Health Sciences, 1-18-1 Kamiyoga, Setagaya, Tokyo, Japan

Yuji Kumagai
Clinical Research Center, Kitasato University School of Medicine, 1-15-1 Kitasato, Minami, Sagamihara, Kanagawa, Japan

Index